Boucher's Prosthodontic Treatment for Edentulous Patients

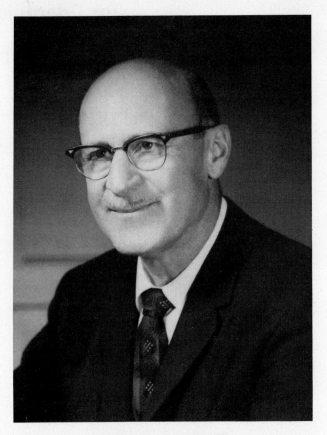

CARL O. BOUCHER

October 14, 1904—March 11, 1975

A respected teacher, a superb clinician,
a gifted editor and author, and a close personal friend.
He enriched the lives of his students,
his colleagues, and his patients.

GEORGE A. ZARB
CHARLES L. BOLENDER
JUDSON C. HICKEY
GUNNAR E. CARLSSON

Boucher's Prosthodontic Treatment for Edentulous Patients

GEORGE A. ZARB, B.ChD. (Malta), D.D.S., M.S. (Michigan), M.S. (Ohio State), F.R.C.D. (Canada)

Professor and Chairman, Department of Prosthodontics,
Faculty of Dentistry, University of Toronto; Section Editor,
The Journal of Prosthetic Dentistry; Member of the School of Graduate Studies,
University of Toronto, Toronto, Ontario, Canada

CHARLES L. BOLENDER, D.D.S., M.S.

Professor and Former Chairman, Department of Prosthodontics,
University of Washington, School of Dentistry, Seattle, Washington

JUDSON C. HICKEY, D.D.S., M.Sc.

Formerly Dean and Professor of Prosthodontics, Medical College of Georgia
School of Dentistry; Member, Graduate Faculty of the Medical College of
Georgia, Augusta, Georgia; Editor, The Journal of Prosthetic Dentistry;
Diplomate, American Board of Prosthodontics

GUNNAR E. CARLSSON, L.D.S., Odont. Dr.

Professor and Chairman, Department of Prosthetic Dentistry,
Faculty of Odontology, University of Göteborg;
formerly, Professor and Chairman, Department of Stomatology,
Faculty of Odontology, University of Göteborg, Göteborg, Sweden

TENTH EDITION

with 979 illustrations and 24 in color

The C. V. Mosby Company

ST. LOUIS • BALTIMORE • PHILADELPHIA • TORONTO   1990

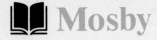

Editor: Robert W. Reinhardt
Assistant Editor: Melba Steube
Manuscript editor: George B. Stericker, Jr.
Book and cover design: Gail Morey Hudson
Production: Ginny Douglas

TENTH EDITION

Previous editions copyrighted 1940, 1947, 1953, 1959, 1964, 1970,
1975, 1980, 1985

Printed in the United States of America

The C.V. Mosby Company
11830 Westline Industrial Drive, St. Louis, Missouri 63146

Library of Congress Cataloging in Publication Data

Prosthodontic treatment for edentulous patients.
    Boucher's prosthodontic treatment for edentulous patients.— 10th
ed. / George A. Zarb . . . [et al.]
      p. cm.
    Rev. ed. of: Boucher's prosthodontic treatment for edentulous
patients. 9th ed. / Judson C. Hickey, George A. Zarb, Charles L.
Bolender. 1985.
    Includes bibliographical references.
    ISBN 0-8016-3310-9
    1. Complete dentures. 2. Edentuous mouth. I. Zarb, George A.
(George Albert), 1938-   . II. Boucher, Carl O. Prosthodontic
treatment of edentulous patients. III. Title. IV. Title:
Prosthodontic treatment for edentulous patients.
    [DNLM: 1. Denture, Complete. 2. Mouth, Edentulous. WU 530 P966]
RK656.P75 1990
617.6'92—dc20
DNLM/DLC
for Library of Congress   89-13106
                                            CIP

C/MV/MV 9 8 7 6 5 4 3 2 1

To our wives
Janet, Mamie, Jean, and Anita
and all students of prosthodontics

Preface

Proper prosthodontic treatment of edentulous patients requires that they be prepared orally, physically, and psychologically before treatment and that these aspects of their health be evaluated during and after clinical treatment. The provision of complete dentures is one important part of the total treatment plan. Every aspect of prosthodontic treatment of edentulous patients, except for certain laboratory procedures, requires clinical skills based on a knowledge and application of basic and behavioral sciences. The purpose of our book is to provide learning experiences that will correlate the basic, behavioral, and clinical skills of the dentist for the most effective comprehensive prosthodontic treatment of edentulous patients.

To accomplish our objectives, this book is so organized that technical considerations are described along with the basic fundamentals that control them. This type of organization allows students to prepare for each step in the treatment procedure and gives them the opportunity to acquire the necessary scientific and mechanical background to make the proper clinical judgments required for the succcessful treatment of their patients.

The clinical phases of denture construction are based on our own experiences in treating edentulous patients.

We recognize that more than one technique can produce good prosthodontic results. For this reason, we have included descriptions of different techniques for certain treatment procedures, such as impression making and the development of the occlusion with different occlusal forms. The choice of method for any patient will be made by the dentist on the basis of the individual conditions and the fundamentals involved.

Edentulous patients require competent, compassionate, and professional dental treatment, even though providing such treatment is difficult and time-consuming. An understanding of people, their problems, and their attitudes is necessary for the successful practice of prosthodontics. The challenge of overcoming the deficiencies of neglect or improper oral health care (for whatever reason) can be the most satisfying aspect of dental practice.

Since the publication of the ninth edition, considerable progress has been made in treating edentulous patients by alternative modalities to complete dentures. The technique of osseointegration as described by Per-Ingvar Brånemark has introduced an exciting, and safe, method for predictably resolving the edentulous problem. The dental faculties at Toronto, Seattle, and Göteborg are only three of several that have undertaken prospective clinical studies confirming the efficacy of osseointegrated implant–supported fixed prostheses, or overdentures.

As a result, this edition reflects the profound shift that is taking place in the treatment of edentulous patients. We anticipate that future editions of this text will include more extensive coverage of implant prosthodontics, as the complete denture is gradually displaced from its preeminent position in treating the edentulous patient.

Many persons have been of great assistance in the preparation of this book, and we wish to acknowledge and thank them for their contributions. Milton Burroughs, medical illustrator, Medical College of Georgia, School of Dentistry, and Steve Burany and Rita Bauer, photographers at the Faculty of Dentistry, University of Toronto, receive our special praise for the art work and photographs they provided. Our thanks to Horst Kroll for laboratory technical services and to Mary P. Faine for her section on nutrition in Chapter 5.

We greatly appreciate the encouragement and patience of our wives, Janet Zarb, Mamie Bolender, Jean Hickey, and Anita Wedel-Carlsson. All others who have helped have our sincere thanks and appreciation.

George A. Zarb
Charles L. Bolender
Judson C. Hickey
Gunnar E. Carlsson

Contents

The edentulous patient

CHAPTER 1

Biomechanics of the edentulous state

It would be inaccurate to state that disease factors such as caries or periodontal disease are the sole causes of patients' becoming edentulous. Some authors actually argue that tooth loss does not bear even a close relationship to the prevalence of dental disease. Although the latter viewpoint is probably equally inaccurate, research has demonstrated that several nondisease factors, such as attitude, behavior, dental attendance, and characteristics of the health care system, do play an important role in the decision to become edentulous. In addition, a significant relationship exists between the edentulous state and low occupational levels. It is therefore reasonable to conclude that edentulism is due to various combinations of cultural and attitudinal determinants, and to treatment received over the past several years.

The heterogenous etiology of edentulism has been tackled on several fronts by the dental profession, resulting in a reported decrease in the numbers of edentulous persons (Fig. 1-1). More recent reviews of tooth loss and edentulism in various parts of North America and European countries predict that treatment of patients with complete dentures will continue to decline in the future while the needs for partial tooth replacement will likely increase in the short term. While these observations may suggest a reduced dental educational commitment to treatment of edentulous patients, at the same time some compelling points must be underscored:

1. Documented evidence supports the idea that, despite projections of declining edentulism, the unmet need for complete denture treatment will remain high.

2. Predictions of several surveys regarding a healthy elderly population indicate that a high percentage of older people will be edentulous. Therefore the effective demand for prosthetic care for this population is likely to increase.

3. The impact of longevity on edentulism has not been fully ascertained. Clinical experience suggests that the cumulative consequences of biologic and chronologic aging will likely confront dentists with a significant increase in the number of difficult edentulous mouths requiring treatment.

Irrespective of precise future population needs, the psychologic and biomechanical implications of tooth loss must never be overlooked.

Most patients regard tooth loss as mutilating and as a strong incentive to seek dental care for the preservation of a healthy dentition and socially acceptable appearance. Dentists, on the other hand, regard tooth loss as posing the hazard of an even greater mutilation—the destruction of part of the facial skeleton and the distortion of soft tissue morphology and function (Fig. 1-2).

The edentulous state represents a compromise in the integrity of the masticatory system that is frequently accompanied by adverse functional and cosmetic sequelae, which are varyingly perceived by the affected patient. Perceptions of the edentulous state may range

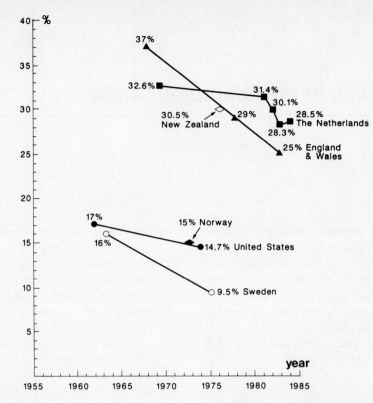

Fig. 1-1 Reports from different countries indicate a gradual reduction in the number of edentulous patients. (Redrawn from Bouma J: Thesis, Rijksuniversiteit te Groningen, 1987.)

from feelings of inconvenience to feelings of severe handicap. When total loss of teeth is regarded as equivalent to loss of a body part, its treatment implies a range of biomechanical problems that involve a wide range of individual tolerances and perceptions.

This text provides an understanding of the effects of the edentulous condition and describes its clinical management.

MECHANISMS OF TOOTH SUPPORT

The masticatory system is made up of morphologic, functional, and behavioral components (Fig. 1-3). The interactions of these closely related components are affected by changes in the mechanism of support for a den-

tition when natural teeth are replaced by artificial ones.

To appreciate the many subtleties associated with the edentulous state and the effects of the transition from a dentulous to an edentulous state, one must compare the mechanisms of tooth support and denture support. Such a review will underscore the nature of the altered environment brought about by the loss of teeth.

The masticatory apparatus is involved in the process of trituration of food. Direct responsibility for this task falls on the teeth and their supporting tissues. The attachment of teeth in sockets is but one of many important modifications that took place during the period when

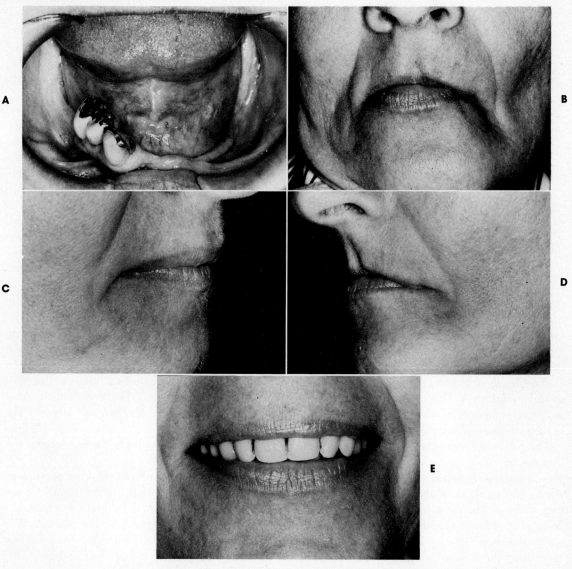

Fig. 1-2   Partial loss of the mandibular dentition, **A,** and complete loss of the maxillary dentition, **B,** have seriously affected this middle-aged patient's appearance, as well as her functional status. Compare the depleted soft tissue support in **B** and **D** to the support obtained by prostheses and the natural teeth, **C** and **E.**

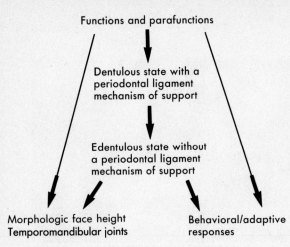

Fig. 1-3   Possible interactions between the various components of the masticatory system in the context of a change in the mechanism of occlusal support.

the earliest mammals were evolving from their reptilian predecessors. The success of this modification is indicated by the fact that it appears to have been rapidly adopted throughout the many different groups of emerging Mammalia. Teeth function properly only if adequately supported. This support is provided by an organ composed of soft and hard connective tissues, the periodontium.

The periodontium attaches the teeth to the bone of the jaws, providing a resilient suspensory apparatus resistant to functional forces. It allows the teeth to adjust their position when under stress. The periodontium comprises hard connective tissues (cementum and bone) and soft connective tissues (the periodontal ligament and the lamina propria of the gingiva), which are covered by epithelium. The periodontium is regarded as a functional unit and is attached to the dentin by cementum and to the jawbone by the alveolar process. Continuity between these two hard tissue components is maintained by the periodontal ligament and the lamina propria.

The periodontal ligament provides the means by which force exerted on the tooth is transmitted to the bone that supports it. The two principal functions of the periodontium are support and positional adjustment of the tooth, together with the secondary and dependent function of sensory perception. The patient needing complete denture therapy is deprived of periodontal support, and the entire mechanism of functional load transmission to the supporting tissues is altered.

The mechanisms of tooth support have received a considerable amount of investigation during the past 25 years, and a number of conclusions have been drawn from observations in human and animal studies. As soon as teeth erupt into the oral cavity and occlusal contact is established, the nonfunctional orientation of the periodontal fibers changes into a functional arrangement. This gives maximal stabilization to the tooth in the alveolar socket and at the same time allows a physiologic range of tooth mobility in all directions.

The occlusal forces exerted on the teeth are controlled by the neuromuscular mechanisms of the masticatory system. Reflex mechanisms with receptors in the muscles, tendons, joints, and periodontal structures regulate mandibular movements. Through normal function the periodontal structures in a healthy dentition undergo characteristic mechanical stress. The most prominent feature of physiologic occlusal forces is their intermittent, rhythmic, and dynamic nature.

Gradual changes in force patterns occur during growth and eruption of the teeth. Abrupt alterations are produced by loss or removal of opposing or adjacent teeth or the placement of fixed or removable prostheses. The position normally occupied by a tooth in the dental arch depends on the balance of all the forces acting on that tooth over an extended time. Sustained alterations in the magnitude or duration of the forces may cause the position of the tooth to change. This change is produced in the structural elements of the periodontium as a result of the position gradually assumed by the tooth in the alveolus.

The precise sequence of events that occur

when force is applied to a tooth and then released is not clear, and likewise the relative importance of the constituent structural elements of the periodontium is not known. It appears, however, that in the healthy state the following factors are involved: (1) magnitude, rate, and duration of the force; (2) biologic status of the periodontal ligament, which is related to the previous loading history during the day; and (3) long-term factors such as the patient's age and general systemic health. Apparently changes in force patterns acting on the teeth over extended periods elicit adjustments in the supporting tissues. Consequently the application of greater loads during mastication tends to cause an increase in the width of the periodontal ligament and in the number and density of principal fibers. Very little change in tooth position occurs, however. More sustained, but smaller, forces cause a change in tooth position; and thus an equilibrium position is reestablished. The specific thresholds of force and time required for these changes are unknown, and they vary in different people.

The greatest forces acting on the teeth are normally produced during mastication and deglutition, and they are essentially vertical in direction. Each thrust is of short duration, and for most people, at least, chewing is restricted to short periods during the day. Deglutition, on the other hand, occurs about 500 times a day, and tooth contacts during swallowing are usually of longer duration than those occurring during chewing. Loads of a lower order but longer duration are produced throughout the day by the tongue and perioral-circumoral musculature. These forces are predominantly in the horizontal direction. Estimates of peak forces from the tongue, cheeks, and lips have been made, and lingual force appears to exceed buccolabial force during activity. During rest or inactive periods the total forces may be of similar magnitude.

During mastication, biting forces are transmitted through the bolus to the opposing teeth whether the teeth make contact or not. These forces increase steadily (depending on the na-

Table 1-1 Calculation of total time during 24 hours when direct functional occlusal force is applied to the periodontal tissues

CHEWING

Actual chewing time per meal	450 sec
Four meals per day	1800 sec
One chewing stroke per sec	1800 strokes
Duration of each stroke	0.3 sec
Total chewing forces per day	540 sec (9 min)

SWALLOWING
Meals

Duration of one deglutition	1 sec
During chewing, three deglutitions per min, one third with occlusal force	30 sec (0.5 min)

Between meals

Daytime: 25 per hr (16 hr)	400 sec (6.6 min)
Sleep: 10 per hr (8 hr)	80 sec (1.3 min)
TOTAL	1050 sec = 17.5 min

From Graf H: Dent Clin North Am **13**:659-665, 1969.

ture of the food fragment), reach a peak, and abruptly return to zero. The magnitude, rise time, and interval between thrusts differ among persons and depend on the consistency of the food, the point in the chewing sequence, and the dental status. The direction of the forces is principally perpendicular to the occlusal plane in normal function, but the forward angulation of most natural teeth leads to the introduction of a horizontal component that tends to tilt the teeth mesially as well as buccally or lingually. Upper incisors may be displaced labially with each biting thrust, and these tooth movements quite probably cause proximal wear facets to develop.

In healthy dentitions, teeth are not in occlusion except during the functional movements of chewing and deglutition and during the movements of parafunction. These various mandibular movements and their significance are described later. It has been calculated that the total time during which the teeth are subjected to functional forces of mastication and deglutition during an entire day amounts to approximately 17.5 minutes (Table 1-1). More than half of this time is attributable to jaw-closing forces applied during deglutition. Thus the total time and the range of forces seem to be well within the tolerance level of healthy periodontal tissues.

MECHANISMS OF COMPLETE DENTURE SUPPORT

The basic problem in the treatment of edentulous patients lies in the nature of the difference between the ways natural teeth and their artificial replacements are attached to the supporting bone.

The unsuitability of the tissues supporting complete dentures for load-bearing function must be immediately recognized. In normal function in the dentulous state, light loads are placed on the mucous membrane. With complete dentures, the mucous membrane is forced to serve the same purpose as the periodontal ligaments that provide support for natural teeth.

Masticatory loads

Masticatory loads are much smaller than those that can be produced by conscious effort and are in the region of 44 lb (20 kg) for the natural teeth. Maximum forces of 13 to 16 lb (6 to 8 kg) during chewing have been recorded with complete dentures, but the average loads are probably much less than these. In fact, maximal bite forces appear to be five to six times less for complete denture wearers than for persons with natural teeth. The forces required for chewing vary with the type of food being chewed. Prosthetic patients frequently limit the loading of supporting tissues by selecting food that does not require masticatory effort exceeding their tissue tolerance.

Mucosa support

The area of mucosa available to receive the load from complete dentures is limited when compared to the corresponding areas of support available for natural dentitions. Researchers have computed the mean denture-bearing area to be 22.96 cm^2 in the edentulous maxillae and approximately 12.25 cm^2 in an edentulous mandible. These figures, particularly the mandibular ones, are in dramatic contrast with the 45 cm^2 of area of periodontal ligament available in each dental arch (Fig. 1-4). It must also be

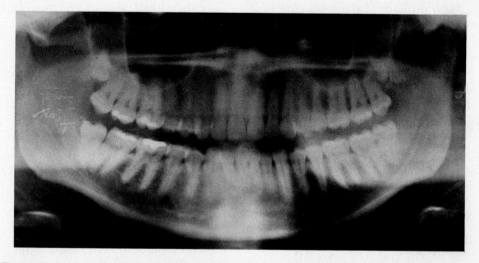

Fig. 1-4 The area of periodontal ligament supporting an intact natural dentition has been computed to be approximately 45 cm^2 in each arch. When teeth are lost and a patient becomes edentulous, quantitative and qualitative aspects of support for an occlusion are severely compromised (see Figs. 1-3 and 1-5).

remembered that the denture-bearing area (basal seat) becomes progressively smaller as residual ridges resorb. Furthermore, the mucosa demonstrates little tolerance or adaptability to denture wearing. This minimal tolerance can be reduced still further by the presence of systemic disease such as anemia, nutritional deficiencies, hypertension, or diabetes. In fact, any disturbance of the normal metabolic processes may lower the upper limit of mucosal tolerance and initiate inflammation.

Residual ridge

The residual ridge consists of denture-bearing mucosa, the submucosa and periosteum, and the underlying residual alveolar bone. Residual bone is that bone of the alveolar process that remains after teeth are lost. When the alveolar process is made edentulous by loss of teeth, the alveoli that contained the roots of the teeth fill in with new bone. This alveolar process becomes the residual ridge, which is the foundation for dentures.

A variety of changes occur in the residual bone after tooth extraction and wearing of complete dentures. They result from three facts: (1) function modifies the internal structure of bone; (2) pressure tends to cause bone resorption; and (3) tension can in some situations bring about bone deposition. Alveolar bone supporting natural teeth receives tensile loads through a large area of periodontal ligament. The edentulous residual ridge receives vertical, diagonal, and horizontal loads applied by a denture with a surface area much smaller than the total area of the periodontal ligaments of all the natural teeth that had been present. Clinical experience underscores the frequently remarkable adaptive range of the masticatory system. On the other hand, edentulous patients demonstrate very little adaptation of the supporting tissues to functional requirements.

One of the few firm facts relating to edentulous patients is that the wearing of dentures is almost invariably accompanied by an undesirable bone loss. The magnitude of this loss is extremely variable, and little is known about which factors are most important for the observed variations (Fig. 1-5). Two concepts have been advanced concerning the inevitable loss of residual bone: One contends that as a direct consequence of loss of the periodontal structures, variable progressive bone reduction occurs. The other maintains that residual bone loss is not a necessary consequence of tooth removal but is dependent on a series of poorly understood factors.

Clinical experience strongly suggests a definite relationship between healthy periodontal ligaments and maintained integrity of alveolar bone; hence the dentist's commitment to preservation and protection of any remaining teeth (Chapters 3 and 25) to minimize or avoid advanced residual ridge reduction. On the other hand, no relationship has been found between periodontal status before tooth extractions and subsequent patterns of residual ridge resorption.

It is apparent that the support for the complete denture is conspicuously limited in its adaptive ability and its inherent capability of simulating the role of the periodontium. The mechanism of support is further complicated by the fact that complete dentures move in relation to the underlying bone during function. This movement is related to the resiliency of the supporting mucosa and the inherent instability of the dentures during function. Almost all "principles" of complete denture construction have been formulated to minimize the forces transmitted to the supporting structures or to decrease the movement of the prostheses in relation to them (Section III). Conclusions regarding denture stability are usually based on clinical experience, but denture instability has the potential of being traumatic to the supporting tissue. Movement of denture bases in any direction on their basal seats can cause tissue damage. In fact it is tempting to construe the recurrent movements of removable prostheses as parafunctional movement and a major factor for residual ridge reduction.

Factors affecting the retention of complete dentures are considered as either physical or

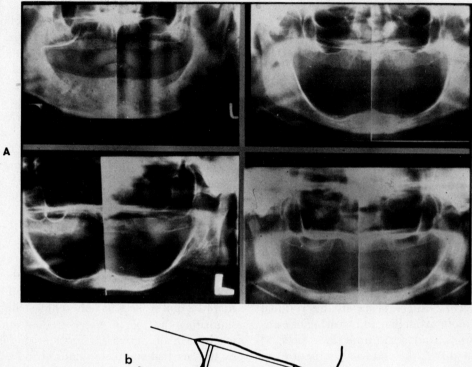

A

B

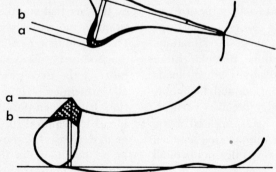

Fig. 1-5 **A,** Panoramic radiographs showing the jaws of four edentulous patients. Residual ridge reduction has occurred to variable extents. In **B,** the rate of ridge reduction is quantified between two stages of observation *(a and b).* The difference, *a − b,* represents the reduction in height of the alveolar ridges between stages of observation. *Shaded area* denotes resorption. (**B** modified from Tallgren A: J Prosthet Dent **27:**120-132, 1972.)

muscular. Three physical factors are involved in denture retention and under the control of the dentist:

1. Maximal extension of the denture base
2. Maximal area of contact between the mucous membrane and the denture base
3. Intimate contact of the denture base and its basal seat

The muscular factors can be used to increase retention (and stability) of dentures. The buccinator, the orbicularis oris, and the intrinsic and extrinsic muscles of the tongue are the key muscles of this activity. Impression techniques, the design of the labial, buccal, and lingual polished surfaces of the denture, and the form of the dental arch should all be considered in balancing the forces generated by the tongue and perioral musculature and the occlusal forces as well.

As the form and size of the denture-supporting tissues (the basal seat) change, the physiologic muscular forces become more important in denture retention. The newly inserted dentures will promote changes in the underlying mucosa and bone.

Psychologic effect on retention

The dentures may have an adverse psychologic effect on the patient, and the nervous influences that result may affect the salivary secretions and thus affect retention. Eventually patients acquire an ability to retain their dentures by means of their oral musculature. This muscular stabilization of dentures is probably accompanied by a reduction in the physical forces used in retaining their dentures. Quite clearly, the physical forces of retention can be improved and reestablished, up to a point, by careful and frequent attention to the denture status. This is done by periodic inspection and by relining and rebasing procedures (Section V).

FUNCTIONAL AND PARAFUNCTIONAL CONSIDERATIONS

The masticatory system appears to operate best in an environment of continuing functional equilibrium. This equilibrium is dependent on the interactions of the many components represented in Fig. 1-3. The substitution of a complete denture for the teeth/periodontium mechanism alters this equilibrium. An analysis of this alteration is the basis for understanding the significance of the edentulous state.

Occlusion

The primary components of human dental occlusion are (1) the dentition, (2) the neuromuscular system, and (3) the craniofacial structures. The development and maturation of these components are interrelated, so that growth, adaptation, and change actively participate in the development of an adult occlusion. The dentition develops in a milieu characterized by a period of dental alveolar and craniofacial adaptability (Fig. 1-6), which is also a time when motor skills and neuromuscular learning are developing. Clinical treatment at this time may take advantage of such responsive adaptive mechanisms; for example, teeth can be guided into their correct alignment by orthodontic treatment.

In a healthy adult dentition, dental adaptive mechanisms are restricted to wear, extrusion, and drifting of teeth. Bony adaptations are essentially of a reparative nature and are slow in their operation. Protective reflexes are learned so one can avoid pain and inefficiency of the masticatory system. If and when an adult dentition begins to deteriorate, the dentist resorts to fixed or removable prosthodontic therapy in attempts to maintain a functional occlusal equilibrium. This period is characterized by greatly diminished dental and reflex adaptation and by pathologic bone resorption. Obviously the presence of tooth loss and disease and the depletion of reparative processes pose a major prosthodontic problem. Finally, in the edentulous state there are few natural adaptive mechanisms left. The prosthesis rests on tissues that will change progressively and irreversibly. The artificial occlusion serves in an environment characterized by constant change that is mainly egressive.

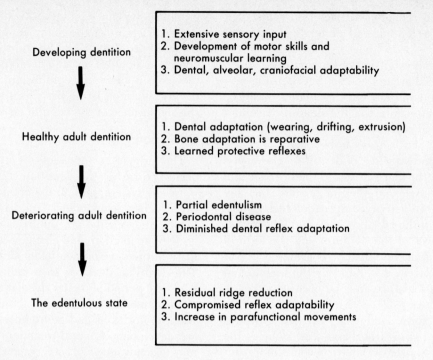

Developing dentition →

1. Extensive sensory input
2. Development of motor skills and neuromuscular learning
3. Dental, alveolar, craniofacial adaptability

Healthy adult dentition →

1. Dental adaptation (wearing, drifting, extrusion)
2. Bone adaptation is reparative
3. Learned protective reflexes

Deteriorating adult dentition →

1. Partial edentulism
2. Periodontal disease
3. Diminished dental reflex adaptation

The edentulous state →

1. Residual ridge reduction
2. Compromised reflex adaptability
3. Increase in parafunctional movements

Fig. 1-6 Development and adaptation of the occlusion. (After Moyers RE: Dent Clin North Am **13:**523-536, 1969.)

The design and fabrication of a prosthetic occlusion have led to fascinating controversies. Dental occlusion was studied first in the field of complete dentures and then in other disciplines. The early workers encountered enormous mechanical difficulties in constructing reasonably fitting dentures that would be both durable and esthetic. Inevitably these dentists had to be mechanically, rather than biologically, minded. Anatomy was the first of the biologic basic sciences to be related to prosthodontic services. Later, histology and physiology were recognized as having an essential role in the treatment of edentulous patients. The emphasis on and application of these basic sciences lifted prosthodontics from the early mechanical art to the applied clinical science it is today.

Currently, complete denture service is characterized by an integration of biologic information with instrumentation, techniques, and use of materials. Narrow beliefs and dogmas are gradually being replaced by enlightened reasoning. Dentists are aware of the need for a better understanding of the physiology of the masticatory system and its application in complete denture service.

Complete dentures are so designed that their occlusal surfaces permit both functional and parafunctional movements of the mandible. Orofacial and tongue muscles play an important role in retaining and stabilizing complete dentures. This is accomplished by arrangement of the artificial teeth to occupy a "neutral zone" in the edentulous mouth so the teeth will occupy a space determined by the functional balance of the orofacial and tongue musculature. Thus the teeth in the dental arch need not necessarily be placed directly over the residual ridges.

Function: mastication and swallowing

Mastication consists of a rhythmic separation and apposition of the jaws and involves biophysical and biochemical processes including the use of the lips, teeth, cheeks, tongue, palate, and all the oral structures to prepare food for swallowing. During masticatory movements the tongue and cheek muscles play an essential role in keeping the food bolus between the occlusal surfaces of the teeth. The control of mastication within the narrow limits of tolerance of the mouth requires considerable sensory information, since deviations from the normal path of mandibular movement can injure the tongue, buccal mucosa, and even the teeth and their supporting tissues. Here, again, the reader's attention must be drawn to the importance of the placement of the arch of artificial teeth in the making of complete dentures. The teeth must be placed within the confines of a functional balance of the musculature involved in controlling the food bolus between the occlusal surfaces of the teeth.

The comminution of much twentieth-century food does not demand a vigorous masticatory performance. Mastication has other functions, however. It is necessary for a full appreciation of the flavor of foods and is therefore indirectly involved in the excitation of salivary and gastric secretions. Since mastication results in the mixing of food with saliva, it facilitates not only swallowing but the digestion of carbohydrates by amylase as well. Amylase activity, of but minor importance while food is in the mouth, is responsible for the continuation of carbohydrate digestion in the stomach, and this phase can account for as much as 60% of the total carbohydrate digestion. Although no reports of quantitative tests on the importance of chewing on the various stages of digestion have appeared, it has been concluded that masticatory efficiency as low as 25% is adequate for complete digestion of foods. Other investigations have noted that loss of teeth can lead to diminished masticatory efficiency. Patients do not compensate for the smaller number of teeth by more prolonged or a larger number of chewing strokes—they merely swallow larger food particles. Although it appears that the importance of a good dentition or denture in promoting digestion and utilization of food has not been adequately demonstrated, clinical experience suggests that the quality of the prosthetic service may have a direct bearing on the denture wearer's masticatory performance.

As mentioned previously, the maximal bite force in denture wearers is five to six times less than in dentulous subjects. Edentulous patients are clearly handicapped in masticatory function, and even clinically satisfactory complete dentures are a poor substitute for natural teeth.

Mandibular movements. The results of studies of mandibular movement patterns of complete denture patients indicate that these movements are similar in denture-wearing patients and persons with natural teeth. Treatment of partially edentulous and edentulous patients therefore might improve their chewing efficiency and masticatory muscle activity, which would be accompanied by a decreased duration of the occlusion phase and contribute to a lessening of elevator muscle activity.

Chewing occurs chiefly in the premolar and molar regions, and both right and left sides are used to about the same extent. The position of the food bolus during mastication is dependent on the consistency of the food, and the tougher the consistency the greater is the person's preference for using the premolar region. The latter observation is apparent even in patients who have worn bilateral, soft tissue–supported, mandibular partial dentures opposing complete upper dentures. It is interesting to note the obvious advantage accruing to a patient by the replacement of missing premolar and molar segments and by the fact that these patients do not chew predominantly in the segments where natural teeth are present.

Reference has been made to the importance

of a complete denture occlusion compatible with the forces developed during deglutition. Tooth contacts while swallowing are fleeting in nature, and they occur many times during a 24-hour day. It has been suggested that the effects of the frequency and duration of tooth contacts while swallowing may be significant in denture base deformation. Swallowing may in the course of a day contribute more to a greater accumulated transfer of energy from the denture base to the underlying mucosa than mastication does.

Both the occurrence of tooth contacts and the observation that the mandible braces itself against the maxillae in denture patients during swallowing suggest that a complete denture occlusion should be compatible with the forces generated by mandibular movements of deglutition. Electromyographic swallowing patterns have been shown to be influenced by changes of natural and complete denture occlusion.

The pronounced differences between persons with natural teeth and patients wearing complete dentures are conspicuous in this functional context: (1) the mucosal mechanism of support as opposed to support by the periodontium, (2) the movements of the dentures during mastication, (3) the progressive changes in maxillomandibular relations and the eventual migration of dentures (described in the discussion of morphologic face height, p. 20), and (4) the different physical stimuli to the sensorimotor systems.

The denture-bearing tissues are constantly exposed to the frictional contact of the overlying denture bases. Dentures move during mastication as a result of the dislodging forces of the surrounding musculature. These movements manifest themselves as displacing, lifting, sliding, tilting, or rotation of the dentures. Furthermore, opposing tooth contacts occur with both natural and artificial teeth during function and parafunction throughout the day and during sleep.

Masticatory investigations have been limited to few subjects, and the occlusal contacts recorded have been in selected experimental areas. Furthermore, the dentures used in the studies have been designed so maximum intercuspation of the artificial teeth would be in centric relation, or the terminal hinge position of the mandible at the selected vertical dimension. Other occlusal concepts that claim other condylar or muscular positions as preferable for complete denture construction have not been investigated for occlusal tooth contact patterns. In all instances the frequency of tooth contact on the nonchewing side has been greater than on the chewing side, irrespective of the side on which the patient chewed or the tooth form or arrangement used.

It has recently been shown that denture wearers with good masticatory performance use a more bilateral muscle effort during chewing whereas those with poor performance employ more of a unilateral effort; the patterns of muscle activity were studied by means of electromyography.

Apparently tissue displacement beneath the denture base results in tilting of the dentures and tooth contacts on the nonchewing side. Also occlusal pressure on the dentures displaces soft tissues of the basal seat and allows the dentures to move closer to the supporting bone. This change of position under pressure induces a change in the relationship of the teeth to each other.

The presence of inanimate foreign objects (dentures) in an edentulous mouth is bound to elicit different stimuli to the sensorimotor system, which in turn influences the cyclic masticatory stroke pattern. Both exteroceptors and proprioceptors are probably affected by the size, shape, position, pressure from, and mobility of the prostheses. The exact role and relative importance of mucosal stimuli in the control of jaw movements need clarification, but it has been clearly demonstrated that control of dentures by muscle activity is reduced if surface anesthetic is applied to the oral mucous membrane. Although it is tempting to assume that there is a correlation between oral stereognosis and purposeful oral motor activity, the results of most investigations up to now indicate that successful denture wearing possibly involves factors other than oral perception and oral performance.

Parafunction

Nonfunctional or parafunctional habits involving repeated or sustained occlusion of the teeth can be harmful to the teeth or other components of the masticatory system. There are no epidemiologic studies about the incidence of parafunctional occlusal stress in normal or denture-wearing populations. However, clinical experience indicates that bruxism is common and is a frequent cause of the complaint of soreness of the denture-bearing mucous membrane. In the denture wearer, parafunctional habits can cause additional loading on the denture-bearing tissues (Table 1-2). The unsuitability of the mechanism of denture support has already been recognized and described.

The neurophysiologic basis underlying bruxism has been studied experimentally both in animals and in humans. The neuromuscular mechanism can be explained by an increase in the tonic activity in the jaw muscles. Emotional or nervous tension, pain or discomfort, the stresses of everyday life, and occlusal interferences are some of the factors that can increase muscle tonus and lead to nonfunctional gnashing and clenching.

The initial discomfort associated with wearing new dentures is known to evoke unusual patterns of behavior in the surrounding musculature. Frequently the complaint of a sore tongue is related to a habit of thrusting the tongue against the denture. The patient is usually unaware of the causal relationship between the painful tongue and its contact with the teeth. Similarly patients tend to occlude the teeth of new dentures frequently at first—perhaps to strengthen confidence in retention until the surrounding muscles become accustomed or because some accommodation in the chewing pattern is usually required and exper-

Table 1-2 Direction, duration, and magnitude of the forces generated during function and parafunction

| | Force generated | |
	Direction	Duration and magnitude
Mastication	Mainly vertical	Intermittent and light
		Diurnal only
Parafunction	Frequently horizontal as well as vertical	Prolonged, possibly excessive
		Both diurnal and nocturnal

imental closure of the teeth is part of the process of adaptation. A strong response of the lower lip and mentalis muscle has been observed electromyographically in long-term complete denture wearers with impaired retention and stability of the lower denture. It is feasible and probable that the tentative occlusal contacts resulting may trigger the development of habitual nonfunctional occlusion.

The mechanism whereby pressure causes soreness of the mucous membrane is probably related to an interruption or a diminution of the blood flow in the small blood vessels in the tissues. These vascular changes could very well upset the metabolism of the involved tissues. *The relationship between parafunction and residual ridge reduction has not been investigated. It is tempting, however, to include parafunction as a possible significant prosthetic variable that contributes to the magnitude of ridge reduction.*

Distribution of stress to the denture-supporting tissues

The need for fulfilling the fundamental objectives of good prosthodontic treatment is underscored by the preceding information. All possible methods should be undertaken to ensure continued tissue health by minimizing the potential traumatic effects of complete denture wear. The capability of the supporting tissues to resist pressure should be improved whenever possible by adequate preparation of both hard and soft tissues. Mucosal health can be promoted by hygienic and therapeutic measures, and tissue-conditioning techniques may be applied when appropriate. Complete denture base extension within morphologic and functional limits will reduce considerably the occlusal load per unit area of mucosa. Resilient denture base lining materials may be used, and the masticatory loading may be decreased by reduction of the area of the occlusal table.

Currently, for practical purposes, denture bases are made of rigid materials. These may be one of various types of resins, metals, or combinations. The dentist must recognize that the prolonged contact of these bases with their underlying tissues is bound to elicit changes in the tissues. Furthermore, the tissues are susceptible to changes caused by the increased longevity of patients and the effects of aging on tissues, as well as by the functional and parafunctional demands that patients make on their denture-supporting tissues. Many dentists have been tempted to equate the prevalent residual ridge reduction in the edentulous population with excessive stresses that are imposed on these ridges. Up to now there has been no specific evidence to indict any one factor as causing advanced ridge reduction. However, strong theoretical evidence exists to justify the development of permanently resilient lining materials in complete dentures. These materials could permit a wider dispersion of forces and result in the transmission of less force per unit area of supporting tissues. Such a soft denture lining material would effectively increase the thickness of the oral tissue by serving as an analogue of the mucoperiosteum, with its relatively low elastic modulus.

The distance increment between the hard denture base and the nonresilient bony support would be increased, with hypothetical salutary long-term results. The Academy of Denture Prosthetics has listed ideas for future research in denture base materials. The list enumerates needed qualities for the improvement of denture base materials and cites the following desirable properties:

1. Possessing variable consistency under varying mouth conditions
2. Selectively resilient—compatible with resiliency of the tissues

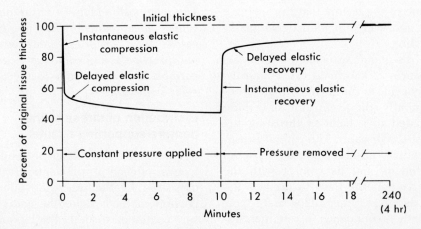

Fig. 1-7   Typical behavior of tissue under a constant pressure load for 10 min. Notice the 90% recovery within 8 min following removal of the pressure. Total recovery requires 4 hr. (From Kydd WL, et al: Int Dent J **21**:430-441, 1971.)

3. Resilient with quick recovery—able to recover shape quickly after deforming forces are removed
4. Compressible on the tissue side but rigid on the occlusal side
5. Shock absorbing
6. Controlling or reducing forces transmitted through the base to the underlying tissue
7. Possessing flexibility that can be controlled and varied in processing as desired

It can be argued that during function and parafunction, pressures are applied by the dentures that displace the soft tissues. These pressures deform the mucoperiosteum and interfere with the circulation of blood, nutrients, and metabolites. Several studies have demonstrated such changes in soft tissue contour as a result of mechanical stress. The viscoelastic character of denture-supporting tissue has been described (Fig. 1-7). There is an initial elastic compression of soft tissues that takes place instantly on application of load. After the elastic phase there is a delayed elastic deformation of the tissue that takes place more slowly and continues to diminish in rate of change as duration of load is extended. An instantaneous elas-

tic decompression occurs when the pressure is removed. This is followed by a continuing delayed elastic recovery. Histologically the stressed oral mucosa has an altered morphologic pattern. The loaded epithelium demonstrates a decrease in the depth of the epithelial ridges, and the connective tissue papillae are obliterated. The extent of these alterations varies with the force and duration of the applied pressure. Human soft tissues may take as long as 4 hours to recover after moderate loading for 10 minutes.

A change in tissue displaceability can also be demonstrated as being a function of age. A longer period is needed for the recovery of displaced mucosa in elderly people (68 to 70 years) than in young adults (21 to 27 years) (Fig. 1-8). It appears that any intraoral prosthesis can be intruded into the denture-supporting oral mucosa by up to 20% of the mucosal thickness with relatively small occluding forces (0.2 g/mm^2). It has also been shown that pressures as small as 0.13 g/mm^2 will displace human soft tissues to 95% of their resting thickness. This indicates that impression materials, for example, must flow readily and with minimal pres-

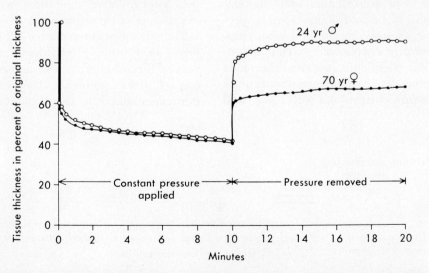

Fig. 1-8 Comparison of responses to tissue loading and removal of the load in an elderly and a young adult. The compression curve is essentially the same. The removal of load shows definite differences in rate of recovery. The load was 11 g/mm^2. (From Kydd WL, et al: Int Dent J **21**:430-444, 1971.)

sure when an impression is being made.

Pressures under complete maxillary dentures have been recorded using a closed fluid system connected to a pressure transducer and recorder to register positive and negative pressures in four subjects at four locations. Each subject performed a number of controlled masticatory and nonmasticatory activities. The findings indicated that a number of nonmasticatory activities (smoking, swallowing, speaking) can create as much positive and negative pressures on the supporting tissues as masticatory activities do, and sometimes more.

It has been observed that people swallow approximately one and a half times per minute while reading, which would total approximately 1500 swallows per day unrelated to eating or drinking. When converted to meter/kilogram units, this amounts to about 1750 N per day from swallowing alone.

The rapid fluctuation from positive to negative pressures indicates a pressure wave beneath the denture. This is attributable to rocking or movement or to a flow of fluid within the vascular channels that possibly creates trauma with each tooth contact. It is tempting to suggest that these pressures could affect the soft tissue and the blood and lymph vessels, perhaps causing sclerosis, diminished blood supply, and the many morphologic variants we encounter in our edentulous patients. The effect of these continually occurring non–masticatory induced pressure changes and waves may well be of greater significance than the effect of mastication.

It appears that pressure may cause tissue damage by occluding the local circulation, subject to a force/time threshold. The harmful effect of pressure can be avoided by diminution or elimination of either factor. The amount of *force* generated by a patient's masticatory system is not controlled by the dentist. The dentist may seek to minimize force distribution by maximizing denture base coverage and developing an optimal denture occlusion. Occlusal surfaces of the artificial teeth can be made smaller, and the patient can be instructed to handle parafunctional habits through education and understanding. Forces can also be reduced or diluted by use of a permanently resilient liner if such materials are readily available (Fig. 1-9). The *time* factor can be controlled to a large extent by frequent rest periods for the denture-supporting tissues. Leaving the dentures out of the mouth during sleeping hours is recommended. Oral tissues were designed to be exposed to oral fluids and to be stimulated by the action of tongue, lips, and cheeks. Nocturnal rest can achieve this objective, along with a quantitative diminution in the duration of exposure of these tissues to stress.

The efficiency of temporary soft or treatment liners in routine prosthodontic practice has proved the value of such an approach in treating soft tissue problems. The contribution of permanent liners to the maintenance of sup-

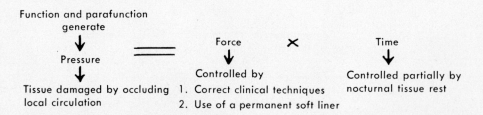
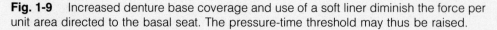

Fig. 1-9   Increased denture base coverage and use of a soft liner diminish the force per unit area directed to the basal seat. The pressure-time threshold may thus be raised.

porting tissue integrity and morphology is still hypothetical, however.

A number of resilient liners with furtive claims to permanency have appeared on the market in recent years. Their major use, however, has been as a therapeutic measure for patients who cannot tolerate the stresses induced by dentures. Clinical experience indicates almost universal tissue tolerance of these materials and acceptable patient reactions. *At present, the materials have to be considered as temporary expedients, since none of the soft liners has a life expectancy comparable to that of the resin denture base.*

The most frequently used liners are usually produced from silicone rubbers or acrylic resins. Recent reports also suggest the possible employment of hydrophilic polymers and fluoropolymers. Research has been in the direction of a material that would be permanently resilient, not absorb fluids, adhere to denture base materials, and be chemically stable. The silicone rubber resilient liners, when properly used, have been found to be the most appropriate of the various types available, but they too are only temporary expedients. They support yeast growth (such as *Candida albicans*) (Fig 1-10) and they must be inspected regularly by the dentist and replaced when unsatisfactory. The use of proper cleansers and home care habits has contributed to the employment of these materials, with significantly beneficial results. It must be emphasized, however, that using these materials does not preclude adherence to the fundamental principles of complete denture construction. Nevertheless, when used intelligently, resilient liners can be an excellent adjunct in prosthodontics.

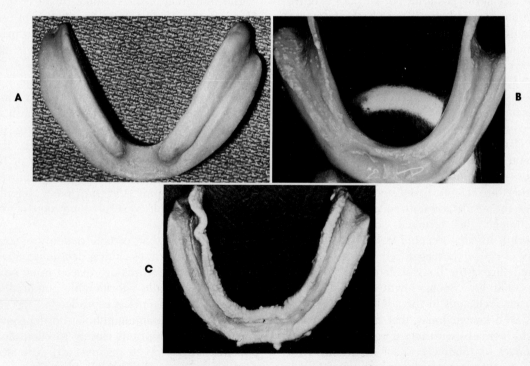

Fig. 1-10   **A,** Recently completed resilient liner on a mandibular denture. **B,** A 6 mo old resilient liner with foci of yeast colonies already apparent. **C,** A neglected 12 mo old resilient liner with almost total coverage by yeast colonies.

CHANGES IN MORPHOLOGIC FACE HEIGHT AND THE TEMPOROMANDIBULAR JOINTS
Face height

Numerous descriptions of TMJ function have evolved as a result of several research methods. The basic physiologic relation between the condyles, the disks, and their glenoid fossae appears to be maintained during maximal occlusal contacts and during all movements guided by occlusal elements. It seems logical that in the treatment with complete dentures, the dentist should seek to maintain or restore this basic physiologic relation. The border movements of the mandible are reproducible and all other movements take place within the confines of the classic "envelopes of motion." Researchers have concluded that the passive hinge movement has a constant and definite rotational and reproducible character. The reproducibility of the posterior border path is of tremendous practical significance in the treatment of prosthodontic patients and is described in Section III. However, this reproducibility has been established in healthy young persons only. It must be recalled that most edentulous patients have experienced a period with variations on the theme of a mutilated dentition. In the course of this period, pathologic or adaptive changes of the TMJs may have occurred. Several authors suggest that structural alterations can take place in the TMJs. These investigations are mainly based on autopsy studies; hence the results are only speculative.

Although the terminal stage of skeletal growth is usually accepted as being at 20 to 25 years of age, it is recognized that growth and remodeling of the bony skeleton continue well into adult life. Such growth accounts for dimensional changes in the adult facial skeleton. It is well known today that morphologic face height increases with age in persons possessing an intact or relatively intact dentition. However, a premature reduction in morphologic face height occurs with attrition or abrasion of teeth. This reduction is even more conspicuous in edentulous and complete denture–wearing patients.

Maxillomandibular morphologic changes take place slowly over a period of years and depend on the balance of osteoblastic and osteoclastic activity. The articular surfaces of the temporomandibular joints are also involved, and at these sites growth and remodeling are mediated through the proliferative activity of the articular cartilages. In the facial skeleton any dimensional changes in morphologic face height or the jawbones as a result of the loss of teeth are inevitably transmitted to the TMJs joints. It is not surprising, then, that these articular surfaces undergo a slow but continuous remodeling throughout life. Such remodeling is probably the means whereby the congruity of the opposing articular surfaces is maintained, even in the presence of dimensional or functional changes in other parts of the facial skeleton.

The reduction of the residual ridges (Fig. 1-11) tends to cause a resultant reduction in total face height and an increase in mandibular prognathism. In complete denture wearers the mean reduction in height of the mandibular process measured in the anterior region may be 6.6 mm, approximately four times greater than the mean reduction occurring in the maxillary process. Cephalometric observations and longitudinal studies support the hypothesis that the vertical dimension of rest position of the jaws does not remain stable and can be altered over time, usurping the previously popular concept of a stable vertical dimension of rest position.

It is obvious that complete dentures constructed to conform to clinical decisions regarding jaw relation records are placed in an environment that retains considerable potential for change. Thus concepts of reproducible and relatively unchangeable mandibular border movements may not apply as closely to edentulous patients as they do to persons with a healthy dentition. Practical methods that recognize these facts are described in subsequent chapters. It must be reemphasized, however, that

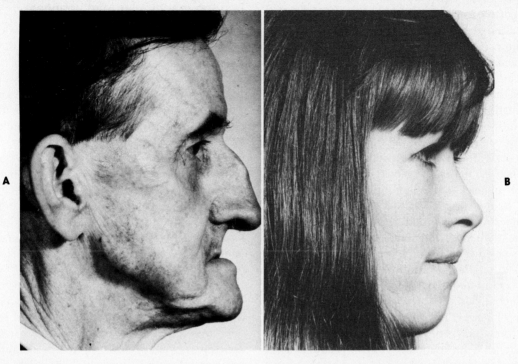

Fig. 1-11   **A,** A 67-year-old man who has worn unserviced dentures for almost 20 years. Notice the reduction in total face height and the increased mandibular prognathism. **B,** Contrast his appearance with that of a 24-year-old woman who recently acquired complete dentures but posed for this picture with her dentures out of her mouth.

the recognition that jaw relations are not immutable does not invalidate the clinical requirement of using a centric relation record as a starting point for developing a prosthetic occlusion.

Centric relation. Concepts of centric relation of the upper and lower jaws have been a dominant factor in prosthodontic thinking on occlusion. Centric relation is defined as the most posterior position of the mandible relative to the maxillae at the established vertical dimension. Centric relation coincides with a reproducible posterior hinge position of the mandible, and it may be recorded with a high degree of accuracy. It is considered the essential relationship in any prosthodontic treatment.

The use of centric relation has its physiologic justification as well. In the vast majority of patients, unconscious swallowing is carried out with the mandible at or near the centric relation position. The unconscious or reflex swallow is important in the developing dentition. The act and frequency of swallowing are important influences in the movement of teeth within the muscle matrix, and this movement determines the tooth position and occlusal relations. The erupting teeth are guided into occlusion by the surrounding musculature (the muscle matrix) whereas the position of the mandible is determined by its location in space during the act of unconscious swallowing. The contacts of inclined planes of the teeth aid in the alignment of the erupting dentition. It must be remembered that in this developmental period most of the mandibular activities have not yet been learned, at least not in their adult form.

The occlusion of complete dentures is designed to harmonize with the primitive and unconditioned reflex of the patient's unconscious swallow. Tooth contacts and mandibular bracing against the maxillae occur during swallowing by complete denture patients. This suggests that complete denture occlusions must be compatible with the forces developed during deglutition to prevent disharmonious occlusal contacts that could cause trauma to the basal seat of dentures. During swallowing the mandible is close to, or in, centric relation or the position of maximum mandibular retrusion relative to the maxillae at the established vertical dimension of occlusion. It is conceded, however, that most functional natural tooth contacts occur in a mandibular position anterior to centric relation, a position referred to as centric occlusion.

In complete denture prosthodontics the position of maximum planned intercuspation of teeth, or centric occlusion, is established to coincide with the patient's centric relation. The centric occlusion position occupied by the mandible in the dentate patient cannot be registered with sufficient accuracy when the patient becomes edentulous. In other words, the muscle memory pattern of the mandibular musculature would not be effective in edentulous patients. Clinical experience supports the conviction that the recording of centric relation is an *essential starting point* in the design of an artificial occlusion.

However, one must realize that an integral part of the definition of centric relation—at the established vertical dimension—has potential for change. This change is brought about by alterations in denture-supporting tissues and facial height morphology and by morphologic changes in the TMJs. An appreciation for the dynamic nature of centric relation in denture wearing patients recognizes the changing functional requirements of the masticatory system. It also accounts for different concepts and techniques of design of occlusions (which are described in Section III).

Temporomandibular joint changes

Several authors claim that impaired dental efficiency resulting from partial tooth loss and absence of, or incorrect, prosthodontic treatment can bring about TMJ pain and dysfunction or even degenerative changes in the joints. Published clinical reports on functional disorders of the masticatory system have included patients who are denture wearers. It is possible that these denture wearers' difficulties started before the offending teeth were removed. However, there are indications also that the impairment of denture quality plays a role in the development of signs and symptoms of TM disorders since such signs and symptoms are often significantly reduced after the insertion of new dentures.

Although the relationship between occlusion and degenerative joint disease (DJD) is not completely clear, the dentist is tempted to believe that a depleted or inadequately cared for dentition obviously loads the temporomandibular joints. Denturer wearers have been shown to suffer from DJD more frequently than persons with a complete natural dentition, but this may be age related rather than due to the state of the dentition. The hypothesis that degenerative joint disease is a process rather than a disease entity has been advanced. The process involves joint changes that cause an imbalance in adaptation and a degeneration that results from alterations in functional demands on or the functional capacity of the joints.

Research strongly suggests that purely dental factors may be important in the etiology of degenerative joint disease of the mandibular condyles. Involvement of the temporomandibular joints in degenerative diseases is well documented; however, it must be appreciated that the onset of degenerative conditions is frequently in the adult years and, since the greater number of denture wearers are adult, the treatment of such conditions is very much the concern of the dentist. Clinical experience and long-term studies indicate that the application of sound prosthodontic principles, accompanied by appropriate supportive therapy, is usually adequate to provide these patients with comfort.

One of the difficulties in managing degenerative joint involvement is achieving joint rest. Because of the necessity for mastication and for the avoidance of tensional habits, voluntary or even enforced rest may be difficult to achieve.

INDIVIDUAL BEHAVIORAL AND ADAPTIVE RESPONSES
Cosmetic changes

There is little doubt that tooth loss can adversely affect a person's appearance. Patients seek dental treatment for both functional and cosmetic reasons, and dentists have been successful in restoring or improving many a patient's appearance (Fig. 1-12).

Table 1-3 lists some of the conspicuous and clinically challenging cosmetic features that frequently accompany the edentulous state. It must be emphasized that one or more of these items can be encountered in persons with intact dentitions, since the compromised facial support of the edentulous state is *not* the exclusive cause of the morphologic changes. In clinical practice we frequently encounter situations in which a patient's weight loss, age, heavy tooth attrition, and so on manifest orofacial changes suggestive of compromised, or absent, dental support for the overlying tissues. Some patients fail to appreciate the fact that aspects of their facial appearance for which they are seeking a solution are merely magnified or else are unrelated to their edentulous predicament.

These patients can cause the dentist considerable frustration. Experience suggests that *early* communication about a patient's cosmetic expectations should be established to avoid later misunderstanding. Patients should be asked to provide photographs of their preedentulous appearance, and relevant details from these photographs should be carefully analyzed·

Table 1-3 Morphologic changes associated with the edentulous state

1. Deepening of nasolabial groove
2. Loss of labiodental angle
3. Decrease in horizontal labial angle
4. Narrowing of lips
5. Increase in columella-philtral angle
6. Prognathic appearance

and discussed with the patient. If this is not possible, photographs of siblings, or of children who resemble the patient, may be helpful.

Careful explanation of prosthodontic objectives and methods is the basis for good communication with all patients. This is particularly so when it becomes apparent to the dentist that the patient's cosmetic desires exceed morphologic or functional realities.

Dietary changes

The effect of prosthetic restorations on masticatory ability has been studied. Optimal complete dentures appear to improve masticatory function, which would suggest an improvement in dietary selection. However, researchers have shown that improved oral function will not in itself lead to changes in dietary selection. It is concluded that dietary changes probably require professional and individually given dietary advice by a trained dietitian.

Adaptive and psychologic responses

The process whereby an edentulous patient can accept and use complete dentures is complex. It requires adaptation of learning, muscular skill, and motivation and is related to patient expectations. It is the patient's ability and willingness to accept and learn to use the dentures that ultimately determine the degree of success of clinical treatment. Helping a patient adapt to complete dentures can be one of the most difficult, but also one of the most rewarding, aspects of clinical dentistry.

Learning means the acquisition of a new activity or change of an existing one. Muscular

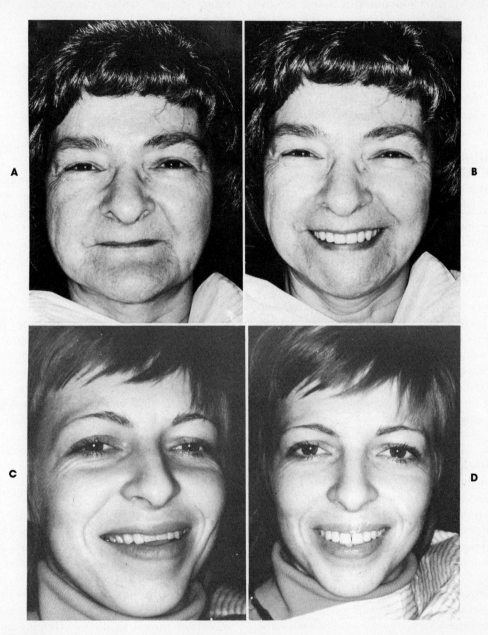

Fig. 1-12   Before, **A,** and after, **B,** clinical views of an edentulous patient who has been treated by construction of complete upper and lower dentures. Before, **C,** and after, **D,** views of another patient whose old cosmetically unsatisfactory dentures were replaced; her youth and appealing smile are brought out by the new tooth arrangement. Notice that several of the features listed in Table 1-3 are readily discernible in **A** and **C.**

skill refers to the capacity to coordinate muscular activity so as to execute movement. The acceptance of complete dentures is accompanied by a process of habituation, which is defined as a "gradual diminution of responses to continued or repeated stimuli." The tactile stimuli that arise from the contact of the prosthesis with the richly innervated oral cavity are probably ignored after a short time. Since each stage of the decrease in response is related to the memory trace of the previous application of the stimulus, storage of information from the immediate past is an integral part of habituation. Difficulty in the storage of information of this type accompanies old age, and this accounts for the difficulties of older patients in getting used to dentures. Furthermore, stimuli must be specific and identical to achieve habituation. This is what probably prevents the transfer of habituation evoked by an old familiar denture to a new denture, which inevitably gives rise to a new range of stimuli. Fish describes several clinical applications of adaptation problems that may be encountered. The patient who has worn a complete upper denture opposing a few natural anterior mandibular teeth will usually find a complete lower denture difficult to adapt to. Such a patient has to contend with altered size and orientation of the tongue. The tongue frequently responds to the loss of posterior teeth and alveolar bone by changing size to bring its lateral borders into contact with the buccal mucosa. The insertion of a new denture introduces a new environment for the tongue, and the intrinsic tongue musculature reorganizes the shape of the tongue to conform to the altered space available. A degree of retraining of tongue activity also takes place. Furthermore, the posterior residual ridges are now exposed to new sensations from the overlying prosthesis. Tactile stimuli from the tongue and frictional contact with food are replaced by pressures transferred via the denture base. Also control of the upper denture frequently must be unlearned, since the posterior part of the tongue is no longer required to counter the dislodging effect on the

denture produced by the remaining mandibular dentition.

It must be realized that edentulous patients expect, and are expected, to adapt to the dentures more or less instantaneously and that the adaptation must take place in the context of the patient's oral, systemic, emotional, and psychologic states.

Facility for learning and coordination appears to diminish with age. Advancing age tends to be accompanied by progressive atrophy of elements in the cerebral cortex, and a consequent loss in the facility of coordination occurs. Certainly patient motivation dictates the speed with which adaptation to dentures takes place. It is imperative that the dentist determine the patient's motivation in seeking treatment, cultivate this motivation, and seek to foster it if it is lacking or absent.

A distinct need exists for dentists to be able to understand a patient's motivation in seeking prosthodontic care and to identify problems before starting treatment. Emotional factors are known to play a significant role in the etiology of dental problems. The interview and clinical examination are obvious ways to observe the patient and form the best treatment relationship. Successful management begins with identification of anticipated difficulties before treatment starts and with careful planning to meet specific needs and problems. Dentists must train themselves to reassure the patient, to perceive the patient's wishes, and to know how and when to limit the patient's expectations. An essential accompaniment of a denture design that is physically compatible with the oral complex is a good interpersonal relationship between dentist and patient. It is up to the dentist to explore the patient's symptoms and tensions. The way the patient handles other illnesses and dental situations will aid in the prediction of future problems. It has been pointed out that the secure patient will adjust readily, cope with discomfort, and be cooperative.

It also has been reported that when a complete denture population was examined for depression most of the depressive symptoms were found to coincide with age groups that included the greatest proportion of denture wearers. An awareness by the dentist of high-risk groups for depression within the patient pool may help explain difficulties in achieving patient satisfaction with dentures, facilitate recognition of a problem, and make possible appropriate referral for diagnosis and treatment of the patient's depression.

The whole area of prosthodontist/patient interpersonal relationships has not been adequately studied or emphasized by the dental profession. Recently, educational programs to modify the often unrealistic expectations of denture patients have shown favorable results. Similarly, programs to modify the knowledge, skills, and habits of denture patients may assist them to adapt more successfully to denture wearing. Although the taking of a health history can be effective, a great deal of experience and training are necessary to conduct a patient interview effectively and profitably. Unfortunately, the rigors of dental practice prevent the majority of dentists from taking the time to carry out a thorough patient interview. Since a connection between emotional problems and denture problems may exist, a health questionnaire should be used as a guide for a structured personal interview with the patient. It is a useful adjunct to establishing a prognosis for the proposed treatment.

Adaptive potential of the patient

The absence of a yardstick to gauge a patient's adaptive potential is one of the most challenging facets of treating edentulism. *The success of prosthetic treatment is predicated not only on manual dexterity but also on the ability of the dentist to relate to patients and to understand their needs.* The importance of empathy on the part of the dentist can hardly be overemphasized. It is the dentist's ability to understand and recognize the problems of edentulous patients and to reassure them that has proved to be of greatest clinical value.

BIBLIOGRAPHY

Atwood DA: A cephalometric study of the clinical rest position. II, The variability in the rate of bone loss following the removal of occlusal contacts, J Prosthet Dent **7**:544-552, 1957.

Atwood DA: The future of prosthodontics, J Prosthet Dent **51**:262-267, 1984.

Berry DC, Mahood M: Oral stereognosis and oral ability in relation to prosthetic treatment, Br Dent J **120**:179-185, 1966.

Blackwood HJJ: Arthritis of the mandibular joint, Br Dent J **115**:317-326, 1963.

Blomberg S, Lindquist L: Psychological reactions to edentulousness and treatment with jawbone anchored bridges, Acta Psychiatr Scand **68**:252-256, 1983.

Bolender CL, Swoope CC, Smith DE: The Cornell Medical Index as a prognostic aid for complete denture patients, J Prosthet Dent **22**:20-29, 1969.

Bouma J: On becoming edentulous. An investigation into the dental and behavioral reasons for full mouth extractions. Thesis, Rijksuniversiteit te Groningen, 1987.

Brill N: Factors in the mechanism of full denture retention, Dent Pract **18**:9-19, 1967.

Brodie AG: Growth pattern of human head from third month to eighth year of life, Am J Anat **68**:209-262, 1941.

Chamberlain BB, Chamberlain KR: Depression: a psychologic consideration in complete denture prosthodontics, J Prosthet Dent **53**:673-675, 1985.

Cohen LK: Dental care delivery in seven nations: the International Collaborative Study of Dental Manpower Systems in relation to oral health status. In Ingle JI, Blair P, editors: International dental care delivery systems. Issues in dental health policies, Cambridge Mass, 1978, Ballinger Publishing Co.

Cutright DE, Brudvik JS, Gay WD, Selting WJ: Tissue pressure under complete maxillary dentures, J Prosthet Dent **35**:160-170, 1976.

Douglass CW, Gammon MD, Atwood DA: Need and effective demand for prosthodontic treatment, J Prosthet Dent **59**:94-99, 1988.

Douglass CW, Gillings D, Sollecito W, Gammon M: National trends in the prevalence and severity of the periodontal diseases, J Am Dent Assoc **107**:403-412, 1983.

Eichner FKW: Recent knowledge gained from long-term observations in the field of prosthodontics, Int Dent J **34**:35-40, 1984.

Ettinger RL, Beck JD, Jakobsen J: Removable prosthodontic treatment needs: a survey, J Prosthet Dent **51**:419-427, 1984.

Farrell JH: The effect of mastication on the digestion of food, Br Dent J **100**:149-155, 1956.

Glaser EM: The physiological basis of habituation, New York, 1966, Oxford University Press Inc.

Graf H: Bruxism, Dent Clin North Am **13**:659-665, 1969.

Hannam AG, De Cou RE, Scott TD, Wood WW: The relationship between dental occlusion, muscle activity and associated jaw movements in man, Arch Oral Biol **22**:25-32, 1977.

Haraldsson T, Karlsson U, Carlsson GE: Bite force and

oral function in complete denture wearers, J Oral Rehabil **6**:41-48, 1979.

Hayakawa I, Kawae M, Tsuji Y, Masuhara E: Soft denture liner of fluoroethylene copolymer and its clinical evaluation, J Prosthet Dent **51**:310-313, 1984.

Hedegård B, Lundberg M, Wictorin L: Masticatory function: a cineradiographic investigation, Acta Odontol Scand **25**:331-353, 1967.

Jemt T, Hedegård B, Wickberg K: Chewing patterns before and after treatment with complete maxillary and bilateral distal-extension mandibular removable partial dentures, J Prosthet Dent **50**:566-570, 1983.

Jemt T, Lundquist S, Hedegård B: Group function or canine protection, J Prosthet Dent **48**:719-724, 1982.

Kydd WL, Daly CH, Wheeler JB: The thickness measurement of masticatory mucosa *in vivo*, Int Dent J **21**:430-441, 1971.

Kydd WL, Mandley J: The stiffness of palatal mucoperiosteum, J Prosthet Dent **18**:116-121, 1967.

Laine P: Adaptation to denture wearing. An opinion survey and experimental investigation, Proc Finn Dent Soc **78**(suppl 2):159-164, 1982.

Laney WR: Processed resilient denture liners, Dent Clin North Am **14**:531-551, 1970.

Lindan P: Etiology of decubitus ulcers: an experimental study, Arch Phys Med **42**:774-783, 1961.

Lönberg P: Changes in the size of the lower jaw on account of age and loss of teeth, Acta Genet Stat Med, suppl, 1951.

Lundberg M, Wictorin L, Hedegård B: Masticatory function; a cineradiographic investigation, Acta Odontol Scand **25**:383-395, 1967.

Lytle RB: Soft tissue displacement beneath removable partial and complete dentures, J Prosthet Dent **12**:34-43, 1962.

Manly RS, Braley LC: Masticatory performance and efficiency, J Dent Res **29**:448-462, 1950.

McNamara J: Neuromuscular and skeletal adaptation to altered orofacial function. Monograph 1, Craniofacial growth series, Ann Arbor Mich, 1972, University of Michigan.

Meskin LH, Brown LJ, Brunelle JA, Warren GB: Patterns of tooth loss and accumulated prosthetic treatment potential in U.S. employed adults and seniors, 1985-1986, Gerodontics **4**:126-135, 1988.

Mohl ND, Zarb GA, Carlsson GE, Rugh JD, editors: A textbook of occlusion, Chicago, 1988, Quintessence Publishing Co Inc.

Sandström B, Lindquist LW: The effect of different prosthetic restorations on the dietary selection in edentulous patients. A longitudinal study of patients initially treated with optimal complete dentures and finally with tissue-integrated prostheses, Acta Odontol Scand **45**(6):423-428, 1987.

Schaub RMH: Barriers to effective periodontal care. Thesis, Rijksuniversiteit te Groningen, 1984.

Smith DE, Kydd WL, Wykhuis WA, Phillips LA: The mobility of artificial dentures during comminution, J Prosthet Dent **13**:839-856, 1963.

Socransky SS, Tanner AC, Goodson JM, Haffajee AD, Walker CB, Ebersole JL, Sornberger GC: An approach to the definition of periodontal disease syndromes by cluster analysis, J Clin Periodontol **9**:460-471, 1982.

Swoope CC Jr, Kydd WL: The effect of cusp form and occlusal surface area on denture base deformation, J Prosthet Dent **16**:34-43, 1966.

Tallgren A: The continuing reduction of the residual alveolar ridges in complete denture wearers: a mixed-longitudinal study covering 25 years, J Prosthet Dent **27**:120-132, 1972.

Thomson JC: Diagnosis in full denture intolerance, Br Dent J **125**:388-391, 1968.

Thomson JC: The load factor in complete denture intolerance, J Prosthet Dent **25**:4-11, 1971.

Tuncay OC, Abadi B, Ellinger C: Cephalometric evaluation of the changes in patients wearing complete dentures. A ten-year longitudinal study, J Prosthet Dent **51**:169-180, 1984.

Weintraub J, Burt B: Oral health status in the United States: tooth loss and edentulism, J Dent Educ **49**:368-376, 1985.

Weintraub JA, Burt BA: Tooth loss in the United States. Presented at the 62nd Annual Session of the American Association of Dental Schools, Las Vegas Nev, 1985.

Woelfel JB, Hickey JC, Allison ML: Effect of posterior tooth form on jaw and denture movement, J Prosthet Dent **12**:922-939, 1962.

Yemm R: Stress-induced muscle activity: a possible etiologic factor in denture soreness, J Prosthet Dent **28**:133-140, 1972.

Zarb GA: Oral motor patterns and their relation to oral prostheses, J Prosthet Dent **47**:472, 1982.

CHAPTER **2**

Tissue response to complete dentures: the aging edentulous patient

A significant percentage of patients seeking complete denture treatment have already worn one or more sets of complete dentures. Their experiences should, of course, be analyzed by the dentist, and the resultant analysis used to design dentures that will significantly increase the possibilities of success with the new treatment. This approach will be reviewed in subsequent chapters. However, it must be emphasized that long-term wear of dentures leads to changes in the oral tissues. Furthermore, these changes, or varying signs in wear and tear of denture-supporting tissues, must be reconciled with concurrent similar or other tissue changes relating to aging. The purpose of this chapter is twofold: to review the most frequently encountered sequelae of long-term denture wearing and to summarize the relevant oral changes associated with the aging edentulous masticatory system.

SOFT TISSUE CHANGES

The response of human skin to everyday wear and tear is to become keratinized and tough. The oral mucosa does not behave in the same manner. Even in the dentulous state, the mucosa demonstrates a low tolerance to injury or irritation. This tolerance is further depleted if systemic disease is present. The mucosa does not appear to be suited to a complete denture load–bearing role and demonstrates little or no ability to respond to this altered function. Denture-bearing mucosal changes are described as bordering on the pathologic but without frank clinical inflammation. A decrease in the keratinization of denture-bearing mucosa and a decrease in mucosal thickness can be seen. Women who wear dentures appear to have a thinner mucosa than men who wear dentures, and they demonstrate a greater predisposition to mucosal injury. Approximately one third of denture wearers with a clinically normal-appearing mucosa show histologic evidence of severe injury. The extent of the injury is also related to the duration of the denture-wearing experience.

Cytologic examination of the denture-bearing mucosa has also demonstrated a depletion in keratinized cell counts. This depletion is related to both habits and duration of wear and to the clinical status of the dentures. The response of the oral epithelium to the placement of prostheses is controversial, however, and some investigators maintain that the tissue response to denture wearing is an individual one. The pathologic significance of the noted changes has not been adequately explained, but it is reasonable to suggest that mucosal inflammation results from denture wear and wherever inflammation is present the process of bone resorption may be accelerated.

It appears that if the tolerance of the mucosal tissues is exceeded (as by an overextended denture border) injury and inflammation will result, and the denture cannot be worn. If, on the other hand, initial tolerance is high and the trauma tolerable, a fibrous response is elicited and the residual ridge is replaced with flabby hyperplastic tissue. Dentures are frequently worn over such tissue without discomfort. In between these two extremes lie the majority of patients, in whom chronic mucosal irritation proceeds quietly and painlessly. Mucosal and underlying bony changes are brought about, often irreversibly. It may be that the character of the underlying bone determines the tolerance and the response of the denture-bearing mucosa.

Changes in both hard and soft tissues under complete dentures are common. They start soon after patients have been treated with such prostheses and include a high incidence of mucosal inflammation within 1 year of denture construction. Consequently a new complete denture with a clinically good fit is no guarantee that mucosal inflammation will not develop in time. Nyquist's classic study underscored the importance of excising hyperplastic ridge tissue before prosthodontic therapy is started. Habits of denture wearers did not influence the incidence of mucosal irritation in this study, but the observation period was of short duration. Round-the-clock denture wearing over a lifetime is conducive to an overloaded mucosal environment, especially when there is nocturnal parafunction.

Clinical observation of many patients who have worn dentures continually reveals that they are more likely to have pseudoepitheliomatous hyperplasia and papillary hyperplasia.

Whereas the adverse effects of insidious and chronic trauma from denture wearing are well documented, recent research also implicates fungal infections (for example, *Candida*) as contributing to pathologic changes associated with denture wearing. Clearly alterations in the stability of the intraoral environment—traumatic, infective, or both—will increase the risk of development of pathologic processes.

Two examples of soft tissue response to long-term denture wearing are frequently encountered: soft tissue hyperplasia and denture stomatitis. Although these conditions are discussed separately, they can and frequently do appear concurrently.

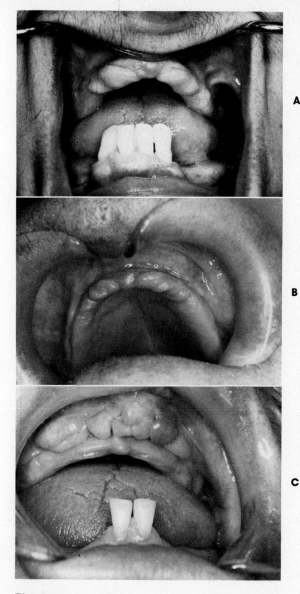

Fig. 2-1 **A,** Anterior maxillary residual ridge hyperplasia extends from one canine area to the other. This patient wore a maxillary denture opposing four natural mandibular teeth. **B,** The entire maxillary alveolar ridge has been replaced by flabby hyperplastic tissue. **C,** The hyperplastic response involves both the ridge and the labial vestibule. Here again, two natural mandibular teeth opposed a complete maxillary denture for several years.

Soft tissue hyperplasia

Hyperplasia of the soft tissues under or around a complete denture is the result of a fibroepithelial response to complete denture wearing. It is often asymptomatic and may be limited to the tissues around the borders of the dentures in the vestibular, lingual, or palatal regions, or it may occur on all or part of the residual ridge (Fig. 2-1). Its etiology is multifactorial, and the following can be listed as probable causes:

1. Changes in the alveolar sockets after extractions
2. Trauma from denture wearing
3. Gradual residual ridge reduction
4. Changes in soft tissue profile and temporomandibular joint function
5. Changes in the relative proportions of both jaws
6. Habits and duration of wear

7. Various aberrant forces to which the supporting tissues are subjected (for example, the natural lower anterior teeth opposing a complete upper denture), including parafunctional mandibular movements (Fig. 2-1, *A* and *C*)
8. Excessive forces on limited segments of the dental arches because of a lack of balancing contacts in eccentric jaw positions

The hyperplasia occurring around the border of a denture may be a fibrous growth referred to as *epulis fissuratum* (Fig. 2-2). It occurs in the free mucosa lining the sulcus or at the junction of the attached and free mucosa. It apparently develops as a result of chronic irritation from ill-fitting or overextended dentures. However, since residual ridges resorb, even the best-fitting dentures gradually develop overextensions as a result of settling into different positions on the basal seat. Clinical exami-

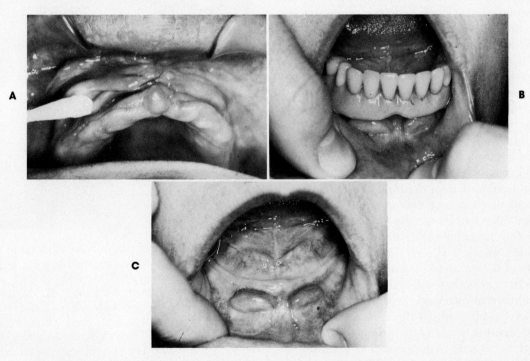

Fig. 2-2　Epulis fissuratum around the border of a maxillary denture, **A,** and around the labial border of a mandibular denture, **B** and **C.**

nation reveals that these tissues are usually hyperemic and swollen. Surgical excision of epulis fissuratum is indicated, but only after a period of prescribed tissue rest to reduce the edema. Experience supports the value of advising patients to rest the irritated/overloaded tissues (keeping the dentures out, with the dentist's reduction of offending flanges) and to institute a program of regular and vigorous massage of the damaged site. Fig. 2-3 demonstrates the efficacy of such an approach. The "home treatment" program for this patient brought about the desired result in 6 weeks and obviated the need for a surgical intervention. Although such a positive result is not always possible, it is clear that the inflammatory reduction makes a conservative surgical intervention possible.

During the surgical procedure all healthy mucous membrane is retained, and great care must be taken to avoid excising any attached mucosa since, otherwise, the depth of the sulcus will be reduced (Fig. 2-4). If attached mucosa is absent over the residual ridge, a graft is usually placed and a splint is then inserted to maintain the patency of the sulcus. Infrequently, the patient's old mandibular denture is modified to serve as a splint that is circumferentially wired into place for the first postoperative week. The modified old denture or a newly fabricated splint is usually lined with a plasticized resin treatment liner. The splint is worn postoperatively until adequate epithelialization has taken place, which usually takes about 6 to 8 weeks. At that time the old dentures can be relined, or new ones can be made. (See Chapter 6.)

Hyperplastic tissue, which may replace the bone of the residual ridge, is incompatible with the demand for healthy denture-supporting tissues and should be excised. The prevalence of denture hyperplasia has been reported as being quite variable (13% to 26%). However, it is frequently encountered in long-term denture wearers, and the anterior part of the jaw is the most common site. Experience supports the value of surgical excision of the hyperplastic tissue in most patients where it exists. Here, again, principles of tissue rest and extreme surgical conservatism are indispensable. The risks of sulcus obliteration are often high, and the need for a vestibuloplasty must always be kept in mind. A high incidence of success for oral sulcus–deepening procedures accompanied by skin graft placement (Fig. 2-5, A) has been reported. The use of the modified old denture or the insertion of a splint after sulcus deepening is similar to that described earlier.

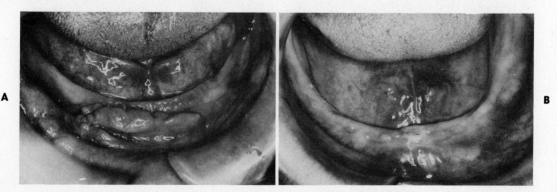

Fig. 2-3   A, In this patient the mucosal response to chronic irritation from a labial flange was treated by reduction of the flange, tissue rest, use of a conditioner, and a program of vigorous and regular finger massage. **B,** Impressive resolution of the soft tissue enlargement 6 wk later.

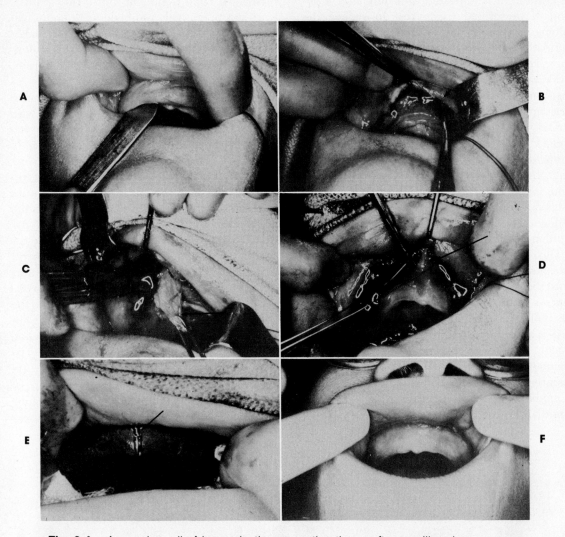

Fig. 2-4 A massive roll of hyperplastic connective tissue after maxillary bone resorption. **A,** Note the tissue between the upper lip and ridge. **B,** An incision is made so as much oral mucosa as possible can be saved. **C,** The tissue is removed. **D,** Ligature wire is passed around the anterior nasal spine to support a splint. **E,** An acrylic resin splint is wired into position *(arrow)*. Wiring the splint is not always essential; however, it should be done when a mucosal or skin graft is used to extend the depth of the vestibule. **F,** Residual ridge 6 months after surgery.

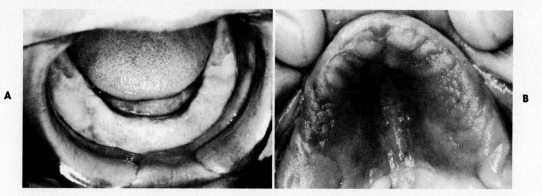

Fig. 2-5 **A,** Enlarged labial and buccal vestibules after a sulcus-deepening procedure with skin graft placement. **B,** Denture stomatitis of the maxillary denture-bearing mucosa. A generalized hyperemic response is present.

Denture stomatitis

Denture stomatitis is a chronic inflammation of the denture-bearing mucosa (the basal seat) that may be localized or generalized in nature (Fig. 2-5, *B*). Some investigators believe that trauma from ill-fitting dentures or a parafunctional habit is the predominant etiologic factor, whereas others believe that nocturnal denture wear is related to denture stomatitis. A hypersensitivity to some component of the denture material with consequent allergic response has also been proposed.

It is possible for denture base materials to acquire antigenic properties as a result of a continuous absorption of such fluids as cleansing agents, foods, or drugs. Also, as dentures become increasingly ill-fitting, tissue trauma is produced that could make tissues more susceptible to any allergen imbibed by the dentures over the years. Infection from poor oral and denture hygiene can aggravate the condition.

Definite conclusions have not been reached concerning the allergic potential of nonmetallic denture base materials. However, a denture that has been worn for some time may absorb fluids that may be capable of promoting an allergic response. The majority of stomatitis conditions are caused by infection, trauma, or mechanical irritation, and less frequently by chemical agents irritating locally or allergens present in the denture base material.

Most patients with denture stomatitis are unaware of their lesion since it is frequently asymptomatic. A small number of patients complain of a burning or itching sensation that is usually related to both the palatal and the glossal mucosa. The inflammation varies in intensity; it may be localized in isolated areas or may involve the entire basal seat. It tends to occur more frequently in the maxillary arch than in the mandibular arch. Occasionally a granular type of palatal inflammation—papillary hyperplasia, or papillomatosis—is seen (Fig. 2-6). Papillary hyperplasia should not be considered an entirely innocuous lesion. Some authors suggest that the best treatment is surgical excision.

The incidence of papillary hyperplasia is related to the presence of relief chambers in dentures (Fig. 2-7) and to the relief-chamber effect that can develop as a result of uneven settling of a maxillary denture. Some authors believe that the chronic irritation resulting from a make-and-break alternating vacuum created under the denture elicits the papillary inflammatory response. The appearance of papillary projections covering variable amounts of the hard palate is characteristic. This lesion is fre-

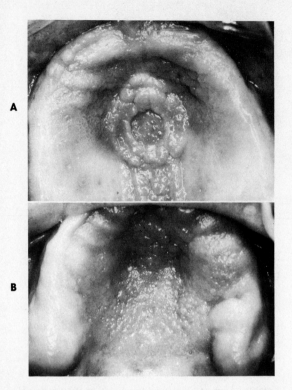

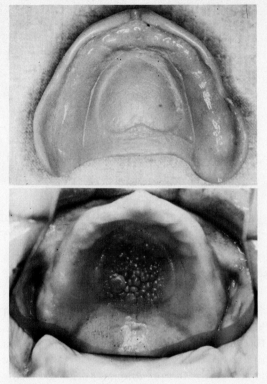

Fig. 2-6 Palatal papillomatosis. **A,** The condition is localized to the midpalatal region as a result of the patient's wearing a maxillary denture with a suction cup. **B,** Notice the papillomatous development in another patient, covering the entire palate and extending distally past where the posterior palatal seal of the denture would be created against the mucosa.

Fig. 2-7 An arbitrary relief chamber in a maxillary denture, **A,** has caused a papillomatous response, **B.** Notice the conformity of the lesion to the outline of the relief areas.

quently camouflaged by a thick mucus-saliva film, and the palatal mucosa should be carefully dried before it is examined. The frequency of papillomatosis appears to be higher in patients who wear their denture throughout the 24-hour day, and patients should be urged to rest the tissues of the mouth by removing their dentures at night or for other comparable periods.

The presence of microbial plaque and yeasts on the fitting surface of the denture base appears to be of critical importance for development and maintenance of denture stomatitis.

Treatment of denture stomatitis. The best treatment for denture stomatitis is to correct the factors that cause it. Good oral and dental hygiene and rest for the tissues of the basal seat are essential, followed by construction of new well-fitting dentures after the achievement of a healthy condition of the mucosa. This is accomplished by the use of tissue conditioners in existing or treatment dentures, indirect relining of existing dentures with autopolymerizing resins, antifungal drugs, a 2% solution of chlorhexidine gluconate, or gingival massage with a toothbrush or fingers.

Several procedures are recommended and may be employed singly or in combination depending on the severity of the condition:

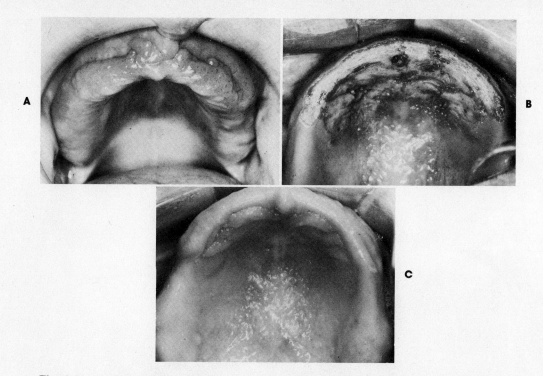

Fig. 2-8   A, Papillomatosis and anterior maxillary ridge hyperplasia have been treated surgically. **B,** Immediate postoperative appearance. **C,** Six weeks later, epithelialization is complete.

1. Oral and denture hygiene accompanied by tissue rest. Tissue rest is achieved by removal of the dentures or by use of a tissue conditioner, occlusal adjustment, and technical improvement of the existing dentures.

2. Antifungal therapy. This can be instituted after an elective verification of *Candida* infection by a palatal smear. A therpeutic dose of one nystatin tablet taken three times a day for 10 to 14 days is usually sufficient to control the infection. Antifungal therapy may be required for up to 4 weeks in some patients. If the dentures are not relined with a tissue conditioner, they must be kept impeccably clean, and a chelating agent with a mixture of enzymes or chlorhexidine may be used. This form of therapy is usually applied when there is generalized stomatitis, especially of a symptomatic nature.

Recent research has demonstrated that nystatin treatment was promptly followed by recolonization of yeasts. Therefore it is suggested that antimycotic drugs not be used in the routine treatment of denture stomatitis. Furthermore patients whose microbial plaque and yeast scores from the denture base decreased when the denture stomatitis healed also showed an accompanying disappearance of their angular cheilitis and glossitis.

3. Surgical excision of papillomatosis (Fig. 2-8). Excision is undertaken only after other methods of treatment have been used. The surgery is easier and more conservative after pretreatment, because of the diminished inflammation. Electrosurgery is frequently used to excise maxillary papillary hyperplasia. Cryosurgery also has been used, with good results. A treatment liner should be placed inside the

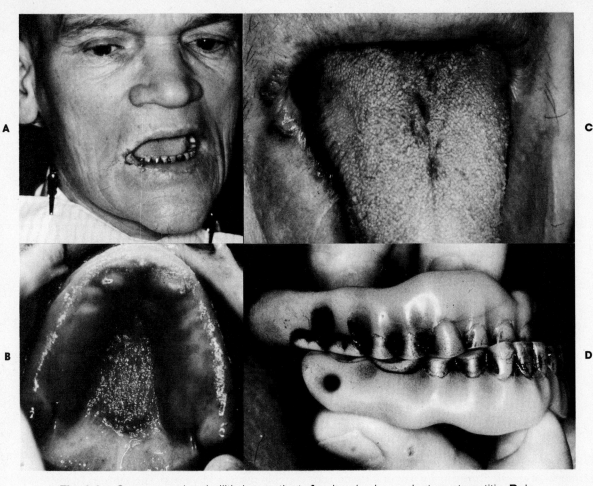

Fig. 2-9 Severe angular cheilitis in a patient, **A,** who also has a denture stomatitis, **B.** In addition, there is a glossitis and a gross loss of vertical dimension, **C** and **D.**

denture postoperatively and changed weekly until epithelialization is completed. It must be emphasized that papillomatosis is an irreversible lesion, which by virtue of its morphology can act as an excellent nidus for the accumulation of plaque and fungal growth. Its surgical elimination is frequently necessary as a prerequisite for optimal hygiene. When it occasionally extends to or past the junction of the hard and soft palate, great care must be paid to its excision, since scar band formation in this area can seriously interfere with the development of a future posterior palatal seal. The maxillary denture may be relined or a new denture constructed when healing is completed after an interval of 6 to 8 weeks.

Denture stomatitis may develop along with an angular stomatitis (a sometimes painful inflammation of the corners of the mouth, also known as angular cheilitis, Fig. 2-9). For years this clinical condition was attributed to a reduction of the vertical dimension of occlusion or to riboflavin and thiamine deficiency. Although either of these situations can predispose to an angular stomatitis, researchers have shown that the condition is usually secondary to a denture stomatitis and usually the result of *Candida* infection from contaminated saliva. Angular stomatitis can respond to antifungal therapy and supplementary antifungal ointment application at the lesion's site (Fig. 2-10). However its recurrence is frequently related to denture stomatitis, and a combined-treatment approach is mandatory.

The interface of skin and oral mucosa at the corner of the mouth, an anatomic landmark known as the angulus oris, is particularly susceptible to inflammation (cheilitis). Whereas the skin on the face is keratinized epithelium (and thus relatively inhospitable to microorganisms), the mucosal surface is unkeratinized (and thus more vulnerable to microbial invasion). Kept moist by saliva and exposed to a large and varied microbial flora, it tends to succumb to any alteration in the stability of the environment, with the consequent development of an angular cheilitis.

Although the exact pathogenesis of angular cheilitis is still unclear, several observations deserve mention:

1. The incidence appears to be higher among women and denture wearers.
2. The inflammation can occur unilaterally or bilaterally and is infrequently accompanied by an atrophic glossitis.
3. Age does not seem to affect its incidence, nor does the duration of the edentulous period.
4. The presence of an angular fold of tissue (frequently encountered in older persons and those wearing dentures), rather than a decreased vertical dimension of occlusion, appears to delay the healing of angular cheilitis.
5. *Candida albicans* and *Staphylococcus aureus* have been isolated from lesions of angular cheilitis; however, this finding does not necessarily mean that the microorganisms are essential for development of the lesions. In fact, no uniform or specific immune responses of angular cheilitis have been identified.
6. Antimicrobial treatment is usually successful, which demonstrates that the infection is significantly persistent.

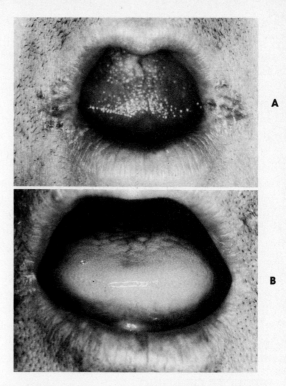

Fig. 2-10 Angular stomatitis that responded to antifungal therapy. **A,** Before and, **B,** after.

7. The lesions recur frequently, which suggests the possible presence of a permanent and vulnerable deficiency in the barrier function of the skin in the region of the anguli ori.

Denture sore mouth

Rarely one encounters mucosal complaints that do not fit into the general description of denture stomatitis. These complaints are conveniently grouped as a "denture sore mouth" syndrome, and the condition is usually determined when the treatment methods just outlined have been unsuccessful. Clinical experience suggests that denture sore mouth is probably the result of an underlying abnormal metabolic or hormonal function or a nutritional deficiency (for example, alcoholism).

Patients with psychologic problems may occasionally fall into this picture. The symptoms are a bizarre spectrum of itching, painful, irritated, and tender denture-bearing mucosa. Clinical findings are frequently negative, and it appears that in such patients mucosal tolerance is extremely low, without any visible clinical or laboratory signs. These symptoms can also be produced by tranquilizers used in the management of psychiatric disorders, and so these drugs may further complicate the diagnosis.

Iron deficiency, insufficient protein, and incomplete intestinal absorption have been cited as contributory factors. Patients presenting with this syndrome should be referred to a physician for a thorough systemic analysis, which may identify the underlying cause or causes of the sore mouth. Medical treatment may consist of a high-protein diet, avoidance of local irritants, slow-release hydrogen chloride supplement in the achlorhydric patient, ascorbic acid tablets dissolved sublingually, and occasionally psychiatric help. Perhaps because of the rather vague nature of denture sore mouth, there is no real consensus about its treatment.

EFFECTS OF AGING

Time leaves its imprint on every living thing, and this principle applies to all the successive levels of organization—molecule, cell, tissue, organ, and organism. The human life-span reveals a period of gradual development of increasing body efficiency in childhood and adolescence until what we call maturity is reached. After a long period of little change, a gradual decline in powers, especially physical ones, occurs. This is commonly referred to as the period of senescence. The time at which age changes become evident is quite variable, and many of the changes can actually occur early. Almost as soon as human beings have passed adolescence, deteriorative changes begin in some tissues. Therefore the curve begins to slope downward slightly from the point of maturation. Degenerative changes in joints have been detected as early as 25 to 30 years of age, and the vascular changes characteristic of old age can be detected almost as early. Other changes (such as reduction in muscle strength) begin later.

Much evidence has accumulated to indicate that this state of ultimate decline is an intrinsic part of the nature of all multicellular organisms. The aging process is insidious and is characterized by individual variation in onset and rate of decline. It includes changes in cardiac output, lowered secretion of digestive juices, a decrease in muscular coordination, and a decline in endocrine activity. On the psychologic level the aging process is characterized by an increase in reaction time, a slowing of the learning process, and a decline in memory and intellectual efficiency. These changes are reflected in a gradual diminution of the individual's adaptability. Homeostasis of the *milieu intérieur* is maintained with greater difficulty. Many aspects of aging have been studied in a representative population, and the inadequacy of any single criterion of biologic age was demonstrated. An assessment of the biologic age in relation to the chronologic age is an important aid to correct treatment planning. A chronologically old person in whom these changes have been delayed is said to be biologically young. If, however, the changes occur comparatively early in life, a patient is described as being biologically old even though he/she may be young in years. The clinician has no alternative but to make subjective judgments, which are imprecise but nonetheless valuable.

Although most living tissues retain a capacity to repair or renew themselves, the dentition is a notable exception. Past surveys in various parts of the world confirm the relatively high percentage of edentulous patients among elderly people; hence, the popular conviction that geriatric dentistry consists largely in the oral rehabilitation of edentulous patients. This situation is changing rapidly though, and current predictions are that there will be a steady decline in edentulism and in the number of missing teeth among elderly persons. It also should be remembered that life expectancy is longer today and there are more people. Patients who started wearing complete dentures in their middle years will pose staggering prosthodontic problems in the future, since time and long-term denture wearing continue to exact a biologic price from the oral supporting tissues.

Oral changes

The oral aspects of aging have received increasing attention. The effects of aging on the edentulous geriatric patient may include (1) oral mucosa and skin changes, (2) residual bone and maxillomandibular relation changes, (3) tongue and taste changes, and (4) salivary flow changes and nutritional impairment. Changes in the psychologic outlook of an individual must also be taken into consideration.

The morphologic changes seen in and around the oral cavity of geriatric patients are frequently quite self-evident. It should be remembered, however, that, although morphologic and biochemical changes in the oral tissues have been demonstrated, changes in normal function are not well documented. In fact, the vast majority of studies on healthy nonmedicated subjects show minimal *age-related changes*. When evidence of change has been observed, the changes could not be regarded as specifically age-related. Clearly there is a need for more research into the physiology of aging, particularly in relation to the edentulous state and the influences of denture wearing, systemic health, nutrition, and medication(s) taken. Some of the more relevant implications of oral aging deserve further discussion.

Mucosa and skin. The clinical picture is one of atrophy. The epithelial layers are less in number, and the mucosa and submucosa show a decrease in thickness. This actual thinning of the tissues, coupled with its depleted repair potential, renders the denture-bearing mucosa of the basal seat friable and easily traumatized (Fig. 2-11). The vulnerability of mucosa may be related to a shift in the water balance from the intracellular to the extracellular compartment of the tissues. Diminished kidney function may also result in dehydration of the tissues. The tissue cells may become nutritionally deficient. Younger edentulous patients tend to have denture-bearing mucosa and submucosa of considerable thickness. On the other hand, edentulous mucosa of the elderly is frequently thin and tightly stretched, and it blanches easily. Mucosa of reduced thickness may be associated with reduced residual ridge height, since epithelial atrophy, which results in a reduction in the number of epithelial cell layers and the

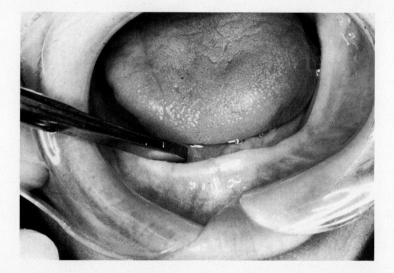

Fig. 2-11   Thin, nonresilient, mandibular denture-bearing mucosa readily blanches and is easily traumatized.

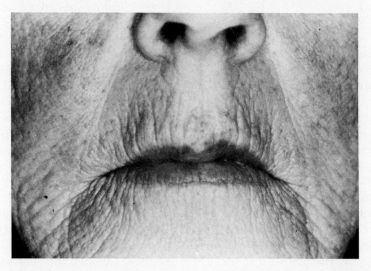

Fig. 2-12   Age changes in the skin around the mouth. A loss of elasticity results in a network of wrinkles that are impossible to camouflage by prosthetic therapy.

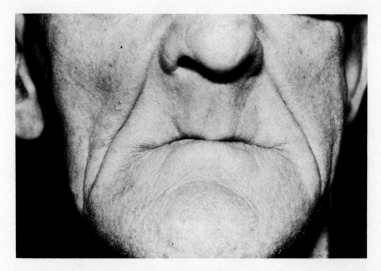

Fig. 2-13   Age changes in the skin of the face. Natural folds and creases are exaggerated and with time become permanent.

thickness of the underlying connective tissues, also manifests itself in a reduction of the surface area of the oral mucosa. This, in turn, applies pressure to the underlying ridge. The externally applied molding force meets more or less resistance from the bone itself, and this is the action involved in the resorption process. The study of age changes in the collagen fibers of the oral mucosa has shown that these fibers shorten to a degree compatible with the concept of a contracting mucosa acting as a molding force on alveolar bone.

An atrophying denture-bearing mucosa is frequently encountered during menopause. The reduction in estrogen output is known to have an atrophic effect on epithelial surfaces. The number of cell layers is reduced as is the potential for keratinization. In addition, there is a reduction in surface area that affects the genital epithelium, oral mucosa, and skin. Clinical experience indicates that hormonal replacement therapy can be beneficial in such patients to create a more favorable oral environment for the dentures.

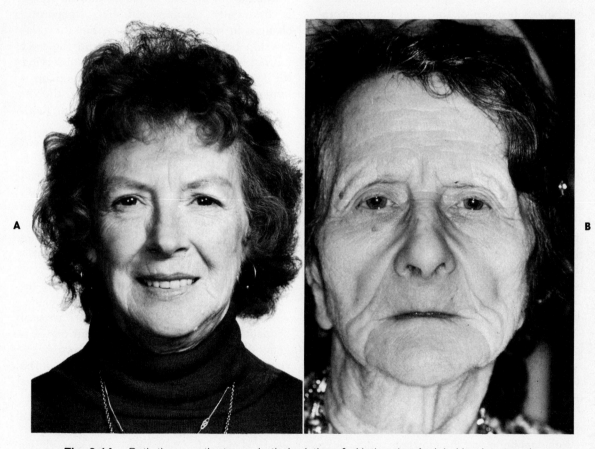

Fig. 2-14   Both these patients are in their sixties. **A,** Notice that facial skin changes do not parallel this patient's chronologic age or the effects of long-term denture wear. The cosmetic aspects of her prosthodontic treatment will not likely be very demanding at a morphologic level. **B,** This patient, on the other hand, combines the cosmetic sequelae shown in Figs. 2-12 and 2-13. Optimal prosthodontics will compensate only minimally for the biologic and chronologic effects of aging.

It must be clear to the reader that the points made earlier, in the discussion of stress distribution to denture-supporting tissues, become particularly relevant when one is dealing with patients with compromised mucosal support. These patients' mucosal tissues need extra care, that is, frequent application of soft liners (tissue conditioners), as well as counseling in tissue handling and cleansing.

Similar changes take place in the skin, which may appear loose and wrinkled, or tight, smooth, and thin. A person's skin is changing throughout life. Young skin is smooth and has a dull sheen because of the almost microscopic pattern of tiny grooves that divide the surface into rhomboidal areas. This network of fine grooves is the outward view of the pattern of the junction between the epithelium and its supporting lamina propria. As the skin ages, its surface loses its fine pattern and the skin loses its elasticity. The concomitant atrophy occurring in the structures beneath the skin leads to even more noticeable changes in the face. The muscles, fat, and connective tissue all diminish in bulk. There is more skin than is needed to cover them, so it droops into folds and exaggerates the creases, which become more obvious (Figs. 2-12 to 2-14). Although the position of these creases is not constant for all persons, there is a certain uniformity in their distribution. As the elastic property of the skin decreases, the lines in the base of the creases become more permanent.

These skin changes cannot be compensated for by prosthodontics, and they can severely compromise the esthetic opportunities of the denture service. The skin changes should be brought to the patient's attention before the denture treatment is started, as mentioned in the previous chapter.

Residual bone and the maxillomandibular relation. The gross reduction of the height of maxillary and mandibular residual ridges is often a result of long-term wear of complete dentures. It has been assumed that ridge resorption is an inevitable accompaniment of denture

wearing, but there is a lack of longitudinal analyses of residual ridge height in edentulous people who have not worn dentures.

Disuse atrophy. Flat residual ridges distal to natural teeth are frequently seen, and several dentists have attributed ridge reduction in these regions to disuse atrophy. However, atrophy of residual ridges has not yet been demonstrated in controlled research. This reinforces the notion that denture wearing is potentially stressful and damaging to the underlying bone.

Changes in the size of the basal seat. Aging is frequently accompanied by osteoporotic changes in the human skeleton, but the relationship between this condition and the jaws has not been adequately studied. By observing the axial inclination of the natural teeth in a human skull, it is possible to envision the direction of residual ridge reduction after tooth loss (Figs. 2-15 to 2-17).

Maxillary teeth generally flare downward and outward, so bone reduction generally is upward and inward. Since the outer cortical plate is thinner than the inner cortical plate, resorption from the outer cortex tends to be greater and more rapid. As the maxillary residual ridges are reduced, the maxillae become smaller in all dimensions and the denture-bearing surface (basal seat) decreases.

The anterior mandibular teeth generally incline upward and forward to the occlusal plane, whereas the posterior teeth either are vertical or incline slightly lingually. The outer cortex is generally thicker than the lingual cortex, except in the molar region. Also, the width of the mandible is greatest at its inferior border. As a result, the mandibular residual ridge appears to migrate lingually and inferiorly in the anterior region and to migrate buccally in the posterior region. Consequently, the mandibular arch appears either to remain static or to become wider posteriorly as resorption progresses. This discrepancy in relative jaw sizes can pose several technical problems for the dentist because failure to place the artificial

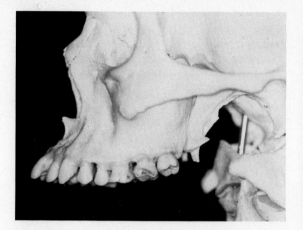

Fig. 2-15   The direction of the roots and alveolar processes of the anterior maxillary teeth can be seen and determines the direction of residual ridge reduction that usually takes place.

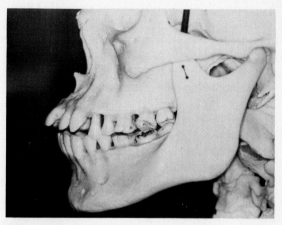

Fig. 2-16   In the mandible the pattern of residual ridge reduction tends to be downward and backward. Relate this to Fig. 1-5, *B,* showing the morphologic pattern of resorption as deduced from longitudinal studies.

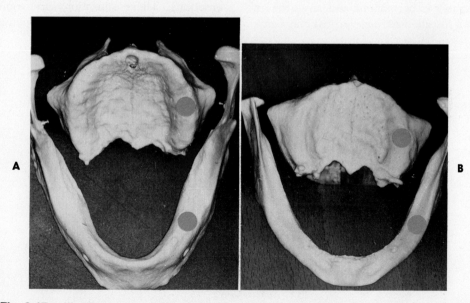

Fig. 2-17   Maxillae and mandible in different stages of resorption. The maxillae become narrower and the mandible wider as progressive resorption modifies jaw morphology. The centers of the ridges are almost aligned in **A,** but not in **B,** after resorption has taken place.

teeth in the positions of the natural teeth can jeopardize denture support and stability. Obviously, any attempt to restore the original arch contour occupied by the natural teeth can be limited by the effects of aging on the adjacent and surrounding tissues.

Maxillomandibular relations. There are changes also in the vertical maxillomandibular relations with the passage of time. Muscle changes occur, and these, coupled with residual ridge reduction, bring about a spatial alteration in the position of the mandible relative to the maxillae. They must be recognized and assessed in the context of the patient's desired or anticipated facial support from new dentures. An accurate assessment must be made of the proposed interarch and interocclusal distances in elderly persons receiving complete dentures.

Such an assessment will take into account the possibility that a certain amount of the reduction of vertical dimension (or increased freeway space) is permanent and any attempt to restore a so-called normal vertical may cause

the patient discomfort. Since denture quality or occlusal support has not been shown to correlate strongly with TMJ dysfunctional problems in elderly persons, however, dentists should be cautious about prescribing prosthetic treatment that will interfere with conventional interpretations of the maxillomandibular relations.

Tongue and taste. A nodular varicose enlargement of the superficial veins on the undersurface of the tongue is commonly seen (Fig. 2-18). There is an association between these sublingual varicosities and the minute spidery nevi that tend to appear on the skin with advancing age, but the varicosities do not have any significant association with cardiac or pulmonary dysfunction and the patient should be reassured about their insignificance.

The tongue may become smooth and glossy or red and inflamed. A variety of symptoms can center on the lingual mucosa, with complaints of soreness, burning, or abnormal taste sensations. These sensations are common in both elderly people and postmenopausal wom-

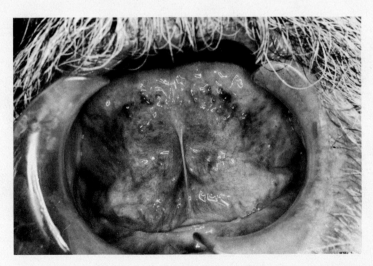

Fig. 2-18 Varicose enlargement of superficial veins on the undersurface of the tongue. They are innocuous.

en. It is not uncommon for the symptoms to be related to the posterior region of the tongue margin (that is, the region of the foliate papillae).

The foliate papillae appear red and projecting and may be a cause for alarm in some patients who must be reassured that they are not a proliferating neoplasm. On the other hand, persistent soreness in this region can occur and is usually eliminated by excision of the sore papillae. Vitamin B therapy has been administered to patients complaining of a sore or burning tongue. The clinical results have often been successful. It must be remembered that the tongue can undergo various changes with age, and there appears to be a tendency for the number of taste buds to diminish. Focal collections of chronic inflammatory cells also are common, and this may be because of ingress of microorganisms or their toxins through the thin epithelium of this region.

Tongue thrusting associated with nervous tension or with attempts to control a lower denture can also lead to a sore tongue. The size of the tongue probably does not vary with age. However, tooth loss can lead to a wider tongue by virtue of an overdevelopment of some parts of the tongue's intrinsic musculature. Constant and habitual attempts to keep a loose maxillary denture in place can cause these changes. The effect of this on subsequent denture wearing must not be overlooked.

Lingual tissue changes may be accompanied by alterations in the sense of taste. Taste bud atrophy can lead to loss of appetite, which in turn can adversely affect tongue comfort as a manifestation of nutritional deficiency. Older patients frequently blame their dentures for a changed sense of taste and a burning sensation of their tongue. Reassurance and diet counseling are necessary to overcome these symptoms. Age-related taste changes are not uniform for all taste qualities, all taste performances, or all populations of elderly individuals.

Current research indicates that aging alters chemosensory sensitivity as well as chemosensory preference. The interrelationship between chemosensory perception and nutrition in the geriatric population is far from clear and may account for the complaints of altered taste perception in some denture-wearing geriatric patients.

Salivary flow and nutritional impairment. A dryness of the mouth may be evident in some patients. This xerostomia can be due to a medication that the patient is taking, usually for gastric complaints or for depression and insomnia. It also may reflect a diminution in salivary flow resulting from atrophy of the salivary glands. Regardless of the cause, it may lead to a diminished facility for mastication, digestive upsets, and sometimes poor retention of the dentures. The dryness of the mucosa renders it more susceptible to frictional irritation from denture movement and may interfere with patients' ability to wear their dentures.

Some older patients, on the other hand, may produce excessive saliva on insertion of new dentures. This effect is transient and can be controlled by explanation of its cause to the patient, reassurance, and antisialagogue administration, if necessary. Until recently, diminished salivary gland performance was regarded as an unavoidable concomitant of geriatric oral health. Current research indicates that changes in oral health suggestive of altered salivary secretion are more likely due to disease and its pharmacologic treatment.

Degenerative changes

The cumulative degenerative changes that develop are often accompanied by a reduced neuromuscular coordination. This manifests itself as impaired adaptability and a consequent reduction of masticatory ability. It is possible that several or all of the biologic changes accompanying aging can be present in one patient. Collectively, they can be the cause of nutritional impairment by altering dietary and nutritional habits.

Dietary problems

Dietary problems in elderly persons generally have numerous causes:

1. Low income and the lack of knowledge of how to spend the money available for food to the best advantage
2. Physical handicaps, debility, and a lack of mobility, which make shopping and food preparation difficult
3. Poor facilities for food preparation
4. Poor dentitions, especially dentures, which may cause the wearer to reject some essential foods that are difficult to chew, without the inclusion of a suitable substitute
5. Existing food habits that may result in the choice of a poor diet
6. Depression, boredom, anxiety, and loneliness, which give little or no incentive for the preparation of nourishing meals

Studies of elderly people have shown that they are susceptible to subclinical, if not frank clinical, malnutrition. The relationship between the integrity of the masticatory system throughout the life-span and the nutritional status of a person has not been thoroughly or conclusively elucidated. However, clinical experience indicates that mucosal tissue intolerance in edentulous patients frequently responds to nutritional supplements and dietary counseling. Patient instruction in the use and the shortcomings of their complete dentures and diet counseling are integral parts of prosthodontic therapy.

Current research suggests that systemic processes are operant in alveolar ridge resorption. Although such resorption can occur in any age group, it tends to be more conspicuous in the elderly edentulous patient. Among the many recognized systemic influences that affect bone resorption and resistance, calcium deficiencies and calcium-phosphorus imbalances have been specifically implicated. The precise role of diet and nutrition in the maintenance of residual ridges is far from clear, and this subject is addressed in Chapter 5.

Psychologic changes

It is important to have some understanding of the psychology of human aging to be able to appreciate the difference between behavioral disorders that are associated with organic brain disease and those that are not. Organic brain damage creates an almost impossible predicament for prosthetic treatment. In senile dementia, for example, an irreversible deterioration of intellectual faculties develops and the patient is frequently hostile, withdrawn, and virtually incapable of adjusting to any prostheses. Such patients are probably best treated by the eradication of oral disease and the institution of dietary changes to accommodate their modified or nonexistent dentition.

Geriatric patients can demonstrate a high incidence of depression and feelings of insecurity, and they may experience vague and often bizarre pains and fears. Nervous habits like tooth clenching can develop, and this places extra stress on tissues that already have a diminished capacity to deal with the loadings. Older patients are also more likely to be using drugs, and care must be taken to understand the dental implications of such use.

Tissue distortion can result from medications taken for edema caused by kidney or cardiac dysfunction, from fatigue, or from changes in fluid intake. Tissue distortion seriously affects impression making, and it is recommended that morning appointments be organized to ensure that there will be minimal distortion from edema.

Reassurance, tolerance, and a versatile clinical approach usually help the elderly person obtain satisfactory prosthodontic results.

BIBLIOGRAPHY

Baum BJ: Salivary gland function during aging, Gerodontics **2**:61-64, 1986.

Bergendal T: Treatment of denture stomatitis. Doctoral thesis, University of Stockholm, 1982.

Budtz-Jørgensen E: Reaktioner i slimhinden hos protesebaerere. Nordisk klinisk odontologi, Copenhagen, 1987, Forlaget for Faglitteratur, vol 21-A-II, pp 1-29.

Budtz-Jørgensen E, Bertram U: Denture stomatitis. I and II, Acta Odontol Scand **28**:71-92, 283-304, 1970.

Budtz-Jørgensen E, Löe H: Chlorhexidine as a denture disinfectant in the treatment of denture stomatitis, Scand J Dent Res **80**:457-464, 1972.

Cawson RA: Denture sore mouth and angular cheilitis, Br Dent J **115**:441-449, 1963a.

Cawson RA: Symposium on denture sore mouth. II, The role of *Candida*, Dent Pract **16**:138-142, 1963b.

Druyon ME: Imbalance in nutrition advice, Gerodontics **4**:176-187, 1988.

Ettinger RL: Diet, nutrition, and masticatory ability in a group of elderly edentulous patients, Aust Dent J **18**:12-19, 1973.

Hölm-Pederson P, Löe H, editors: Geriatric dentistry, Copenhagen, 1986, Munksgaard International Publishers Ltd.

Kapur K, Shklar G: The effect of complete dentures on alveolar mucosa, J Prosthet Dent **13**:1030-1037, 1963.

Koopmans ASF, Kippuw N, de Graaff J: Bacterial involvement in denture-induced stomatitis, J Dent Res **67**:1246-1250, 1988.

MacEntee MI, Weiss R, Morrison BJ, Waxler-Morrison NE: Mandibular dysfunction in an institutionalized and predominantly elderly population, J Oral Rehabil **14**:6, 523-529, 1987.

Mäkilä E: Prevalence of angular stomatitis; correlation with composition of food and metabolism of vitamins and iron, Acta Odontol Scand **27**:655-680, 1969.

Massler M: Oral aspects of aging, Postgrad Med **49**:179, 1971.

McMillan DR: The cytological response of palatal mucosa to dentures, Dent Pract **22**:302-304, 1972.

Miles AEW: Changes in oral tissues with advancing age, Proc R Soc Med **65**:801-806, 1972.

Nyquist G: A study of denture sore mouth, Acta Odontol Scand **10**(supp 9):11-154, 1952.

Öhman SC: Angular cheilitis. Doctoral thesis, University of Göteborg, 1988.

Olsson KA, Bergman B: A comparison of two prosthetic methods for the treatment of denture stomatitis, Acta Odontol Scand **29**:745-753, 1971.

Österberg T, Steen B: Relationship between dental state and dietary intake in 70-year-old males and females in Göteborg, Sweden, J Oral Rehabil **9**:509-521, 1982.

Palinquist S: Oral health patterns in a Swedish country population aged 65 and above. Doctoral thesis, University of Göteborg, 1986.

Shaffer WG, Hine MK, Levy BM: Oral pathology, ed 2, Philadelphia, 1974, WB Saunders Co.

Shepherd RW: Prosthetic treatment for the older patient, Aust Dent J **12**:339-342, 1967.

Sreeburg LM, Schwartz SS: A reference guide to drugs and dry mouth, Gerodontology **5**:75-99, 1986.

Turrell ASW: Aetiology of inflamed upper denture-bearing tissues, Br Dent J **118**:542-546, 1966.

von Wowern N: Pattern of age-related bone loss in mandibles, Scand J Dent Res **88**:134-146, 1980.

Wallenius K, Heyden G.: Histochemical studies of flabby ridges, Odontol Rev **23**:169-179, 1972.

Weiffenbach JM: Taste perception mechanisms. In Ferguson DB, editor: The aging mouth, Front Oral Physiol **6**:151-167, 1987.

Wical KE, Brusse P: Effects of calcium and vitamin D supplement on alveolar ridge resorption in immediate denture patients, J Prosthet Dent **41**:4-11, 1979.

Wical KE, Swoope CC: Studies of residual ridge resorption. II, The relationship of dietary calcium and phosphorus to residual ridge resorption, J Prosthet Dent **32**:13-22, 1974.

Winkler S: The geriatric complete denture patient, Dent Clin North Am **21**:403-425, 1977.

Preparing the patient for complete dentures

CHAPTER 3

Diagnosis and treatment planning for the patient with some teeth remaining

Dentists have been very successful in treating edentulous patients with complete dentures. However, the profession's commitment to avoiding the edentulous state continues, and this commitment has led to expanded knowledge and clinical skills. As a result, earlier and improved operative and prosthodontic treatment, combined with the effectiveness of modern endodontic and periodontal therapy, usurped the old myth that tooth loss inevitably accompanies old age. The same therapeutic modalities can also be applied to persons who, as a result of earlier neglect, come for treatment with broken-down dentitions. These patients can frequently have their masticatory systems restored to near normal without having to consider prosthodontic intervention as an interim postponement of the edentulous state.

Patients with some teeth remaining who request complete dentures should be carefully diagnosed to ensure that treatment alternatives to complete dentures are thoroughly considered. The decision to retain or remove even one tooth is serious, and all alternatives must be explored before a final decision is made. The removal of teeth is an irreversible procedure, underscoring the significance and importance of a correct diagnosis.

Diagnosis consists of planned observations to determine and evaluate the existing conditions, which lead to decision making based on the conditions observed. All the facts must be known before they can be correlated in such a way that judgments and decisions can be

made. Only then can treatment plans be developed to best serve the needs of each individual patient.

Those patients with some teeth remaining who may need complete denture service tend to fall into the following three groups, each of which poses special problems and decisions:
1. Patients with severely depleted dentitions characterized by extensive caries or advanced periodontal disease (Fig. 3-1); immediate dentures are usually prescribed for such patients, and this topic is described in Chapter 26
2. Patients with depleted dentitions (Fig. 3-2) or, infrequently, failed reconstructions with one or more teeth that can serve as overdenture abutments; these potential abutments may require minimal preparation or else entail several procedures (such as endodontic or periodontal therapy or gold coping) to enhance their longevity

   The objective in retaining teeth under complete dentures is alveolar bone preservation (Fig. 3-3) and is discussed in Chapter 25. The overdenture or tooth-supported complete denture concept has led to a dramatic increase in the number of patients who have been spared the edentulous predicament.
3. Patients who are edentulous in only one arch, most frequently the maxillary; a characteristic clinical picture emerges in such patients and includes one or more of

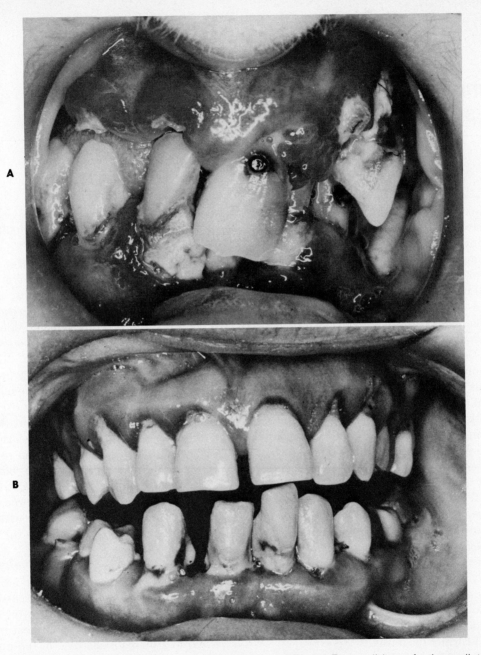

Fig. 3-1 Advanced neglect makes both patients, **A** and **B,** candidates for immediate denture therapy. The full-mouth radiographic survey, **C,** of the patient in **B,** combined with an assessment of poor patient motivation, confirms the decision to prescribe total extraction for this individual.

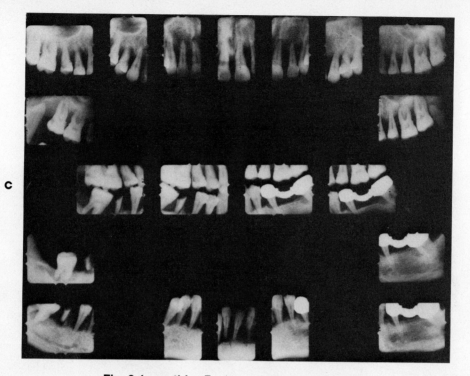

c

Fig. 3-1, cont'd   For legend see opposite page.

the following: (a) few anterior mandibular teeth present, (b) variable hyperplastic replacement of the anterior maxillary ridge secondary to anterior upward settling of the maxillary denture, (c) the presence of pendulous enlarged maxillary tuberosities, or (d) loss of the vertical dimension of occlusion (Figs. 3-4, 3-7, and 3-9)

Infrequently an intact or restored maxillary dentition is opposed by an edentulous mandible, and in these patients

the mandible appears to be very susceptible to residual ridge resorption (Fig. 3-5). In previous editions of this text, we favored sacrificing the remaining teeth in such situations. However, experience has demonstrated that such drastic action is only rarely needed, and modifications in technique and the materials used allow for a more conservative approach. The single denture opposing a natural dentition is discussed in Chapter 27.

Text continued on p. 58.

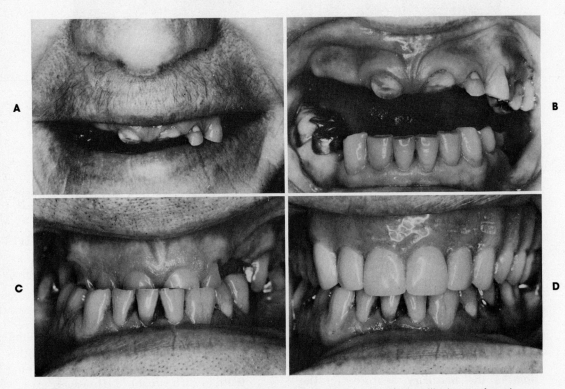

Fig. 3-2 **A** and **B,** This middle-aged patient had complaints of mandibular dysfunction and dissatisfaction with his appearance. Recovery of the lost vertical dimension of occlusion and bilateral function was easily accomplished by treatment with overdentures. **C** and **D,** The results of such treatment in another patient are illustrated.

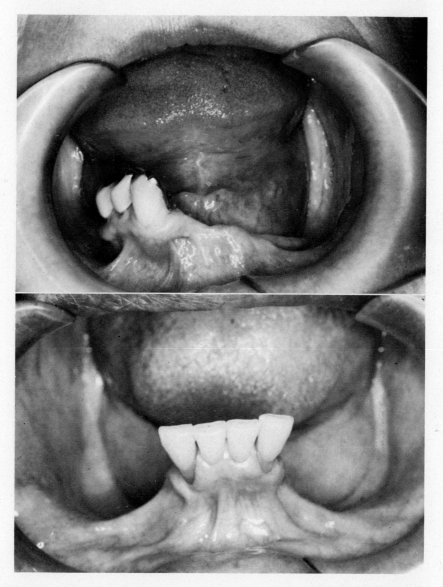

Fig. 3-3   The level of alveolar bone around retained teeth contrasts dramatically with the absence (due to resorption) of bone around the site of the former natural teeth.

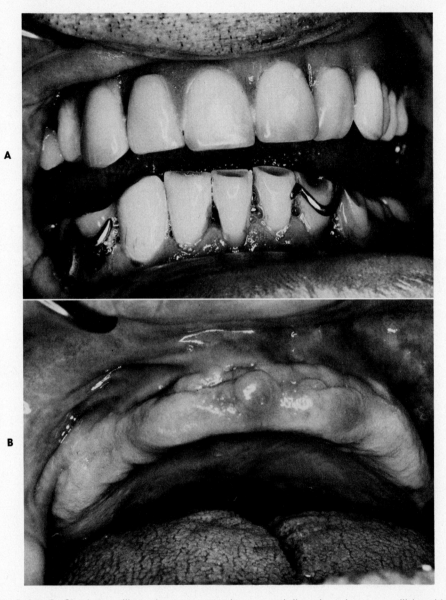

Fig. 3-4 **A,** Single maxillary denture opposing a partially edentulous mandible with an unserviced bilateral distal extension prosthesis. **B,** The vertical dimension of occlusion has collapsed, and the anterior maxillary ridge is now replaced by hyperplastic tissue.

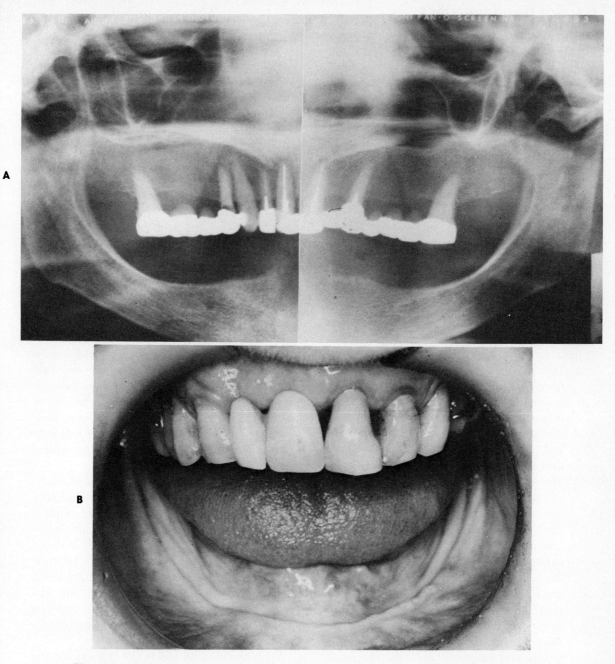

Fig. 3-5   A, This patient never wore a lower denture, and the edentulous mandibular ridge opposed a restored maxillary dentition for several years. Usually the mandibular ridge demonstrates advanced resorption in such patients, especially if a denture is worn, **B.** (See Chapter 27.)

DIAGNOSTIC PROCEDURES

To make correct decisions, the dentist needs to follow certain steps in an orderly sequence, and this is preferably done in two appointments. The first appointment should allow the dentist and the patient to become acquainted with each other and allow the dentist to obtain essential information from the patient. This information consists of a thorough history, a radiographic survey, and diagnostic casts. After thorough consideration of the diagnostic information, the dentist discusses the proposed treatment with the patient at the second appointment, along with the sequence in which this treatment will be carried out and the anticipated fee for service.

The first contact of the patient with the dental office is usually by telephone. The call may be received by an assistant, a secretary, a receptionist, or the dentist. At this time certain general, but important, information can be obtained, such as the following:

1. The patient's name, address, and telephone number are important for making future contacts as may be necessary. This information also can be an indication of the socioeconomic status of the patient and may provide a clue to the desires and expectations of the patient.
2. The means by which the patient selected you as the dentist is important. Was the patient referred by a dentist? Another patient? A physician? Or was your name obtained from the telephone book or other listing? The information about the way the patient found you will guide you in discussions regarding office policy, arrangement of appointments, and the type of service that will be expected. If the patient was referred by a dentist, radiographs and diagnostic casts may be available from that dentist. If not, the patient may wish to have that dentist make them so that they will be available to you at the first appointment. Otherwise, these records should be made at the first appointment with you.
3. The type of treatment the patient is seeking will make it possible to arrange adequate time for the first appointment. If it is treatment for a toothache, an emergency visit can be arranged. If it is for new dentures, an appointment for making preliminary records can be made.

The first appointment

The purpose of the first appointment is to allow the dentist to become acquainted with the patient so an evaluation of the problems involved in diagnosis and treatment can begin. It also provides an opportunity for the patient to become acquainted with and evaluate the dentist. Since the success or failure of prosthodontic treatment depends greatly on mutual confidence and rapport between the dentist and the patient, this appointment is extremely important. The things that are said and the questions that are asked and answered will determine to a great extent the way the dentist and patient will react to each other. Therefore the first contact should be pleasant but serious and dignified. The dentist's attitude should be one of kindness and concern for all patients and their problems. A planned office procedure will help to put patients at ease and develop the mutual respect that is essential.

The patient is met by the receptionist, assistant, or dentist at the reception room and conducted to the dental chair. After being comfortably seated, the patient is asked for the information that is necessary for the business records. This will verify or correct the information that had been received by telephone when the appointment was made. At this time the patient can supply information about age and general health by filling out a questionnaire devised for this purpose (Fig. 3-6).

When the dentist meets the patient for the first time, the receptionist or assistant makes the necessary introduction. Then the dentist carries on some conversation on general topics for a few moments and tries to avoid answering questions about the patient's dental problems at this time. Instead, this time is for making certain observations of the patient. These include the *apparent* age (i.e., physiologic age rather than chronologic age), facial appearance and expression (esthetics), speech (phonetics), lip support, vertical jaw relations, and general health and attitude of the patient as determined from an analysis of the health questionnaire. Each of these observations will be taken into consideration as the diagnosis is made.

Temporomandibular joint disorders. Signs and symptoms associated with TMJ disorders or problems of mandibular dysfunction are frequently encountered in patients with depleted dentitions. Although the cause of mandibular dysfunction appears to be multifactorial, it seems that occlusion is a contributory factor that can be best controlled and adjusted by the dentist. Research suggests that the temporomandibular joints of patients who are candidates for immediate or tooth-supported complete dentures often demonstrate arthritic or degenerative changes. Although hard research evidence is lacking to support the claim that occlusal therapy by itself is of value in the treatment of all types of mandibular dysfunction, an understanding of the pathogenesis of degenerative arthritis gives strength to the belief that the arthritic process is influenced by adverse joint loading, which can result from depleted dentitions.

A nonarthritic mandibular dysfunction is diagnosed on the basis of reported symptoms and clinical findings (Table 3-1). A degenerative arthritis is similarly recognized but usually is confirmed by means of TMJ radiographs. The dentist's treatment strategies will generally emphasize rest for the masticatory system plus the elimination of occlusal discrepancies and the restoration of support for the vertical dimension of occlusion. Quite frequently, recording jaw relations accurately will be a problem with these patients, and this fact must be taken into consideration when the treatment plan is made and appointments are scheduled. Recommended strategies are fairly routine, and tend to include (1) symptomatic treatment, (2) con-

Table 3-1 Common symptoms associated with TMJ disorders

Reported by patient	Clinical findings
Joint noise(s)	Clicking, crepitation
Pain in face, jaw, ears; headache	Pain, tenderness with palpation of masticatory muscles and TMJ
Pain on mouth opening	TM arthralgia
Difficulty opening wide and chewing	Impaired mandibular mobility; irregularity or deviation of opening; locking of mandible

trol or reduction of contributory factors, and (3) treatment of pathologic sequelae. A relatively simple and reasonable way to achieve these objectives is by patient counseling about the nature of TMJ disorders and by the use of a bite plane.

The making of maxillomandibular relation records is one of the most critical procedures in providing prosthodontic treatment for patients. The health of the temporomandibular joints is a key factor in the assessment of the ability of patients to cooperate with the dentist when jaw relation records are made. The health of the temporomandibular joints can be estimated by a simple test. The patient is asked to open the mouth wide and relax, then to move the jaw to the left and relax, and finally to move the jaw forward and relax. If the patient has difficulty coordinating these movements or following the instructions correctly, problems in recording the jaw relations can be anticipated.

The next test consists in placing a fingertip on the face over each of the condyles and instructing the patient to open the mouth slightly and move the jaw rapidly from side to side and then to open wide and close rapidly. Any possible clicking or crepitus in the joints can be detected by the fingers. If these conditions exist, more difficulty in recording jaw relations can be anticipated. Naturally, this means that more time will be required for making jaw relation records and that changes in maxilloman-

Text continued on p. 64

Instructions:

   This history is designed to assist us in finding out more about you and your problems (if any). Please circle the correct answer YES or NO. We will check your answers with you.

Mr. Mrs. Miss Ms_____

Address_____

City_____Zone_____

Phone (HOME)_____(BUSINESS)_____

Occupation_____Age_____

Bus. Address_____Birth date_____

Referring doctor_____

Address & phone_____

Name of spouse_____

Occupation_____

Number of children_____

Ages_____

Family physician: (name, address, tel.)_____

_____

When did you last see him and why?_____

Do you take any medication? (how much and why)_____

Other doctors?_____

SECTION I   MEDICAL

Has a doctor ever told you that you have a heart condition (heart murmur, heart leakage, heart attack . . .   NO   YES
or angina pectoris, for example)?

Have you ever had rheumatic fever or rheumatic heart disease?. . . . .   NO   YES

Have you ever been told that your blood pressure is too high? Too low? . . . .   NO   YES

Have you ever been told that you have diabetes?. . . . .   NO   YES

Do you bleed abnormally following a cut, a tooth extraction, or other operation? . . . .   NO   YES

Do you have any allergies (hay fever, asthma, for example)? . . . .   NO   YES
Are you allergic to any drug or medicine (aspirin, sulfas, penicillin, or Novocaine, for example)?   NO   YES

Have you ever had a lung, liver, or kidney disease? . . . .   NO   YES

Have you ever had syphilis? . . . .   NO   YES

Fig. 3-6   Sample of a health questionnaire.

SECTION II   CARDIOVASCULAR

Do you get out of breath easily?	NO	YES
Do you have difficulty breathing when you are lying down?	NO	YES
Are your ankles often badly swollen?	NO	YES
Have you ever had a stroke?	NO	YES

Nervous system

Have you ever been treated for an emotional disturbance?	NO	YES
Have you ever been treated for epilepsy?	NO	YES
Have you fainted more than twice in your life?	NO	YES
Have you ever been treated for any other disease of the nerves?	NO	YES

Respiratory system

Have you ever had a sinusitis?	NO	YES
Have you ever coughed up blood?	NO	YES
Have you ever lived with anyone who had tuberculosis?	NO	YES

Gastrointestinal

Do you have frequent spells of diarrhea?	NO	YES
Have you ever vomited blood?	NO	YES
Have you suffered from any other stomach trouble?	NO	YES
Have you ever had jaundice?	NO	YES

Endocrine system

Does a blood relative of yours have diabetes?	NO	YES
Have you ever taken thyroid tablets?	NO	YES
Are you taking, or have you ever taken, ACTH or cortisone?	NO	YES

Blood

Have you ever had anemia?	NO	YES
Are you a hemophiliac?	NO	YES
Have you ever had any other blood diseases?	NO	YES

Bones and joints

Do you have arthritis?	NO	YES
Have you ever had more than one fractured bone?	NO	YES
Have you ever had more than one dislocation?	NO	YES
Have you ever had a bone infection?	NO	YES
Have you gained or lost much weight recently	NO	YES
Has your doctor given you a special diet?	NO	YES

Fig. 3-6, cont'd   Sample of a health questionnaire.   *Continued.*

Bones and joints—cont'd

Have you ever had radiation treatments for any disease? . . . .   NO   YES

Have you ever had a tumor or cancer? . . . .   NO   YES

Have you ever had an operation? . . . .   NO   YES

Do you smoke? . . . .   NO   YES

Alcoholic beverages? . . . .   NO   YES

Physical activities? . . . .   NO   YES

(Women) Are you pregnant? . . . .   NO   YES

Do you feel you are in good health at the present time? If not, please specify:_____   NO   YES

Summary of medical history

Do you have dental insurance?
Carrier _____   Group Policy No. _____   Cert. or Soc. Ins. No._____

Dental history:
How often do you brush your teeth? . . . .   NO   YES

What kind of toothbrush and toothpaste do you use? . . . .   NO   YES

Do you use anything else? . . . .   NO   YES

Do you wear a prosthesis: (denture or bridge)? . . . .   NO   YES

Complete upper   Partial upper   Bridges   Upper   Right

Complete lower   Partial lower   Lower   Left

Have you received treatment by a dentist in the past year? . . . .   NO   YES

Have you ever experienced prolonged bleeding following a tooth extraction? . . . .   NO   YES

Have you ever experienced dizziness, or have you ever fainted, while undergoing dental treatment?

. . . .   NO   YES

Have you ever experienced any difficulty when dental anesthetics (such as Novocaine) were administered?

. . . .   NO   YES

Have you ever been treated for a gum disease (such as pyorrhea or trench mouth)? . . . .   NO   YES

Fig. 3-6, cont'd   Sample of a health questionnaire.

CURRENT COMPLAINT, HISTORY OF PRESENT CONDITION, PAST DENTAL HISTORY

_____
_____
_____
_____
_____
_____
_____
_____
_____
_____

ON EXAMINATION (Extra-oral, functional analysis, soft and hard tissues, prostheses)

_____
_____
_____
_____
_____
_____
_____
_____

IMPRESSION AND DIAGNOSIS   **PROPOSED TREATMENT AND PROGNOSIS**

_____   _____
_____   _____
_____   _____
_____   _____
_____   _____

Fig. 3-6, cont'd   Sample of a health questionnaire.

dibular relations may occur after the dentures have been in use for some time. Such changes are especially likely if the patient reports tenderness when fingertip pressure is applied by the dentist.

Dental history. It is important that the dentist know about the patient's dental history, and this can be determined when the right kinds of questions are asked. Some of these are general, and some are specific. Some will reveal simple but important facts, and others will stimulate or encourage the patient to discuss dental problems, troubles, and complaints. Any significant comments should be noted on the patient's record card for further study and consideration at the next appointment. Up to this point, the questions are preliminary.

After the preliminary conversation, in which the patient is encouraged to talk and the dentist and assistant are good listeners, the discussion can be directed toward the patient's present dental problem by the question, What do you have in mind for us to do for you? The response will indicate considerations that are of major concern to the patient. It may be to obtain new dentures for one or more reasons such as to improve his/her appearance or to eat better. These should be carefully noted because they could influence the diagnosis and the treatment procedures to be used. For example, if a patient's major concern is appearance, it will most likely require more time to solve the problem at the try-in stage than if the concern is only about eating.

As each of the patient's objectives or complaints is mentioned, it should be carefully noted on the patient's chart, but the dentist should refrain from making any comments about them in relation to the previous treatment received by the patient.

Intraoral examination. With this background information recorded, the dentist should carry out an intraoral examination. The remaining teeth are charted to show their location and condition. If the patient is wearing removable prostheses, the occlusion of these restorations should be observed before they are removed.

Any disharmony in the occlusion or between centric relation and centric occlusion should be noted because it could explain some of the difficulties that the patient has been experiencing. These observations also provide information about the patient's coordination and ability to move his mandible to the centric position as well as to perform multidirectional contact movements when instructed to do so.

Existing prostheses should be cleaned and laid aside while the teeth and oral cavity are examined. The mobility of the remaining teeth should be tested, and the depth of the gingival sulcus should be measured. The clinical crowns should be inspected visually and by use of a sharp explorer. If teeth have restorations, the margins of the restorations, the occlusal surface contours, the general shape of each tooth and its restorations, and the materials of which the restorations are made should be observed and recorded. This information provides evidence of the quality of home care and professional care that the teeth and mouth have received. If this care has been inadequate, the decision to retain or remove remaining teeth becomes easier to make. If the patient cannot be trained and motivated to give his teeth adequate care, their restoration by crowns, inlays, and other operative dentistry procedures will be futile. This problem should be thoroughly discussed with the patient so that a similar observation and evaluation can be made at the second appointment, at which time the final decision can be made.

Diagnostic casts and a radiographic survey are essential for the completion of the diagnosis.

Diagnostic casts. Diagnostic casts that may be used as part of the preextraction records are essential if the correct decisions are to be made. Therefore diagnostic casts must be available before the final decision is made regarding the removal of any teeth. The impressions for making diagnostic casts can be made in alginate (irreversible hydrocolloid) impression material in stock trays.

The making of the impressions for diagnostic

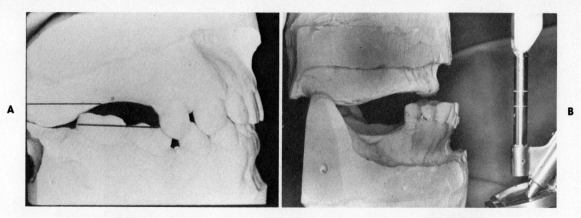

Fig. 3-7 Mounted diagnostic casts reveal existing conditions and potential problems. **A,** The mandibular occlusal plane is unfavorable and needs to be leveled; the tuberosity encroaches on the interarch space. **B,** A Class III jaw relationship is evident. Notice that this mounting on a semiadjustable articulator necessitated the use of occlusion rims.

casts is an important diagnostic procedure in itself. It will reveal unusual sensitivity of the mucous membranes, a tendency toward gagging, tolerance of the patient to procedures in the oral cavity, coordination of tongue activity, and other factors important to the diagnosis.

When teeth remain in both dental arches, the casts made in these impressions are preferably mounted on a simple hinge articulator. A wax interocclusal record can serve for relating the casts to each other on the instrument. If the impressions and interocclusal record are made at the first appointment, the casts can be mounted and studied before the second appointment (Fig. 3-7). When bilateral centric stops are absent, an articulator mounting is impractical and casts can be examined in a hand-held relationship.

Perhaps the most important diagnostic information to be obtained from mounted diagnostic casts is related to the occlusion. This information is essential because it will determine for many patients whether teeth that might be saved should be saved. For example, periodontal therapy may be able to save some teeth that actually should be removed to develop a favorable occlusal plane or to avoid rotating or tipping forces on opposing, usually maxillary, dentures.

A third molar that is tipped forward can exert horizontal forces against its opposing tooth in eccentric occlusions, and this can dislodge a maxillary denture (Fig. 3-7). If the occlusal surface cannot be reshaped so it is parallel to and on the occlusal plane, the tooth should be removed. This can be done by grinding on its occlusal surface or by making a full coverage crown. Endodontic therapy may be necessary if the tooth is to be saved.

Interarch space problems. Diagnostic casts, which are mounted or hand held, will reveal the amount of interarch space. This is important information because a lack of space in this part of the mouth has caused many dentures to fail. If a tooth is so extruded that its occlusal surface is above the occlusal plane, it should be removed unless it can be shortened sufficiently to be on the same plane with the other teeth in that dental arch.

Extremely large maxillary tuberosities make it necessary to locate the back end of the occlusal plane too low, to omit some posterior teeth, or more frequently to shorten the denture bases from their correct border extent and

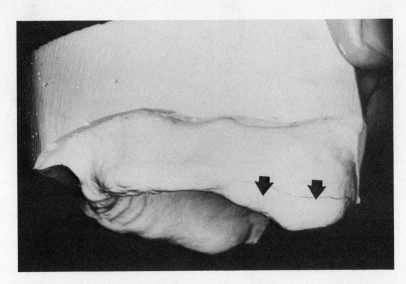

Fig. 3-8 Retention of this large tuberosity *(arrows)* would compromise the occlusal plane and distal extension of a mandibular denture. If reduction is feasible, it should be done.

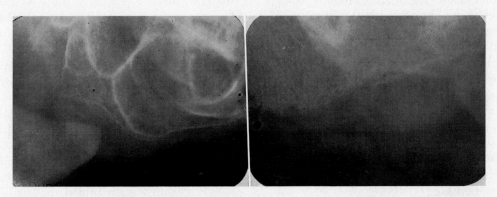

Fig. 3-9 A thick layer of fibrous connective tissue on the tuberosity does not provide a firm foundation for a denture. The bulk of the tissue will cause interference between the denture bases and prevent proper location of the back end of the occlusal plane. These films also emphasize the fact that the external ridge contours (as observed in Fig. 3-8) are not necessarily reflected in an identical morphology of the underlying bone.

contour (Fig. 3-8). If there is insufficient space between the residual ridges, the denture bases will interfere with each other and cause the dentures to tip away from the basal seats in the anterior part of the mouth. In this situation the lower denture base will wear away over the retromolar pads and holes will be worn through the maxillary denture base, leading to reduced retention in both dentures. The fact that a patient may have been wearing dentures does not rule out this difficulty.

Although lack of adequate space between the ridges is easily recognized on the mounted casts, radiographs will show whether large tuberosities are bone or are simply an overgrowth of fibrous connective tissue in the tuberosity region (Fig. 3-9).

The large fibrous tuberosity can usually be moved from side to side when grasped by a thumb and forefinger. If it is movable in this test, it should be removed.

If the tuberosity is firm and hard and radiographs show that it is composed of a thin layer of soft tissue over bone, it may have to be accommodated in the design of the denture. If it seems necessary to shorten a large bony tuberosity, care must be taken to avoid opening into the maxillary sinus. Such a surgical procedure may be contraindicated by a patient's systemic health.

The problem of insufficient interarch space in the posterior part of the mouth can be avoided for most people if the soft tissue distal to the last upper and lower molars is excised at the same time those teeth are removed.

Radiographs. Radiographs are essential for evaluating the conditions existing in every patient needing prosthodontic service. The dentist must know the conditions under the mucous membrane and the condition of the surfaces that can be seen.

The presence of abnormalities in edentulous jaws or in the edentulous segments of partially edentulous jaws is most often unsuspected because of the absence of clinical signs or symptoms. Abnormalities can and do occur, however, and have been demonstrated in a high percentage of patients on radiographic examination. These may be foreign bodies, retained tooth roots, unerupted teeth, or varied pathoses of developmental, inflammatory, or neoplastic origin (Fig. 3-10). Of these, the retained root is most commonly present. A histologic survey of a series of retained tooth roots suggests that in the absence of clinical or radiographic abnormality, the retained tooth root can be regarded as having been accepted by the tissues. The decision to extract such roots preprosthetically tends to be an elective one. However, some situations are specific indications for their removal (for example, the root's occupying a superficial submucosal position after progressive alveolar ridge resorption).

Radiographs also confirm the depth of periodontal pockets and provide information about pulpless teeth. They can show the amount of bone lost around the remaining teeth and in the edentulous regions (Fig. 3-10). They also can show the relative thickness of the submucosa covering the bone in edentulous regions, the location of the mandibular canal, and the mental foramen in relation to the basal seat for dentures. They can give an indication of the quality of the bone that supports the teeth and will support the dentures, though this is not as reliable as it should be because of variations in radiographic techniques, since variations in exposure time and developing procedures cause difficulty. In general, however, the more dense (radiopaque) the bone appears to be, the better the bony foundation and the less likelihood there is for rapid change in the basal seat when dentures are worn.

Sharp spicules of bone on ridge crests are also apparent on properly exposed dental radiographs, and these conditions may affect decisions about the location of the occlusal plane and about the types of impressions and denture base design that have to be used. A panoramic radiograph should be taken routinely. It is also

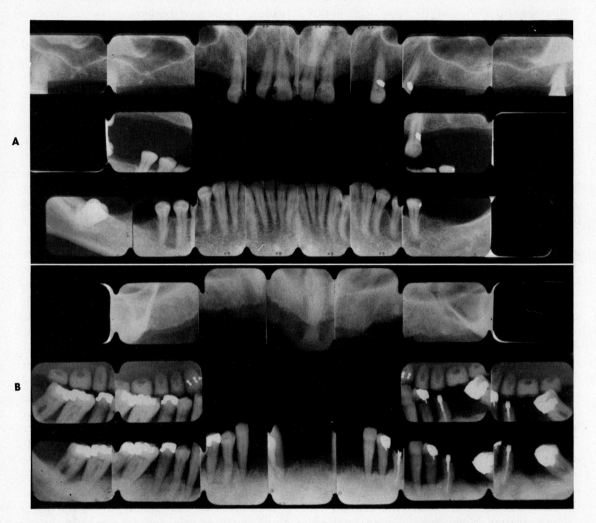

Fig. 3-10 Radiographic evidence can be combined with clinical observations to enable the dentist to prescribe optimal treatment. The patients in **A** and **B** are both partially edentulous and each requested complete denture treatment. In **A,** it is clear that all the teeth can be retained and removable partial dentures can be prescribed rather than complete dentures. In **B,** a minimum of two bilaterally located and suitable abutments to support an overdenture are not present. This mandible was therefore treated with an immediate denture.

advisable to compensate for the unreliability of radiographic interpretation of the anterior regions where distortions frequently occur. This can be achieved by adjunctive use of periapical or standard occlusal films.

TREATMENT PLAN

Once all the intraoral and general physical and mental conditions have been noted on appropriate record cards or sheets, the treatment plan can be developed. This includes which teeth are to be saved and how, the sequence in which teeth should be removed, the amount and type of oral surgery that might be required, and the type of prosthesis that is indicated. Should it be an overdenture, an immediate overdenture (some teeth are extracted at the same time as the immediate denture is inserted), or an immediate denture? Or should all of the teeth be removed and a waiting time arranged so that the tissues can heal somewhat before impressions are made or the dentures are inserted? Only in the rare cases of serious systemic health problems is the latter treatment chosen. (See Chapter 26.)

Deciding whether to extract the remaining teeth

The loss of all remaining teeth can be a terrible psychologic shock to patients, even though some of them may not admit it. Consequently the dentist should be empathic for patients who must lose their teeth. Every possibility for saving them should be explored. It is when patients recognize that the dentist does not want them to lose their teeth that the necessary feeling of confidence can be developed.

Even patients who say that they want to get rid of their teeth so that they will not have to see dentists anymore really do not want to lose their teeth. They are only trying to prepare their defenses against future difficulties they do not understand. If the dentist removes the teeth without adequate reason, physical, mental, and even legal problems may arise.

The answer so far as the dentist is concerned is simple: to get all the facts and consider all possibilities before making the decision to remove the remaining teeth. Many diagnostic factors are involved. To ignore or fail to recognize any of them could lead to incorrect decisions.

The facts to be learned before the remaining teeth are removed include the following:

1. General health of the patient

    This will determine the extent and sequence of any surgical procedures that may be necessary. In most instances it may be more desirable for the patient to retain loose or broken teeth than to have them removed. In other patients it may be that their health can be improved if infected teeth are removed.

2. Age of the patient

    This can be a determining factor in the decision to have the remaining teeth removed. If the patient is young and the bone is not fully calcified, the remaining teeth should probably be saved regardless of the cost of restoring them or the attitude of the patient toward the discomfort involved. The experience of many edentulous young people is that they lose much too much alveolar bone in a short time after they lose their teeth.

    If the patient is old and feeble, it may be better to save the few remaining teeth. If, however, elderly persons have loose, extruded teeth that are endangering their health, the teeth should be removed.

3. Tooth mobility

    Highly mobile teeth that have been extruded from their sockets and teeth with radiographic evidence of infection either at their apices or along their sides should be removed.

It is essential that natural teeth not be removed unless there is a valid reason for doing so. These reasons may include one or more of the conditions listed on the next page.

1. Advanced periodontal disease with severe bone loss around the teeth
2. Severely broken-down clinical crowns (subgingival) that cannot be adequately restored; fractured roots
3. Periapical or lateral abscesses that cannot be successfully treated
4. Unfavorably tipped or inclined teeth that pose problems for their use as abutments for fixed or removable prostheses
5. Extruded or tipped teeth that interfere with the proper location of the occlusal plane

It must be emphasized that a number of techniques and skills are available to the dentist to cope with conditions 4 and 5, reducing the numbers of candidates for total extractions and immediate dentures. There has been a corresponding increase in the number of overdenture patients as a result, attesting to the profession's growing awareness that alveolar bone must be preserved at all costs.

Preextraction records

No patient should ever be made completely edentulous or treated with complete overdentures without first having preextraction records of the existing dental and facial conditions made. It requires only a few minutes to make diagnostic impressions and casts if these have not been made before. The diagnostic casts may or may not be mounted on an articulator, but failure to make them is a serious breach of the trust placed in the dentist by the patient. In fact, it is probably valid to suggest that failure to make preextraction records may constitute professional negligence.

The color of the natural teeth should be recorded on the patient's record card. This will reassure the patient of the dentist's interest in the patient's well-being, but equally important, this record made before the teeth are removed will be valuable to the dentist. It will save time and help to avoid errors in tooth color selection when the dentures are made.

Photographs of the patient will be most helpful when the prosthetic work is completed, and they will be even more helpful as years go by and the patient needs modification or replacement of the dentures. The photographs are easily made in the dental office. Most useful are the following: (1) full face with the lips closed, (2) full face with a smile, (3) close-up with the teeth together and the lips separated, (4) full face with the mouth open wide, and (5) profile of the face with the teeth in centric occlusion and the lips relaxed.

BIBLIOGRAPHY

Axelsson G: Orthopantomographic examination of the edentulous mouth, J Prosthet Dent 59:592-598, 1988.

Carlsson GE, Kopp S, Oberg T: Arthritis and allied diseases. In Zarb GA, Carlsson GE, editors: Temporomandibular joint—function and dysfunction, St. Louis, 1979, The CV Mosby Co, Chapter 10.

Herd JR: The retained tooth root, Aust Dent J 18:125-131, 1973.

Rugh JD: Psychological factors in the etiology of masticatory pain and dysfunction. In Report of the President's Conference on the Examination, Diagnosis, and Management of Temporomandibular Disorders, J Am Dent Assoc 106:75-77, 1982.

Zarb GA, Bergman B, Clayton JA, MacKay HF, editors: Prosthodontic treatment for partially edentulous patients, St. Louis, 1978, The CV Mosby Co.

CHAPTER 4

Diagnosis and treatment planning for the patient with no teeth remaining

The procedures used in diagnosis and treatment planning for a patient who has no teeth are similar to those used for one who still has some teeth at the time treatment begins. These basic procedures have been discussed in Chapter 3. The same sequence of appointments should be followed, and the same diagnostic aids used. There are, however, some additional observations to be made. These are critical because the problems faced by dentists in treating edentulous patients are progressively more difficult to solve after the last teeth have been removed.

Treatment with fixed partial prosthodontics is somewhat simplified by the fact that restorations are cemented to retained teeth. Removable partial prostheses are retained by clasps or internal attachments. Complete dentures are maintained in position by muscular coordination and the physical forces of adhesion, cohesion, and interfacial surface tension, which are in turn dependent on the dentures' adaptation to supporting and surrounding structures of the edentulous oral cavity.

For this adaptation to be effective, the procedures used in making the dentures must be coordinated with the residual ridges' basic anatomy; but, equally important, the procedures used must be coordinated with the individual variations within the mouth of each patient.

Clinical experience proves the importance of developing refined *mechanical skills*, the *unavailability* of a panacea for all edentulous patient problems, and above all the importance of *treating the patient* instead of just constructing dentures for the patient. We can hardly overemphasize the importance of such an objective. It is probably far easier to acquire the skills of complete denture construction (challenging as these may be) than to acquire those necessary to treat a patient's aspirations and expectations; but both skills must be mastered if our patients are to be happier and if we are to receive greater satisfaction and pleasure from our work. Whereas in this text, we describe the diagnostic and clinical skills for treating the edentulous patient, we must reiterate our commitment to treating the whole patient and not just the mouth. Clinical skills alone, without compassion or awareness, distort the image of a true professional.

THE PATIENT RECENTLY MADE EDENTULOUS

Patients who have had their teeth removed less than 6 months previously have problems different from those who have had some denture-wearing experience. Likewise, the problems faced by dentists in treating recently edentulous patients are different from the problems in treating patients who have been edentulous for a long time.

The first difference is in the patients' awareness of the difficulties involved and in their expectations regarding dentures, and the second is in the biologic aspects of the treatment.

New problems of the recently edentulous patient

Patients who are edentulous and have never attempted to wear dentures face problems that they do not know exist. At best, they are not aware of any difficulties and assume that the dentures will be placed in their mouth and that they will continue to use the same eating habits as with their natural teeth. In a few people—the delicate eaters—this may be true. Most people will find it necessary to reduce the size of the portions of food taken at one time and to reduce the amount of force applied on the dentures during mastication. Patients should be made aware of the fact that chewing should be *into* the food, rather than *through* the food. The education of patients as to these facts should begin with the second examination appointment and continue through the entire treatment sequence.

The patient's concept of the permanence of dentures

Many recently edentulous patients expect their new teeth to last them the rest of their lives. Some even believe that by obtaining complete dentures they will no longer require the services of dentists. Of course, this is not true or possible. Changes occur in the basal seats for the dentures, and these will allow the positions of the dentures to change in relation to their foundation and to each other.

When teeth are removed, there remain the cavities in the bone (alveoli), which contained the roots of the teeth, and sharp ridges around each alveolus. Blood clots will form in the alveoli and form a matrix for the deposition of new bone in the tooth sockets. It would be nice if the new bone would entirely fill the alveolus, but this does not happen often.

At the same time that bone is forming in the tooth socket, the bony edge of the socket is resorbing in its attempt to become rounded. When these two processes proceed ideally, the resultant residual ridge is considered to be favorable, with a more or less flat crest and nearly vertical sides. When the residual ridge assumes this form, it provides good support for vertical forces applied through the dentures and resistance to horizontal forces that tend to cause the dentures to skid, slide, or rotate on their basal seats.

Unfortunately, in many people the tooth sockets do not completely fill with new bone, and the edges of the sockets do not always round off as desired (Fig. 4-1). These conditions can cause problems for both the dentist and the patient. The mucosa covers the edges of bone around the sockets, but this tissue will be pinched between the denture base and the bone during mastication or whenever tooth contacts are made. These tissues can be tender and even painful when closing pressure is applied on new dentures. In time, the bone will change enough to eliminate the sharp points and tender spots.

The residual ridges may have undercuts after tooth extraction, and these make the insertion and removal of impressions and dentures painful and sometimes difficult. At the time of the second examination appointment, the dentist must determine whether surgical reduction of the undercuts is necessary. This can best be determined by palpation of the tissues *and* a survey of the diagnostic casts. The cast placed on a surveyor can be tipped to reveal the most

Fig. 4-1 **A** and **B,** Radiographic evidence of failure of the maxillary sockets to round off. Contrast this with the well-healed mandibular ridges *(arrows).* Clinical evidence of gentle, **C,** to more conspicuous, **D,** residual ridge discrepancies. Both these situations can be treated conservatively, but alternate strategies (such as the use of soft liners or preprosthetic surgery) may be initiated if healing of the underlying bone is unfavorable, and particularly if symptoms persist.

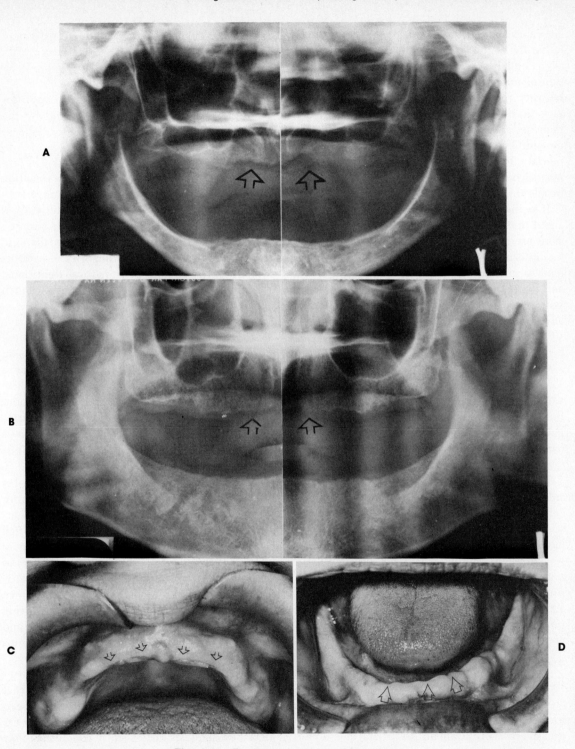

Fig. 4-1   For legend see opposite page.

favorable angle of insertion for the denture. It is hardly ever necessary to remove any bone from the labial side of the ridges. Some reduction of undercuts may be necessary in the tuberosity region, but only rarely is this necessary in the premolar region. No more bone than is absolutely necessary should be removed. The resiliency of the mucosa will compensate for most undercuts. Then time and normal bone changes will continue to ease the problem.

It is important that the patient be informed about inevitable changes *before* any impressions are made. To postpone giving the patient this information until later will almost certainly lead to misunderstanding between the dentist and the patient, who will look on such information as excuses. The patient must be warned in advance that the dentures will become progressively looser as the residual ridges change their form.

Changes in the bone supporting the basal seat continue as long as the patient lives. They vary greatly in amount from patient to patient, but they are unavoidable. Recent-extraction patients should be warned of these changes, which are more rapid in the first year after teeth are removed than they will be later on.

The same basic observations and diagnostic aids are used for partially edentulous and recently edentulous patients. Radiographs are essential for making diagnoses for people who have lost their teeth, and diagnostic casts often reveal problems that would not otherwise be noticed before too late. As for other types of prosthodontic patients, the critical observations and decisions are made at the second examination appointment when all the diagnostic aids are available.

THE PATIENT EDENTULOUS FOR A LONG TIME

When patients have been edentulous for a long time, the problems they present are progressively more difficult to treat, and these must be recognized before adequate treatment procedures can be planned.

Mental attitudes

Traditionally, prosthodontic therapy for edentulous patients could be depicted by the following equation:

Clinical skill + Knowledge = Successful care

Some dentists have even enlarged the equation to Clinical skill + Knowledge + Prompt payment of professional fees = Successful care, a cynical and semifacetious formula for success. Although clinical experience does actually support such a formula for the majority of patients who require care for their natural dentitions, the prosthodontic experience demands a much more profound understanding of the patient as a whole. During the past few years there have been strong and exciting initiatives in dental education to place the patient's well-being alongside the dentist's clinical expertise as a major educational and treatment objective. The modern equation for prosthodontic treatment now includes both technical and patient management skills, with the latter being based on a keen understanding of the patient's mental attitude.

Attitude studies on satisfied denture patients are not available, but psychologic inventories have been used to assess the personality characteristics of the difficult denture patient. Such studies have shown that a high proportion of these patients score highly on indices of neuroticism. Neurosis is regarded as a chronic anxiety state at the physiologic level and is known to affect the performance of tasks requiring neuromuscular coordination. Both learning and skilled performance show optimal relationships with moderate levels of anxiety whereas levels of anxiety that are too high or too low appear to be incapacitating. Although this suggests that only the most anxious patients should experience difficulty with their dentures, clinical experience suggests that such a conclusion may be a narrow and restrictive one. It should be pointed out, however, that cheerful extroverts are rarely found in the ranks of difficult denture patients who frequently complain unceasingly, although no causative factors can be found for their problems.

The House classification. Many years ago Dr. Milus House proposed a general classification of patients' mental attitudes. This classification is based on extensive clinical experience rather than on scientific yardsticks or psychologic inventories. It has stood up well to the test of time and deserves discussion at some length.

Philosophic. Patients in the philosophic class are willing to accept the judgment of their dentists without question. They accept their oral situation and know that their dentist will do the best that can be done. They have an ideal attitude for successful treatment, provided the biomechanical factors are reasonably favorable.

Indifferent. Indifferent patients have little concern for their teeth or oral health. They have little appreciation for the efforts of their dentists and often seek treatment because of the insistence of their families. They will give up easily if problems are encountered with their new teeth. Indifferent patients require more time for their instruction on the value and use of dentures. Their attitude can be very discouraging to dentists who treat them.

Critical. Patients in the critical group are those who find fault with everything that is done for them. They were never happy with their previous dentists, and this is usually because the previous dentists did not follow their instructions. They may bring with them a collection of dentures made by a number of dentists and will tell their new dentist exactly what is wrong with each one. Careful observation and listening will reveal that the big mistakes had been the result of dentists' trying to follow the directions of the patient.

Critical patients may try the temper of any dentist attempting to treat them. A failure to recognize critical patients during diagnosis is certain to cause the inexperienced dentist many problems. A firm control of these patients is essential. They must not be allowed to even think that they are directing the treatment. The dentist must be the doctor who directs all treatment and decisions. These patients can be traumatic in a dental practice if they are not properly controlled, but their successful treatment can be most rewarding. The first and most important phase of treatment is accomplished at the first professional contact. These people can be helped, despite themselves, when one identifies them early and works for a revision of their attitude. Many of these patients are in poor health, which affects their personalities and makes them tend to look for trouble. Often consultation with their physicians will provide information to explain their attitudes. Medical consultation is always advisable for critical patients before treatment is started.

Skeptical. Patients who may be classed as skeptical are those who have had bad results with previous treatment and are therefore doubtful that anyone can help them. They are often in poor health, with severely resorbed residual ridges and other unfavorable conditions. They have tried to be good patients, but their problems seemed insurmountable. Often they will have had a recent series of personal tragedies such as the loss of a spouse, business problems, or other things not directly related to their denture problems. They think the world is against them and simply doubt the ability of anyone to help them with problems that are greater than anyone else has to bear. They need kind and sympathetic help as much as they need new dentures.

A careful and thorough examination can be the start of successful treatment. The dentist should take more time than usual in making examinations of skeptical patients, since care and attention to detail at this time will help the patient begin to develop confidence in the new dentist. A hurried or cursory examination will destroy the confidence and trust that is essential for satisfactory treatment. These patients can be made into excellent patients if dentists recognize them and handle them properly, but it will take extra time before, during, and after treatment.

Application of the House classification. Obviously, not the least important factor in the diagnosis of patients needing complete denture service is their mental attitude. This is not a mechanical problem or a biologic problem. It is one that requires an understanding of people and the ways in which they may react to the situations they face. Dentists, with their background education in psychology, can learn to detect patient attitudes and reactions during diagnostic appointments. They can then so modify their own attitudes and reactions that mutual confidence, which is essential, can be established.

In this process dentists must establish within themselves empathy for the patient. If they are unable to do so, the results of any treatment they prescribe are most likely to be less than successful. Dentists must have a sense of real concern for the health, comfort, and welfare of their patients to establish the necessary mutual confidence. Clinical experience has proved the merits of a "tender loving care" approach to dental patients. This should be done before treatment is started and continued throughout the treatment planning and the treatment itself.

Desires and expectations

To establish rapport and confidence, the dentist must find out just what the patient's desires and expectations are. Inquiries should be made into the history of the patient's denture experience and these should be coupled with careful listening to the patient's comments and complaints. Questions such as "What difficulties are you having with your present dentures?" may stimulate the patient to tell of looseness, soreness, or difficulty in eating or talking. An evaluation by the dentist of the existing dentures in relation to the patient's complaints can reveal much information about the patient's mental attitude toward dentures and dentists. This can guide the dentist in what things to say and what things not to say to gain the confidence of the patient without promising more than is possible.

The question by the dentist "Are you happy with the way you look with your present dentures?" may prompt a flood of comments that will be helpful later on in the arrangement of teeth for esthetics. This question should be asked during the examination appointment rather than after treatment has been started.

DIAGNOSIS OF THE PATIENT WITH NO TEETH REMAINING

The examination of edentulous mouths should be visual, palpatory, and radiographic, and it should be made after some preliminary questioning by the dentist.

The questions should relate primarily to the patient's oral, dental, and general health. The answers will often reveal the causes for difficulties the patient may have had with previous dentures and will point to the use of procedures that might avoid these same problems. In addition, the answers will often reveal the mental attitudes of patients and thus bring out the real problems of some individuals. This is discussed in more detail later in the chapter.

Examination charts and records

As information about each patient is accumulated, a record must be made and kept for further study and later use. The information gained will be helpful in determining the method of treatment, but equally important from a practical viewpoint, it will determine the fee to be charged that is fair to both patient and dentist. Since there are great variations in the difficulty of treating different patients, it is essential that the differences be recorded for future reference.

Many types of examination records are used

by dentists for edentulous patients. Two are shown in Fig. 4-2. Other forms can be used equally well. Some of these are more complicated than the examples shown, and some are less detailed. Many dentists may prefer to write out the conditions they observe and dictate their observations to their assistant at the same time. This procedure has certain advantages: (1) the records can be less detailed than those recorded by the dental assistant, (2) patients are made aware of their dental problems in a single operation, and (3) the dental assistant is made aware of the necessary variations from a basic time schedule for complete denture service.

Remember that the type of record system used is less important than the fact that a record system is used in the course of making a diagnosis.

General observations affecting diagnosis

Age. The age of the patient has a definite bearing on diagnosis for complete dentures. A young person will be more adaptable to new situations such as new dentures than an older person. The facility for learning and coordination appears to diminish with age, probably as a result of progressive atrophy of elements of the cerebral cortex. The oral and facial tissues become progressively less elastic and resilient as a person grows older, and they become more easily injured by the necessary manipulation for making impressions and other records.

With advancing age, people have more difficulty adapting to new situations and learning new skills. This increases their problems in learning how to use their new teeth. Older patients also have a reduced coordination, which complicates the problems faced by dentists who provide complete denture service. If the patient has a hearing loss along with advancing age, the communication of instructions becomes more difficult.

The characteristic loss of tissue tone with age makes the problems of tooth arrangement and positioning more difficult than they would have

been when the patient was younger.

Although these conditions should be recognized by the dentist, it is not always wise to discuss them in detail with patients because of the psychologic effect. Many patients know of the changes in their physical condition and ability, but they may resent being told about them. Instead, the dentist should recognize the conditions, make allowance for them in the scheduling by allocating more time to certain critical steps in the procedures, and adjust the fees to cover the extra time the treatment will require.

General health. The general health of the patient may or may not be correlated with the patient's age. Poor health may cause the physiologic age of the patient to be far beyond the chronologic age. The effects are the same. Poor health causes the same kinds of problems as advanced age, and corresponding changes in procedures and scheduling are necessary.

The general health of patients can be estimated by observation of their posture and gait when they enter the dental operatory. However, these judgments may be incorrect, and further information is essential. This additional information can be obtained by use of a health questionnaire, by questioning of the patients, or by consultation with their physicians.

Questions relating to the health of the patient must be carefully worded to avoid arousing a feeling of distrust in the mind of the patient or stirring up resentment at the dentist's impertinence. The questions should be dignified and professional in character and tone. They should stimulate the patient to volunteer the information that is essential for the dentist to know.

It is relatively simple to get patients to talk about their health if the questioning is done in a strictly professional manner. After the usual general conversation mentioned in Chapter 3, it is logical to ask "How is your general health?" or "How have you been feeling?" Most of the time the responses to these questions will not be very revealing, but sometimes they

DIAGNOSTIC CHART

STUDENT_____ PATIENT'S NAME_____

Extraction history:

Maxillary   Periodontal disease ____   Caries ____   Both ____   Year ____

Mandibular Periodontal disease ____   Caries ____   Both ____   Year ____

Earlier denture experience: None ____   Previous set(s) ____

    Good ____   Poor ____

Age of present denture: ____   Duration of edentulism ____

Type of denture: U & L ____   Upper ____   Other ____

Immediate denture(s):   Upper ____   Lower ____   Both ____

Denture worn: Constantly ____   Intermittently ____   Day only ____   Rarely or never ____

Tooth material: Resin ____   Porcelain ____

Tooth form: Cusped ____   Cuspless ____

Denture base material: Resin ____   Other ____

Further prosthetic treatment since last dentures were made: Yes ____   No ____

If yes, explain: _____

_____

Patient evaluation: (subjective)

Comfort	Good ____	Fair ____	Poor ____
Chewing efficiency	Good ____	Fair ____	Poor ____
Esthetics	Good ____	Fair ____	Poor ____
Articulation	Good ____	Fair ____	Poor ____
Soreness	Good ____	Fair ____	Poor ____
Food trapping	Good ____	Fair ____	Poor ____

Clinical assessment of prostheses (if present)

Interocclusal distance	Adequate ____	(+) ____	(−) ____
Stability	Satisfactory ____	Defective ____	
Occlusion	Correct ____	Incorrect ____	
Articulation	Correct ____	Incorrect ____	

Total assessment:

Maxillary denture

1	2	3	4	5

Poor   Excellent

Mandibular denture

1	2	3	4	5

Poor   Excellent

Clinical data (use numerical code below)

Facial expression: Changed ____   Unchanged ____

Lips: Thin ____   Full ____   Short ____   Long ____   Tense ____   Active ____

Resorption   Slight U ____   Uneven U ____   Extensive U ____

    L ____   L ____   L ____

Ridge relation: Normal ____   Protruded ____   Retruded ____

Floor of mouth: Favorable ____   Unfavorable ____

Border tissue: Attachments   Maxillary ____   Mandibular ____

Oral mucosa: Upper   1. ____   2. ____   3. ____   4. ____

    Lower   1. ____   2. ____   3. ____   4. ____

Resiliency of   Upper   1. ____   2. ____   3. ____   4. ____   5. ____

mucosa: Lower   1. ____   2. ____   3. ____   4. ____   5. ____

Undercuts: Upper ____   Lower ____

Tongue: Favorable ____   Unfavorable ____

Saliva: Serous ____   Mucous ____

Throat form: Favorable ____   Unfavorable ____

*Radiographic assessment*_____

*Explain preprosthetic surgical treatment (if recommended)*_____

_____

*Prognosis explained to patient: probable outcome of treatment and adjustment period*_____

_____

*Probable future treatment necessary*_____

_____

Clinical instructor_____

Code:

Oral mucosa

1. Clinically normal—no signs of inflammation, no granulation
2. Local inflammation—cases with red or small inflamed regions in otherwise normal tissue
3. Diffuse reddening—diffuse hyperemia with practically a smooth surface
   Slight trauma induces hemorrhage
4. Granulated—denture-bearing mucosa degenerates into a nodular, usually greatly hyperemic surface

Resiliency of denture supporting alveolar process

1. Firm—mucosa taut over bone
2. Slight mobility of most ridges—localized
3. Slight mobility of most ridges—generalized
4. Half or more of ridge height is mobile—localized
5. Half or more of ridge height is mobile—generalized

Fig. 4-2   For legend see opposite page.

REMOVABLE PROSTHODONTIC EXAMINATION FORM

Patient_____ Chart No._____

1. Cornel Medical Index results

    Last page_____Section I_____Total_____
    Interview results (agree-disagree) with CMI
    results

2. Previous denture experience
    Type   Years   Reason for replacement
           Worn   (Problems and/or criticism)

    ☐ Additional comments on back

3. Evaluation of current dentures
    (S = Satisfactory, U = Unsatisfactory)
    Speech_____ Esthetics_____
    Occlusion_____
    Extension_____
    Retention_____
    ☐ Additional comments on back, including
       specific patient request(s) for change

4. Habits with current dentures
    Tongue_____ Clenching or bruxing_____
    Dentures worn at night_____

5. Mouth opening (large-small-medium)

6. Arch size
    Maxillary (large-medium-small)
    Mandibular (large-medium-small)

7. Contour of ridge—in cross section
                 Anterior   Posterior
    Max. (U-V-bulbous-flat) (U-V-bulbous-flat)
    Mand. (U-V-bulbous-flat) (U-V-bulbous-flat)

8. Contour of vault (flat-high-U)

9. Contour of soft palate
    (favorable-unfavorable)

10. Maxillary posterior palatal seal area
     Width (wide-narrow-average)
     Displaceability (marked-average-slight)

11. Torus palatinus (present-absent)

12. Torus mandibularis (present-absent)

13. Resorption
     Maxillary (slight-moderate-severe)
     Mandibular (slight-moderate-severe)

14. Mucosa (thickness and resilience)
     Outline areas 2, 3, or 4 type mucosa

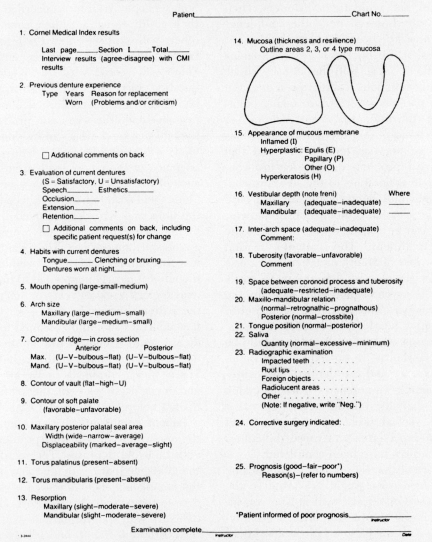

15. Appearance of mucous membrane
     Inflamed (I)
     Hyperplastic: Epulis (E)
                   Papillary (P)
                   Other (O)
     Hyperkeratosis (H)

16. Vestibular depth (note freni)   Where
     Maxillary   (adequate-inadequate) _____
     Mandibular (adequate-inadequate) _____

17. Inter-arch space (adequate-inadequate)
     Comment:

18. Tuberosity (favorable-unfavorable)
     Comment

19. Space between coronoid process and tuberosity
     (adequate-restricted-inadequate)

20. Maxillo-mandibular relation
     (normal-retrognathic-prognathous)
     Posterior (normal-crossbite)

21. Tongue position (normal-posterior)

22. Saliva
     Quantity (normal-excessive-minimum)

23. Radiographic examination
     Impacted teeth . . . .
     Root tips . . . .
     Foreign objects . . . .
     Radiolucent areas . . . . . .
     Other . . . .
     (Note: If negative, write "Neg.")

24. Corrective surgery indicated: _

25. Prognosis (good-fair-poor*)
     Reason(s)-(refer to numbers)

*Patient informed of poor prognosis_____
                                         Instructor

Examination complete_____
                           Instructor   Date

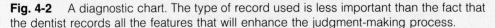

Fig. 4-2   A diagnostic chart. The type of record used is less important than the fact that
the dentist records all the features that will enhance the judgment-making process.

will open the floodgates and an extensive story of bad health will come out. Much of what will be said is of no real concern to the prosthodontic treatment, but some of it will be. It is at this time, particularly, that dentists must be good, careful, and sympathetic listeners. Their attitude at this time can build the confidence that is essential for successful treatment.

Responses to the question "Are you taking any medicines?" will tell the dentist much more than the previous leading questions. For example, if patients say they are taking chlordiazepoxide (Librium), diazepam (Valium), or some other tranquilizer, the dentist will know there is some nervous tension involved that may be a real problem during denture construction or in adaptation to the new prostheses. The medicines being taken can also indicate possible personal problems of the patient, which later can be reflected in criticism of the prosthetic treatment. The patient's marital problems or loss of family members can cause problems for the dentist that are more easily handled if the psychologic trauma faced by the patient is known. The existence of diabetes, hypertension, heart problems, allergies, chronic diseases, and other disorders should be known by the dentist so procedures can be altered if necessary and the dentist can be prepared for possible emergencies. Patients taking hormones, digitalis, nitroglycerin, or other drugs have special problems that can affect construction procedures and cause difficulties after the dentures have been completed.

It is important that these health problems be recognized *before* treatment is started so the difficulties they may cause will not be considered as excuses if troubles do arise. Certainly, consultation with the patient's physician should be obtained before certain surgical procedures are prescribed. If the patient's health is endangered by the surgical shortening of a tuberosity, for example, the prosthodontic procedures should be altered to avoid the dangers, even though the result might not be as satisfactory.

Social training. The life-style or social training of patients must be considered when the diagnosis is made. Some people will expect more of their new dentures than others, and the expectations of the patient must be determined before a treatment plan is proposed. Some people will be concerned only about their ability to eat and their comfort, whereas others will want their new teeth to defy detection by their family, friends, and associates. Some will accept whatever is done without question, but others will insist on the impossible. Some will be concerned about their appearance and others will not, probably because they do not know what can be done. Some patients will want no change whatever in the appearance of their new teeth from the appearance of the dentures they have been wearing. Others will wish to have their face lifted and all the lines and wrinkles removed by their new teeth, even though to do this would give them a grotesque appearance. They want the "bloodless face-lifting" and the "wrinkle removers" though it is clearly impossible to turn the physiologic clock back 20 years or so, just because the patient desires it (Fig. 4-3). Instead, the new dentures should be planned to restore the dignity and harmony of the mouth region with the conditions found in the rest of the face. These special problems must be determined and recognized by *both* the patient and the dentist before any treatment is started.

Patient complaints. Patients must be given the opportunity to tell what problems they had with their old dentures. The reason for this is the guidance that the dentist may receive from the complaints about the area of greatest concern to the patient. Is it comfort, ability to eat, difficulty with speech, looseness, gagging? Is it the attitude of friends and relatives or the appearance of their teeth or their face? When this is known, the dentist will know which procedures or parts of a procedure will be most critical, how to overcome the difficulty if possible, and thus how to adjust the time schedule and fee properly.

If the chief concern is appearance, the den-

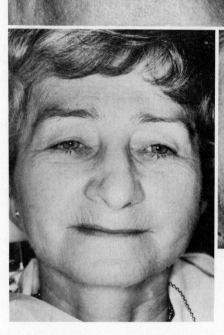

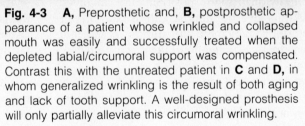

Fig. 4-3   **A,** Preprosthetic and, **B,** postprosthetic appearance of a patient whose wrinkled and collapsed mouth was easily and successfully treated when the depleted labial/circumoral support was compensated. Contrast this with the untreated patient in **C** and **D,** in whom generalized wrinkling is the result of both aging and lack of tooth support. A well-designed prosthesis will only partially alleviate this circumoral wrinkling.

tist should make a personal assessment for comparison with that of the patient. In other words, is the patient's judgment correct or is it misdirected? To make an assessment, the dentist should observe the color and size of the teeth on the existing dentures and determine their harmony, or lack of it, with the patient's face and features. The basic position of the teeth should be observed, along with the amount of teeth exposed when the patient talks and smiles. The dentist should judge whether the irregularities of the teeth are natural or unlikely to be found in natural teeth.

Lip support. If the tissue around the mouth has wrinkles (Fig. 4-3) and the rest of the face does not, significant improvement can be expected. If the existing anterior teeth are set too far lingually or palatally, the lips will lack the necessary support, and plans can be made to bring the new teeth further forward and thus provide the necessary support to help eliminate the wrinkles. If the wrinkles, especially the vertical lines in the lower half of the lip, are long-standing, they will not disappear at once and patients should be warned about this. Also, they should be told that for a short time

their mouth might appear to them to be too full because of the sudden change. The real danger insofar as the dentist is concerned is that too much support for the lips might be provided in an attempt to eliminate the vertical lines in the upper lip. Extra time will be needed at the tryin of the wax dentures and should be planned for.

Questions about the prominence of the natural upper anterior teeth may reveal that surgery was done when the teeth were removed—"to get rid of the buck teeth I never liked." Attempts to reduce the horizontal overlap of anterior teeth by setting the teeth back "under the ridge" and by surgery usually lead to a lack of lip support that produces the vertical lines as tissue tone deteriorates later in life.

Lip thickness. Patients with thin lips present special problems. Any slight change in the labiolingual tooth position makes an immediate change in the lip contour. This can be so critical that even overlapping of teeth may distort the surface of the lip. Both the arch form and the individual tooth positions are involved. Thick lips give the dentist a little more opportunity for variations in the arch form and individual tooth arrangement before the changes are obvious in the lip contour.

Lip length. Patients with a short upper lip will expose all the upper anterior teeth and much of the labial flange of the denture base as well. This means that special attention and care must be given to the color and form of the denture base.

Lip fullness. The fullness of the lip is directly related to the support it gets from the mucosa or denture base and the teeth in back of it. Lip fullness should not be confused with lip thickness, which involves the intrinsic structure of the lip. An existing denture with an excessively thick labial flange could make the lip appear to be too full rather than displaced. The problem with lip fullness is in the patient's reaction to changes. If the existing dentures have the teeth set too far palatally, the patient may feel that the new and corrected tooth arrangement makes the lip too full.

Profile and contour of features. Observation of the facial profile gives an indication of the relative size of the upper and lower jaws and of the vertical jaw relations. A receding chin and convex profile mean that the upper jaw is larger than the lower, and the occlusion will have a characteristic Class II disharmony in the centric position (Fig. 4-4, *A* and *B*).

If the chin is prominent, the profile will be concave and the occlusion will have a characteristic Class III disharmony (Fig. 4-4, *C* and *D*), unless the appearance is created because the vertical separation of the jaws is too small. This reduced occlusal vertical dimension can result from loss of bone from the basal seats or from errors in the construction of the existing dentures. If the latter have occurred, improvement in the patient's appearance can be expected. If the variation from an ideal straight profile was developmental, only restoration of the profile similar to the one with natural teeth present can be expected.

Tone of the facial tissues. A close inspection of the skin of the face will reveal the tone of the facial tissues. This is important because two factors affect tissue tone. First, the age and health of the patient influence the intrinsic structures of the facial tissues. These must be accepted as two of the conditions under which the dentist must work, unless the patient's general health can be improved. The tone of facial tissues may indicate limitations on what might be done to improve the patient's facial contours. A face that has poor tissue tone, with loose or wrinkled tissues throughout, cannot be made to appear youthful by new dentures. Second, poor tissue tone may be the result of inadequate support by the intraoral structures. This condition can be improved by new dentures if the existing ones are inadequate. The arch form and placement and the denture base contours are the keys to supplying adequate, but not excessive, support for facial tissues. It should be remembered, however, that the facial tissues around the mouth should be supported only to their original positions and that

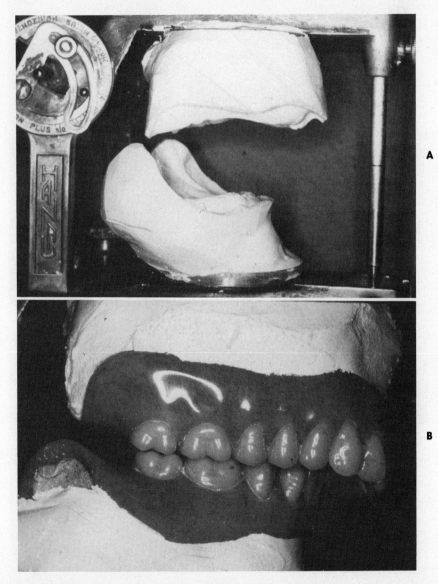

Fig. 4-4   A and **B,** The upper jaw is much larger than the lower. Since the teeth must be correctly related to each of the residual ridges, a large horizontal overlap is necessary.

Continued.

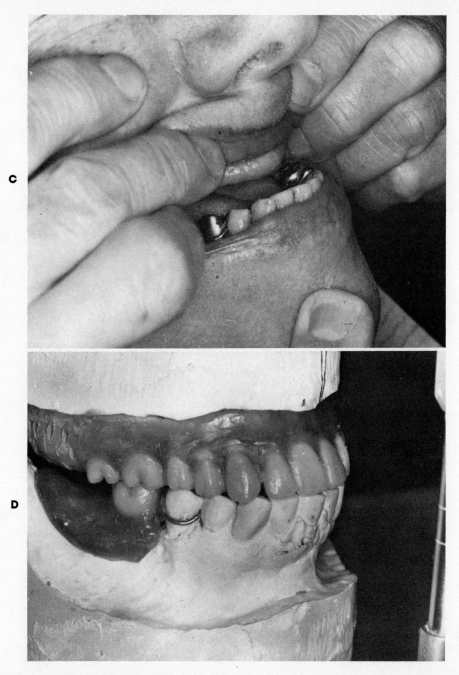

Fig. 4-4, cont'd   C and **D,** The lower jaw is much larger than the upper. In this case treatment with dentures can modify the appearance of the Class III disharmony.

the tone of the skin should be comparable throughout the face.

Vertical face length. General observation of the patient's face while in conversation or while the esthetic possibilities and limitations are considered should be directed to the length of the patient's face. This dimension is directly related to the vertical height of the dentures. If the dentures permit the jaws to close too far when the teeth are in contact, the muscles of mastication and facial expression are affected and the tone of the facial tissues in the lower third of the face is not maintained. A judgment made at this time (that is, during the examination) may be more effective than one made while new teeth are being constructed. A general appearance of the chin being too intimate with the nose can be apparent with the old dentures in place, and this should be observed.

Some patients may suggest that the occlusal vertical dimension be increased to eliminate wrinkles around the mouth. Care should be taken to avoid excessive denture height for these people. Usually, the cause of the wrinkles is a lack of anteroposterior support for the lips, and the dentist should not be led into using the patient's judgment in this regard. Misunderstandings regarding vertical jaw relations and vertical face length can consume much construction time later if the problems are not recognized.

Radiographic and intraoral examination

The health of the oral tissues should be thoroughly studied as soon as the existing dentures are removed from the mouth. This evaluation should be both radiographic and intraoral. The reason for doing this at once is that the dentist may be able to distinguish between damage being caused by the old dentures and damage from underlying conditions that may be observed. Superficial inflammation caused by the dentures may disappear quickly, but the results of long-term irritation by dentures will cause more lasting problems for both dentist and patient. To decide on the best treatment,

one should observe, palpate, and evaluate many conditions.

Advantages of a radiographic examination. Reference was made in Chapter 3 to the indispensability of a radiographic study of the jaws as an integral part of any clinical assessment for prosthetic treatment. Figs. 4-1 and 4-5 illustrate some radiographic evidence that should enable the dentist to diagnose or anticipate possible denture wearing problems. Regrettably, edentulous patients are not always examined radiographically prior to the initiation of prosthodontic treatment, although several studies have demonstrated positive radiographic findings in 30% to 40% of surveyed edentulous patients. Apart from information about variations in edentulous morphology, the most frequently observed findings are root fragments, unerupted teeth, radiopacities, radiolucencies, and foreign bodies.

Current clinical wisdom endorses the use of a panoramic radiographic view of both arches, supplemented by periapical or occlusal views where necessary to enhance the merits of this diagnostic service. Although the objective is a thorough assessment of anatomic landmarks and the absence or presence of abnormal jaw bone changes, patient radiation exposure should be kept to a minimum. Since radiation association with a panoramic exposure is significantly less than that with a full mouth periapical survey, panoramic views should be prescribed routinely and periapical or occlusal views selectively and adjunctively.

All too frequently clinically observed ridge morphology does not reveal the true anatomy of the underlying bone. Autopsy studies have verified that the intraoral appearance of ridge contours bears little resemblance to the bony ridge exposed in the dissection. It must be emphasized that the diagnostic yield from a radiographic assessment is high and the expected radiation-induced risk is low.

The intraoral examination

Color of the mucosa. The color of the mucosa will reveal much about its health. The differ-

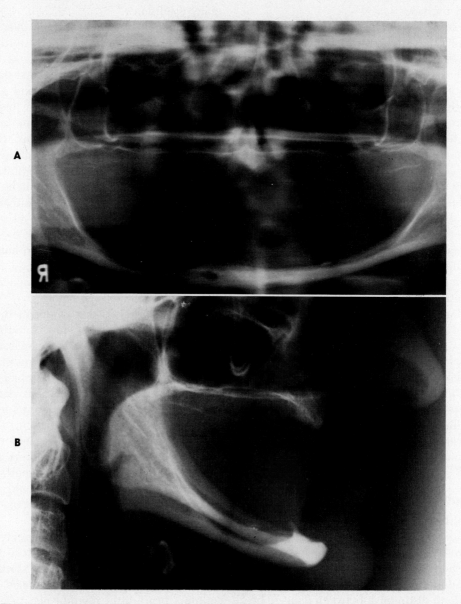

Fig. 4-5 Panoramic, **A,** and lateral cephalometric, **B,** views of an edentulous patient. Although both are essential when a preprosthetic surgical procedure is being planned, only the panoramic view is mandatory for a screening examination. Both views demonstrate the advanced residual ridge resorption that has taken place. Notice the superficial orientation of the inferior alveolar canals and the large cancellous spaces in the right mandibular canine region.

ences in appearance between a healthy pink mucosa and red inflamed tissue are apparent. The problem is how to get all the oral mucosa into a healthy state. The solution will vary because of differences in the causes of inflammation and the length of time the tissues have been irritated. Some tissues will recover with simple rest (keeping the dentures out of the mouth); others will require the use of tissue-conditioning resins inside existing or treatment dentures. Still others will require surgery of the mouth to make them as healthy as possible.

Regardless of the problem and its treatment, the oral tissues *must* be healthy before impressions for new dentures are made. To fail to see that the tissues are healthy is to invite trouble from a continuing inflammation or from new dentures that become loose because the inflammation disappears after the new dentures are in service. The treatment plan and schedule must provide for the necessary procedures to be done and for complete recovery of the tissues from the preparatory treatment used.

Abrasions. Abrasions, cuts, or other sore spots may be found in any location under the basal seats of the existing dentures or at the borders. They may be the result of overextended or underextended borders, or malocclusion may cause them. At the time of the examination the causes should be removed to allow the tissues an opportunity to heal before impressions are made.

Pathoses. Many types of pathologic lesions can be found in the oral cavity, including lesions of the mucous membrane or of tissues under it. They may be in the bone or glandular tissue, on the soft palate, hard palate, cheeks, tongue, or floor of the mouth, or in the throat. Like mechanical cuts and abrasions, pathologic lesions should be diagnosed and treated before impressions are made. Among the more common lesions found in the mouth of edentulous patients are pseudoepitheliomatous hyperplasia, papillary hyperplasia, aphthous ulcers, lichen planus, hyperkeratosis and leukoplakia, and epulis fissuratum.

Other lesions may be more serious: lumps and ulcers that could be evidence of malignancies. These may be found in the floor of the mouth and on the tongue, throat, and palate. If they are not detected, serious consequences can result for the patient and for the dentist. If suspicious lesions are found, adequate steps must be carried out to determine the precise cause. These include biopsy and referral for further tests. Oral malignancies are most common in people who are old enough to be likely to need complete dentures, but they may occur in people of all ages. Dentists' obligations in maintaining health do not end when the last teeth are gone. Instead, they become more important.

The maxillary basal seat (Plate 4-1). Each basal seat has some tissues that are harder than others, and these should be located so the dentures will distribute occlusal and limiting forces where they should be. This consideration is discussed in detail in Chapter 7, but the observations are made at the time of the examination. Some hard tissues such as the torus palatinus should be relieved of pressure from the denture. Likewise, soft tissues such as the incisive papilla should be protected from pressure that would impinge on the blood vessels and nerves lying under them.

An ideal basal seat for a maxillary denture is one that has a more or less uniform layer of soft tissue over the bone. The ideal tissue will be quite firm, but still slightly resilient. When the tissue covering the bone is too thin, it will be easily damaged by the pressure from the denture and will be more difficult to fit with the denture base. When the tissue is too thick, it will be too soft and permit the denture to move more than it should under occlusal pressure.

The maxillary tuberosities are often enlarged with movable fibrous tissue. Obviously, freely movable soft tissues will not provide as good support for the denture as will firm ones. It may be desirable to remove large fibrous tuberosities if they are movable, even though they may not interfere with the location of the

Plate 4-1   An extensive range of morphologic and tissue health variables must be diagnosed before treatment planning is finished and complete denture fabrication is started. Six different edentulous maxillae underscore some of the frequently encountered variables.

A, This residual ridge shows minimal resorption and is covered by firm healthy soft tissues. Hamular notches are well defined, and no adhesions are present. This maxillary basal seat area offers an excellent morphologic prognosis.

B, This residual ridge, though substantial, is irregular, with bony undercuts and small exostoses present. The left tuberosity is pendulous and mobile, and a large torus is present. A denture can be built on these foundations, but surgical considerations should also be addressed to optimize the basal seat area.

C, Anterior localized ridge resorption has occurred and been replaced by hyperplastic tissue. This tissue is usually excised prior to impression making. When a patient's health precludes this option, a modified impression technique is employed.

D, Home care and a regular recall program were not instituted for this patient. Consequently the basal seat area became inflamed and an epulis resulted. Tissue rest, massage, and the prescription of a treatment liner should precede a surgical assessment in this patient.

E, Advanced residual ridge resorption is evident, with low mobile peripheral tissue attachments and obliteration of the hamular notches. As a result, compromise in both peripheral and posterior palatal seals will not improve the prognosis for a retentive and stable denture.

F, A morphologic picture similar to the one in **E** has been rectified by a preprosthetic sulcus deepening with skin graft placement. This prescription is more frequently used in the mandible.

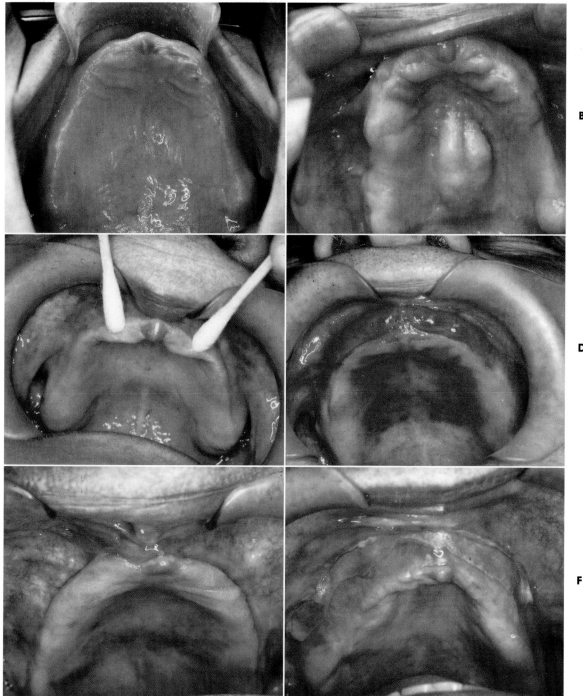

Plate 4-1   For legend see opposite page.

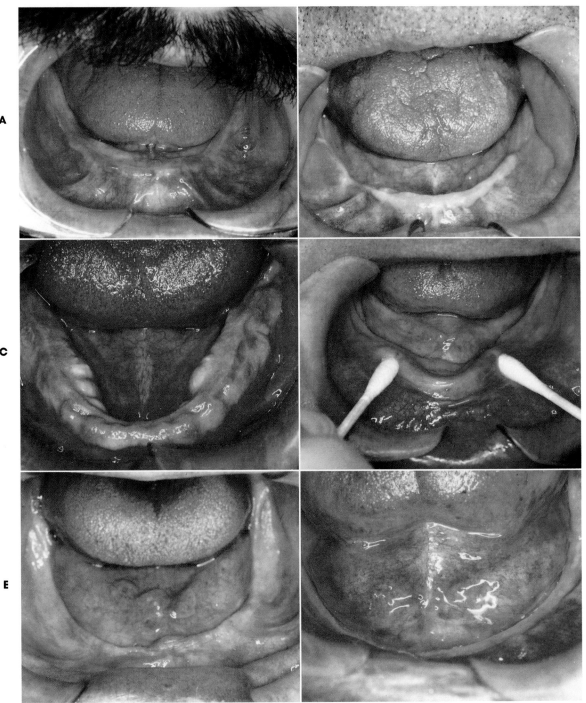

Plate 4-2 For legend see opposite page.

Plate 4-2   Six diverse edentulous mandibular morphologic outcomes.

A, A firm, broad, and well-developed ridge accompanied by a favorable tongue size and position suggests a good prognosis.

B and **C,** Alveolar ridge undercuts are present, though ridge size differs substantially. Surgical removal of the undercuts can be readily avoided by prudent relief of the denture base. However, tender areas over the exostoses and/or the tori in **C** may have to be treated surgically to ensure a comfortable prosthetic experience.

D to **F,** Hyperplastic replacement of the entire residual ridge does not usually provide a firm denture-bearing area. However, surgical excision may result in a significantly reduced basal area, as in **E.** Extension of the denture's posterior lingual flanges will usually allow for a stable denture in **E.** This objective may not be fulfilled in **F,** because of the unfavorably high attachment of the floor of the mouth. Also notice the virtual continuity of mobile mucosa in the floor of the mouth and the labial/buccal vestibule. They are separated by a thin mobile fibrous band. From a morphologic point of view, this does not provide a favorable prognosis. Preprosthetic surgery for placement of osseointegrated implants is likely to be needed in these situations.

occlusal plane or the denture base material (Chapter 6). (See Figs. 3-8 and 3-9.)

An even more hazardous condition affecting stability and support for maxillary dentures is the hyperplastic or flabby maxillary ridge. This large mass of easily movable and displaceable tissue occupies the space where the residual alveolar (bony) ridge formerly was. It may extend from one tuberosity to the other, or it may be only in the anterior part of the maxillary arch. The best treatment is to remove it by surgery. The foundation for the denture will appear to be smaller; but, in fact, it is not. The bone is the same after surgery and is more effective in its support of the mucosa that supports the denture.

When the patient who has this condition is examined for dentures, other factors also must be considered in the decision to remove the hyperplastic tissue. If the patient's general physical health is not good, if his age is such that physical tolerance is low, or if there is a recent history of a number of general surgical operations, it may be wise to alter the impression procedure and avoid or postpone further oral surgery. In this situation the patient must understand that the dentist is using an alternate procedure that is more difficult than the usual one and that the results may not be as good as could be expected from the regular procedure. The dentist is choosing the lesser of two evils in a bad situation.

Whether the hyperplastic tissue is surgically removed or not, the maxillary bones will be smaller than before the hyperplasia developed, producing unfavorable leverages on the maxillary denture base and more difficulty in developing occlusal harmony. These factors must be recognized at the time the diagnosis is made so adjustments can be incorporated into the treatment schedule and the fee for the denture service.

One other hard area found in some patients is the zygomatic process of the maxillary bone as it crosses the buccal vestibule on each side. When the top of the buccal vestibule is pal-

pated in the molar region, this bony process may be seen to be low in relation to the crest of the residual ridge. When the soft tissue is thin over the zygomatic process, the denture may tend to rock over these hard tissues on each side and thus be loosened. This difficulty can be anticipated when the mouth is examined, and the correction is simple when the cause is known.

Torus palatinus. A torus palatinus is a bony enlargement found at the midline of the hard palate. It is not found in all patients, and it varies in size from a small pea to a huge enlargement that may even fill the palate to the level of the occlusal plane. Palatine tori are covered with a thin layer of soft tissue, and consequently they are very hard. In fact, they are much less resilient than the fibrous tissues on the crest of the residual ridge, which provide the primary support for the maxillary denture. Therefore the torus palatinus must be relieved of pressure from the denture, or it may be removed by surgery (Chapter 6).

Generally surgery to remove a torus palatinus should be avoided, but if the torus is so large that it extends beyond the vibrating line and over part of the soft palate, it should be removed or reduced in size. When the torus extends too far back, it may interfere with the development of a posterior palatal seal (Fig. 6-7).

A palatine torus is easily relieved of pressure by placement of an appropriately thick sheet of lead foil over it on the cast when the denture is processed. The size of the relief will coincide with the size of the convexity in the hard palate. The thickness of the relief will vary with the relative hardness of the torus, which is usually increased in larger tori.

Adhesions. Adhesions between the residual ridge and the cheek may occur in either the maxillary or mandibular basal seats. Usually, a notch or notches in the impression and in the denture base will accommodate these adhesions, but if they attach close to the crest of the residual ridge, it is best to remove them before the impression is made. When they are "clipped" or removed, a stent must be used to keep the soft tissue parts separated while healing occurs; otherwise, the cut surfaces will grow together again, and the situation will be worse than before the surgery.

The mandibular basal seat (Plate 4-2). The hard tissues in the mandibular basal seat are either favorable (as on a broad residual ridge crest) or unfavorable (as a torus mandibularis, a series of hard sharp points, or a sharp bony ridge). Each of these must be handled in a different way.

The torus mandibularis is a bony bulge or knob found on the lingual side of some mandibular residual alveolar ridges in the region of the premolar teeth. Mandibular tori form while the teeth are present and remain after the

teeth are lost unless they are removed. They range in size from a small pea to half a hazelnut or larger. They occur singly or in rows just above the floor of the mouth (Fig. 4-6). They are usually removed long before impressions for complete dentures are made. They are thinly covered by soft tissue, which means that this tissue is more sensitive to pressure from dentures than the other tissue of the basal seat.

The torus itself has a thin covering of cortical bone, and the interior of the torus is made up of cancellous bone. When the cortical bone is removed, pressure from a denture will be against cancellous bone unless there is adequate healing time for a new cortical plate to be formed. This takes from 2 to 6 months.

It is practically impossible to provide relief

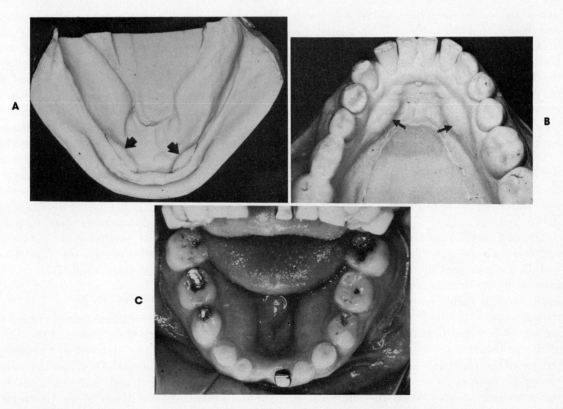

Fig. 4-6 Mandibular tori. **A** and **B,** Average size. **C,** Extremely large. (See also Fig. 9-15.)

for mandibular tori inside a denture. The tori are too close to the floor of the mouth, and attempts to take pressure off them will break the border seal so necessary for mandibular dentures. However, some mandibular tori can be accommodated by carefully planned relief of the denture.

Two other hard tissues are of practical significance: the hard points of attachment of the mentalis muscles that exist near the crest of badly resorbed residual ridges (which can be relieved by modification of the denture bases without surgery) and the crest of the residual mandibular ridge (a relatively hard surface compared with the tissue covering the broad area of the buccal shelf, provided that unfavorable resorption has not occurred).

The buccal shelf is on the body of the mandible between the buccal frenum and the retromolar pad and between the residual ridge crest and the external oblique line. It has a good cortical bone surface, but it also has a covering of the suctorial pad and the inferior attachment of the buccinator muscle, as well as free gingiva on its superior surface. These soft tissues are more easily displaced than those found on the crest of the residual ridge unless there has been severe bony ridge resorption.

Diagnostic procedures should be used to determine the relative thickness of these soft tissues and the condition of the residual ridge itself. Radiographs are essential for making such determinations.

The soft tissues include the retromolar pad, which is both soft and easily displaceable. The pad does not support the denture but must be covered by the denture if a border seal is to be maintained. It should not be displaced from its normal relaxed position, since some movable structures enter or pass through it. These include the buccinator muscle, the superior constrictor of the pharynx, the pterygomandibular raphe, fibers from the temporalis tendon, and some mucous glands. When the diagnosis is made, plans should include full coverage of the retromolar pads.

Fibrous cordlike ridges. Some patients with a severely resorbed mandible have cordlike soft tissue ridge crests (Fig. 4-7, *A*). These are fibrous tissue and usually extend from one retromolar pad to the other. They are easily displaced labially, buccally, or lingually, and they do not supply stability or support for dentures. They must not be displaced when impressions are made since they will be painful when the dentures are worn and will tend to lift the denture when the teeth are not in contact.

Surgery can improve this situation by removing the movable tissue, but the procedure has its hazards as well. In many patients the surgical removal of a fibrous ridge crest detaches the mucosa from the mandible, so the mucous membrane over the residual ridge crest can be pulled forward by the lip and backward by the tongue. This disastrous condition is, of course, avoided by combining the tissue "trim" with a vestibuloplasty (Fig. 4-7, *B* to *E*).

Absence of tuberosities and loss of the pterygomaxillary notch. Advanced bone resorption or excessive surgical reduction can lead to absence of one or both tuberosities. Such a morphologic feature is frequently accompanied by obliteration of the pterygomaxillary (hamular) notch, which is essential for ensuring the maximum breadth to the posterior palatal seal of the denture. When this condition is encountered, the patient should be informed since the maxillary denture will not be as resistant to posterior downward dislodgment when incising takes place. Our oral surgical colleagues can sometimes improve the site for the prosthesis by creating a localized vestibuloplasty.

Biomechanical considerations

A number of biomechanical factors influence the choice of methods to be used and the difficulties that will be encountered in providing complete denture service. These factors must be recognized even though not much can be done to eliminate the causes of the problems. Instead, it is necessary to make alterations in the technical procedures that will help reduce

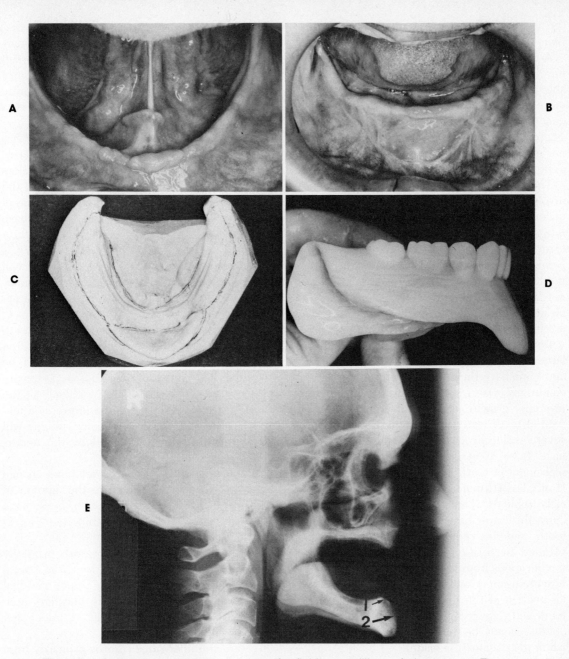

Fig. 4-7   A, This residual ridge consists of a flabby, cordlike, soft tissue crest. The attached mucosa is limited and mobile. In **B** to **D** a similar situation was treated surgically and the new labial sulcus can be filled by a significant labial denture extension. **E,** This is possible because the origin of the mentalis has been severed at *1* and the depth of the labial sulcus is now at *2*.

the adverse effects of the unfavorable conditions.

Arch size. The size of the mandible and the maxillae determines the ultimate support available for complete dentures. Large jaws provide more support than small jaws, and the difference is directly proportional to their sizes. Therefore a patient with small jawbones should not expect to put as much closing force on the dentures as a person with large jawbones.

The size of the maxillae and mandible is also involved in the margin for error in impression making. If the jaws are small, the impressions must be as accurate as possible because a small error would be relatively larger than the same error in an impression of a large mouth. This is not to say that impressions of large jaws should not be as accurate as those of small jaws. Instead, impression requirements for small jaws are more critical than those for large ones.

Disharmony in jaw sizes. Some patients have large maxillary jaws and small mandibular jaws, and some have the opposite disharmony. These conditions arise from genetic factors and from improper growth and development. When the natural teeth were present, these patients had severe malocclusions, which may or may not have been treated orthodontically. The replacement of teeth for people who had a Class II or Class III malocclusion presents some special problems. The artificial teeth should occupy the same basic positions as the natural teeth, and this requires that the occlusion be planned in relation to the disharmony. The modifications from an ideal occlusion to a crossbite occlusion or one with an excessive horizontal overlap of the upper teeth over the lower teeth will require time to develop. These difficulties should be recognized and anticipated when the diagnosis is made.

Ridge form. The cross-section contour of the ridge has an important influence on the selection of the impression procedure. Resorption of the residual ridge after the removal of teeth radically changes its cross-section form. When the teeth are first removed, the ridge is broad at its occlusal surface; but as resorption occurs, the residual ridge becomes progressively narrower and shorter. The ideal ridge has a broad top and parallel sides. As the ridge becomes narrower, it becomes sharper and consequently is unable to withstand as much force as a broader ridge.

When the mandibular ridge is sharp and has sharp bone spicules, it is best to use a selective pressure impression (that is, one that selectively "unloads" the ridge crest) so more of the occlusal force is placed on the cortical bone of the buccal shelf on either side of the sharp crest.

When the sharp ridge has disappeared, it is best to use an impression procedure that will distribute occlusal forces more evenly. A minimum pressure procedure is best in this situation.

When severe undercuts exist after the teeth have been removed, some surgical alteration may be necessary. However, this should be minimal. The undercuts may not be as severe as they seem because of the resiliency of the mucosa. Occasionally an elastic impression material (such as Thiokol or silicone rubber) will overcome the difficulty caused by the undercuts.

Ridge relations. The ridge relations change as shrinkage occurs. Therefore the amount of resorption that has occurred after teeth have been lost affects this relationship (see Fig. 2-17).

The bones of the maxillae resorb primarily from the occlusal surface and from the buccal and labial surfaces. Thus the upper residual ridge becomes shorter and the maxillary arch becomes narrower from side to side and shorter anteroposteriorly.

The mandibular ridge resorbs primarily from the occlusal surface. As this occurs, the ridges in the posterior part of the mouth, in effect, move progressively farther apart. It appears as though the mandibular arch becomes broader while the maxillary arch becomes narrower. The mandible changes in this way because its inferior border is broader from one side of the jaw to the other than its occlusal part. The cross-section shrinkage in the molar region is downward and outward. The cross-section shrinkage in the anterior region at first is downward and backward. Then as shrinkage continues, the anterior part of the basal seat for the mandibular denture moves forward.

These changes must be noted at the time of the examination to plan for the resultant problems of leverage, occlusion, and tooth position for esthetics.

Arch shape. The shape of the residual arch from the occlusal surface should be noted so the dentist can anticipate, in a general way, the form of the teeth to be used and can estimate the relative development of the lower third of the face. This may guide the arrangement of the teeth. If the arches are asymmetric, some problems of tooth arrangement and occlusion may occur.

Sagittal profile of the residual ridge. Closely related to the factor of parallelism of residual ridges is the problem of the upward slope of the distal part of the mandibular residual ridge. In making the intraoral examination, the dentist should observe the mandibular residual ridge by palpation to determine the location where the ridge slopes up toward the retromolar pad and the ramus. This upward slope is important because occlusal contacts immediately above the incline at the back part of the residual ridge will cause a complete denture to skid forward. Plans must be made to avoid this kind of dislodging force on mandibular dentures. Unfavorable ridge slopes are not often found in recent extraction situations, but they are common in patients whose posterior teeth have been out a long time.

Shape of the palatal vault. Palatal vaults vary considerably from patient to patient. The most favorable vault form is one that has a medium depth with well-defined rugae in the anterior part of the palate.

A flat palatal vault can present some difficulties if the bone in the anterior region is se-verely resorbed. The problem is insufficient resistance to forward movement of the maxillary denture. Such a loss of stability will cause a loss of retention of the denture, especially during masticatory function. Dentures in a mouth with a flat palatal vault can resist removal by a direct downward pull, but they can be easily dislodged by a laterally or anteriorly directed or a rotating force. Therefore particular attention must be paid to balancing the occlusion.

A high, narrow, V-shaped vault is also unfavorable for the retention of dentures. The tighter the denture presses against the sides of the palatal vault, the faster it will loosen and slip out of place. In most mouths with a V-shaped vault, the residual ridges also are V-shaped in cross section. Thus the problem is complicated. The solution involves the development of the border seal, border thickness, and shape of the polished surfaces so the cheeks and buccinator muscles can automatically perfect the border seal and mechanically aid in the retention of the denture. The necessary additional time and care should be planned at the time of the examination.

Muscular development. The muscular development of the tongue, cheeks, and lips is a significant factor influencing impression making and the ability of patients to use their dentures after they have been completed. The tongue can be very troublesome if it is overly large or small.

The tongue seems to become larger and more powerful when a person has been wearing loose or otherwise inadequate dentures. Apparently it is used to hold the upper dentures in place; other persons even masticate their food by pushing it against the roof of the mouth with their tongue. Persons who have worn a complete upper denture against eight or ten lower anterior teeth are especially prone to develop these habits. Also, when lower molar teeth have been missing for some time, the tongue tends to fill the space vacated by the teeth, and often the sublingual glands are forced over the crest of the residual ridge into

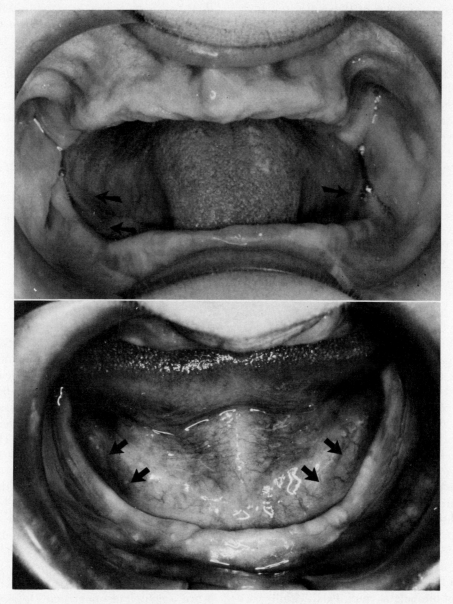

Fig. 4-8 A large tongue and sublingual glands (shown here in two patients) may occupy the space *(arrows)* needed for denture placement. In such cases it is necessary to push the tongue and glands aside with a finger so the tray can be placed in the mouth and an impression made and so the denture can subsequently be inserted. Usually also a reduction in lingual flange dimensions is necessary.

the place occupied by the denture. This problem must be recognized at the initial examination so adequate time can be scheduled to handle a difficult situation (Fig. 4-8).

A small tongue will cause difficulty for the person wearing a complete mandibular denture. Usually the small tongue will drop back away from the lower anterior teeth and thus break the border seal. Proper training can help patients to learn the proper location of the tongue for the best results. Time should be alloted for this training at each step of the construction procedure. If the training is to be effective, it must be done while the dentures are being made rather than after they are completed.

Saliva. The amount and consistency of saliva will affect the stability and retention of dentures and the comfort with which a patient can wear them.

Excessive saliva will complicate impression making and be an annoyance to the patient. This problem is usually much worse when dentures are new. The new dentures may feel like foreign objects and stimulate the flow of saliva. In time, the feeling and the flow of saliva will decrease. Patients need assurance about this.

A lack of saliva, xerostomia, presents some more serious problems. Moisture is necessary for the usual factors of retention to act, and if saliva is absent the possibility of reduced retention for dentures increases. Furthermore, the absence of saliva often causes the cheeks and lips to stick to the denture base in an uncomfortable manner. Petroleum jelly applied over the surface of the denture can alleviate the latter problem.

Saliva that is thick and ropy can cause problems. It is made up of heavy secretions of mucus from the palatal glands under the maxillary denture. The very thickness of the mucus is often sufficient to force the dentures out of their correct position. The thick saliva also complicates impression making by forming voids in the impression surface while the impression material sets. Thick ropy saliva is also a factor

in causing a patient to gag while impressions are made and after the placement of new dentures. The palatal surface should be wiped free of saliva and the mucous glands should be massaged with a piece of gauze just before the final impression is made to eliminate as much of the mucus as possible.

Ideally, there should be a moderate flow of serous-type saliva, which seems to be the situation most frequently found.

Cheeks and lips. The muscles in the cheeks and lips have a critical function in successful use of dentures. The denture flanges must be properly shaped so they can aid in maintaining the dentures in place without conscious effort on the part of the patient. This involves the development of the correct arch form and tooth positions as well as the shape of the polished surfaces and the thickness of the denture borders.

Patients with very thick cheeks may present severe technical problems during impression making and jaw relation recording. Thick cheeks often do not allow easy manipulations at the proper time for border molding of impression materials or for manipulation of the mandible into the desired position for certain jaw relation records.

Muscle tonus. The tone of the facial tissues is critical to several steps of denture construction. If the muscles are too tense, cheek and lip manipulations will be difficult; if too slack, the lips and cheeks may be easily displaced by the dentures. Either too firm or too weak a tissue tone is unfavorable, and this means that extra time will be needed to overcome the difficulties.

Muscular control. Good muscular control and coordination are essential to the effective wearing of complete dentures. For example, if tongue movements are used for border molding the lingual flanges of a mandibular impression, the timing, direction, and amount of movement are critical to the success of the molding. If the tongue movements are too slow, too fast, too little, too great, or in the wrong direction, the effort is wasted and more time will be required to complete the operation successfully.

To make an observation of muscular control, the dentist asks the patient to open about half way and then to put the tongue into the right cheek and into the left cheek, to stick it out, and to put it up and back inside the mouth. The ability, or lack of ability, to do these things on demand will be apparent, and the work schedule can be modified accordingly.

Jaw movements. The ability, or lack of ability, of a patient to move the mandible to the right place at the right time will reveal problems in making jaw relation records before they are attempted. If the patient cannot move the mandible as instructed, problems of recording jaw relations can be expected that could affect the scheduling of treatment appointments.

Temporomandibular joint problems. Patients presenting with one or more of the following symptoms are usually considered to be suffering from a TMJ disorder. The symptoms include (1) pain and tenderness in the region of the muscles of mastication and the temporomandibular joints, (2) sounds during condylar movements, and (3) limitations of mandibular movement. Quite logically, the temporomandibular joints should be healthy before new dentures are made. Unhealthy temporomandibular joints complicate the registration of jaw relation records and sometimes even preclude them completely. If it is to be a functional position, centric relation depends on the structural and functional harmony of osseous structures, the intraarticular tissue, and the capsular ligaments. If these specifications cannot be fulfilled, the patient will not have a centric relation or for that matter provide the dentist with a recordable one; hence the importance of the routine evaluation of a patient's TM function as an integral part of complete denture treatment. If symptoms are present, they must be treated. The treatment usually takes the form of a soft diet, improvement in fit and occlusion of the prosthesis, recovery of overt loss of vertical dimension of occlusion in the old prosthesis, and prescription of appropriate medication when necessary. Simple but accurate explanation of the dysfunction, its multifactorial etiology, and its consequences, treatment, and prognosis should also be provided for the patient. Furthermore, when there is reason to believe that organic joint pathosis exists, radiographs of the temporomandibular joints should be made.

Gagging. A patient's protective gag reflex can compromise a dental treatment plan if the reflex is an active one. The exaggerated gag reflex, though not common, can frustrate both patient and dentist. A thorough history and oral examination will reveal the presence of such a reflex early in the patient-dentist relationship. The dentist can then assess the possible cause of the problem as being attributable to iatrogenic factors, organic disturbances, anatomic anomalies, biomechanical inadequacies of existing prostheses, or psychologic factors. Effective management of the gagging problem tends to be based on experience and anecdote, with combinations of clinical techniques, prosthodontic management, medication, and psychologist referral being regarded as the most successful approaches. Usually reassurance and kind handling of the patient prove to be useful therapeutic adjuncts. However, patients who gag need the services of trained specialists, and the dentist should be vigilant about seeking help for these individuals.

DEVELOPMENT OF THE TREATMENT PLAN

After all the indicated observations have been made, it is time to develop the treatment plan and to inform the patient about it. The decisions are based on an analysis of the information collected during the diagnosis.

The dentist should review each item in relation to its effect on procedures that might be used and in relation to the amount of time the item will require during and after the treatment. The amount of time is important because it will determine the estimate of the cost of the treatment to the patient. In this regard, certain minimum costs to the dentist in time and money are unavoidable, and the unfavorable factors found in the examination will add to the dentist's costs.

Once the methods, procedures, materials, and time requirements are known, a fairly accurate estimate of the cost to the patient can be presented, but only after all these factors have been considered should the dentist discuss the proposed treatment or fees with the patient.

BIBLIOGRAPHY

Bolender CL, Swoope CC, Smith DE: The Cornell Medical Index as a prognostic aid for complete denture patients, J Prosthet Dent 22:20-29, 1969.

Conny DT, Tedesco LA: The gagging problem in prosthodontic treatment. I, Identification and causes; II, Patient management, J Prosthet Dent 49:601, 757, 1983.

Friedman N, Landesman HM, Wixler M: The influences of fear, anxiety, and depression on the patient's adaptive responses to complete dentures. I, J Prosthet Dent 58:687-689, 1986; II, J Prosthet Dent 59:45-48, 1988.

Gilboe DB: Centric relation as the treatment position, J Prosthet Dent 50:685, 1983.

Jones JD, Seals RR, Schelb E: Panoramic radiographic examination of the edentulous patient, J Prosthet Dent 53:535-539, 1985.

Keur JJ, Campbell JP, McCarthy JF, Ralph WJ: Radiological findings in 1135 endentulous patients, J Oral Rehabil 14:183-191, 1987.

Landt H: Oral recognition of forms and oral muscular coordination ability in dentulous subjects of various ages, Svensk Tandlak Tidskr 69(suppl 5), 1976.

Levitt EE: The psychology of anxiety, London, 1971, Paladin Books.

McGivney GP, Haughton V, Strandt JA, Eichholz JE, Lubar DM: A comparison of computer-assisted tomography and data-gathering modalities in prosthodontics, Int J Oral Maxillofac Implants 1:(1)55-68, 1986.

Nairn RI, Brunello DL: The relationship of denture complaints and the level of neuroticism, Dent Pract 21:156-157, 1971.

Smith JP: A survey of referred patients experiencing problems with complete dentures, J Prosthet Dent 60:583-586, 1988.

Wright SM: The radiographic examination of edentulous patients, J Prosthet Dent 50:164-166, 1983.

CHAPTER 5

Communicating with the patient

Successful management of an edentulous patient requires both the clear communication of any problems identified during the examination appointment and a careful explanation of how the problems will be managed. As described in Chapter 4, the examination appointment involves the gathering of information on (1) the current oral conditions and (2) the condition of the patient's present dentures. It is also essential that the patient be given an opportunity to openly discuss problems and concerns that he/she is experiencing. This information is recorded for future reference in developing the treatment plan and consultation report.

This chapter will focus on the following areas: nutrition care, identification and management of the patient with problems, use of a consultation report, and the economics of prosthodontic service.

NUTRITION CARE OF THE DENTURE PATIENT*

The enjoyment of food is regarded as an important determinant of the quality of life. Loose teeth, edentulousness, or ill-fitting dentures may preclude the consumption of favorite foods as well as limit the intake of essential nutrients. Conversely, the nutritional health of a denture patient affects the condition of the oral tissues and how well the patient adapts to a new prosthesis. A set of dentures may be well designed and constructed but may prove to be unsatisfactory in the mouth because of poor tissue response.

Clinical symptoms of malnutrition are often observed first in the oral cavity. Because of rapid cell turnover in the mouth, a regular and balanced intake of essential nutrients is required for the maintenance of the oral epithelium. The diet of the denture wearer frequently consists of soft foods. This diet limits the variety of foods eaten and increases the risk of not obtaining necessary amounts of specific nutrients. Long-term inadequate nutrition may be associated with angular cheilitis, glossitis, and slow tissue healing. Alveolar bone resorption following tooth extractions also may be influenced by low calcium and vitamin D intakes.

Nearly half of older individuals have clinically identifiable nutrition problems. Nutritional risk increases with advancing age; persons over 70 years tend to have poorer diets. Since the majority of edentulous adults are of advanced age, a large number of denture patients can be expected to have problems with nutrition. In addition to the condition of the dentition and dietary patterns, the nutritional status of a denture wearer is influenced by socioeconomic factors, the presence of degenerative diseases, medication regimens, and dietary supplementation practices (Fig. 5-1). An understanding of the nutritional requirements, eating problems of older adults, and symptoms of malnutrition will assist dentists in identifying those denture patients at risk of malnutrition. Dietary guidance based on assessment of the edentulous patient's nutrition history and diet should be an integral part of comprehensive prosthodontic treatment. Adequate nutritional status will improve the tolerance of the oral mucosa to new dentures and reduce rejection

---

*Mary P. Faine, BS, MS, RD.

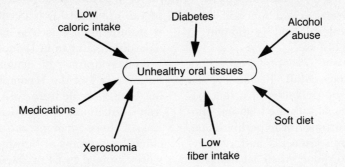

Fig. 5-1   Poor adaptation to new dentures, cracking at the corners of the lips, and persistent soreness of the tongue and oral mucosa may be related to a low intake of essential nutrients, reduced nutrient absorption, or altered nutrient metabolism because of medications or alcohol abuse.

of dentures. Since denture construction requires a series of appointments, dietary analysis and counseling can be easily incorporated into the treatment sequence.

Nutritional needs and status of the elderly

The nutrient needs of older persons are determined by their rate of aging, health status, and level of physical activity. Thus it is difficult to generalize about energy, vitamin, and mineral requirements appropriate for all older adults. Depending on level of body functioning, an individual may need greater or lesser amounts of nutrients than the Recommended Dietary Allowance (RDA) for his chronologic age.

Because of a reduction in basal metabolism and physical activity, energy needs decline with age. With aging, lean body mass is replaced by fat; this leads to a decrease in metabolic rate. The onset of chronic disease usually induces a decline in physical activity. Cross-sectional surveys show that the average energy consumption of 65-year-old women is about 1300 to 1400 kilocalories and 1800 kilocalories for men. This is lower than the mean RDA (1600 Kcal for women, 2400 Kcal for men) but may be appropriate if body weight is being maintained. When caloric intake is low, foods of high nutrient density (such as vegetable soups, fruit desserts, dairy foods, and whole-grain breads and cereals) must be consumed. Obesity results when caloric intake is not reduced to balance energy expended. Maintaining ideal body weight is especially important for older individuals with diabetes, hyperlipidemia, hypertension, arthritis, or gout. Weight control is the primary therapy for these chronic conditions.

The best means of reducing caloric intake is to replace foods high in fat with complex carbohydrates. In fact, complex carbohydrates should be the mainstay of the elderly person's diet. In contrast to pastries, luncheon meats, salad dressings, and frozen desserts that are high in fat, whole-grain breads, cereals, pasta, fruits, vegetables, beans, and legumes contain little fat and are important sources of vitamins, minerals, and fiber. Denture patients who select soft foods (such as pastries, cakes, and cookies, which are high in simple sugars and fat) should be advised of the superiority of complex carbohydrates. There are two reasons for this recommendation: (1) Blood glucose levels are often elevated in older people, and complex carbohydrates cause less rise in these levels than simple sugars do. (2) An important component of complex carbohydrates is fiber, which promotes normal bowel function, may reduce serum cholesterol, and is thought to prevent diverticular disease.

Fats contribute about 37% of total calories in the diet of the average adult. Because of the growing epidemiologic evidence of a link between dietary intakes of saturated fat and cholesterol and the occurrence of hyperlipidemia, heart disease, certain cancers, and obesity, adults are advised to reduce their fat intake to 30% of total calories. Fats vary in degree of saturation. The American Heart Association recommends dividing fat intake equally among saturated (10%), monounsaturated (10%), and polyunsaturated (10%) fats. Animal fats are highly saturated, and most liquid oils of vegetable origin are highly polyunsaturated.

Because physiologic stresses are associated with age-related degenerative diseases, protein needs of older adults are thought to be slightly higher than for younger persons. It is recommended that 12% to 14% of total calories or 1 gm/kg of body weight come from protein. Surveys show that protein intake declines with age, but a protein deficiency seems unlikely among healthy elderly persons in Western countries. This conclusion is based on studies of serum albumin levels and nitrogen balance studies in older adults. The protein intake of denture wearers is lower than that of dentate adults, but above the 1980 RDA.

Currently vitamin requirements for elderly persons are being established. Vitamin deficiencies in the elderly are apt to be subclinical, but any body stress may result in an individual's developing detectable symptoms. Individuals who have low caloric intake, ingest multiple drugs, or have disease states that cause malabsorption are at greatest risk of hypovitaminosis. Low intakes of vitamin D, vitamin B_6, and folic acid are most often reported.

Vitamin D deficiency may occur in elderly persons who are housebound and receive minimal exposure to sunlight. Because of the importance of vitamin D in calcium metabolism, adequate intake is crucial. The primary dietary source of vitamin D is fortified dairy products. If an individual is lactose intolerant and avoids dairy foods, a vitamin D supplement is needed.

Oral symptoms of malnutrition are usually due to a lack of the B complex vitamins. Burning tongue or denture sore mouth may result from nutritional deficiencies, especially the lack of these vitamins and iron. In one study clinical symptoms of burning mouth syndrome were resolved in 24 of 28 patients with proved vitamin deficiency when vitamin B complex supplementation was given. Pyridoxine and folic acid play an important role in red blood cell formation, and anemia results from long-term inadequate intake of vitamin B_{12}. Many drugs and alcohol negatively affect pyridoxine and folic acid absorption and metabolism. Individuals with a marginal intake of folic acid and under chronic drug therapy are at greatest risk of developing a deficient state. Pyridoxine is found in whole grain breads and cereals and animal products. Oranges, dark green leafy vegetables, and asparagus are good sources of folic acid.

Anemia and neurologic damage can be due to vitamin B_{12} deficiency. Pernicious anemia, resulting from a lack of gastric intrinsic factor, leads to vitamin B_{12} deficiency. Achlorhydria, common in the elderly, also results in decreased B_{12} absorption. Vitamin B_{12} is found only in animal products but also is synthesized by gut bacteria.

Although vitamin C intakes in elderly people are generally high, low plasma levels of ascorbic acid have been reported. Heavy smokers, alcohol abusers, or persons with high aspirin intake have a higher daily requirement for vitamin C. The denture patient should be encouraged to have a vitamin C–rich food (such as citrus fruits, berries, melons, tomatoes, broccoli, or peppers) daily.

Two minerals, calcium and zinc, are of particular concern in older adults. (Calcium is discussed under its own heading.) Mild zinc deficiency is suspected to occur among some U.S. elderly, with reported intakes below the RDA and serum levels lower than in younger adults. Tissue healing and immune function are affected by zinc status. Good sources of bioavailable zinc are animal products.

Iron needs of women decline at menopause. Iron deficiency is uncommon among U.S. elderly, except in individuals who have diseases that cause blood loss (such as ulcers). A high intake of aspirin can lead to gastric bleeding.

Alcohol abuse is a serious health problem among some U.S. elderly. Although the actual incidence is unknown, estimates are that 5% to 10% of persons over 60 may be heavy drinkers. Most often, alcoholism is undetected and untreated. Loneliness, depression, retirement, loss of status, and reduced income all contribute to excess alcohol intake by older adults. In the United States, alcoholism is the single most important cause of malnutrition among adults. Substitution of alcoholic drinks, which contain no nutrients, for food usually results in multiple nutrient deficits. Deficiencies of thiamine, niacin, pyridoxine, and folate (all B complex vitamins) and of ascorbic acid are commonly seen in alcoholics. Osteopenia in males without a history of bone disease may be due to chronic alcohol intake. When all efforts to resolve tissue intolerance of a prosthesis are unsuccessful, the possibility of misuse of alcohol should be considered.

Impact of wearing dentures on dietary intake

Nutrient intake of older adults is closely linked to dental status and masticatory efficiency. Although an intact dentition is not a prerequisite for maintaining nutritional health, the loss of teeth in adults often leads to selecting softer diets that are lower in nutrient density. Recently investigators in Sweden and the United States have found that adults with compromised dentition are overrepresented in groups with poor-quality diets.

A large number of healthy denture wearers were among the elderly persons surveyed by researchers at the USDA Human Nutrition Research Center on Aging in Boston. Nutrient intakes of denture wearers were lower than those of dentate subjects, and male denture wearers had poorer intakes than did female. Specifically, mean intakes of calories, protein, vitamin A, ascorbic acid, pyroxidine, and folic acid were lower among male denture wearers than among dentate men, and calcium and protein intakes among female denture wearers were inferior to those among dentate women.

Similar findings have been reported in a study of institutionalized elderly. A significant association was found between denture wearing and low protein intakes: Women denture wearers had lower vitamin A, pyridoxine, folate, and vitamin B_{12} intakes, and men with complete dentures had lower calorie, protein, and calcium intakes, than did adults with a natural dentition.

Earlier studies had shown no association between dental status and nutrient intake. These contradictory findings may have been due to the fact that sample size was too small, detailed diet analysis was not done, or the effects of socioeconomic status and physical or psychologic impairment were not compensated in the earlier studies. Although biochemical tests have been used to validate dietary histories and detect subclinical malnutrition, measurement of nutrient levels in body tissues of denture wearers to verify nutritional status has not been reported.

An individual's masticatory ability is determined by age and the number of natural teeth in the mouth. There is general agreement that masticatory function of denture wearers is greatly inferior to that of persons with an intact dentition. Although a great deal of individual variation exists, the chewing efficiency of the average denture wearer is about 20% that of an adult with a complete natural dentition. Denture wearers must complete a greater number of chewing strokes before reaching the swallowing threshold. Even with additional chewing, the average denture wearer cannot reduce foods to as small a particle size as a person with natural teeth can. The chewing ability of individuals with a complete denture in only one arch against a natural dentition appears to be reduced to nearly the same extent as in persons with a complete denture in both arches.

The purpose of mastication is to reduce food particles to a size that can be swallowed and to increase the surface of food exposed to digestive juices and enzymes. Individuals with poor masticatory ability often swallow larger pieces of food. Thus there is a risk of choking on improperly masticated food. It has been shown that gastric distress and use of laxatives were reduced when ill-fitting dentures were replaced with new dentures having good retention and balanced occlusion.

Because of impaired chewing ability, texture and hardness rather than taste and smell are what determine the acceptability of a food for many denture patients. Generally the intake of harder foods (such as raw vegetables or fruits, fibrous meats, hard breads, seeds, and nuts) is reduced while that of soft foods (ground beef, soft breads, cereals, and pastries, and canned fruits and vegetables) is increased. Whether these changes negatively affect nutritional status depends on the nutrient density of the foods substituted. (For instance, replacing steak with ground beef provides similar nutrients, but substituting applesauce for a green salad results in lower nutrient intake.)

Studies in Finland have shown that the insertion of dentures in persons who had had no teeth for several years improved the quality of their diets. Fruit, raw vegetables, bread, cheese, and meat were eaten more frequently after denture placement. The condition of a person's dentures also may influence food selection. When new complete dentures replace old ones with poor retention, patients report that masticating performance improves; they can chew better and chew different foods.*

Inability to distinguish the sensory qualities of food reduces a person's enjoyment of eating and may lead to a reduced caloric intake. A decrease in taste and smell acuity is part of aging; therefore it is difficult to separate the effects of aging and of denture wearing on sensory acuity. Nearly all denture patients report a decline in taste acuity when dentures are first inserted. This is attributed to covering the hard palatal area. However, the condition is usually temporary and for most persons the ability to taste returns a few months after denture insertion. When compared to dentate adults or partial denture wearers, however, complete denture wearers have lower perceptions of the acceptability of taste and texture and a lower perceived ease of chewing.

Calcium and bone health

Bone loss, a normal part of aging, affects the maxilla and mandible as well as the spine and long bones. Several factors are thought to contribute to age-related bone loss that leads to osteoporosis: genetics, hormonal status, bone density at maturity, a disturbance in the bone remodeling process, a low exercise level, loss of teeth, and inadequate nutrition. Because of the loss of estrogen at menopause and a smaller skeleton, osteopenia affects women earlier than men. Bone loss begins at about 35 years of age or whenever estrogen secretion ceases. Skeletal sites where trabecular bone is more prominent than cortical bone are affected first. With extensive loss of mineral content, sites that are primarily trabecular bone (vertebrae, wrist, and neck of the femur) become so weak that they fracture. The diagnosis of osteoporosis is usually not made until a fracture has occurred.

Dietary calcium intake is critical to maintaining the body skeleton. The most important means of preventing metabolic bone disease is acquiring a dense skeleton by the time of maturation. Calcium accumulation in bone occurs until about 30 to 35 years of age. Adequate calcium intake during the teenage and early adult years will result in a high peak bone mass for

---

*In the study by Gunne and Wall (1985), however, nutrient intake was not improved.

women. A woman who has a dense skeleton at 35 years will retain proportionately more skeletal mineral content and be less susceptible to fracture after menopause. Estrogen replacement therapy is thought to be the primary means of limiting bone loss after menopause.

With aging the alveolar bone, which is primarily trabecular, undergoes irreversible loss of mineral. It has been proposed that alveolar bone loss may precede loss of mineral from the vertebrae and long bones. The dentist may be the first health care provider to detect loss of bone mass. The amount of bone found in the mandible correlates with total body calcium and the bone mass of the vertebrae and wrist of postmenopausal women. Osteoporotic women tend to retain less alveolar bone than healthy women.

Resorption of the alveolar ridge is a widespread problem among denture patients and results in unstable dentures. A greater reduction in ridge height occurs among women than among men. Bone loss is accelerated in the first 6 months following tooth extractions, with resorption much greater in the mandible than in the maxilla. The loss of alveolar bone makes it difficult to construct a mandibular denture that has good stability and retention.

Experimental data concerning the relationship of calcium deficiency to alveolar bone health are limited. Investigations have been hampered because there has been no reliable method of quantifying small changes in mandibular bone mass. Still, it has been found that mandibular bone resorption in animals fed a low-calcium high-protein diet is significantly greater than in animals receiving the opposite diet. Denture patients with excessive ridge resorption report lower calcium intakes and poorer calcium/phosphorus ratios than do other edentulous subjects. It also has been suggested that calcium and vitamin D supplementation significantly reduce alveolar ridge resorption following tooth extractions and placement of immediate dentures. Although a generous calcium intake by older adults will not result in

restoration of bone mass, it may slow the rate of bone loss.

After age 35, about 75% of U.S. women have inadequate calcium intakes. A chronically low intake of calcium results in negative calcium balance. To maintain serum calcium levels, calcium is mobilized from the bones, and this leads to demineralization of the skeleton. Thus a negative calcium balance produces a negative bone calcium balance. A high calcium intake can reverse the situation.

The importance of a high calcium intake throughout life was clearly demonstrated in a study of women living in different regions of Yugoslavia. Women from the region where calcium intake was traditionally high had denser bones and fewer fractures than did women living in an area where mean dietary calcium intakes were low.

Other foods and nutrients also affect calcium balance. Adequate vitamin D intake is important for calcium absorption in the intestine. Serum levels of vitamin D decline with age because intakes are lower and the rate of conversion to the active metabolite in the liver and kidney takes place more slowly. Vitamin D–fortified milk and formation of the vitamin in the skin are the primary means of obtaining vitamin D. If adults expose their arms and face to sunlight for 10 to 15 minutes two or three times a week, adequate vitamin D is synthesized in the skin. Because vitamin D is a fat-soluble vitamin, caution must be exercised in recommending a supplement. Intakes should not exceed 1000 IU per day.

It has been proposed that a high phosphorus intake negatively affects calcium balance. However, human studies show that neither a high phosphorus intake nor the dietary Ca/P ratio has much effect on calcium balance. The trace element fluoride, being used in the treatment of osteoporosis, can reduce urinary losses of calcium and increase spinal bone mass. However, adverse side effects to high fluoride doses (nausea, vomiting, stomach irritation, and joint pain) have limited its use. The status of the alveolar bone in persons living in fluoridated communities has not been determined. Phytates and fiber found in whole grain products may form insoluble complexes with calcium; therefore, high intake of unrefined cereals may bind calcium from other sources eaten at the same meal, thus reducing calcium availability. High intakes of caffeine and alcohol increase calcium losses in the urine.

About three fourths of the calcium in American diets is obtained from dairy foods. Major sources are milk, cheese, yogurt, and ice cream. Dairy foods are also a source of protein, riboflavin, vitamin A, and vitamin D. Collard greens, broccoli, oysters, canned salmon, sardines, and tofu made with a calcium coagulant are nondairy foods containing substantial amounts of calcium.

The recommended dietary calcium intake for adults is 800 mg. However, this is probably inadequate for adult women. Both aging and menopause lead to reduced calcium absorption and less body adaptation to changes in dietary content. At a Consensus Development Conference on Osteoporosis sponsored by the National Institutes of Health in 1984, researchers proposed that women need to increase their calcium intakes to prevent osteoporosis. The recommended intake for premenopausal women and postmenopausal women receiving estrogen replacement therapy is 1000 mg of calcium. For postmenopausal women taking no estrogen, 1500 mg of calcium is recommended. This far exceeds the usual dietary calcium intake of American women, which is only 450 to 550 mg/day.

To receive 1000 to 1500 mg of calcium, women must drink three or four glasses of milk per day, eat 5 to 7 ounces of hard cheeses, or consume large quantities of nondairy foods. Lactose-intolerant adults who avoid milk may find yogurt or cheese acceptable. This amount of dairy foods represents a significant number of calories. Women with low caloric intakes should be encouraged to obtain at least half their calcium needs from food sources and the balance from calcium tablets.

For women who consume minimal amounts of dairy products, calcium supplementation may be appropriate. Supplements are easy to take and inexpensive, and they have few side effects. The most common are calcium carbonate, calcium citrate, calcium lactate, calcium gluconate, and calcium diphosphate. Body absorption of these salts seems to be similar. The most practical supplement to prescribe is calcium carbonate because it contains the highest concentration of elemental calcium—40%. Calcium supplements that contain vitamin D to enhance absorption of calcium in the gut are useful if vitamin D is not obtained from other sources. A dosage of 1000 mg of calcium carbonate spaced over the day is commonly prescribed. Five 500 mg tablets of $CaCO_3$ will provide 1000 mg of calcium. Bone meal and dolomite calcium supplements should be avoided because they may be contaminated with heavy metals (lead or mercury).

Few adverse affects of calcium supplementation have been observed. Some older women have reported nausea, bloating, or constipation. Increasing calcium intake results in higher urinary levels of calcium. A small percentage of the population, mainly men, is susceptible to forming kidney stones. Calcium supplements should be used under a physician's supervision by these persons.

Vitamin supplementation

The use of vitamin and mineral supplements is widespread among Americans, especially the elderly. In fact, nutrient supplements are the most common nonprescription pharmaceuticals used in the United States. The reported prevalence of nutritional supplement use by healthy older adults ranges from 30% to 70%. Many reasons are reported for using vitamin-mineral supplements to increase energy level, to extend life, to prevent the onset of degenerative diseases, to relieve the symptoms of chronic diseases, and to make up deficits caused by unbalanced diets. Most elderly people are interested in a means of maintaining or enhancing health, and a large percentage of the supplements ingested are self-prescribed and unrelated to any particular physiologic need. Family, friends, self-help books, health magazines, and health professionals all influence individuals to take nutritional supplements. There is concern among nutritionists as to the appropriateness and potential toxicity of these pills. Self-medication by individuals may lead to a delay in seeking diagnosis and treatment for a curable condition.

On the basis of current knowledge, the best way to achieve a well-nourished state is to eat a variety of foods, which will contain the macronutrients (fiber, complex carbohydrate, protein, and essential fatty acids) and micronutrients essential to health. Use of supplements, which contain no energy and only a few micronutrients, may foster a false sense of security in the prosthodontic patient.

The only time a nutrient supplement is useful is when there is a vitamin or mineral deficiency state. The best means of determining whether a nutrient deficiency exists is to do a biochemical test. Iron status is routinely monitored by blood analysis. Vitamin nutriture is best assessed by measuring the concentration of the vitamin or metabolites of the vitamin in different body fluids or measuring enzyme activity. For instance, vitamin C nutriture is determined by measuring leukocyte content of ascorbic acid. This is not a routine procedure in the medical clinic. If clinical signs of malnutrition are detected in the oral tissues of denture patients, referral to a physician for definitive diagnosis should occur (Table 5-1). However, it may be reasonable to prescribe a low dose multivitamin-mineral tablet for certain denture patients even if clinical signs are not present. Persons at greater risk of the development of malnutrition include those consuming less than 1200 Kcal per day and those eating an unbalanced diet that lacks fruits, vegetables, or protein foods. Low income or physical disabilities that hinder mobility may limit a person's access to food. Vitamin and mineral bioavailability in adults is also affected by preexisting disease, medications, fiber intake, emotional status, and

Table 5-1 Possible oral signs of nutrient deficiencies

Oral symptom	Nutrient deficiency
Decreased salivary flow	Protein
Enlarged parotid glands	Protein
Lips:	
Cheilosis	Vitamin B complex*
Angular stomatitis	Vitamin B complex*, Iron
Angular scars	Vitamin B complex*, Iron
Tongue:	
Edema	Vitamin B complex*
Magenta tongue	Vitamin B complex*
Atrophy of filiform papillae	Vitamin B complex*, Iron
Glossitis	Vitamin B complex*, Iron Tryptophan
Gingiva:	
Tender, Edematous	Vitamin C
Bleeding	Vitamin C

*Includes thiamine, riboflavin, niacin, pyridoxine, folic acid, and vitamin B_{12}.

environmental stress. The heavy smoker has increased vitamin C needs. A person ingesting aspirin several times a day may need more iron, vitamin C, and folic acid. Individuals taking corticosteroids have increased calcium needs.

The older adult often selects a pill that does not include the nutrients most likely to be missing in his diet. Vitamin C and vitamin E are the supplements most frequently used by the elderly. Regular use of iron and vitamin B_{12} supplements is also reported. Inadequate dietary intake of these nutrients is uncommon, and thus supplementation is unnecessary. In contrast, low intakes of calcium, zinc, vitamin B_6, and folacin are reported among the elderly and thus a multivitamin-mineral supplement containing these nutrients may be justified.

To assure that nutrients are present in the proper ratio, a multivitamin-mineral supplement is preferable to tablets containing a single nutrient. For patients at risk of nutritional deficits, the American Medical Association (1987) recommends a multivitamin-mineral supplement that contains 50% to 150% of the U.S. Recommended Dietary Allowance. For prosthodontic patients a generic one-a-day tablet that includes zinc, folacin, and vitamin B_6 may be recommended. If intake of dairy foods cannot be increased to meet daily needs, a calcium supplement is advised; but, because it is bulky, calcium must be taken in a separate tablet.

The use of megadoses of vitamins or minerals by the elderly is a practice of great concern. When a high dose of a vitamin is taken, it no longer functions as a vitamin but becomes a chemical with pharmacologic activity. However, the elderly person may not consider vitamins and minerals drugs. Vitamins and minerals ingested in large doses have been popularized by salespeople, health promoters, or other public figures; but adverse reactions from such megadoses of nutrients are likely, despite the lack of studies on nutrient toxicity in the elderly. Also older adults metabolize drugs less efficiently and excrete them more slowly.

High doses of any nutrient are potentially toxic; but because the fat-soluble vitamins (A, D, E, and K) are stored in the body, they are considered toxic at lower levels of intake.

Vitamin D is toxic at the lowest doses. Women taking a multivitamin with vitamin D or a calcium supplement with vitamin D may exceed the maximum safe intake of the vitamin, 1000 IU. Megadoses of vitamin D can induce a disturbance in calcium metabolism leading to calcification of soft tissues. Vitamin A, the second most commonly ingested nutrient supplement, is often reported toxic. Long-term ingestion of vitamin A supplements containing 5 to 25 times the RDA have resulted in skin and bone disorders and disturbances in blood clotting.

Although water-soluble vitamins are considered nontoxic, well-documented toxicity syndromes have been associated with megadoses of niacin, vitamin B_6, and ascorbic acid.

Chronic intake of vitamin C megadoses can induce a copper deficiency anemia, cause false-positive readings for glucose in the urine, and increase the risk of urinary stone formation in susceptible individuals. Rebound scurvy may occur if high doses are stopped abruptly. Peripheral neuropathies have resulted from high vitamin B_6 intakes.

Zinc supplementation can reduce iron absorption and availability. A high fiber intake may bind calcium, zinc, and iron. Thus the denture patient should be cautioned against indiscriminate use of megadoses of any nutrient or fiber.

Nutrition counseling

One expectation of persons seeking new dentures is that they will be able to eat a greater variety of foods. Thus denture patients are often receptive to suggestions aimed at improving the quality of their diets. However, a single structured nutritional interview is not apt to result in much behavior change. Nutrition care must begin at the first appointment so counseling and follow-up can occur during the course of treatment. With continued guidance and encouragement from the dental team, patients are more apt to make permanent changes in their food patterns. Nutrition care can be provided by the dentist and dental hygienist, who have backgrounds in basic nutrition. Costs of nutrition care should be built into the fee for the denture.

The main objective of diet counseling for prosthodontic patients is to correct imbalances in nutrient intake that may interfere with maintenance of the oral tissues. It is often difficult to identify patients in need of nutritional care based on a visual inspection or an interview. Most will tell the dentist that they eat a balanced diet. In the United States clinical signs of malnutrition are not seen very often. However, certain denture patients are known to be at greater risk of being malnourished. Dietary evaluation and counseling should be included in treatment if patients have any of the following risk factors: greater than 75 years of age, low income, physical isolation (living alone), oral lesions (glossitis, cheilosis, denture sore mouth), significant bone resorption, daily use of more than three prescription drugs, disease of the joints that limits movement, use of high doses of dietary supplements, ingestion of an unbalanced diet, adherence to a fad diet.

The dentist is expected not to diagnose specific nutrient deficiencies but to determine the general adequacy of the diet. If the patient reports a recent weight loss of greater than 10 pounds or an untreated or poorly controlled hypertensive or diabetic state, or presents with oral tissue changes suggestive of malnutrition, referral to a physician should be made. Patients who express concern about obesity or low body weight or who report poor adherence to a diabetic, reduced-sodium, or low-cholesterol diet can be referred to a consulting registered dietitian.

Providing nutrition care for the denture patient entails the following steps:

Obtaining a nutrition history and an accurate record of food intake over a 3-, 4-, or 5-day period
Evaluating the diet
Teaching about the components of a diet that will support the oral mucosa as well as bone health and total body health
Guidance in the establishment of goals to improve the diet
Follow-up

To learn about a patient's food intake, one needs a nutrition history and food diary (Fig. 5-2). Dietary questions can be incorporated into

---

DEPARTMENT OF PROSTHODONTICS
NUTRITION HISTORY

Name: _____ Date: _____
Age: _____ Height: _____ Weight: _____ Desirable Weight: _____

Food Habits:

1. Do you consider your appetite to be: Good _____ Fair _____ Poor _____
2. How many meals do you eat each day? _____
   When are your meals eaten? _____
   Where are most meals eaten? _____
3. Do you eat alone? _____ , with family _____ , with friends _____
4. Do you usually snack between meals?   Everyday _____ Seldom _____ Never _____
   What time of day? _____ List: _____
5. Do you use gum, mints, cough drops? _____
   What kind? _____
6. How much sugar do you add to coffee or tea? _____
   What other beverages do you like? _____
7. Are you on a special diet?   Yes _____ No _____
   If yes, what kind? _____
   Who recommended the diet? _____
8. Are there any foods you cannot eat?   Yes _____ No _____
   List: _____
9. What kind of medication, food supplements, or vitamin-mineral pills do you use, if any?
   [   ] Medications: _____

   [   ] Vitamins, minerals, other supplements: _____

   [   ] Antacids, laxatives, others: _____
10. Does your mouth get dry?   Yes _____ No _____ When: _____
    What do you eat or drink to moisten your mouth? _____

Fig. 5-2 A nutrition history questionnaire that could be completed by the patient at the time the health history is obtained.

DIET EVALUATION SUMMARY   ID no._____

Food groups	Portion size/serving	1st day	2nd day	3rd day	4th day	5th day	Recommended 5-day total	5 day total	Difference
Milk group (milk, cheese)	2 cups ice cream 8 oz milk 1 1/2 oz cheddar cheese 1 1/2 slices American cheese 1 1/2 cup cottage cheese						10 15* 20†		
Meat group (meat, fish, poultry, egg, dried peas or beans)	2-3 oz cooked lean meat, fish poultry 2 eggs 4 Tbsp peanut butter 1 cup cooked dry beans or lentils						10		
Vegetable/fruit group	1 orange 1/2 med grapefruit 4 oz (1/2 cup) fruit juice						5		
Vitamin A	1/2 cup cooked dark green or yellow vegetable fruit						3		
Other	1 med apple, pear, banana 1/2 cup cooked peas, beans, corn						12		
Bread/cereal group	1 pancake 1 slice bread 3/4 cup dry cereal 1/2 cup cooked cereal, rice, noodles, macaroni						20		

*Women 20-50 yr   †Women after menopause

Fig. 5-3 Form for evaluating a 5-day food diary submitted by the patient. The average number of servings per day of each food group is compared to the recommended daily intake.

the medical history form or in a separate nutrition questionnaire administered at the first appointment. Any patient reporting nutritional risk factors is then instructed to prepare a food record. The dental counselor records the past 24 hours' food intake on the record. The patient is instructed to record 2 or more days, which should include a weekend day, at home. The purpose of diet counseling must be clearly understood. Cooperation can be gained by advising the patient that dietary habits influence how well the oral tissues will adjust to the new denture. The food record is returned by mail or brought to the next appointment.

When the food diary is received, the quality of a patient's diet is assessed by classifying reported foods into the four basic groups and comparing the total reported servings to the recommended number of the four groups (Fig. 5-3). Recommendations are two or more servings each from the dairy* and meat groups and four servings each from the fruit-vegetable and bread-cereal groups. Within the fruit and vegetable group, one serving of a citrus fruit is needed daily and one serving of a vitamin A rich food (such as deep yellow or dark green fruits and vegetables) should be included every other day. The 2-2-4-4 food group plan will provide about 1200 Kcal. Servings of processed foods high in sodium and fat should be noted. After informing patients of food group deficiencies and excess high salt and high fat foods in their diets, ask them to propose more desirable foods that can be substituted. Fish, ground meat, poultry, peanut butter, and soups or casseroles made with beans or legumes are high quality sources of protein.

If a detailed food record is obtained, nutrient analysis can be accomplished on a computer. Numerous software programs are available for dietary analyses.

At the second appointment the relationship of diet to the health of the oral tissues and evaluation of the patient's diet can be discussed. This will take 30 to 45 minutes. Nontechnical terms should be used when teaching about the diet–oral health relationship. Two concepts are to be stressed: First, the epithelial cells in the mouth have a rapid turnover. Cells lining the gingival sulcus are renewed every 3 to 7 days; therefore a constant supply of nutrients used in cell synthesis (protein, vitamin A, vitamin C, and vitamin B_6) must be present. Second, the health of the mandible and maxillae is dependent on a constant supply of calcium and vitamin D. Lack of calcium may accelerate bone resorption. The patient's own radiograph can be used to illustrate the amount of bone remaining in the mandible. This is usually enlightening for patients because they have probably not considered the systemic role of nutrients in maintaining the oral tissues.

When discussing the quality of a patient's diet, always begin by pointing out positive aspects. Identify which food group quotas are being met. If the diet is generally poor, focus on one or two of the most critical deficiencies. Low intakes of calories, protein, or calcium or the excessive use of fat-soluble vitamin supplements would be of primary concern. Do not overwhelm the patient with information or alarm him by presenting a long list of dietary weaknesses. Older denture patients are often sensitive to possible threats to their health and may feel disconcerted. If serious dietary problems are detected, referral to a physician or registered dietitian is advisable.

Nutrition goals for the denture patient are to eat a variety of foods, including protein sources, dairy foods, and complex carbohydrates and to limit the intake of salt, fat, and sugar (Table 5-2). The dentist can suggest desirable nutrient-dense foods to improve the diet, but the patient must establish his own dietary goals. Ask the patient to describe what foods he can add or substitute in his diet to im-

---

*Three servings of dairy foods for premenopausal women or estrogen-treated women and four servings for postmenopausal women who are not taking estrogen will fulfill the recommendations of the NIH Consensus Development Conference on Osteoporosis.

Table 5-2 Guidelines for nutrition counseling

1. Eat a variety of foods
2. Build diet around complex carbohydrates—fruits, vegetables, whole-grain breads and cereals
3. Include citrus fruit or juice containing vitamin C everyday
4. Select fish, poultry, lean meat, or dried peas and beans everyday
5. Obtain adequate calcium
6. Limit intake of bakery products high in fat and simple sugars
7. Limit intake of processed foods high in sodium and fat
8. Consume eight glasses of water daily

prove the nutritional balance. Small changes that are possible within the patient's budget and respect for food preferences are more likely to be accepted. When it is determined what food changes can be made to improve the patient's diet, write these down on a diet prescription that the patient can take home (Fig. 5-4). The results of the diet assessment and the diet prescription should also be recorded in the patient's dental chart so all members of the dental team can reinforce the dentist's goals.

Compliance with dietary advice is more likely if follow-up is provided. Patients need a trial period to try new foods and eating patterns. Dietary progress should be discussed at

Diet prescription

NAME: DATE:

ANALYSIS OF YOUR DIET:

TO IMPROVE YOUR DIET:

Drink plenty of fluids (8 glasses each day)

Try: fruit juices   cocoa
           milk shakes   soups
           frappes   water
           egg nog   milk
           chocolate milk   buttermilk

Fig. 5-4 A diet prescription form.

future appointments. Roadblocks to modifying a diet can be identified and addressed. Progress may be slow, but modest dietary changes should be praised. Small steps are more likely to result in permanent dietary improvement.

Conclusions

Denture wearers represent a segment of the older population especially vulnerable to poor nutritional health. Nutritional deficiencies may result from a combination of low caloric intake, poor masticatory efficiency, and the presence of chronic disease, economic hardship, and psychologic problems. The ability of the oral tissues to withstand the stress of dentures is greater if the patient is well nourished. Dietary assessment must be an integral part of treatment for the denture patient.

Early in treatment the dentist can assess the general adequacy of the diet and address major deficiencies. An older person will probably not make sweeping dietary changes but may add nutritionally important foods if the need is clearly explained. If dietary improvement is to occur, the patient must participate in developing nutrition goals.

Community-based nutrition programs for the elderly include food stamps, home-delivered meals, and congregate meals. Nutrition education as well as food is provided. These services can have a significant impact on the nutrient intake and nutritional status of participating older adults, and dental providers can refer patients to them.

• • •

IDENTIFICATION AND MANAGEMENT OF THE PATIENT WITH PROBLEMS

Years of clinical experience have provided insight into common characteristics of patients who have a high potential for encountering difficulty adjusting to new dentures or for presenting management problems. Some of these characteristics will be described in the hope that the reader can avoid unpleasant experiences associated with trial and error learning. It is hoped that the reader will return to this chapter if a major problem is encountered to determine whether sufficient warning signs were present to have prevented the unhappy encounter.

In dealing with difficult denture patients, a better than 50% chance of success should exist before the dentist begins to make new dentures. When there are many indications that success cannot be achieved, the facts must be clearly explained to the patient. This will occasionally cause a patient to become angry and storm out of the dental office, but facing reality and discussing honestly the chances for success will prove to be the best approach. If the prognosis is poor, a general dentist should seriously consider referring the high-risk patient to a prosthodontist.

BASIC RULES TO FOLLOW TO AVOID PROBLEMS

Always conduct a comprehensive examination

The first step in avoiding problems is always to conduct a comprehensive examination of *every* patient who is treated. Every area on the examination forms discussed in Chapter 4 must be carefully evaluated. Occasionally, a patient will demand that definitive treatment begin immediately, for a variety of reasons—pain, expiring dental insurance benefits, or impending social engagements. Usually this type of patient has been squeezed into an already busy schedule, which does not allow sufficient time for a comprehensive examination. The tendency is to respond to the patient's urgent request to proceed rapidly with treatment, failing to follow the established office procedure. Emergency types of treatment can usually relieve the primary problem (a temporary restoration, tooth extraction, replacement of a missing or fractured tooth in the denture, or a temporary reline). Yielding to the patient's demands to proceed with definitive care prematurely can force you into decisions that you later regret.

Make no final recommendation at the examination appointment

The purpose of the examination appointment is to gather information. It is essential that a follow-up consultation appointment be made so you will have some time for thinking after evaluating the examination data. To determine whether the patient is interested and able to proceed, it is acceptable and even advisable to give general fee estimates for general treatment possibilities. However, the final treatment plan and exact fees should not be presented at the initial examination but should be given at the consultation appointment, preferably in a written consultation report.

Complete all indicated correctional procedures prior to making dentures

It is essential that you carefully plan what will be necessary to achieve success. This includes such items as corrective surgery, elimination of inflammation, or correction of a poor diet. If the patient refuses to accept the recommended procedures, you must decide whether treatment can still be successful with these limitations. This is the crucial time to establish who is in control of the situation. If you decide to yield to the patient's desires, it is essential to place a statement, signed by the patient, in the chart indicating that the patient assumes full responsibility for any adverse effects resulting from failure to accept the procedure recommended.

PATIENT BEHAVIOR CHARACTERISTICS OBSERVED DURING THE EXAMINATION APPOINTMENT THAT MAY INDICATE FUTURE MANAGEMENT PROBLEMS*

Disrupting your regular office routine

The patient may refuse to complete the office registration form or a medical history questionnaire, which are normal parts of the new patient evaluation.

---

*Any given patient may exhibit one of these characteristics and still have a favorable prognosis. However, if several are manifested, it may be better not to proceed with treatment.

The patient may talk continuously and make it impossible to conduct the examination in an efficient and orderly manner.

The patient may be available only at specific times that are not compatible with your scheduling policy.

The patient may not leave the office at the conclusion of the appointment but continue to talk with the receptionist after it has been made clear that it is time to depart.

Overreacting to normal examination procedures

For example, the patient may complain of great discomfort when the lips are stretched during the examination, of intense pain when the oral tissues are palpated, or of distress when the fit of a preliminary alginate impression tray in the mouth is being checked. Such behavior could be caused by a lowered pain threshold, which might be alterable through an improved diet or the resolution of an inflammatory response. On the other hand, it might be the result of an emotional disorder. This, of course, would have to be resolved before proceeding.

Downgrading or criticizing treatment provided by a previous dentist

This becomes particularly significant if the patient is critical of more than one dentist. It usually indicates an inability to assume some of the responsibility for the success of dental treatment.

Refusing to divulge the name of a previous dentist or dentists

It is essential to determine why the patient has this attitude. It may be due to failure to pay for the previous care, to an action underway by the local dental society grievance committee, or to a pending lawsuit.

Not having paid for previous dental care

This information is difficult to secure if the patient is not open about his/her previous experience. Failure to pay the fee may or may not have been justified. It is important for you to determine the circumstances before deciding to proceed with treatment.

Dissatisfaction with existing dentures that does not coincide with your evaluation of the dentures

The patient may complain of a lack of retention, yet retention is adequate. This could indicate that the patient's demands for retention are unrealistic and impossible to achieve.

The patient may complain of extreme pain, with no visible cause that can be related to the dentures.

Numerous sets of dentures made in a short time (for example, three in 2 years)

It is essential that the previous dentures be evaluated for major faults. If only minor technical defects are present, be cautious about proceeding with the making of new dentures.

Unrealistic desires to change facial appearance

For example, the patient may want to erase wrinkles around the mouth (the result of aging) by positioning the denture teeth abnormally to the labial or buccal or by adding an unreasonable amount of bulk to the flanges. This could cause problems with retention and stability. It also might be an indication that the patient is unable to face the reality of aging. This type of patient is frequently a 40+ woman who is fearful of her declining appearance, and as a result may be difficult to satisfy. Before accepting such a patient you may find it useful to agree on the number of tryins to be included in the fee. Also you might suggest a plastic surgery consultation.

Recent major catastrophe in the immediate family (such as a death, divorce, or severe illness)

This is usually a poor time to begin a major dental procedure since the patient is likely to be subjected to abnormal stress. It is more appropriate to perform minor procedures that can make the patient comfortable (adjustment or a repair or temporary reline of an existing denture). Discussing the wisdom of delaying treatment with the patient is essential. Waiting several months or even a year before proceeding may increase the likelihood of success.

Legal action pending with the former dentist

In general, this is not an appropriate time for initiating extensive dental care even if it appears needed. Usually the patient has considerable hostility toward the previous dentist, which, unfortunately, may be transferred to you. The chances of success under these conditions are remote. The only reasonable action is to counsel the patient regarding the inadvisability of proceeding before the legal action has been completed. **Note:** The patient may be considering involving you in a court hearing relative to the quality of care provided by the previous dentist. If treatment is initiated at this time, it should be with the clear realization that involvement in a law suit may become a reality. A conversation with the previous dentist can provide considerable insight about the patient's behavior and may reveal whether the patient has given a distorted view of treatment rendered previously.

History of severe gagging and inability to wear dentures

The chances of success are poor without some major change occurring. Frequently emotional problems and/or excessive alcohol consumption coupled with heavy smoking can precipitate a severe gagging problem. Changing the underlying cause of these habits may be impossible.

Occasionally the patient has forced the previous dentist to grossly underextend the upper denture in an attempt to eliminate the gagging problem. Do not be misled into thinking that making new dentures will eliminate the gagging without first testing adequate extension with a baseplate or some other desensitizing procedure.

Crying during discussion of previous dental experiences

This is unusual and generally involves an emotionally unstable woman. It should cause concern because it may be a clear indication of major underlying problems that will not be eliminated simply by making new dentures.

Evidence of excessive smoking

Consuming one or more packs of cigarettes a day is an indication that the patient may be experiencing considerable stress. It decreases the chances of success with new dentures. In addition, it tends to cause an adverse soft tissue response. Usually the tissues of an excessive smoker respond poorly to the stress of denture wearing, and this can contribute to a gagging problem.

Evidence of severe bruxing and/or clenching

This habit is usually the result of anxiety or tension. Since it subjects the underlying tissues to excessive pressures, the chances of gaining comfort with new dentures are remote. In addition, the denture teeth will usually wear rapidly.

Restlessness in the dental chair

This is occasionally seen with elderly people, individuals with brain damage, or those suffering from orofacial dyskinesia. Unless the problem can be controlled, the chances of successfully treating such a patient are remote.

When and how to refer the patient to a specialist for treatment

It is appropriate to refer a patient to a specialist when (1) the patient exhibits numerous characteristics that indicate future problems, (2) the treatment called for is beyond your capabilities, or (3) you do not feel comfortable about assuming responsibility for the necessary care.

Background information. As mentioned earlier, a careful examination, diagnosis, and treatment planning of each patient is absolutely essential. Of primary importance is determining a *realistic* prognosis for whatever care you are considering. If you do not feel confident in dealing with all the complications that the patient presents, tell the patient exactly that. Explain that both you and the patient will be better off if the patient goes to a specialist.

The reason for this is that there is usually only one good chance to successfully treat a patient; once the patient has been treated unsuccessfully, the chances that another dentist will succeed drop significantly. Part of this is due to the psychologic effect of experiencing failure relative to an anticipated outcome. In addition, dental insurance coverage limitations complicate the situation. In the United States and Canada most insurance carriers will pay for new dentures only once every 5 years. With the exception of a reline or a denture adjustment, prosthodontic care is not approved during the intervening time. Insurance coverage of other areas of dentistry (restorative, endodontic, periodontal) varies from carrier to carrier; however, the 5-year limit on removable or fixed prostheses seems to be standard.

There has been a general reluctance to refer difficult prosthodontic patients, probably because many dentists believe that no irreversible damage will occur if treatment is unsuccessful. Unfortunately, this is not true, since damage does occur in several areas:

1. The patient's attitude toward and confidence in wearing new dentures can be seriously undermined, which will complicate later treatment.
2. Inadequate base extension, occlusion, etc. can damage the residual ridges.
3. Treating patients beyond one's capability invites frustration in dealing with the problems.
4. There is a great loss of time and money to both the patient and the dentist when treatment is not successful.

Procedure
1. Send a note to the specialist with all of the background information that has been compiled. In addition, make it clear that the patient is being referred for total care. If radiographs have been made, send them to the specialist. All available information should be provided, to enhance the chances for success and to prevent needless duplication of questions, radiographs, questionnaires, etc.
2. Explain to the patient that he/she is being sent to a well-qualified specialist in whom you have great confidence and that he can feel comfortable following the recommendation.
3. Make it easy for the patient to get to the specialist. Many patients appreciate having the receptionist call and make the ap-

pointment while they are still in the office. The receptionist can quickly explain the reason for the referral and set up the initial appointment.

If the patient is to make the appointment, it is a good idea to tell him/her to delay the appointment until sufficient time (usually a week) has elapsed for your note and radiographs to reach the specialist's office.

USE OF A CONSULTATION REPORT

It is helpful to schedule a separate consultation appointment as soon as possible after the examination appointment. The patient will be given the written report to read upon arrival. After allowing sufficient time for him to look it over, you should personally meet with him to review its contents and to answer any questions the patient may have. It is helpful to point out unusual items (an unerupted tooth, extreme bone loss, low tuberosities, etc) on the panoramic radiograph or diagnostic casts. Occasionally, if there are alternate treatment possibilities, the patient will be asked to decide which approach will be taken. In this case the original report can be given to take home and will provide an opportunity for family members to review the findings and the recommended treatment. A copy of this is placed in the patient's chart for future reference. Having a written document minimizes the chances that misunderstanding will develop at a later time. The receptionist has ready access to this written report, which includes the financial agreement.

Some dentists have found that it works better for their office routine to mail the consultation report to the patient and have the patient call with any questions. Although this is acceptable, it is not as trouble free as the approach just described. Frequently when an insurance company representative calls to clarify a predetermination-of-benefits request or an insurance claim request, the receptionist is able to secure the needed information from the consultation report and this avoids having to bother you for details.

Contents of the report

Whether you use a written report or rely on only a verbal discussion, the following points must be covered:

1. Description of the patient's problems and complaints
2. The main findings from the examination appointment
3. Specific description of the work to be completed
4. List of any limitations—be specific; this is not a time for reluctance about being open and honest with the patient
5. Listing of the fees for all care to be provided
6. Description of how the fees are to be paid
7. Clarification of how much follow-up care is included with the quoted fee—be very specific

An actual consultation report is reproduced for your reference (Fig. 5-5).

ECONOMICS OF PROSTHODONTIC SERVICE

It is only after the diagnosis is complete and the treatment plan has been made that a fee for complete denture service can be determined. A uniform or standard fee for dentures is unrealistic. The conditions in patients' mouths vary so much that a fixed fee for this service would be unfair to the patient in some cases and unfair to the dentist in others. The patient who has favorable ridges and jaw relations and a favorable mental attitude will require less time to treat than one who has unfavorable conditions. Therefore with a standard fee the patient with uncomplicated conditions would, in effect, be paying for the treatment of a patient with more complicated problems. This is unfair to all concerned. The fee should be determined on an individual basis for each patient according to the time and difficulties involved in the treatment.

There is, however, a basic cost to each dentist for the production of complete denture ser-

April 16, 1989

(Edentulous Male)
Age - 55

Mr. Complete Denture Patient
1100 97th Ave. W.
Any City, U.S.A.
Re: Consultation Report

Dear Mr. Patient:

During the examination I made on March 19, 1989, you indicated that you had been wearing complete dentures for approximately twenty-seven years. Your present dentures were made six years
ago. You indicated that the primary problems you are currently experiencing were
   1. <u>Soreness</u> of your lower ridge at all times
   2. <u>Looseness</u> of the lower denture (you have to place denture adhesive in the lower denture to
      be able to wear it)
   3. <u>Appearance</u> of the lower denture (you feel the lower teeth are not visible at any time now)
      Note: The photograph that you brought showing your natural teeth confirms your obser-
                vation.

During the examination, I noted the following problems:
   1. Generalized inflammation of the gum tissues covering your upper and lower ridges
      Note: The inflamed tissue will probably return to a normal appearance if you follow the
                recommendations in this report.
   2. Sharp prominences of the bone are present on the inside of your lower ridge on both sides
      toward the back (they are covered with very thin gum tissue that can be easily irritated)
      Note: These prominences should be reduced by surgery to improve the chances of your
                being comfortable wearing a lower denture.
   3. The band of tissue attaching your lower lip to your lower ridge on both the right and left sides
      is very high (this is probably one cause of the poor fit of your lower denture)
      Note: These bands of tissue should be lowered surgically.
   4. You have lost considerable bone from your lower ridge (which makes it difficult to provide re-
      ally good retention for a complete lower denture)

<u>EXAMINATION OF PRESENT DENTURES</u>
Your upper denture appears to fit fairly well, while your lower denture fits very poorly. Your lower denture does not adequately cover your lower ridge in the back. The appearance is poor, with your lower
front teeth hidden from view. The teeth are severely abraded, possibly from a clenching or grinding
habit.

<u>HABITS</u>
You indicated that you wear your dentures day and night. Unfortunately, many individuals tend to
grind or clench their teeth together, especially at night, which results in excessive pressures being
transmitted to the ridges. <u>It would be ideal</u> if you could develop the practice of taking the dentures out
of your mouth at night. This allows the gum tissues to relax and recover from the day's use. It also
prevents clenching or grinding. <u>As an alternative,</u> you should try leaving the lower denture out at
night. If even that is out of the question, it is essential that you find a time each day to take both of the
dentures out of your mouth . During this time, the dentures should be placed in a soaking cleanser to
kill all of the bacteria as well as to remove stains. This requires a minimum of thirty minutes; however,
I would strongly encourage you to leave the dentures out of your mouth for at least one hour each
day.

Fig. 5-5   An actual consultation report written for a denture patient needing corrective
surgery before new dentures were made.

RADIOGRAPHIC FINDINGS

The panoramic X-ray of your mouth shows the resorption (bone loss) that has occurred on your lower ridge. About half of your lower ridge has resorbed away. All other areas appear to be within normal limits.

DIET

Since you have experienced sore gum tissue and bone resorption, I felt that it would be worthwhile to have you complete a five-day diet survey so we could evaluate your diet. Sore spots and excessive bone resorption can be caused by inadequate vitamin and mineral intake.

At the time this report is being written, I have not yet received your diet survey.

GENERAL HEALTH

Several aspects of your health may affect your ability to adjust to wearing new dentures.

1. <u>Drug treatment for your heart problem</u>—Occasionally, medication taken for a heart problem can cause a person's mouth to become dry, which can create difficulty in wearing dentures. Fortunately, I did not notice a saliva problem when I conducted the examination; however, it is possible that you might encounter this problem in the future.
2. <u>Age</u>—Unfortunately, a person's adaptability tends to decrease with age. This means that you will probably encounter much more difficulty adjusting to wearing new dentures than you did when your first set of dentures was made twenty-seven years ago.
3. <u>Smoking</u>—You also indicated that you are a heavy smoker (e.g., one and a half packs per day).
   Note: I would strongly encourage you to completely stop smoking since smoking can cause many serious life-threatening health problems. In addition, it tends to increase the problems encountered with wearing dentures. For one thing, gum tissues of a heavy smoker usually respond poorly to the stress of dentures. The soreness that you are experiencing with wearing your lower denture may be aggravated by your heavy smoking.

RECOMMENDATIONS

It appears that you would benefit from having new upper and lower dentures made. If you can accept the limitations that the previously discussed factors will impose, I will accept you as a patient. The following preparatory work should be done:

1. Evaluate your diet and provide nutrition counseling. We will identify food group deficiencies and suggest ways to improve your diet.
2. Refer you to an oral surgeon to have the bands of tissue lowered that attach your lower lip to your lower ridge and to reduce the sharp prominences of bone on the inside of your lower ridge toward the back.
   Note: The oral surgeon will place a temporary lining inside your lower denture at the time of surgery. This will enable you to wear your dentures after surgery.
3. Approximately one week after surgery, I will properly extend your lower denture with hard plastic and then place a soft treatment lining in both dentures to improve the fit. This will allow the tissue to relax and be in a more normal position.
4. The lining in the lower denture may have to be changed at least once depending on the amount of tissue change that occurs during healing. We will want to wait a <u>minimum of six weeks</u> following surgery before proceeding with final impressions for new dentures. When you can manage your old dentures and your ridge tissues are comfortable and free of any inflammation, we can proceed with making new dentures.
5. We will teach you how to effectively massage the gums covering both upper and lower ridges. This will improve the tissues' ability to withstand the forces from your dentures.
6. If you are comfortable with the soft temporary treatment lining in your lower denture, you might consider having a soft lining (processed silicone rubber) in your new lower denture. It will probably give you some added comfort. The life of this material is three to four years, so periodic replacement of the lining will be necessary. Paying strict attention to home care instructions tends to increase the life expectancy of the lining.

Fig. 5-5, cont'd

Continued.

FEES

The fees for the treatment I will provide are listed below.

	Examination	$
	Panoramic X-ray	$
	Consultation	$
	Extend lower denture with hard plastic	$
	*Temporary treatment lining in lower denture	$
	*Temporary treatment lining in upper denture	$
	**New upper and lower dentures	$
(Optional)	Processed silicone lining in lower denture	$

TOTAL: $ _____

The fee <u>does not</u> include the oral surgery. The fee does include all adjustments to the new dentures for a period of sixty days following delivery. An office visit charge will be made for adjustments after that period of time. The fees quoted are valid for a six-month period starting from the date of this report.

*The temporary treatment linings may have to be replaced if they deteriorate. There would be a fee for replacement of the lining if required.

**I will provide up to two tryin appointments (evaluating the placement of teeth while they are in wax) for the fee listed. If additional appointments are requested by you, an additional fee will be charged based on the amount of time required.

TERMS:

Half of the total fee will be due when we place the temporary treatment linings in your dentures. The balance will be due at the tryin appointment (when the teeth are aranged in wax).

INSURANCE BENEFITS

As a courtesy to you, we will assist you in preparing any insurance forms that you may require. All insurance benefits will be paid directly to you by your insurance company.

FUTURE CARE

The new dentures should be checked at twelve-month intervals and adjusted to maintain good tissue adaptation and good tooth contacts. There is a charge for these recall visits, but you will find them to be a good investment since periodic adjustment of the dentures tends to increase their life.

Sincerely yours,

John Q. Dentist, D.D.S.

JQD/ef

Fig. 5-5, cont'd

vice that is based on the minimum time it takes to render the service. This cost must include the time spent in diagnosis, treatment planning, basic treatment procedures, installation of the dentures, and adjustment after the dentures have been completed. The time spent in these activities will vary with the difficulties presented by the patient. Other costs will include office overhead and maintenance, payroll for office assistance, and laboratory service. All these items together establish the actual cost of rendering complete denture service. They represent the basis for the minimum fee for service to any patient, but the fees for patients with difficult problems that will take more time to treat should be greater than the minimum fee. This variation should be based on the amount of time required for the solution of the problems. If the impressions are difficult to make, they will require more of the dentist's time, and this should be reflected in the fee quoted to the patient.

As mentioned earlier in this chapter, the patient is entitled to know the cost of treatment before it is started. The cost can be estimated with assurance if the diagnosis is thorough and the treatment plan has been carefully worked out.

When the fee is quoted to the patient, the arrangement for its payment should be explained at the same time. The most satisfactory arrangement is for half the fee to be paid when the treatment sequence begins and the balance paid at the clinical tryin appointment (when the teeth are arranged in wax). Fortunately, complete denture service is an elective service and can be postponed if necessary.

A failure to make definite arrangements for both the amount of the fee and the method of its payment can lead to misunderstandings and unhappiness. This part of complete denture service is a business arrangement between the dentist and the patient, and it must be handled on a businesslike basis so good rapport can be maintained. Once these details have been agreed on, a series of appointments for providing the service should be made.

BIBLIOGRAPHY

American Medical Association, Council of Scientific Affairs: Vitamin preparations as dietary supplements and as therapeutic agents, JAMA **257**:1929-1936, 1987.

Barboriak JJ, Rooney CB: Alcohol and its effect on the nutrition of the elderly. In Watson WR, editor: Handbook of nutrition in the aged, Boca Raton Fla, 1985 CRC Press Inc, p 215.

Chauncey HH, Muench ME, Kapur KK, Wayler AH: The effect of the loss of teeth on diet and nutrition, Int Dent J **34**:98-104, 1984.

Dawson-Hughes B, Jaques P, Shipp C: Dietary calcium intake and bone loss from the spine in healthy postmenopausal women, Am J Clin Nutr **46**:685-687, 1987.

Druyan ME: Imbalance in nutrition advice, Gerodontics **4**:176-187, 1988.

Gordon SR, Kelley SL, Sybyl JR, Mill M, Kramer A, Jahnigen DW: Relationship in very elderly veterans of nutritional status, self-perceived chewing ability, dental status, and social isolation, J Am Geriatr Soc **33**:334-339, 1985.

Gunne HJ, Wall AK: The effect of new complete dentures on mastication and dietary intake, Acta Odontol Scand **43**:257-268, 1985.

Hartsook EI: Food selection, dietary adequacy, and related dental problems of patients with dental prostheses, J Prosthet Dent **32**:32-40, 1974.

Hartz SC, Otvadovec CL, McGandy RB, Russell RM, Jacob RA, Sahyoun N, Peters H, Abrams D, Scura LA, Whinston-Perry RA: Nutrient supplement use by healthy elderly, J Am Coll Nutr **7**:119-124, 1988.

Heaney RP, Gallagher JC, Johnson CC, Neer R, Parfitt AM, Whedon GD: Calcium nutrition and bone health in the elderly, Am J Clin Nutr **36**:986-1013, 1982.

Kapur KK, Soman SD: Masticatory performance and efficiency in denture wearers, J Prosthet Dent **14**:1054-64, 1964.

Kribbs PJ, Smith DE, Chestnut CH III: Oral findings in osteoporosis. II, Relationship between residual ridge and alveolar bone resorption and generalized skeletal osteopenia, J Prosthet Dent **50**:719-724, 1983.

Lamey PJ, Allam BF: Vitamin status of patients with burning mouth syndrome and response to replacement therapy, Br Dent J **160**:81-83, 1986.

Lappalainen R, Nyyssonen V: Self-assessed chewing ability of Finnish adults with removable dentures, Gerodontics **3**:238-241, 1987.

Marcus R: Calcium intake and skeletal maturity: is there a critical relationship? J Nutr **117**:631-635, 1987.

Matkovic K, Kostial K, Simonovic I, Buzina R, Brodarec A, Nordin BEC: Bone status and fracture rates in two regions of Yugoslavia, Am J Clin Nutr **32**:540-549, 1979.

McGandy RB, Russell RM, Hartz SC, Jacob RA, Tannenbaum S, Peters H, Sahyoun N, Otradovec BL: Nutritional status of survey of healthy noninstitutionalized elderly: energy and nutrient intakes from three-day diet records and nutrient supplements, Nutr Res **6**:785-798, 1986.

Mudassir SS, Santa CA, Nicar MJ, Schiller LR, Fordtran JS: Gastrointestinal absorption of calcium from milk and calcium salts, N Engl J Med **317**:532-536, 1987.

Munro HN, Suter PM, Russell RM: Nutritional require-

ments of the elderly, Annu Rev Nutr 7:23-49, 1987.

National Institutes of Health: Consensus Development Conference statement. Osteoporosis, cause, treatment, and prevention, NIH Publ 86-2226, revised 1986.

Natow AB, Heslin J: Counseling and compliance. In Nutritional care of the older adult, New York, 1986, MacMillan Publishing Co Inc, pp 65-76.

Nizel AE, Pappas AS: Nutrition in clinical dentistry, ed 3, Philadelphia, 1989, WB Saunders Co.

Osterberg T, Steen B: Relationship between dental state and dietary intake in 70-year-old males and females in Goteborg, Sweden: a population study, J Oral Rehabil 9:509-521, 1982.

Peterkin BB, Rizek RL, Posati LD, Harris SS: When, where, with whom, and what older Americans eat, Gerodontics 3:14-19, 1987.

Ranta K, Tuominen R, Paunio I, Sepponen R: Dental status and intake of food items among an adult Finnish population, Gerodontics 4:32-35, 1988.

Sandstead HH: Nutrition in the elderly, Gerodontics 3:3-13, 1987.

Sones AD, Wolinsky LE, Dratochvil FJ: Osteoporosis and mandibular bone resorption: a prosthodontic perspective, J Prosthet Dent 56:732-736, 1986.

Spencer H, Kramer L: Osteoporosis, calcium requirement, and factors causing calcium loss, Clin Geriatr Med 3:389-402, 1987.

Wayler AH, Chauncey HH: Impact of complete dentures and impaired dentition on masticatory performance and food choice in healthy elderly men, J Prosthet Dent 49:427-433, 1983.

Wical KE, Brussee P: Effects of a calcium and vitamin D supplement on alveolar ridge resorption in immediate denture patients, J Prosthet Dent 41:4-11, 1979.

Wical KE, Swoope CC: Studies of residual ridge resorption. II, The relationship of dietary calcium and phosphorus to residual ridge resorption, J Prosthet Dent 32:13-22, 1974.

CHAPTER 6

Improving the patient's denture foundation and ridge relations

The vast majority of patients for whom complete denture therapy is prescribed have already been wearing dentures. As suggested earlier, there is a risk in wearing dentures for prolonged periods. This risk, or biologic price, manifests itself in a number of adverse changes in the dentures' foundations. Consequently several conditions in the edentulous mouth should be corrected or treated before the construction of complete dentures. Often patients are not aware that tissues in their mouth have been damaged or deformed by the presence of old prostheses. Other oral conditions may have developed or be present that must be altered to increase the chances for success of the new dentures. The patient must be made cognizant of these problems, and a logical explanation by the dentist, supplemented with radiographs and diagnostic casts, will usually convince the patient of the necessity for the suggested treatment.

The methods of treatment to improve the patient's denture foundation and ridge relations are usually either nonsurgical or surgical in nature, or a combination of both methods.

NONSURGICAL METHODS

Nonsurgical methods of edentulous mouth preparation include (1) rest for denture-supporting tissues, (2) occlusal and vertical dimension correction of old prostheses, (3) good nutrition, and (4) conditioning of the patient's musculature.

Rest for the denture-supporting tissues. Rest for the denture-supporting tissues can be achieved by removal of the dentures from the mouth for an extended period or the use of temporary soft liners inside the old dentures. Both procedures allow deformed tissue of the residual ridges to recover normal form. Clinical reports and experience also support the merits of regular finger or toothbrush massage of denture-bearing mucosa, especially of those areas that appear edematous and enlarged.

It has been demonstrated that tissue abuse caused by improper occlusion can be made to disappear and redevelop at will by (1) withholding the faulty dentures from the patient, (2) substituting properly made dentures, and then (3) allowing the patient to reuse the faulty dentures with the improper occlusal relations. In these cases it is necessary to allow the soft tissues to recover by removing the dentures for 48 to 72 hours before impressions are made for the construction of new dentures. However, it generally is not feasible to withhold a patient's dentures for an extended period while the tissues are recovering. Therefore temporary soft liners have been developed as tissue treatment or conditioning materials. These soft resins maintain their softness for several days while the tissues recover. Tissue conditioners consist of a polymer powder and an aromatic ester-ethanol mixture. They have been widely used in dentistry for years, and provide the dentist with an expanded scope for short-term resolution of patient problems.

The major uses of these tissue-conditioning

materials are tissue treatment, liners for surgical splints, trial denture base stabilizers, optimal arch form or neutral zone determinants, and functional impression materials. Clinical experience indicates that soft liners can also be used as functional impression materials when refitting complete dentures.

It is well recognized that denture-bearing tissues demonstrate microscopic evidence of inflammation, even if they appear clinically normal. Consequently, tissue rest for at least 24 hours and the use of tissue treatment resins are essential preliminaries to each prosthetic appointment. Tissues recover rapidly when the dentures are not worn or when treatment liners are used. The method of achieving optimal health of the denture-bearing tissues is not as important as the result (the tissues' being made healthy). Many dentures fail because the impressions or registrations of the relations are made when the tissues are distorted by the old dentures. The same error is frequently commited when dentures are relined without adequate denture-bearing tissue rest or tissue treatment.

Occlusal correction of the old prostheses. An attempt should be made to restore an optimal vertical dimension of occlusion to the dentures presently worn by the patient by using an interim resilient lining material. This step enables the dentist to prognosticate the amount of vertical facial support that the patient can tolerate, and it allows the presumably deformed tissues of the temporomandibular joints to recover. The decision to create room inside the denture depends on its fit and the condition of the tissues. The tissue treatment material also permits some movement of the denture base so its position becomes compatible with the existing occlusion, apart from allowing the displaced tissues to recover their original form. Consequently, ridge relations are improved and this improvement facilitates the dentist's eventual relation-registration procedures.

It may also be necessary to correct the extent of tissue coverage by the old denture base so all usable supporting tissue is included in the treatment. This correction can be easily achieved by use of one of the resin border-molding materials combined with a tissue conditioner.

Good nutrition. A good nutritional program must be emphasized for each edentulous patient. This program is especially important for the geriatric patient whose metabolic and masticatory efficiency have decreased. (See Chapter 5.)

Conditioning the patient's musculature. The use of jaw exercises can permit relaxation of the muscles of mastication and strengthen their coordination as well as help prepare the patient psychologically for the prosthetic service. If at the initial appointment the dentist observes that the patient responds with difficulty to instructions for relaxation and coordinated mandibular movement, a program of mandibular exercises may be prescribed. Experience indicates that such a program is usually beneficial and the subsequent clinical appointment stages of registration of jaw relations are facilitated.

SURGICAL METHODS

Frequently, certain conditions of the denture-bearing tissues require edentulous patients to be treated surgically. These conditions

Table 6-1 Objectives of preprosthodontic surgical prescriptions

1. Correcting conditions that preclude optimal prosthetic function
    Localized or generalized hyperplastic replacement of resorbed ridges
    Epulis fissuratum
    Papillomatosis
    Unfavorably located frenular attachments
    Pendulous maxillary tuberosities
    Bony prominences, undercuts, and ridges
    Discrepancies in jaw size relationships
    Pressure on mental foramen
2. Enlargement of denture-bearing area(s)
    Vestibuloplasty
    Ridge augmentation
3. Provision for placing tooth root analogues by means of osseointegrated dental implants

are the result of unfavorable morphologic variations of the denture-bearing area, or more commonly may follow long-term wear of ill-fitting dentures. The objectives of prescribing a preprosthetic surgical procedure are listed in Table 6-1.

Correcting conditions that preclude optimal prosthetic function

Hyperplastic ridge, epulis fissuratum, and papillomatosis. The surgical treatment of these conditions is described in Chapter 2. The premise underscoring surgical intervention is that mobile tissues (such as a hyperplastic ridge), tissues that interfere with optimal seating of the denture (an epulis), or tissues that readily harbor microorganisms (a papillomatosis) are not conducive to firm healthy foundations for complete dentures. Whenever possible, these tissues should be rested, massaged, and/or treated with an antifungal agent prior to their surgical excision. If the patient's health precludes surgical intervention, the less invasive protocol that routinely precedes a surgical

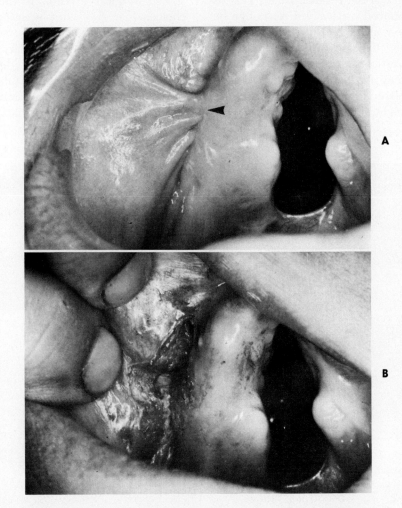

Fig. 6-1   A, Preoperative and, **B,** postoperative views of the maxillary buccal frenum *(arrowhead)* in an edentulous patient with an unrepaired palatal cleft. Excision allowed for optimal extension of the denture flange into this area.

prescription is undertaken prior to denture construction.

Frenular attachments and pendulous maxillary tuberosities. Frena, or fibrous bands of tissue attached to the bone of the mandible and maxillae, are frequently superficial to muscle attachments. If the frenum is close to the crest of the bony ridge (Fig. 6-1), it may be difficult to obtain the ideal extension and border of the flange of the denture. The upper labial frenum may be composed of a strong band of fibrous connective tissue that attaches on the lingual side of the crest of the residual ridge. This tissue can be removed surgically. Frena often become prominent as a result of reduction of the residual ridges. If muscle fibers are attached close to the crest of the ridge when the frenum is removed, they are usually detached and elevated or depressed to expose the amount of desired ridge height. The frenectomy can be car-

ried out before prosthetic treatment is begun, or it can be done at the time of denture insertion when the new denture can act as a surgical template. The former is preferred because the patient will not have to contend with postoperative discomfort along with adjustment to the dentures.

Pendulous fibrous maxillary tuberosities (Fig. 6-2) are frequently encountered. They occur unilaterally or bilaterally and may interfere with denture construction by excessive encroachment on or obliteration of the interarch space. Surgical excision is the treatment of choice (Fig. 6-3), but occasionally maxillary bone must be removed. Care must be used to avoid opening into the maxillary sinus. In those instances in which the sinus dips down into a pneumatized and elongated tuberosity, it may be possible to collapse the sinus floor upward without danger of opening into it. This tech-

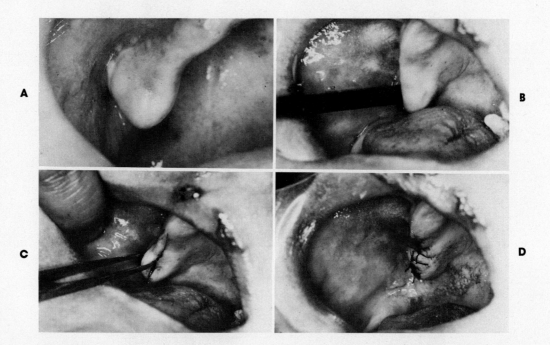

Fig. 6-2 **A,** A pendulous, fibrous, mobile right maxillary tuberosity that is easily displaced, **B,** Two elliptic incisions undermine the mass, **C,** and allow for approximation of the mucosal surfaces, **D,** over a firm bony base.

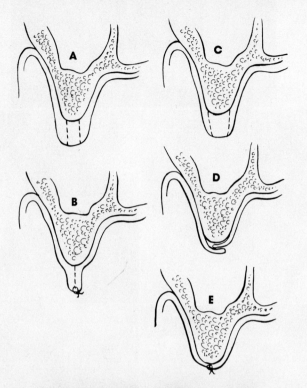

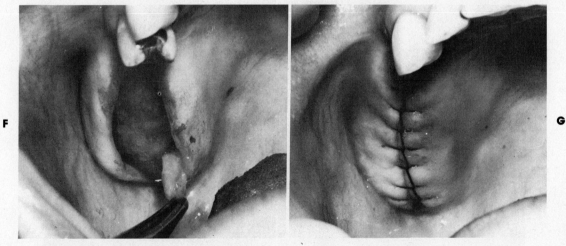

Fig. 6-3   Procedure for reducing the vertical height of a maxillary tuberosity. **A,** Incisions are made in the fibrous tuberosity. **B,** A wedge of fibrous tissue is removed. The tuberosity is less bulky but is still as long vertically as before. **C,** Incisions made just under the mucosa permit removal of all unwanted fibrous connective tissue. **D** and **E,** Thin mucosal flaps are fitted, trimmed, and sutured. This technique decreases vertical length of the tuberosity. **F** and **G** are clinical views of **C** and **E.**

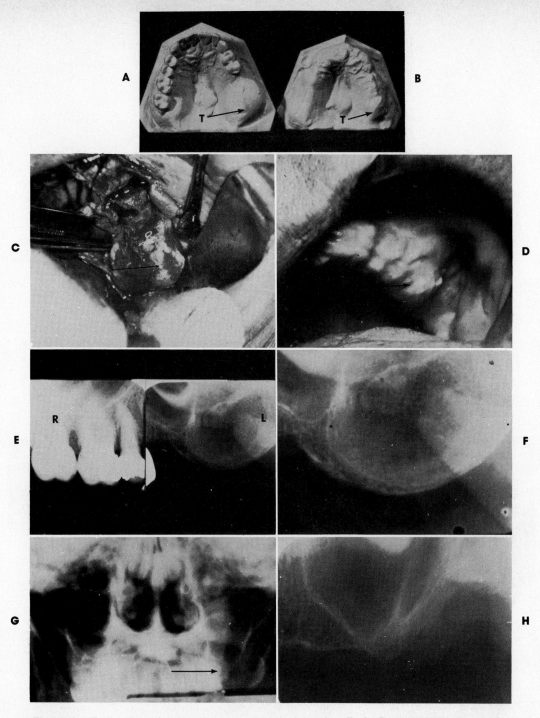

Fig. 6-4 Reduction of a huge pneumatized tuberosity, *T*. **A,** Preoperative diagnostic cast. **B,** Cast made 2 years after surgery. **C,** Clinical view of the enlarged tuberosity. **D,** The tuberosity 2 years after surgery. **E,** Dental radiographs of the patient's right and left maxillary molar regions. **F,** Radiograph of the enlarged pneumatized tuberosity. **G,** Radiograph showing the buccal undercut of a pneumatized sinus *(arrow)*. **H,** Another radiograph 2 years after surgery.

nique is also employed when a bony undercut exists on the buccal side of the tuberosity and the sinus has pneumatized into the undercut (Fig. 6-4).

Bony prominences, undercuts, spiny ridges, and nonparallel bony ridges. Mandibular tori are usually removed to avoid undercuts and to make possible a border seal beyond them against the floor of the mouth (Fig. 6-5). They generally occur so close to the floor of the mouth that a border seal cannot be made. On the other hand, maxillary tori are infrequently

removed. Satisfactory dentures can be made over most of them. The indications for the removal of maxillary tori are as follows:

1. An extremely large torus that fills the palatal vault and prevents the formation of an adequately extended and stable maxillary denture (Fig. 6-6)
2. An undercut torus that traps food debris, causing a chronic inflammatory condition; surgical excision is necessary to create optimal oral hygiene

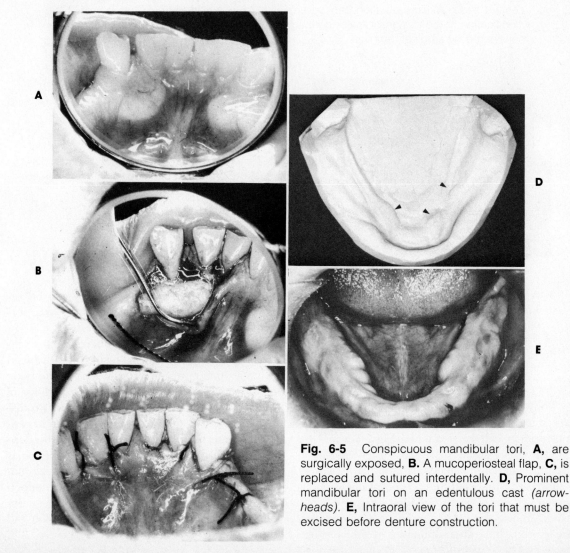

Fig. 6-5 Conspicuous mandibular tori, **A,** are surgically exposed, **B.** A mucoperiosteal flap, **C,** is replaced and sutured interdentally. **D,** Prominent mandibular tori on an edentulous cast *(arrowheads).* **E,** Intraoral view of the tori that must be excised before denture construction.

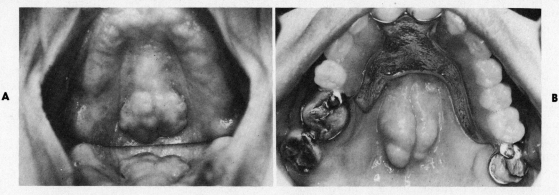

Fig. 6-6 The sheer bulk of a torus may prevent conventional palatal coverage by the denture base, **A.** This situation can be ameliorated in a partially edentulous mouth by modification of the design of major connectors, **B,** or (less frequently) the torus may be considered for surgical removal.

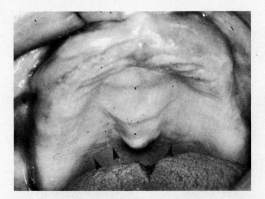

Fig. 6-7 A large maxillary torus that extends distally past the proposed posterior palatal seal area.

3. A torus that extends past the junction of the hard and soft palates and prevents the development of an adequate posterior palatal seal (Fig. 6-7)
4. One that causes the patient concern (because of a cancerphobia)

Bony exostoses may occur on both jaws but are more frequent on the buccal sides of the posterior maxillary segments (Figs. 6-8 and 6-9). They may create discomfort if covered by a denture and are usually excised. It must be emphasized that routine excision of mandibular exostoses is not recommended (Fig. 6-8, *B),* since all alveolar ridge surgery is accompanied by varied, but often dramatic, residual ridge

reduction. Frequently the denture can be relieved to accommodate the exostoses, or a permanent soft liner can be employed.

Sometimes the genial tubercles are extremely prominent as a result of advanced ridge reduction in the anterior part of the body of the mandible (Fig. 6-10). If the activity of the genioglossus muscle has a tendency to displace the lower denture or if the tubercle cannot tolerate the pressure or contact of the denture flange in this area, the genial tubercle is removed and the genioglossus muscle detached. If it is clinically necessary to deepen the alveololingual sulcus in this area, the genioglossus muscle is sutured to the geniohyoid muscle below it (Fig. 6-10).

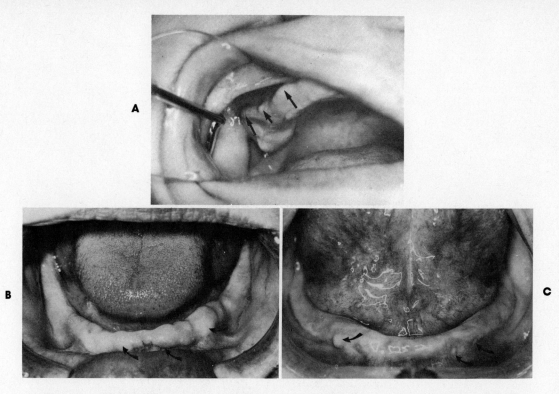

Fig. 6-8   Bony exostoses *(arrows)* on the right buccal aspect of the maxillary residual ridge, **A,** and on the labial and buccal aspects of the anterior mandibular ridge, **B** and **C.**

Residual alveolar ridge undercuts (Fig. 6-11) are rarely excised as a routine part of improving a patient's denture foundations. Usually a complex path of insertion and withdrawal of the prosthesis or careful adjustment of a denture flange enables the dentist to utilize the undercuts for extra stability. Diagnostic casts can be surveyed as a guide in the assessment of the minimal amount of tissue to be removed. Considerable evidence exists that residual ridge surgery causes excessive bone reduction. This matter is discussed at length in Chapter 26. However, the dentist may comfortably elect to remove a severe undercut that occurs opposite the lingual side of mandibular second and third molars and is tender to palpation (Fig. 6-12). Such an undercut is caused by a sharp mylohyoid ridge that (usually) is covered by very thin mucosa. When painless undercuts occur in this

area, they can help achieve added stability with a lower denture (Fig. 6-13). The path of insertion in such a situation is altered to allow for distal placement of the lingual flanges with a downward and forward final seating movement.

Discrepancies in jaw size. Impressive advances in surgical techniques of mandibular and maxillary osteotomy have enabled the oral surgeon to create optimal jaw relations for prosthetic patients who have discrepancies in jaw size. The prognathic patient frequently places considerable stress and unfavorable leverages on the maxillary basal seat. This may cause excessive reduction of the maxillary residual ridge. Such a condition is even more conspicuous when some mandibular teeth are still present. A mandibular osteotomy in these cases can create a more favorable arch align-

Text continued on p. 137.

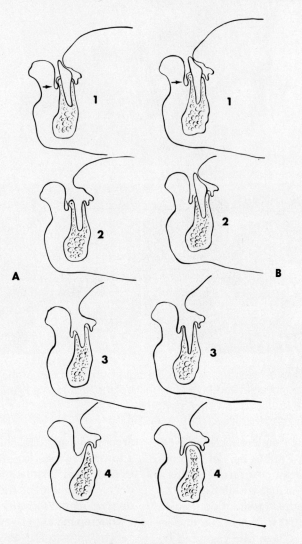

Fig. 6-9   Incorrect, **A,** and correct, **B,** methods for trimming an exostosis of the crest of the alveolar process labial to the mandibular incisors. The exostosis should be removed *before* the incisor teeth are removed. (In **A** an undesirable loss of bone occurs if a labial undercut is trimmed *after* the tooth is removed. *1,* Tooth in position. Notice the labial bony prominence. *2,* The removed tooth leaves an undercut. *3,* Removal of the undercut shortens the labial plate of bone. *4,* The end result is a lingually placed sharp residual ridge. The correct method, **B,** is to remove a labial undercut *before* the teeth are removed. This conserves bone and leaves a larger and more desirable residual ridge. *1,* Tooth in position, with a labial bony prominence. *2,* The bony prominence is removed, but the height of bone is retained. *3,* Tooth removed. *4,* The resulting residual ridge is favorable.)

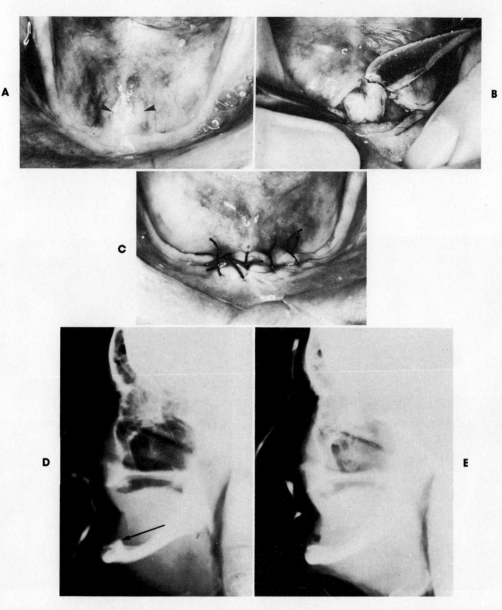

Fig. 6-10   A prominent and painful superior genial tubercle, **A** *(arrowheads),* is surgically exposed, **B,** and excised, **C.** Cephalometric radiographs, **D** and **E,** show the thinness of the mandible. In **D,** notice that the superior genial tubercle *(arrow)* is higher than the crest of the bony ridge. Notice also the extreme interarch distance at the rest position. **E,** After the tubercle had been removed.

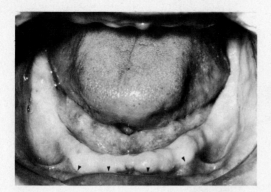

Fig. 6-11 Anterior mandibular alveolar ridge undercuts *(arrowheads)* are rarely excised; they can even be used to enhance denture stability.

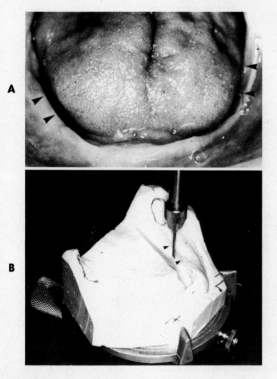

Fig. 6-12 Undercuts frequently occur on the lingual of the mandibular second and third molars. Occasionally they are very tender, and a sharp mylohyoid ridge of bone must be excised, **A** *(arrowheads)*. In **B** a surveyor is used to emphasize the undercut that such a ridge can create.

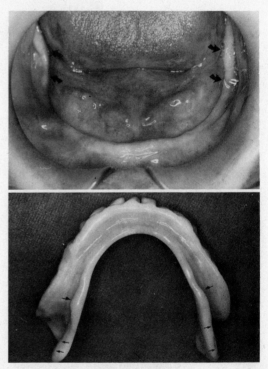

Fig. 6-13 Posterior mandibular lingual undercuts, **A** *(arrows)*, occur frequently and can be used to enhance mandibular denture stability, **B.**

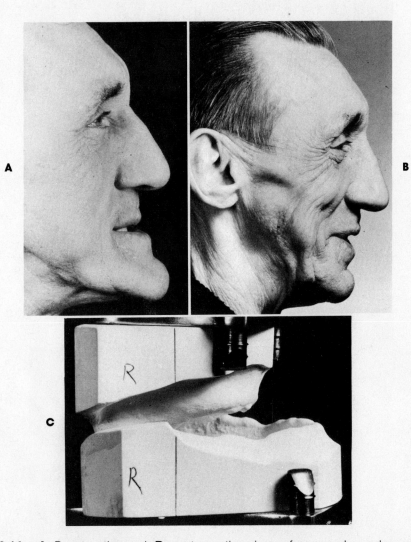

Fig. 6-14   **A,** Preoperative and, **B,** postoperative views of a man who underwent mandibular osteotomy. **C,** The preoperative diagnostic cast.

Continued.

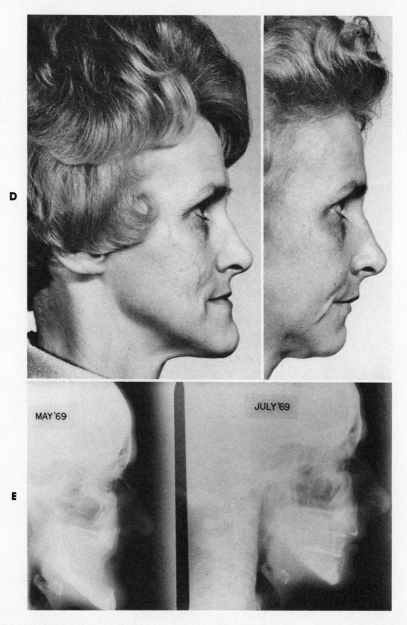

Fig. 6-14, cont'd   D and **E,** Preoperative and postoperative profiles and cephalometric views of a woman treated in a similar manner. (Courtesy Dr. P. Smylski.)

ment and improve cosmetics as well (Fig. 6-14). However, changes in the soft tissues of the face tend to be accentuated by such a procedure (as evidenced by the patient in Fig. 6-14). Usually an adjunctive face-lifting procedure in this type of patient produces impressive results.

Pressure on the mental foramen. If bone resorption in the mandible has been extreme, the mental foramen may open near or directly at the crest of the residual bony process (Fig. 6-15). When this happens, the bony margins of the mental foramen are usually more dense and resistant to resorption than the bone anterior or posterior to the foramen is. This causes the margins of the mental foramen to extend and have very sharp edges 2 to 3 mm higher than the surrounding mandibular bone. Pressure from the denture against the mental nerve exiting the foramen and over this sharp bony

edge will cause pain. Also, pressure against the sharp bone will cause pain because the oral mucosa is pinched between the sharp bony margin of the mental foramen and the denture. The most suitable way of managing this is to alter the denture so pressure does not exist. However, in some instances it may be necessary to trim the bone to relieve the mental nerve of pressure. Pressure on the mental nerve is reduced by increasing the opening of the mental foramen downward toward the inferior border of the body of the mandible. Such a change permits the mental nerve to exit the bone at a point lower than it had previously, thereby taking pressure off the nerve.

Occasionally the anterior part of the residual ridges becomes so resorbed that it is extremely thin labiolingually, and it may have a sharp knife-edge with small spicules of bone protruding from it (Fig. 6-16). Careful denture relief in these areas frequently overcomes this problem. If, however, constant irritation develops as a result of the soft tissue's being pinched between the denture and the bone, the spicules and the knife-edged ridge must be reduced.

A lack of parallelism between the maxillary and mandibular ridges can be encountered and, on occasion, may require surgical repair. This lack of parallelism may be caused by a lack of trimming of the tuberosity and ridge behind the last maxillary tooth when it is removed or may be the result of jaw defects, unequal ridge reduction, or abnormalities of growth and development. Most clinicians favor parallel ridges for their denture foundations, since the resultant forces generated are directed in a way that tends to seat the denture rather than dislodge it. Also, the height of the occlusal plane of the upper denture can be elevated posteriorly to improve the denture esthetically. Virtually all the surgical procedures described necessitate the use of a surgical template. The patient's old dentures can usually be modified with a soft treatment resin to function as such. The use of a lined template protects the operated area from trauma and enables the patient to con-

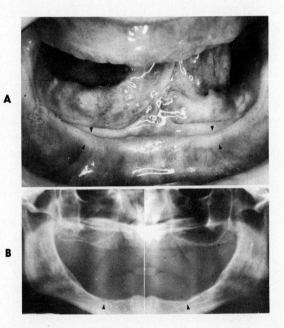

Fig. 6-15 Intraoral, **A,** and radiographic, **B,** views of an edentulous mandible with superficially placed mental foramina *(arrowheads)* secondary to extensive residual ridge reduction. The foramina are usually quite palpable in such situations.

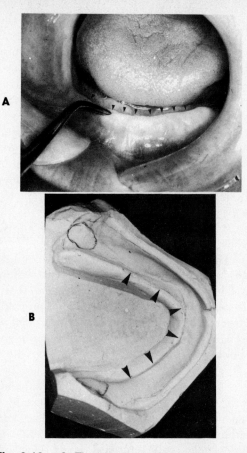

Fig. 6-16 **A,** The slender knife-edge mandibular alveolar ridge is covered by a thin and nonresilient mucosa. **B,** The working cast clearly demonstrates the knife-edged character of the ridge *(arrowheads).*

tinue wearing the dentures. All the surgical interventions mentioned in this chapter must be considered in the context of their potential effects on residual ridge resorption. It must be underscored that extensive surgical preparation of the edentulous mouth is rarely necessary and that any required surgical procedure should be as conservative as possible.

Enlargement of denture-bearing areas

Vestibuloplasty. The reduction of alveolar ridge size is frequently accompanied by an apparent encroachment of muscle attachments on the crest of the ridge. These so-called high (mandibular) or low (maxillary) attachments serve to reduce the available denture-bearing area and to undermine denture stability. The anterior part of the body of the mandible is the site most frequently involved: the labial sulcus is virtually obliterated, and the mentalis muscle attachments appear to "migrate" to the crest of the residual ridge (Fig. 6-17). This usually results in the dentist's arranging the teeth more lingually than the position of the former anterior teeth. Such lingual crowding (Chapter 14) may not be tolerated by the patient; and when the absent sulcus is accompanied by little or no attached alveolar mucosa in this area, it is virtually impossible for a lower denture to be retained. Myoplasty accompanied by sulcus deepening has been carried out in an attempt to improve denture retention. With this operation the oral surgeon detaches the origin of

Fig. 6-17 Sagittal sections through the lower lip and anterior part of the mandible, **A** and **B,** show the space available for a labial flange and the effect of the mentalis, *M,* on this space. The muscle originates on the bone and inserts into the skin. Contraction of the muscle lifts the lip and reduces the space available for the flange of a denture. A lateral cephalogram, **C,** shows the contour of the residual alveolar ridge immediately after tooth extraction, *1,* and the origin of the mentalis (simulated at *2*). When *1* resorbs to its present level, the relative locale of origin of this muscle now obliterates the labial sulcus. **D** and **E,** A mandibular vestibuloplasty provides for dramatic increase in the labial flange extension. (**A** and **B** courtesy Dr. A.L. Martone.)

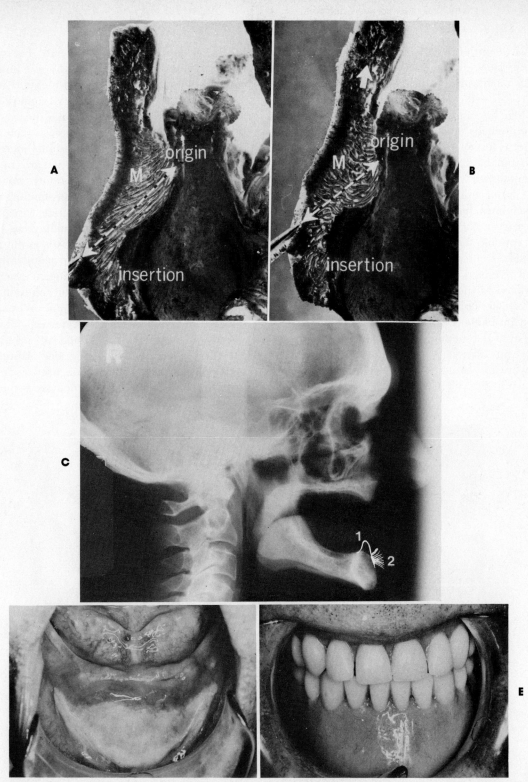

Fig. 6-17 For legend see opposite page.

muscles on either the labial or the lingual, or both, sides of the edentulous residual ridges. This enables the prosthodontist to increase the vertical extensions of the denture flanges. When horizontal bony shelving is present in the mentalis muscle region, the surgical procedure is less successful and its relative efficacy is attributable to the modification of the powerful mentalis muscle's activity.

Close cooperation between the two involved disciplines has resulted over the years in a clearer understanding of what the surgical intervention should achieve. A wide and deep sulcus is not essential for success (Fig. 6-18, *A* and *B*), and the vestibuloplasty can be restricted to the interpremolar region, since the buccinator muscles are not the major cause of the problem (Fig. 6-17, *D* and *E*). Displacement of the mentalis muscle and adjacent muscle slips allows for the production of a looser lower lip, along with a wound margin low down in the sulcus and an increase in both sta-

bility and depth of the labial flange. The situation varies in the maxillae, where a muscle comparable to the action of the mentalis in its unstabilizing potential is not encountered. A broader vestibuloplasty is indicated here.

Although a lingual vestibuloplasty can provide for a major denture dimensional increase, the procedure is traumatic, particularly in frail and elderly patients, and therefore not frequently recommended. The long-standing clinical impression that free skin grafts lose resiliency and develop nuisance crinkling has been confirmed in several reports. Skin grafts tend to have a noticeable increase in parakeratosis, with subsequent clinical sogginess. Furthermore, they seem to exhibit poor cohesion and adhesion compared with mucosa. Whenever possible, mucosal grafts are preferred.

Current research has aimed at providing substitutes for homologous grafts. Heterologous collagen grafts have been used as a biologic dressing, with the denuded areas quickly

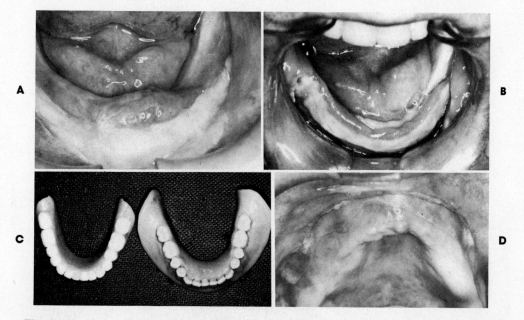

Fig. 6-18   **A** and **B,** A deepened facial mandibular sulcus with skin graft in place. Current procedures do *not* aim at achieving such a wide area of operation. **C,** Mandibular dentures before and after sulcus deepening are compared. **D,** Maxillary vestibuloplasty.

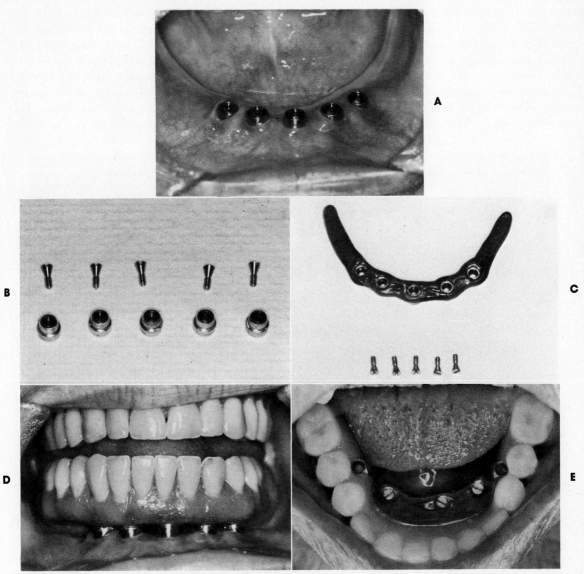

Fig. 6-19   A, After two preprosthetic surgical stages the osseointegrated implants are used as abutments for an electively removable fixed prosthesis. **B,** Prosthetic cylinders are matched to the implants and joined together via a wax scaffolding, **C,** which is cast to provide support for the final prosthesis, **D** and **E.** Notice that access to the retaining screws allows for ready removal of the prosthesis and that the gingival surface design allows for hygiene maintenance as with standard fixed prostheses.

becoming covered by normal mucous membrane. It appears that collagen xenografts may prove to be a suitable alternative for split skin or mucosal grafts. The use of acrylic resin templates or the modified previous denture to support vestibuloplasty in the mandible is essential. These templates must be fastened to the mandible with circummandibular wires for 1 week. Carefully designed splints will reduce inflammation, reduce postoperative scarring,

and maintain muscles in the desired position, thereby improving the result. The effect of mandibular vestibule-extension surgery on muscle activity and prosthesis retention has been investigated. The electromyographic activity of the mentalis and inferior orbicularis was shown to undergo only slight changes despite the mentalis muscle's being severed completely from its origin in the mandible. This minor change was presumed to be caused by

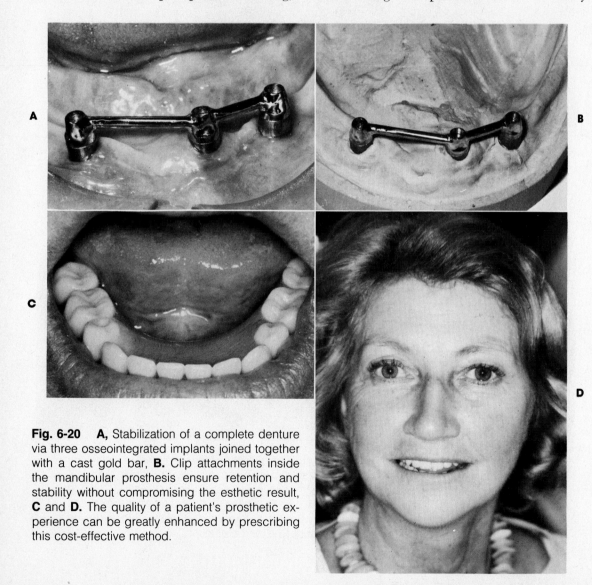

Fig. 6-20 **A,** Stabilization of a complete denture via three osseointegrated implants joined together with a cast gold bar, **B.** Clip attachments inside the mandibular prosthesis ensure retention and stability without compromising the esthetic result, **C** and **D.** The quality of a patient's prosthetic experience can be greatly enhanced by prescribing this cost-effective method.

the fact that the mentalis was given a new origin in the lower lip, with mainly the same activity pattern.

One other result of excessive alveolar bone loss or reduction is obliteration of the hamular notch. This anatomic cul-de-sac, with its potential for displacement, makes it an important part of the posterior palatal seal of the maxillary denture. Its absence can severely undermine retention of the denture, and a small localized deepening of the sulcus in this area is then indicated. The patient's old denture or a surgical template is employed after the surgery to help retain the patency of the newly formed sulcus, or notch.

Ridge augmentation. For many years surgeons have attempted to restore mandibular bulk by placing onlay bone grafts from an iliac or rib source above or below the mandible. Unfortunately, follow-up reports suggest that the result generally leaves much to be desired with respect to ridge height. Current research in the area of alveolar ridge deficiencies and nonabsorbable alloplastic materials such as hydroxyapatite indicates cause for optimism, but longitudinal studies in several treatment centers must be analyzed before the approach is accepted as an integral part of preprosthetic surgical strategies. Other methods of dimensional increase of the mandible (as by means of a "visor" or "sandwich" osteotomy) also have been proposed, and some reports suggest optimism for this procedure. However, caution is recommended because it is a formidable undertaking for elderly patients.

Replacing tooth roots by osseointegrated dental implants

Whenever complete dentures are prescribed, the optimization of a denture-bearing area is a logical and compelling objective. However, complete dentures are *not* the only method available for treating edentulous patients. Recent research has provided irrefut-

able evidence of both the desirability and the feasibility of osseointegrating tooth root replicas or analogues in edentulous jaws. This scientific advance has ushered in a new era for the treatment of edentulism by virtue of the fundamental change in its applied concept of preprosthetic surgery. In this technique, a number of cylindrically shaped screws, made of specific materials and conforming to specific designs, are buried inside the selected host bone sites. They are left to heal in situ for 4 to 6 months while osseointegration occurs. The screws, or tooth root analogues, are uncovered at a second surgical procedure, when an elective removable fixed bridge is attached to the implants (Fig. 6-19). The technique also improves the scope for use of supporting overdentures (Fig. 6-20) and is discussed further in Chapter 30.

BIBLIOGRAPHY

Björlin G, Palmquist J, Ahlgren J: Muscle activity and denture retention after vestibular extension surgery, Odontol Rev **18**:179-190, 1967.

Boos RH: Preparation and conditioning of patients for prosthetic treatment, J Prosthet Dent **9**:4-10, 1959.

de Koomen HA, Stoelinga PJW, Tideman H, Huybers JM: Interposed bone-graft augmentation of the atrophic mandible, J Maxillofac Surg **7**:129, 1979.

Harrison A: Temporary lining materials. A review of their uses, Br Dent J **151**:(12):419-422, 1981.

Kent JN, Quinn JH, Zide MF, Singer IM, Jarco M, Rothstein SS: Correction of alveolar ridge deficiencies with nonresorbable hydroxylapatite, J Am Dent Assoc **105**:993-1001, 1982.

Lytle RB: The management of abused oral tissues in complete denture construction, J Prosthet Dent **7**:27-42, 1957.

Lytle RB: Complete denture construction based on a study of the deformation of the underlying soft tissues, J Prosthet Dent **9**:539-551, 1959.

Mitchell R: A new biological dressing for areas denuded of mucous membrane, Br Dent J **155**:346-348, 1983.

Møller JF, Jolst O: A histologic follow-up study of free autogenous skin grafts to the alveolar ridge in humans, Int J Oral Surg **1**:283, 1972.

Quayle AA: The atrophic mandible: aspects of technique in lower labial sulcoplasty, Br J Oral Surg **16**:169-178, 1979.

Taylor RL: A chronological review of the changing concepts related to modifications, treatment, preservation, and augmentation of the complete denture basal seat, Aust Prosthodont Soc Bull **16**:17-39, 1986.

Rehabilitation of the edentulous patient

Complete dentures are artificial substitutes for living tissues—teeth and their supporting structures—that have been lost. They must replace the form of the living tissues as nearly as possible; and, more important, they must function in harmony with the remaining tissues that both surround and support them. It is therefore logical and convenient to regard a denture as having three surfaces: the impression or fitting surface, the occlusal or chewing surface, and a polished surface (Fig. 8-1). The polished surface is made up of the facial and lingual/palatal surfaces that join the impression and occlusal surfaces together. To achieve a harmonious coexistence between the living oral tissues and the nonliving substitutes (dentures), the dentist must fully understand the anatomy and physiology of the tissues that support and influence the design of complete dentures. In this section, applied principles of relevant anatomic and physiologic information are reconciled with esthetic considerations, to enable the dentist to rehabilitate edentulous patients.

CHAPTER 7

Biologic considerations for maxillary impressions

If dentures and their supporting tissues are to coexist for a reasonable length of time, the dentist must fully understand the macroscopic and microscopic anatomy of the supporting and limiting structures involved, for these are the foundation of the denture-bearing areas. A thorough understanding of their role will determine (1) the selective placement of forces by the denture bases on the supporting tissues and (2) the form of the denture borders that will be harmonious with the normal function of the limiting structures around them. To enable the dentist to produce a laboratory analogue, or working cast, of the denture-bearing area (DBA), both the proper placement of selective pressures by the denture base and the form of its borders are developed during preliminary and final impression procedures. It is convenient to regard the impression or fitting surface of a denture as comprising two areas: a stress-bearing or supporting area and a peripheral or sealing area. Each of these will be discussed separately but, like the sides of a coin, they are inseparable.

MACROSCOPIC ANATOMY OF SUPPORTING STRUCTURES

The foundation for dentures (DBA) is made up of bone covered by mucous membrane—mucosa and submucosa. In the submucosa are the vessels that carry blood to the basal seat and the nerves that innervate it. The microscopic anatomy of the basal seat is discussed later in this chapter. The macroscopic structures involved in supporting maxillary dentures will be considered first.

Each type of tissue found in the oral cavity has its own characteristic ability to resist external forces. This is important to the maintenance of health of the tissues of the basal seat and to the stability and support of dentures. For example, nature has placed fibrous connective tissue in places where external forces are applied, and these tissues are firmly attached to the bone underneath. Glandular tissues, on the other hand, are not found in locations where external forces are to be applied. Therefore the distribution of forces applied to the basal seat by dentures should be planned in relation to the types of tissues found in various parts of the basal seat.

Support for the maxillary denture

The ultimate support for a maxillary denture is the bone of the two maxillae and the palatine bone. The palatine processes of the maxillae are joined together at the midline in the median suture (Figs. 7-1 and 7-2). The two palatine processes of the maxillae and the palatine bone form the foundation for the hard palate and provide considerable support for the denture. More important, however, they support soft tissues that increase the surface areas of the basal seat.

A cross section of the hard palate readily shows that the palate is bone covered by tissues of varying depths. A study of these sections further reveals how important it is to em-

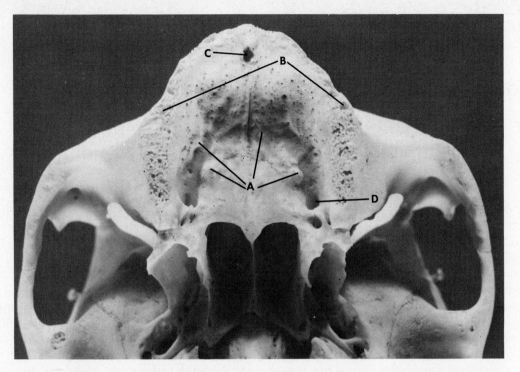

Fig. 7-1   Both the maxillae and the palatine bone provide support for an upper denture. Individual differences in form determine how forces should be directed to these bones during function with complete dentures. *A,* Spiny projections that would irritate tissues under a denture; *B,* rough and irregular bone of the maxillary ridges; *C,* incisive foramen; *D,* greater palatine foramen.

ploy an impression technique that equalizes the pressure distribution. The center of the palate may be very hard because the layer of soft tissues covering the bone in the region of the median palatal suture is extremely thin. If the hard palate is less resilient than the soft tissues (submucosa) covering the residual ridges, it should be relieved to prevent a tendency of the denture to rock or the development of soreness in this region when vertical forces are applied to the teeth. The relief for the median palatal suture and its overlying raphe can be developed in the impression-making or denture-processing procedure or after the denture has been completed. These alternatives are discussed in Chapter 8. The various regions in the

mouth that have special responsibilities for stress distribution are seen in Fig. 7-3.

The alveolar processes develop as the teeth are formed and erupt. The maxillary deciduous, or primary, teeth develop in the maxillae, and this stimulates the alveolar processes to grow. Such development continues as the permanent teeth and the alveolar processes are formed. The alveolar processes then support the natural teeth. The socket surrounding the root of each natural tooth is the alveolus, and the bony ridge that supports the teeth is the alveolar ridge. The bony process remaining after teeth have been lost is the residual alveolar ridge, which also includes the mucous membrane that covers the bone. The thickness of

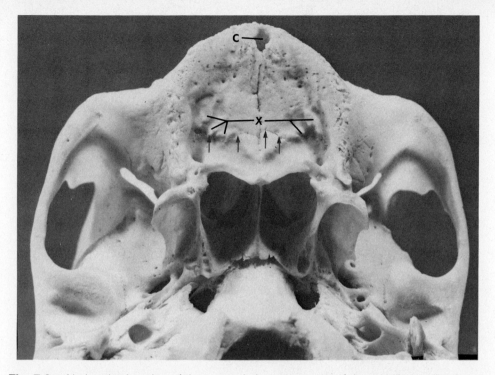

Fig. 7-2   Notice the junction of the two palatine processes of the maxillae and palatine bone *(arrows)*. *X,* Sharp bony spines present in the palate are covered with soft tissue; they frequently are an obscure cause of soreness under denture pressure. Because of increased resorption of the residual alveolar ridge, the incisive foramen, *C,* is nearer the crest of the ridge than the incisive foramen in Fig. 7-1 is. The location of the incisive papilla (covering the incisive foramen) in relation to the crest of the ridge is a guide to the amount of resorption that has occurred.

the soft tissues covering the bone is different in different parts of the maxillary basal seat. The nature and relative thickness of the soft tissues in different parts of the basal seat determine the amount of support these tissues can provide for a denture.

Residual ridge

The shape and size of the alveolar ridges change when the natural teeth are removed. The alveoli become mere holes in the jawbone and begin to fill up with new bone, but at the same time the bone around the margins of the tooth sockets begins to shrink away. This

shrinkage, or resorption, is rapid at first, but it continues at a reduced rate throughout life.

The resorption of the alveolar process causes the foundation for the maxillary denture to become smaller and otherwise change shape.

If a denture is made soon after the teeth are removed, the apparent foundation may be large but it also may be tender to pressure. This is the result of incomplete healing and a lack of cortical bone over the crest of the residual alveolar ridge.

If the teeth have been out for many years, the residual ridge may become quite small and the crest of the ridge may lack a smooth corti-

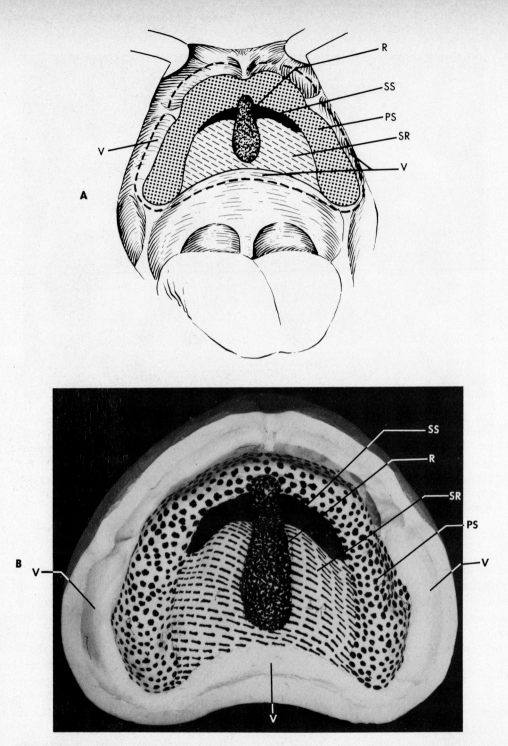

Fig. 7-3 Various areas of primary function of the maxillary basal seat are indicated on, **A,** a drawing of an edentulous upper jaw and, **B,** a cast impression. *PS,* Primary stress-bearing area; *SS,* secondary stress-bearing area; *SR,* secondary retentive area; *R,* relief area; *V,* peripheral or valve seal area.

cal bony surface under the mucosa. There may be large nutrient canals and sharp bony spicules (Figs. 7-1 and 7-5). These conditions limit the amount of pressure that can be applied on a denture without creating pain.

Stress-bearing areas

The residual ridge and most of the hard palate are considered the major or primary stress-bearing area in the upper jaw (Fig. 7-3). The crest of the residual alveolar ridge (after healing from the surgery) is covered with a layer of fibrous connective tissue, which is most favorable for supporting the denture because of its firmness and position. The artificial teeth will be placed near this ridge so leverage will be minimal.

The rugae in the anterior part of the hard palate are irregularly shaped rolls of soft tissue that serve no function in humans. They should not be distorted in an impression technique, since rebounding tissue tends to unseat the denture. In the rugal area the palate is set at an angle to the occlusal plane of the residual ridges and is rather thinly covered by soft tissues (Fig. 7-3). This area contributes to the stress-bearing role as well as to retention, though in a secondary capacity.

The third area of special concern is the glandular region on each side of the midline in the posterior part of the hard palate. This region should be covered by the denture so it can aid in retention, but it should not provide significant support for the denture because of the relatively higher resiliency at this site. The mucous glands in this region are relatively thick, and they cover the blood vessels and nerves coursing forward in the palate from the greater palatine foramen. These vessels and nerves anastomose with vessels and nerves passing through the nasopalatine canal and into the region of the basal seat at the incisive papilla.

Incisive papilla

The incisive papilla covers the incisive foramen and is located on the line immediately be-

hind and between the central incisors (see Fig. 7-6). Its position varies in different patients (Figs. 7-1 to 7-5). It is located on the center of the ridge after resorption has occurred in mouths that have been edentulous for a long time.

The incisive papilla covers the incisive foramen (the opening of the nasopalatine canals, which carry the nasopalatine vessels and nerves). Relief for the papilla should be provided in every denture to avoid any possible interference with the blood and nerve supply.

Posterior palatal area

The posterior palatine foramina are so thickly covered by soft tissue that they do not need to be relieved except in extreme cases of resorption. A study of the bony portions of the palate reveals many sharp spines, which are a source of trouble in ridges with extreme resorption and loss of the palatal glands. These bony spines are difficult to locate when they are covered by soft tissues of the palate (Fig. 7-1).

Bone of the basal seat

The configuration of bone that forms the basal seat for the maxillary denture varies considerably with each patient. Factors that influence the form and size of the supporting bone of the basal seat include (1) its original size and consistency, (2) the patient's general health and resistance, (3) forces developed by the surrounding musculature, (4) severity and location of periodontal disease, (5) forces accruing from the wearing of dental restorations, (6) surgery at the time of removal of the teeth, and (7) the relative length of time different parts of the jaws have been edentulous. Important components of the bone of the basal seat for the maxillary denture that will be described include the incisive foramen, the zygomatic process, the maxillary tuberosity, sharp spiny processes, and the torus palatinus. The pterygomaxillary (hamular) notch is discussed under macroscopic anatomy of limiting structures.

Incisive foramen. The incisive foramen is lo-

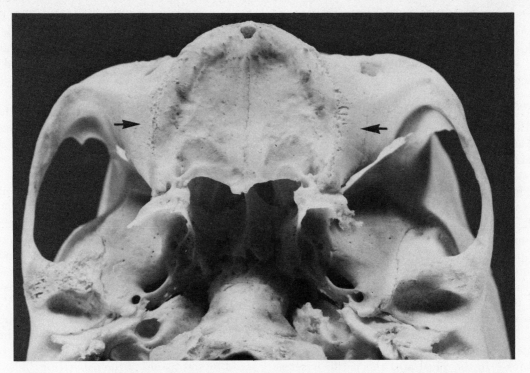

Fig. 7-4 The zygomatic process *(arrows)* is close to the crest of the residual alveolar ridge in the molar region because of an excessive amount of resorption of the alveolar ridge. The process is thinly covered by mucous membrane and may likely require relief of the denture border to prevent or eliminate soreness.

cated in the palate on the median line at the lingual gingiva of the anterior teeth; it comes nearer to the crest of the ridge as resorption progresses (Figs. 7-1 and 7-2). Relief for the incisive foramen should be provided in the denture to prevent impingement on the nasopalatine nerves and blood vessels as they pass through the foramen. The location of the incisive papilla gives an indication as to the amount of resorption of the residual ridge and thus is an aid in determining vertical dimension and the proper position of the teeth.

Zygomatic process. The zygomatic, or malar, process, which is located opposite the first molar region, is one of the hard areas found in mouths that have been edentulous for a long time (Fig. 7-4). Some dentures require relief over this area to aid retention and prevent soreness of the underlying tissues.

Maxillary tuberosity. The tuberosity region of the maxilla often hangs abnormally low because, when the maxillary posterior teeth are retained after the mandibular molars have been lost and not replaced, the maxillary teeth extrude, bringing the process with them. Often the low-hanging tuberosity is complicated by an excess of fibrous connective tissue (see Fig. 3-9). This excess soft tissue can prevent proper location of the occlusal plane if it is not removed. In addition, rough and irregular bone can be irritated by the denture base (Fig. 7-5).

Sharp spiny processes. Frequently there are sharp spiny processes on the maxillary and palatal bones that are deeply covered with soft tissue (Figs. 7-1 and 7-2). However, in patients with considerable resorption of the residual alveolar ridge, these sharp spines irritate the soft tissues left between them and the denture

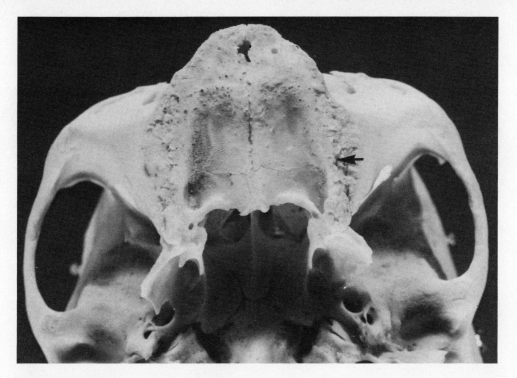

Fig. 7-5   Notice the rough and irregular bone on the crest of the residual alveolar ridge, particularly the left maxillary tuberosity *(arrow)*.

base. The canal leading from a posterior palatine foramen often has a sharp spiny overhanging edge that may cut and irritate the palatal soft tissues overlying it as a result of pressures from the maxillary denture (Fig. 7-1).

Torus palatinus

A hard bony enlargement that occurs in the midline of the roof of the mouth is called a torus palatinus (Figs. 6-6 and 6-7). It occurs in about 20% of the population. One type is almost entirely soft tissue and is loose and flabby; the other has a thin layer of mucosal tissue covering the bone. The extent of the torus can be determined by palpation, and an arbitrary relief shape that disregards the extent of this hard area should not be used. Such a relief shape may rob the denture of part of its support area (see Fig. 6-6). The relief provided in the palate

should conform accurately to the shape of the hard area. Generally, the more convex the hard area the more relief will be required.

MACROSCOPIC ANATOMY OF LIMITING STRUCTURES (peripheral or sealing area of a denture)

The functional anatomy of the mouth determines the extent of the basal surface of a denture. The denture base should include the maximum surface possible within the limits of the health and function of the tissues it covers and contacts. This means that a denture should be made in such a way that covers all the available basal seat tissues without causing soreness at the denture borders and without interfering in the action of any of the structures that contact or surround it.

To follow the basic principle of impression

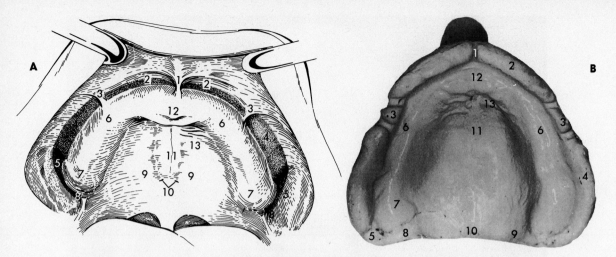

Fig. 7-6   Correlation of anatomic landmarks. **A,** Intraoral drawing of the maxillary arch. *1,* Labial frenum; *2,* labial vestibule; *3,* buccal frenum; *4,* buccal vestibule; *5,* coronoid bulge; *6,* residual alveolar ridge; *7,* maxillary tuberosity; *8,* hamular notch; *9,* posterior palatal seal region; *10,* foveae palatinae; *11,* median palatine raphe; *12,* incisive papilla; *13,* rugae. **B,** Maxillary final impression showing the corresponding denture landmarks; *1,* Labial notch; *2,* labial flange; *3,* buccal notch; *4,* buccal flange; *5,* coronoid contour; *6,* alveolar groove; *7,* maxillary tubercular fossa; *8,* pterygomaxillary seal; *9,* posterior palatal seal; *10,* foveae palatinae; *11,* median palatine groove; *12,* incisive fossa; *13,* rugae. (Based on Fig. 17 in Martone AL: J Prosthet Dent **13:**4-33, 1963.)

making—extend the impression to cover the maximum area possible within the limits of the health and function of the tissues of the basal seat—one must possess a thorough knowledge of the functional anatomy of the basal seat and its limiting structures. The anatomy to be considered is the anatomy in function, rather than descriptive anatomy. Certain definite anatomic limitations for dentures exist in both jaws. Their details vary from patient to patient, but the location and function of the various structures are basically the same for all edentulous patients.

The limiting structures of the maxillary basal seat can be analyzed in different regions (Fig. 7-6). The anterior region extends from one buccal frenum to the other on the labial side of the maxillary ridge and is called the labial vestibular space. In this region three objectives are apparent. First, the impression must supply

sufficient support to the upper lip to restore the relaxed contour (or appearance) of the lip. This means that the thickness of the labial flange of the upper tray and the final impression must be developed according to the amount of bone that has been lost from the labial side of the ridge. Second, the labial flange of the impression must have sufficient height to reach to the reflecting mucous membrane of the labial vestibular space without distorting it. Third, there must be no interference of the labial flange with the action of the lip in function.

Labial frenum

The maxillary labial frenum is a fold of mucous membrane at the median line. It contains no muscle and has no action of its own. This band of tissue starts superiorly in a fan shape and converges as it descends to its terminal at-

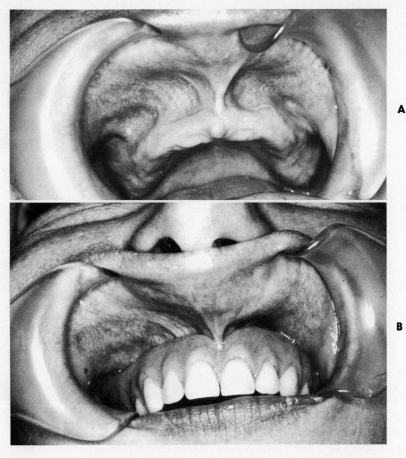

Fig. 7-7   A, A broad maxillary labial frenum. **B,** The labial flange must fit snugly around the frenum.

tachment on the labial side of the ridge (Fig. 7-7, *A*). The labial notch in the labial flange of the denture must be just wide enough and just deep enough to allow the frenum to pass through it without manipulation of the lip (Fig. 7-7, *B*). This fact should be taken into consideration in the relief for this attachment. The denture borders should not only be cut lower but also have less thickness adjacent to the labial notch in the border of the denture. A shallow bead can be formed in the denture base around the notch to help perfect the seal.

Orbicularis oris

The orbicularis oris is the main muscle of the lips, lying in front of and resting on the labial flange and teeth of the denture. Its tone depends on the support it receives from the thickness of the labial flange and the position of the arch of teeth.

The fibers of the orbicularis pass horizontally through the lips and anastomose with fibers of the buccinator muscle. Since they run in the direction they do, the orbicularis oris has only an indirect effect on the extent of an impres-

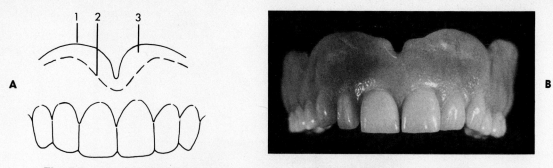

Fig. 7-8 Maxillary labial flange. **A,** **1,** Correct contour of the flange; **2,** incorrect contour of the denture border; **3,** tissue that should have been covered. **B,** Properly formed labial notch and flange in a complete denture.

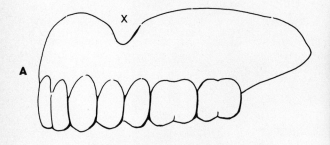
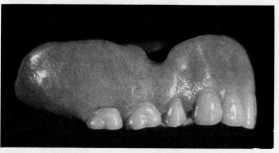

Fig. 7-9 Maxillary buccal notch. **A,** Notice that in the region of the buccal frenum the notch, **X,** is wide to allow frenal movement. The frenum moves posteriorly as a result of buccinator action and anteriorly because of forward movement of the modiolus and the corner of the mouth. **B,** Properly formed notch in an upper complete denture. Its size and form will vary with the individual patient.

sion and the denture base. This muscle and its action are discussed in more detail in Chapter 19.

Buccal frenum

The denture border between the labial and buccal frena is known as the labial flange (Fig. 7-8). The buccal frenum is sometimes a single fold of mucous membrane, sometimes double, and, in some mouths, broad and fan shaped. It requires more clearance for its action than the labial frenum does. The caninus (levator anguli oris) attaches beneath and affects the position of the buccal frenum. The orbicularis oris pulls

the frenum forward, and the buccinator pulls it backward. The buccal notch in the denture must be broad enough to allow this movement of the buccal frenum (Fig. 7-9). The border of the denture should be functionally molded to fit exactly the depth and width of this frenum when it is in function, being moved by the three muscles associated with it (orbicularis oris, buccinator, and caninus). The buccal frenum is part of the continuous band of tissue going from the maxilla through the modiolus in the corner of the mouth to the buccal frenum on the mandible. Inadequate provision for the buccal frenum or excess thickness of the flange

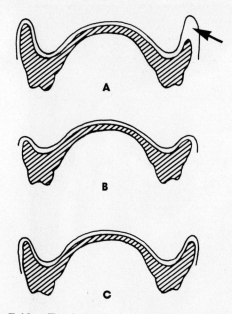

Fig. 7-10   The buccal vestibule. **A,** High; **B,** low; **C,** medium. *Arrow* denotes the space improperly filled by the denture base, with a consequent loss of tissue coverage and border seal.

distal to the buccal notch can cause dislodgment of the denture when the cheeks are moved posteriorly as in a broad smile.

Buccal vestibule

The buccal vestibule is opposite the tuberosity and extends from the buccal frenum to the hamular, or pterygomaxillary, notch (Fig. 7-6, A, 4). This space between the ridge and the the buccal flange of the maxillary denture, which should fill but not overfill it. However, the size of the buccal vestibule varies with the contraction of the buccinator, the position of the mandible, and the amount of bone lost from the maxilla. The thickness of the distal end of the buccal flange of the denture must be adjusted to accommodate the ramus and coronoid process and the masseter as they function. When the mandible moves forward or to the opposite side, the width of the buccal vestibule is reduced. When the masseter contracts under

heavy closing pressures, it also reduces the size of the space available for the distal end of the buccal flange. The extent of the buccal vestibule can be deceiving because the ramus obscures it when the mouth is wide open during examination. Therefore it should be examined with the mouth as nearly closed as possible. This space usually is higher than any other part of the border (Fig. 7-10). The size and shape of the posterior part of the buccal vestibule are altered by the lateral movements of the mandible. The distal end of the flange must not be too thick or the ramus will push the denture out of place during opening or lateral movements of the mandible.

Distal to the buccal frenum, the zygomatic process is often unyielding and needs relief (Fig. 7-4).

Pterygomaxillary (hamular) notch

The hamular notch is situated between the tuberosity of the maxilla and the hamulus of the medial pterygoid plate (Fig. 7-11). It is used as a boundary of the posterior border of the maxillary denture back of the tuberosity. The posterior palatal seal must be placed through the center of the deep part of the hamular notch, since no muscle or ligament is present at a level to prevent the placement of extra pressure.

Palatine fovea region

The foveae palatinae (Figs. 7-12 and 7-24) are indentations near the midline of the palate formed by a coalescence of several mucous gland ducts. They are close to the vibrating line and always in soft tissue, which makes them an ideal guide for the location of the posterior border of the denture.

Vibrating line of the palate

The vibrating line is an imaginary line drawn across the palate that marks the beginning of motion in the soft palate when the patient says "ah." It extends from one pterygomaxillary notch to the other. At the midline it usually passes about 2 mm in front of the foveae palati-

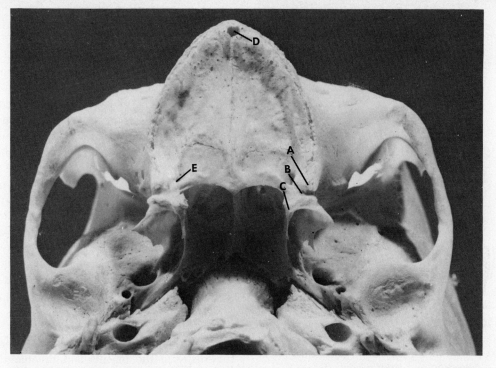

Fig. 7-11 *A,* Maxillary tuberosity; *B,* pterygomaxillary (hamular) notch; *C,* hamular process of the pterygoid plate; *D,* incisive foramen; *E,* greater palatine foramen.

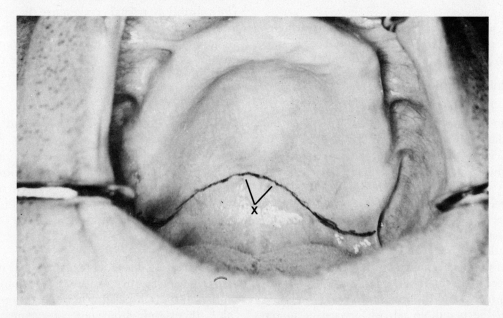

Fig. 7-12 Vibrating line indicated by indelible marks. Notice the two foveae palatinae, *X,* in the middle of the soft palate just behind the marked area.

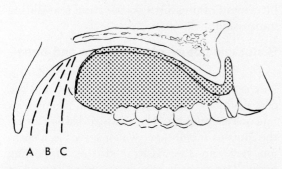

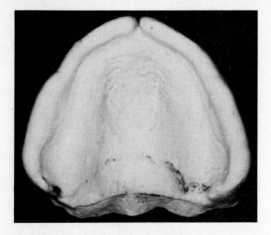

Fig. 7-13 *A,* Soft palate form that allows a broad posterior palatal seal area; *B,* form that allows a medium-width posterior palatal seal area; *C,* form with a very narrow posterior palatal seal area.

Fig. 7-14 The posterior palatal seal on the tray displaces the tissue across the palate on both sides of the vibrating line to form a posterior palatal seal on the denture.

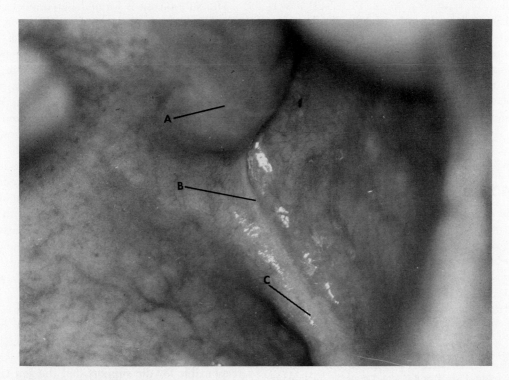

Fig. 7-15 The pterygomandibular raphe, *B,* pulls forward when the mouth is opened wide. *A,* Maxillary tuberosity; *C,* retromolar pad.

nae (Fig. 7-12). The vibrating line is not to be confused with the junction of the hard and soft palates, since the vibrating line is always on the soft palate. This is not a well-defined line and should be described as an area rather than a line. The direction of the vibrating line usually varies according to the shape of the palate (Fig. 7-13); the higher the vault, the more abrupt and forward the vibrating line. In a mouth with a flat vault, the vibrating line is usually farther posterior and has a gradual curvature, affording a broader posterior palatal seal area.

The distal end of the upper denture must extend at least to the vibrating line. In most instances the denture should end 1 or 2 mm posterior to the vibrating line. However, when the anterior teeth are to be placed well anterior to the residual ridge, it may be possible to extend the denture farther posteriorly, provided the patient can tolerate it. The denture must cover the tuberosities and extend into the pterygomaxillary or hamular notches (Fig. 7-14). Overextension at the hamular notches will not be tolerated because of pressure on the pterygoid hamulus and interference with the pterygomandibular raphe, which extends from the hamulus to the top inside back corner of the retromolar pad. When the mouth is opened wide, the pterygomandibular raphe is pulled forward (Fig. 7-15). If the denture is too long at these places, the mucous membrane covering the raphe will be injured by the denture.

MICROSCOPIC ANATOMY*

The clinical procedures used in making impressions are directly related to gross anatomic structures of the oral cavity and their function. However, the response of the individual cellular components that make up the basal seat determines the ultimate success of the dentures in terms of preservation of the residual ridges and comfort to the patient. Thus a constant

awareness of the microscopic anatomy of the mucous membrane and bone that form the residual ridge is essential in the development of border form and length and in the selective placement of pressures on the basal seat during impression making.

Histologic nature of soft tissue and bone

The bones of the upper and lower edentulous jaws are covered with soft tissue, and the oral cavity is lined with soft tissue known as mucous membrane. The denture bases rest on the mucous membrane, which serves as a cushion between the bases and the supporting bone. The mucous membrane is composed of two layers, the mucosa and the submucosa.

The mucosa in the oral cavity is formed by stratified squamous epithelium (often keratinized on its outer surface) and a subjacent narrow layer of connective tissue known as the lamina propria.

The submucosa is formed by connective tissue that varies in character from dense to loose areolar tissue and also varies considerably in its width or thickness, depending on its location in the mouth. The submucosa may contain glandular, fat, or muscle cells and transmits the blood and nerve supply to the mucosa. When the mucous membrane is attached to bone, the attachment occurs between the submucosa and the periosteal covering of the bone.

The nature of the mucous membrane in different parts of the mouth varies between patients and within the same patient. The keratinized layer of the epithelium (stratum corneum) may be totally absent in some instances and extremely thick in others. The presence of dentures in the mouth does not always have the same effect on the amount of keratinization in different patients.

Although the importance of the mucosa (epithelium and lamina propria) from a health standpoint cannot be neglected, the thickness and consistency of the submucosa are largely responsible for the support that the soft tissues (mucous membrane) afford the dentures, since

*We wish to acknowledge the assistance of Dr. Steve Kolas, Professor, Department of Oral Pathology, Medical College of Georgia School of Dentistry, Augusta.

in most instances the submucosa makes up the bulk of the mucous membrane.

In a healthy mouth the submucosa is firmly attached to the periosteum of the underlying bone of the residual ridge and will usually successfully withstand the pressures of dentures. When the submucosal layer is thin over the bone, the soft tissue will be nonresilient and small movements of the dentures will tend to break the retentive seal. When the submucosal layer is loosely attached to the periosteum of the residual ridge or is inflamed or edematous (excess fluid present), the tissue is easily displaceable and the stability and support of the dentures are adversely affected. Impression making often requires modification to accommodate these variations in the submucosa.

The histologic nature of the bone in different parts of the residual ridge also varies between patients and within the same patient. The amount and location of resorption can often be difficult or impossible to predict. Normally certain parts of the jaws are made up of compact bone, as opposed to spongy or trabeculated bone. Impression procedures should take advantage of these differences. A knowledge of the normal microscopic anatomy of the oral cavity can be the key to effective biologic impression procedures.

Classification of oral mucosa

Most classifications divide the oral mucosa into three categories depending on its location in the mouth: masticatory, lining, and specialized mucosa.

In the edentulous patient the *masticatory* mucosa covers (1) the crest of the residual ridge, including the residual attached gingiva firmly adherent to the supporting bone, and (2) the hard palate. Masticatory mucosa is characterized by a well-defined keratinized layer on its outermost surface that is subject to changes in thickness depending on whether dentures are worn and on the clinical acceptability of the dentures.

The *lining* mucosa is generally found to cover the mucous membrane in the oral cavity that is not firmly attached to the periosteum of the bone. The lining mucosa forms the covering of the lips and cheeks, the vestibular spaces, the alveololingual sulcus, the soft palate, the ventral surface of the tongue, and the unattached gingiva found on the slopes of the residual ridges. Lining mucosa is normally devoid of a keratinized layer and is freely movable with the tissues to which it is attached because of the elastic nature of the lamina propria.

The *specialized* mucosa covers the dorsal surface of the tongue. This mucosal covering is keratinized and includes the specialized papillae on the upper surface of the tongue.

Microscopic anatomy of supporting tissues

The microscopic anatomy of the supporting tissues of the upper impression will be described for the crest of the residual ridge, the slopes of the residual ridge, and the palatal tissues.

The mucous membrane covering the crest of the upper residual ridge in a healthy mouth is firmly attached to the periosteum of the bone of the maxillae by the connective tissue of the submucosa (Fig. 7-16). The stratified squamous epithelium is thickly keratinized. The submucosa is devoid of fat or glandular cells, and it thus does not become edematous, but is characterized by dense collagenous fibers that are contiguous with the lamina propria. The submucosal layer, though relatively thin in comparison to other parts of the mouth, is still sufficiently thick to provide adequate resiliency for primary support of the upper denture. The mucous membrane covering the crest of the edentulous ridge is comparable to the attached gingiva in the dentulous mouth, except that the submucosal layer in the edentulous mouth is usually thicker than is found in the attached gingiva of the dentulous mouth.

The outer surface of the bone in the region of the crest of the upper residual ridge may be

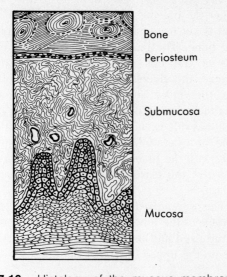

Bone

Periosteum

Submucosa

Mucosa

Fig. 7-16 Histology of the mucous membrane covering the crest of the residual ridge. Notice that the submucosal layer is sufficiently thick to provide resiliency for support of complete dentures and that bone covering the crest of the upper ridge is often compact. Thus the crest is the primary stress-bearing area for an upper denture.

compact in nature, being made up of haversian systems. This compact bone, in combination with the tightly attached mucous membrane, makes the crest of the upper residual ridge histologically best able to provide primary support for the upper denture. One should take advantage of the nature of this tissue when providing for additional stress to be placed on the crest of the ridge of the upper jaw during final impression making.

As the mucous membrane extends from the crest along the slope of the upper residual ridge to the reflection, it tends to lose its firm attachment to the underlying bone. This change marks the end of the residual attached mucous membrane (Fig. 7-17). The more loosely attached mucous membrane in this region has a nonkeratinized or slightly keratinized epithelium, and the submucosa contains loose connective tissue and elastic fibers. This loosely attached tissue will not withstand the forces of mastication or other stress transmitted

through the denture bases and the firmly attached mucous membrane over the crest of the ridge. Less stress is placed on the movable tissue of the slope of the ridge during making of the final impression because the impression material in that region is closer to the escapeways (border of the impression tray) than the material over the crest of the ridge is (Fig. 7-18). This follows the principle that in a semiconfined container, impression material farthest from the escapeways is under the greatest pressure.

The soft tissue covering the hard palate varies considerably in consistency and thickness in different locations even though the epithelium is keratinized throughout. Anterolaterally, the submucosa of the hard palate contains adipose tissue (Fig. 7-19) and posterolaterally it contains glandular tissue (Fig. 7-20). These tissues should be recorded in a resting condition, because when they are displaced in the final impression they tend to return to normal form within the completed denture base, creating an unseating force on the denture or causing soreness in the patient's mouth. Proper relief of the final impression tray aids in recording these tissues in an undistorted form. In addition, the secretions from the palatal glands can be an important factor in the selection of the final impression material.

The submucosa in the region of the median palatal suture of the maxillary bones is extremely thin. The mucosal layer is practically in contact with the underlying bone (Fig. 7-21). For this reason, the soft tissue covering the median palatal suture is nonresilient. Little or no stress can be placed in this region during the making of the final impression or in the completed denture lest the denture tend to rock over the center of the palate when vertical forces are applied to the teeth. In addition, this part of the mouth is highly sensitive, and excess pressure can create excruciating pain. Proper relief in the impression tray or the completed denture is essential for accommodation of the histologic nature of this tissue.

Histologic section through the incisive pa-

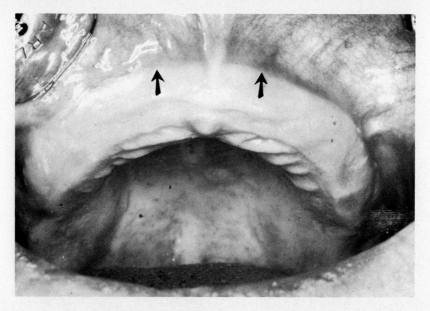

Fig. 7-17 *Arrows* denote the line of demarcation between the attached and unattached residual mucous membrane. Attached mucous membrane is desirable for support of complete dentures; however, the peripheral area is what contributes to the denture's seal. Notice the prominent incisive papilla anteriorly at the center of the residual alveolar ridge. It overlies the incisive foramen.

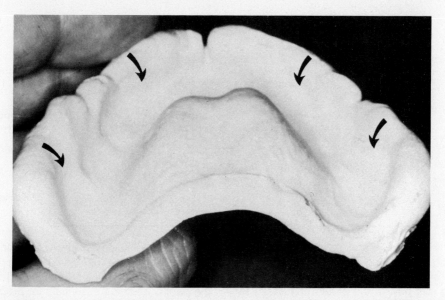

Fig. 7-18 Impression material near the borders of the impression tray *(arrows)* can flow out of the tray relatively easily during making of a final impression. Thus less pressures are placed on tissues near the borders of the impression than on the crest of the ridge during making of a final impression. This is desirable.

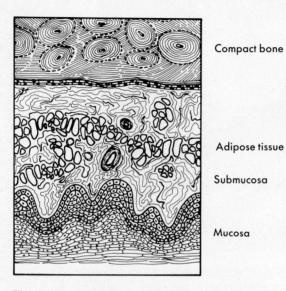

Compact bone

Adipose tissue

Submucosa

Mucosa

Fig. 7-19 Histology of the mucous membrane in the anterolateral part of the hard palate. Notice that the submucosa contains abundant adipose tissue.

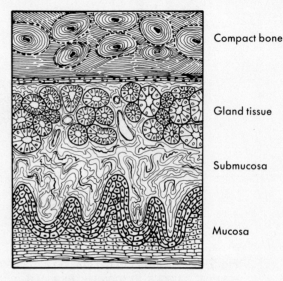

Compact bone

Gland tissue

Submucosa

Mucosa

Fig. 7-20 Histology of the mucous membrane in the posterolateral hard palate. Notice the abundant glandular tissue.

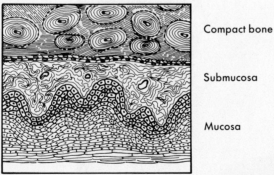

Compact bone

Submucosa

Mucosa

Fig. 7-21 Histology of the mucous membrane covering the median palatal suture. The submucosal layer is thin or may be practically nonexistent, making this part of the mouth unsuitable for support of an upper denture.

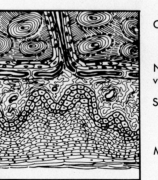

Compact bone

Nasopalatine vessel and nerve

Submucosa

Mucosa

Fig. 7-22 Histology of the region near the incisive papilla. Notice the nasal palatine vessels and nerves contained in the submucosa. The nature of the papilla makes it essential that proper relief be provided in the completed denture.

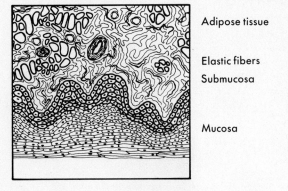

Adipose tissue

Elastic fibers
Submucosa

Mucosa

Fig. 7-23   Histology of the mucous membrane lining the vestibules. The loose areolar tissue and elastic fibers in the submucosa permit a relatively large movement of the tissues at the reflection.

pilla and the nasopalatine canal will reveal that the submucosa contains the nasopalatine vessels and nerves (Fig. 7-22). Relief should be provided for the incisive papilla in both the final impression and the completed denture to prevent pressure on the nasopalatine vessels and nerves.

Microscopic anatomy of limiting structures

The microscopic anatomy of the limiting tissues of the upper denture will be described for the vestibular spaces, the hamular notches, and the posterior palatal seal area in the region of the vibrating line.

A histologic section of the mucous membrane lining the vestibular spaces depicts a relatively thin epithelium that is nonkeratinized. The submucosal layer is thick and contains large amounts of loose areolar tissue and elastic fibers (Fig. 7-23). The nature of the submucosa in the vestibular spaces makes this tissue easily movable. Thus the labial or buccal flanges of the upper impression can easily be overextended or underextended. A knowledge of the size of the space in the vestibule available for dentures is the key to proper determination of the length and form of the flange. The procedures for molding the borders of an impression to allow for natural muscle activity in the lips and cheeks are important in the development of properly formed flanges that will be in har-

mony with the histologic limitations of these tissues.

The submucosa in the region of the vibrating line on the soft palate contains glandular tissue similar to that in the submucosa in the posterolateral part of the hard palate (Fig. 7-24). However, because the soft palate does not rest directly on bone, the tissue for a few millimeters on both sides of the vibrating line can be repositioned in the impression to improve the posterior palatal seal. The secretion of the palatal glands during making of the final impressions can affect the choice of impression material.

The submucosa of the mucous membrane contained within the hamular notch (the space between the posterior part of the maxillary tuberosity and the pterygoid hamulus) is thick and made up of loose areolar tissue (Fig. 7-25). Additional pressure also can be placed on this tissue at the center of the notch to complete the posterior palatal seal. Space is provided in the final impression tray except in the region of the vibrating line and through the hamular notches before the final impression is made. Thus the tray itself contacts the soft tissue in this region when the impression is made (Fig. 7-26). In this manner, additional pressure by the denture can be placed on these palatal tissues because the histologic nature of the mucous membrane allows it to be displaced without trauma.

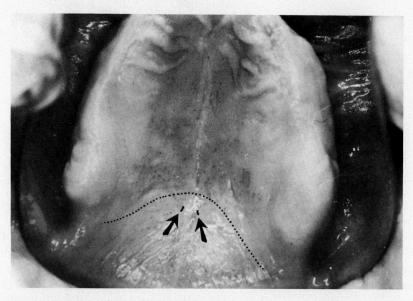

Fig. 7-24 *Dotted line* indicates the approximate location of the vibrating line, which is the first point of movement of the soft palate in relation to the hard palate. *Arrows* point to the foveae palatinae (accentuated by *black marks*). Notice that the reflections posteriorly follow the curvature of the maxillary tuberosities and blend into the hamular notches. This anatomic form should be incorporated into the borders of the impression.

Fig. 7-25 Histology of the mucous membrane in the hamular notch. The loose areolar connective tissue in the submucosa can be displaced without trauma by the complete denture to improve the posterior palatal seal.

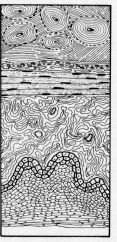

Compact bone

Tensor veli palatini tendon

Loose areolar connective tissue

Mucosa

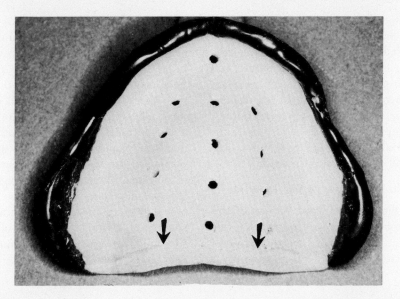

Fig. 7-26   The posterior part of the impression tray *(arrows)* contacts and displaces the soft tissue in the region of the vibrating line and hamular notches during making of the final impression to develop a posterior palatal seal. Space has been provided in the remainder of the tray for final impression material. Holes have been drilled to avoid any buildup of pressure from trapped impression material in the center of the tray.

CLINICAL CONSIDERATIONS OF MICROSCOPIC ANATOMY

A knowledge of the microscopic anatomy of the oral mucous membrane has direct clinical implications for dentists and directly affects their success when they treat edentulous patients.

Histologic studies of the effect of wearing dentures on the keratinization of the mucosa of the crest of the residual ridges and the palate have produced conflicting results. However, most studies indicate that wearing dentures does not seem to be harmful to the epithelium even though keratinization is of reduced thickness and the stratum corneum is thinner in patients who wear them. Cytologic studies indicate that increased amounts of keratinized material are present in edentulous ridges when the clinical quality of the dentures is good, an indication that good-fitting dentures may be important in maintaining the normal histologic condition of the mouth. Stimulation of the mu-

cosa of the residual ridge through toothbrush physiotherapy also increases the presence of keratinized material. Histologically, removing the dentures from the mouth for 6 to 8 hours a day, preferably during periods of sleep, allows keratinization to increase and the signs of inflammation, often found in the submucosa when dentures are worn, to be dramatically reduced.

The aging process is accountable for a number of important unfavorable histologic changes in the oral mucous membrane. Nerves in the mucous membrane of the residual ridges in elderly edentulous persons are greatly reduced, and those present are confined mostly to the lamina propria adjacent to the underlying bone. Alveolar and gingival arteries show signs of sclerosis. Age also plays a major role in the ability of the oral mucous membrane to recover from compression loading caused by pressures from the denture base. In the child or young person, recovery of deformed mucosa occurs in terms of seconds whereas in the elderly person it may require hours or eventually result in irreversible changes. The immediate changes in the form of the supporting mucous membrane by pressures from the denture base seriously compromise correction of the occlusion of dentures in the patient's mouth or correction of parts of final impressions by the addition of impression material directly to the defect rather than a remaking of the total impression.

Cross-sectional anatomy of the maxillae

A study of the soft and hard tissues of the edentulous mouth in cross section reveals many important facts in relation to complete denture construction. The idea is all too prevalent that the bony contours of the ridge are covered with a more or less uniform thickness of soft tissue. The vast difference in depth of tissue in different parts of the palate may not be abnormal. A comparison of the bony outline with the soft-tissue outline will usually show a moderate amount of fibrous connective tissue over the crest of the ridge and an increasing depth of glandular tissue toward the higher portion of the vault, with a decreasing amount of submucosal tissue over the median suture of the maxillary bones. This tissue has (1) a layer of epithelium, (2) a layer of fibrous and loose connective tissue, (3) a layer of glandular tissue, and (4) periosteum that attaches these tissues to the bone.

CHAPTER 8

Maxillary impression procedures

The capability of the mucous membrane of the basal seat to withstand stress from the denture base varies greatly because of the histologic makeup of different parts of the residual ridge. For example, the crest of the healthy maxillary residual ridge is often designated as a primary or major stress-bearing area for dentures because the submucosa is formed by a layer of thick fibrous connective tissue that is attached firmly to compact bone. This combination provides favorable support for the denture. On the other hand, the much thinner nonresilient mucous membrane and underlying bone of the median palatal suture often requires relief for the denture base. Because of these variations, impressions of edentulous ridges must selectively place pressures on the mucous membrane and bone in amounts that are compatible with the histologic tolerances of the supporting tissues for each patient. When this important biologic principle is violated, dentures lose retention, stability, and support; create soreness; or cause resorption of the underlying bone. It becomes obvious that for successful treatment to occur the dentist must (1) understand the histology and pathology of the living tissues that make up the basal seat and (2) use a clinical technique in making impressions that will selectively distribute pressures to the basal seat to meet the needs of each edentulous patient.

PRINCIPLES AND OBJECTIVES OF IMPRESSION MAKING

The basic objective of a maxillary or mandibular impression is to record all the potential denture bearing surface available. To a large extent this surface is readily identified if the biologic considerations of impression making are correctly understood. However, the denture's retention is enhanced considerably if the denture extends peripherally to harness the resiliency of most of the surrounding limiting structures. Therefore clinical techniques and, above all, judgment must be reconciled if the objectives of impression making are to be fulfilled.

Although impression techniques, methods, and materials of choice are constantly changing, they nevertheless should be selected on the basis of biologic factors. Techniques too often follow shortcuts, perhaps to satisfy the patient's desire for immediate results, without a consideration of the future destruction that such procedures may induce.

The objectives of an impression are to provide retention, stability, and support for the denture. An impression also may act as a foundation for improved lip esthetics and at the same time should maintain the health of the oral tissues.

Retention for a denture is its resistance to removal in a direction opposite that of its insertion. It is the quality inherent in a denture that resists the force of gravity, the adhesiveness of foods, and the forces associated with the opening of the jaws. Retention is the means by which dentures are held in position in the mouth. When the soft tissues over the bones are displaced under pressure, the denture bases may lose their retention because of the change in adaptation of the basal surface of the denture to its basal seat.

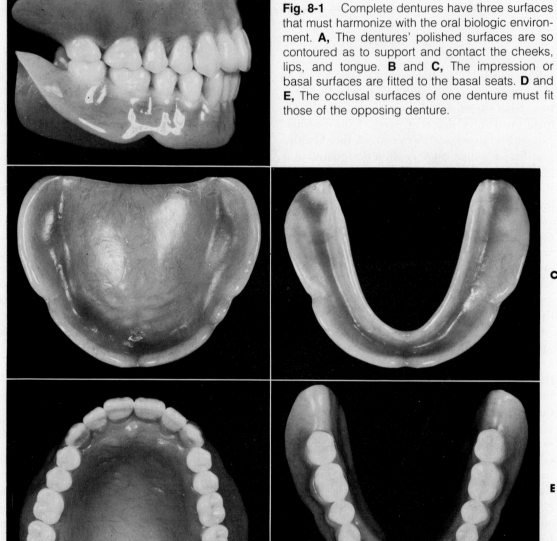

Fig. 8-1 Complete dentures have three surfaces that must harmonize with the oral biologic environment. **A,** The dentures' polished surfaces are so contoured as to support and contact the cheeks, lips, and tongue. **B** and **C,** The impression or basal surfaces are fitted to the basal seats. **D** and **E,** The occlusal surfaces of one denture must fit those of the opposing denture.

Stability of a denture is its quality of being firm, steady, and constant in position when forces are applied to it. Stability refers especially to resistance against horizontal movement and forces that tend to alter the relationship between the denture base and its supporting foundation in a horizontal or rotatory direction. The size and form of the basal seat, the quality of the final impressions, the form of the polished surfaces, and the proper location and arrangement of the artificial teeth play a major role in the stability of the dentures (Figs. 8-1 and 8-2).

Support is the resistance of a denture to the vertical components of mastication and to occlusal or other forces applied in a direction toward the basal seat. Support is provided by the maxillary and mandibular bones and their covering of mucosal tissues. It is enhanced by selective placement of pressures that are in harmony with the resiliency of the tissues that make up the basal seat (see Fig. 7-3).

Biologic principles of tissue health must be adhered to before a final impression is made. These principles were described in Chapter 7. The following concepts incorporated in any impression procedure will enhance the retention, stability, and support of a denture (which are all interrelated features):

1. The impression extends to include all of the basal seat within the limits of the health and functions of the supporting and limiting tissues.
2. The borders are in harmony with the anatomic and physiologic limitations of the oral structures.
3. A physiologic type of border-molding procedure is performed by the dentist or by the patient under the guidance of the dentist.
4. Proper space for the selected final impression material is provided within the impression tray.
5. Selective pressure is placed on the basal seat during the making of the final impression.
6. The impression can be removed from the

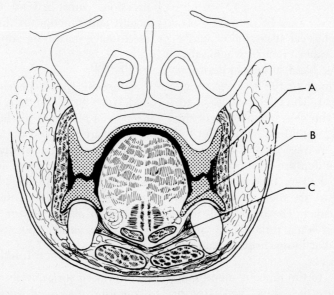

Fig. 8-2 Frontal section showing dentures properly filling the available space. *A,* The buccinator. *B,* The lingual flange and border are placed under the tongue. *C,* The mylohyoid. Notice that both upper and lower dentures are so shaped that the action of the tongue and cheeks tends to seat rather than unseat them. If posterior artificial teeth are too wide buccolingually, the form of the dentures will be changed and the tongue and cheeks will tend to unseat them.

mouth without damage to the mucous membrane of the residual ridge.

7. A guiding mechanism is provided for correct positioning of the impression tray in the mouth.
8. The tray and final impression are made of dimensionally stable materials.
9. The external shape of the final impression is similar to the external form of the completed denture.

The two most important factors in making satisfactory impressions for complete dentures are a properly formed and accurately fitting final impression tray and proper positioning of the final impression tray on the basal seat in the mouth.

FACTORS OF RETENTION OF DENTURES

A number of forces and factors combine to retain complete dentures in the mouth. Not all these factors act at the same time. Instead, some act only when they are needed to meet or resist a certain dislodging force.

Adhesion

Adhesion is the physical attraction of unlike molecules for each other. It acts when saliva wets and sticks to the basal surface of dentures and, at the same time, to the mucous membrane of the basal seat. The effectiveness of adhesion depends on the close adaptation of the denture base to the supporting tissues and the fluidity of the saliva. A watery saliva is quite effective, provided the denture base material can be "wetted." Some denture base materials allow water (or saliva) to stick to them and spread out in a thin layer. These materials have greater potential for being retained by adhesion than materials that cause drops of water to form over their surfaces.

Adhesion of saliva to the mucous membrane is no problem because the saliva "wets" it very effectively. Saliva that is thick and ropy adheres well to both the denture base and the mucosa; but since much of it is produced by the palatal glands under the maxillary basal

seat, it builds up and literally pushes the denture out of position. The forces of adhesion still act on both surfaces, but the hydraulic pressure produced by the thick mucus secretions may overpower them.

Adhesion is also the molecular attraction between the surfaces of unlike bodies in contact. This type of adhesion is observed between denture bases and the mucous membranes of patients with xerostomia. The denture base materials seem to stick to the dry mucous membrane of the basal seat and of the cheeks and lips. Such adhesion is not very affective for retaining dentures, and it is annoying to patients when it sticks the denture base to the cheeks and lips. A mouthwash of Cepacol and glycerin can be helpful in this situation.

The amount of retention supplied by adhesion is directly proportionate to the area covered by the denture. Patients with small jaws (basal seats) cannot expect retention by adhesion to be as effective as patients with large jaws can. Thus the dentures (and hence the impressions) must extend to the limits of the health and function of the oral tissues if they are to have maximum adhesion and retention.

Cohesion

Cohesion is the physical attraction of like molecules for each other. It is a retentive force because it occurs in the layer of saliva between the denture base and the mucosa. It is effective in direct proportion to the area covered by the denture, if other factors are equal. Since saliva is a liquid, the layer of saliva must be thin if it is to be effective for retention. Therefore the adaptation of the denture base to the mucosa must be as close as possible.

Interfacial surface tension

Interfacial surface tension is the resistance to separation possessed by the film of liquid between two well-adapted surfaces. It is found in the thin film of saliva between the denture base and the mucosa of the basal seat and is quite similar in its action to cohesion and to capillary attraction, or capillarity. It is also effective in direct proportion to the size of the basal surface of dentures, if other things are equal. One of its requirements is minimal distortion or displacement of the soft tissues by the impression and, of course, the denture. A perfect fit is essential.

Capillary attraction

Capillary attraction, or capillarity, is a force (developed because of surface tension) that causes the surface of a liquid to become elevated or depressed when it is in contact with a solid. It is what causes a liquid to rise in a capillary tube, since surface tension tends to form a round surface on the liquid. When the adaptation of the denture base to the mucosa on which it rests is sufficiently close, the space filled with a thin film of saliva acts like a capillary tube and helps retain the denture. This force, like the others, is directly proportionate to the area of the basal seat covered by the denture base.

Atmospheric pressure

Atmospheric pressure can act to resist dislodging forces applied to dentures. It has been called "suction" because it is a resistance to the removal of dentures from their basal seat; but there is no suction, or negative pressure, except when another force is applied. Atmospheric pressure itself is supplied by the weight of the atmosphere, and it amounts to 14.7 lb/in^2. This means that the retentive force supplied by atmospheric pressure is directly proportionate to the area covered by the denture base. For atmospheric pressure to be effective, the denture must have a perfect seal around its entire border. Atmospheric pressure is an "emergency" retentive force. If the other retentive forces are being overpowered, atmospheric pressure may be able to keep a denture in position. Suction alone applied to the soft tissues of the oral cavity for even a short time would cause serious damage to the health of the soft tissues under negative pressure.

Oral and facial musculature

The oral and facial musculature can supply supplementary retentive forces, provided (1) the teeth are positioned in the neutral zone between the cheeks and tongue and (2) the polished surfaces of the dentures are properly shaped. This is not to say that patients must hold their teeth in place by conscious effort, only that the shape of the buccal and lingual flanges must make it possible for the musculature to fit automatically against the denture and reinforce the border seal (Figs. 8-1 and 8-2). If the buccal flanges of the maxillary denture slope up and out from the occlusal surfaces of the teeth and the buccal flanges of the mandibular denture slope down and out from the occlusal plane, the contraction of the buccinators will tend to seat both dentures on their basal seats.

The lingual surfaces of the lingual flanges should slope toward the center of the mouth so the tongue can fit against them and perfect the border seal on the lingual side of the denture. The base of the tongue is guided on top of the lingual flange by the lingual side of the distal end of the flange, which turns laterally toward the ramus. This part of the denture also helps perfect the border seal at the back end of mandibular dentures. All this reinforcement is automatic, without conscious effort on the part of the patient.

The base of the tongue serves also as an emergency retentive force for some patients. It rises up at the back and presses against the distal border of a maxillary denture during incision of food by the anterior teeth. This is done without conscious effort when the experienced denture wearer bites into an apple or sandwich or other food. It is seldom that a patient needs to be told how to do this. For the oral and facial musculature to be most effective in providing retention for complete dentures, the following conditions must be met: (1) denture bases must be properly extended to cover the maximum area possible without interfering in the health and function of the structures that surround the denture; (2) the occlusal plane must be at the correct level; and (3) the arch form of the teeth must be in the neutral zone between the tongue and cheeks.

HEALTH OF THE BASAL SEAT TISSUES

It is essential that the oral tissues be healthy before impressions are made. A careful diagnosis will reveal pathosis in the oral cavity of a startling number of edentulous patients who wear dentures. In a study of responses to variations in denture techniques, 41 of 64 edentulous denture-wearing patients selected from the general population required special treatment to restore abused oral tissues to a healthy condition. Oral lesions and their causes must be treated before impressions are considered. Simple observation of the oral mucosa provides important information about the health of the tissues. Some conditions require immediate attention before impressions are made.

Inflammation of the mucosa. Because of the nature of inflammation, the soft tissues are not their natural size. The swelling, which is a characteristic result of inflammation from either trauma or disease, changes the gross form of the surface to be recorded in the impression. All inflammation must be eliminated before the new impressions are made lest the new dentures not fit the tissues after they are no longer distorted by the swelling. Treatment is accomplished by surgery or proper medication or by keeping the old dentures out of the mouth until the tissues are healthy. Soft resin treatment (tissue-conditioning) materials may be used in the old dentures to reduce the period in which the dentures must be left out of the mouth (Chapter 6). However, the old dentures must be kept out of the mouth at least 24 hours before the impressions are made.

Distortion of the denture-foundation tissues. The denture that the patient is wearing may appear to have good retention and stability, but at the same time it may not fit the true form of the oral structures. In such a situation, the denture has molded the soft tissues to its own shape. This molding may have progressed slowly over a period of years, and the patient's resistance may have been such that little or no inflammation occurred in the process. The distortion of the oral tissues can be corrected when the old dentures are left out of the mouth for 1, 2, or more days before the impressions are made. A combination of leaving the dentures out and the use of conditioning materials that allow tissues to assume more normal form within the confines of the denture base can be an effective treatment. Some patients will object to leaving their dentures out of the mouth, but their objections can be overcome by careful explanation, insistence by the dentist, use of conditioning material, and selection of a convenient time for scheduling their appointments.

Excessive amounts of hyperplastic tissue. Since the maxillae and the mandible (the bones) are the real foundations for dentures, their soft tissue covering must be firm. Excessive amounts of movable soft tissue will permit the dentures to move in relation to the bone, and many types of difficulties (such as looseness, tipping, malocclusion of the dentures, and difficulty in recording jaw relations accurately) may result. The best treatment is finger massage on a daily basis or surgical removal of the hyperplastic tissue followed by sufficient time for complete healing. The apparent ridge size can be reduced by this procedure, but the real foundation will be the same size and much more effective (Chapter 6).

Insufficient space between the upper and lower ridges. Usually the insufficient space is found in the tuberosity region. It may be caused by an excessive amount of fibrous connective tissue covering the tuberosity (Fig. 3-9), which will be disclosed by dental radiographs. Intraoral radiographs or small dental films are more effective than panoramic radiographs for this purpose (Chapter 6). Mounted diagnostic casts will disclose potential interference by the excess fibrous tissue over the tuberosities with the correct location of the occlusal plane. This determination should be made before the impressions are started. Excess fibrous tissue should be removed surgically, and time allowed for complete healing before impressions are made.

IMPRESSIONS FOR THE EDENTULOUS PATIENT

Impressions are made with many types of materials and techniques. Some materials are more fluid than others before they harden or set. The softer materials displace soft tissues less and require less force in their molding than do materials that flow more sluggishly. These variations in the working properties of materials make it possible to devise many types of techniques for controlling the position and shape of the oral tissues. Some techniques are intended to record the shape of the tissues with a minimum of displacement; others are intended to displace the border tissues to a predetermined extent. Still others are devised to obtain the advantages of placement or control of the border tissues with a minimal displacement of the tissues under the denture. The choice is made by the dentist on the basis of the oral conditions, concept of the function of the tissues surrounding the denture, and ability to handle the available impression materials.

Impression trays

Regardless of the type of impression being made, the tray is the most important part of the impression-making procedure. If it is too large, it will distort the tissues around the borders of the impression and will pull the soft tissues under the impression away from the bone. If it is too small, the border tissues will collapse inward onto the residual ridge. This will reduce the support for the denture and prevent the proper support of the lips by the denture flange.

A properly formed tray can carry the impression material to the mouth and control it without distorting the soft tissues that surround it.

An improperly formed tray will make impossible the registration of the true negative form of the basal seat tissues on which the denture must rest. The tray must not distort or displace the tissues and structures that are to fit against the borders and polished surfaces of the denture.

"Individual" or "custom" trays are made of different materials (usually acrylic resin) with borders that can be adjusted so they control the movable soft tissues around the impression but do not distort them. At the same time space is provided inside the tray so the shape of the tissues covering the residual alveolar ridge may be recorded with minimal or selective displacement.

The next most important part of impression making, after the tray, is proper positioning of the tray on the basal seat in the mouth. This is best accomplished by using guiding factors incorporated into the tray and by practicing proper placement of the tray in the mouth before actually making the final impression.

Final impression materials

Many different types of materials have been used successfully for making final impressions.

Plaster of Paris, zinc oxide–eugenol paste, irreversible hydrocolloid, silicone, polysulfide rubber, polyether, and tissue-conditioning material have been used for this purpose. Each has its advantages and its disadvantages.

The setting time of plaster of Paris must be accelerated and is often modified so the molding time will be increased. It absorbs some of the mucous secretions from the palate while it sets, but requires the use of a separating medium before the cast is formed in it. Plaster of Paris has enough body to support itself up to 1.5 mm beyond the border of a tray.

Zinc oxide–eugenol paste accurately records surface detail and does not require a separating medium. It does not absorb the mucous secretions that are produced in the palate and can cause defects in the palatal part of the impression. The borders of the tray must be accurately formed because the material is fluid. The borders of the tray should be so adjusted that they reach to within 1 mm of the reflecting tissues.

The irreversible hydrocolloids record detail accurately if they are properly controlled and confined, and they do not require the use of a separating medium. They do not absorb the mucous secretions from the palate, which can produce defects in the palatal part of the impression. However, because the irreversible hydrocolloids lose moisture and consequently change their size so rapidly, the casts must be poured into them immediately or the record will be distorted. The weight of the artificial stone of the cast may be sufficient to distort the borders of the impressions, and removal of the impressions from the mouth without distortion presents some difficulties.

Tissue-conditioning materials have been shown to be sufficiently accurate for making final impressions. They are resilient and continue to flow under stress for periods of up to 24 hours. They are useful for making functional impressions that record the basal seat and border tissues in their functional state.

The silicone, polysulfide rubber, and polyether impression materials can record the shape of the soft tissues accurately if they are adequately supported by the tray. The polysulfide rubbers must be closely confined to the soft tissues, lest they produce an inaccurate impression. They are particularly useful for making impressions of thin high mandibular ridges with soft tissue undercuts. The elasticity of the rubber and its tear strength, which is higher than that of silicone or polysulfide materials, allow the impression to be removed from the cast without fracture of the delicate ridge on the cast. The polyether impression materials (1) have sufficient body to make up discrepancies between tray borders and the reflecting vestibular tissues of up to 4 or 5 mm, (2) can be shaped by the fingers, and (3) are accurate in reproducing detail. Since these materials are

opaque, however, it is more difficult to detect pressure spots in the impressions than it is with other impression materials. Pressure spots are places where the tray shows through the impression material, and they indicate a displacement of tissues by pressure from the tray.

IMPRESSION TECHNIQUES

Three techniques are described in this chapter. They are all variations on a theme: the use of custom-made impression trays. The first and second techniques involve making a preliminary impression in a stock metal tray with alginate (irreversible hydrocolloid) impression material. The final impression is then made in a border-molded special tray. In the first technique a thermoplastic material is used for border molding. In the second technique a polyether impression procedure is used. In the third technique a custom tray is made from a stone cast that has been poured from the patient's "corrected" or improved previously worn complete denture.

The same diagnostic and treatment-planning procedures are followed for each patient regardless of the impression technique. Proper preparation of the oral tissues is essential and is completed as described previously.

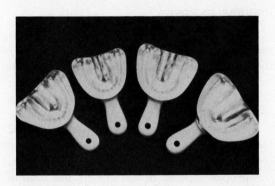

Fig. 8-3   Selection of different sizes of properly designed stock metal trays for maxillary impressions.

First technique—border-molded special tray

Preliminary impression. The space available in the mouth for the upper impression is studied carefully by observation of the width and height of the vestibular spaces with the mouth partway open and the upper lip held *slightly* outward and downward.

An edentulous stock metal tray that is approximately ¼ inch (6 mm) larger than the outside surface of the upper residual ridge is selected (Fig. 8-3). The dentist places the tray in

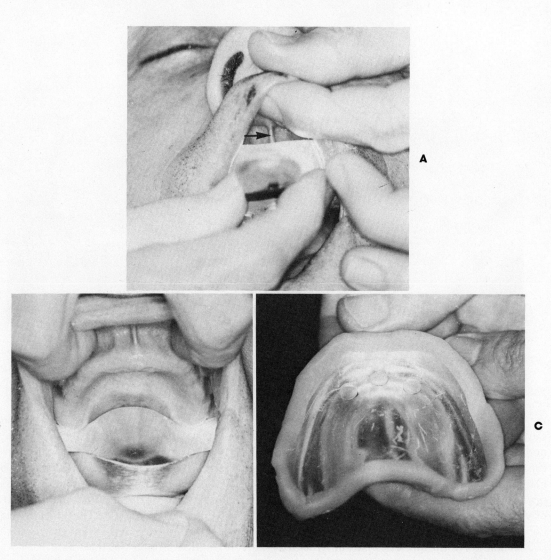

Fig. 8-4   A stock metal tray must be of proper size and must be correctly positioned in the mouth. **A,** The tray is inserted and centered by positioning the labial notch over the labial frenum (*arrow*). **B,** The tray covers the hamular notches and the vibrating line posteriorly. **C,** A strip of boxing wax lines the borders of the tray.

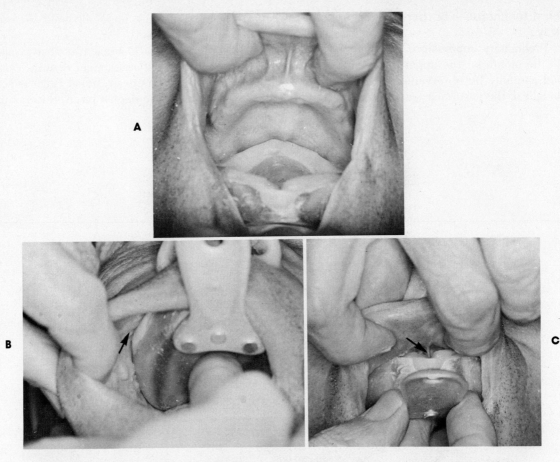

Fig. 8-5 **A,** Wax across the posterior border of the tray is adapted to the tissue of the posterior palatal seal area. **B,** Space for the buccal frenum is provided by wax lining the tray (*arrow*). **C,** Space for the labial frenum is also provided (*arrow*).

the mouth and initially positions it by centering the labial notch of the tray over the labial frenum (Fig. 8-4, *A*). The posterior extent of the tray relative to the posterior palatal seal area is maintained, and then the handle is dropped downward to permit visual inspection. Posteriorly the tray must include both the hamular notches and the vibrating line (Fig. 8-4, *B*).

The borders of the stock tray are lined with a strip of soft boxing wax so a rim is created to help confine the alginate (irreversible hydrocolloid) impression material (Fig. 8-4, *C*). The tray is returned to the mouth, and the wax across

its posterior border is adapted to the tissue of the posterior palatal seal area by careful elevation of the tray in this region with the anterior part of the tray in the proper position (Fig. 8-5, *A*). Again the borders of the tray are observed visually relative to the limiting anatomic structures (Fig. 8-5, *B* and *C*). The objective is to obtain a preliminary impression that is slightly overextended around the borders.

Before making the preliminary impression, the dentist should practice placing the preliminary tray in position on the upper residual ridge. The tray is first centered below the up-

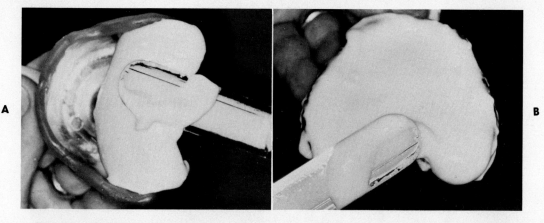

Fig. 8-6   A, Impression material is placed in the tray from the posterior border. **B,** The impression material is evenly distributed throughout the tray, care being taken to prevent air from becoming trapped.

per residual ridge. The upper lip is elevated with the left hand, and the tray is carried upward into position, with the labial frenum used as a centering guide. When the tray is located properly anteriorly, the index fingers are placed in the first molar region on each side of the tray, and with alternating pressure they seat the tray upward until the wax across the posterior part of the tray comes into contact with the tissue in the posterior palatal seal area. The fingers of one hand are shifted into the middle of the tray, and border molding is carried out with the other hand.

The tissue surface and borders of the tray, including the rim of wax, are painted with an adhesive material to ensure that the irreversible hydrocolloid adheres to the tray. The irreversible hydrocolloid is mixed according to manufacturer's instructions and is placed in the tray and evenly distributed to fill the tray to the level of its borders (Fig. 8-6). A small amount of irreversible hydrocolloid is placed in the area of the rugae of the hard palate to help prevent air from being trapped in this part of the preliminary impression (Fig. 8-7, *A*), and the loaded tray is positioned in the mouth in a manner similar to that during the practice sessions (Fig. 8-7, *B* to *D*) The tray is left in the

mouth for 1 minute after the initial set of the irreversible hydrocolloid. The impression is removed from the mouth in one motion and inspected to ensure that all the basal seat is included (Fig. 8-7, *E*).

The dentist should now determine the borders of the custom tray. Two choices are available: (1) the periphery can be outlined with a disposable indelible marker at chairside or (2) the outline can be approximated on the poured cast in the laboratory and the correct location of the tray periphery reassessed when the tray is subsequently tried in the mouth. We recommend that both choices be undertaken. The completed impression is observed next to the patient's mouth, and the junction of attached and unattached mucosal tissue is visually identified on the border of the impression (Fig. 8-8). The accuracy of its location reflects the dentist's understanding of the biologic principles of maxillary impression making. The impression is poured in artificial stone, and the custom tray outline should now be evident on the cast. If the tray outline on the impression is not clearly visible, it can be penciled on the cast. However, then, with the patient not present for a correlation between anatomic features and the inanimate cast, it becomes an educated guess

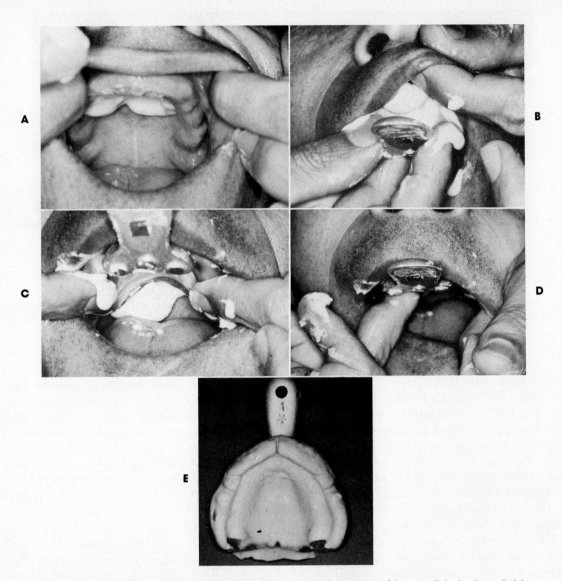

Fig. 8-7 **A,** With a finger the dentist places a small amount of irreversible hydrocolloid on the patient's palate. **B,** The tray, containing the impression material, is carried to position anteriorly. The labial frenum must be carefully observed in relation to the labial notch of the tray. **C,** The tray is seated posteriorly by the index fingers in the region of the first molars. **D,** It is held steadily until the impression material has set. Notice the position of the finger on the palatal part of the tray. **E,** All of the basal seat is included in the preliminary impression. The palatal wax periphery showing through the impression material is not significant, since any displaced tissue at this stage can be corrected in the custom tray. Furthermore, this wax will protect the peripheral tissues from the stock tray's hard edges.

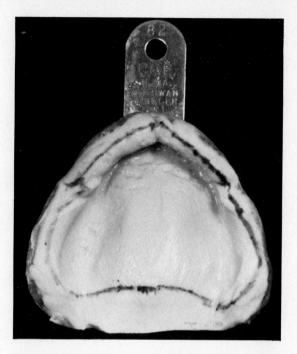

Fig. 8-8 All the basal seat is in the preliminary impression. The clinically determined proposed denture base outline is penciled on with a disposable indelible marker (if possible).

or estimate. A wax spacer is placed within the outlined border to provide space in the tray for the final impression material (Fig. 8-9, *A* and *B*). The posterior palatal seal area on the cast is not covered with the wax spacer. Thus the completed final impression tray will contact the upper residual ridge across the posterior palatal seal, and additional stress can be placed here during the making of the final impression. In addition, this part of the tray will act as a guiding stop to help position the tray properly on the residual ridge during the impression procedure. Baseplate wax approximately 1 mm thick is placed on the cast as designated by the previously drawn outline (Fig. 8-9, *B*).

A self-curing acrylic resin tray material is mixed and uniformly adapted over the cast so the tray will be 2 to 3 mm thick (Fig. 8-9, *C*). A resin handle is attached in the anterior region of the tray to facilitate removal of the final impression. The handle is placed in the approximate position of the upper anterior teeth so it will not distort the upper lip when the tray is in the mouth (Fig. 8-9, *D*). The premise in pre-

scribing a custom tray is that the denture bearing (tissue-contacting) area of the denture will be reflected in the tray's extension at this stage. The next step is to complete the tray for the final impression by developing/confirming the peripheral or sealing part of the tray.

Preparing the final impression tray. When the acrylic resin final impression tray is removed from the preliminary cast, the wax spacer is left inside the tray. The spacer allows the tray to be properly positioned in the mouth during border-molding procedures (Fig. 8-10, *A*).

Border molding is the process by which the shape of the borders of the tray is made to conform accurately to the contours of the buccal and labial vestibules. This essential refinement of the tray's fit ensures an optimal peripheral seal. It has often been erroneously referred to as "muscle trimming."

It begins with manipulation of the border tissues against a moldable impression material that is properly supported and controlled by the tray. The amount of support supplied by

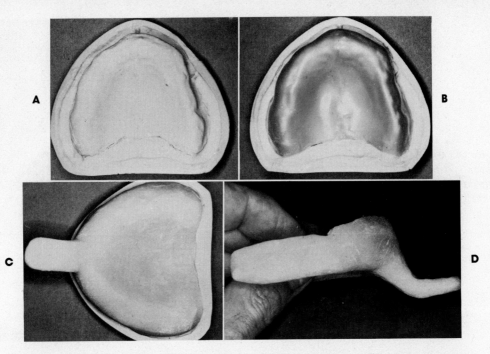

Fig. 8-9 **A,** Outline for the wax spacer drawn in pencil on the cast that was poured in the preliminary impression. **B,** Relief wax covers the basal seat area, except for the labial and buccal reflections and the posterior palatal seal area. The reflections are not covered; thus the proper length and width of the borders of the tray will be maintained as determined by the preliminary impression or as desired. **C,** Final impression tray with self-curing acrylic resin; the resin should be approximately 2 to 3 mm thick. **D,** The handle on the final upper tray should not interfere with the normal position of the upper lip during making of the final impression.

the tray and the amount of force exerted through the tissues vary according to the resistance or viscosity of the impression material.

After the available space for denture flanges is again checked in the patient's mouth, the buccal and labial flanges of the impression tray are marked in pencil and reduced until they are short of the reflections (Fig. 8-10, *B* and *C*).

Stick modeling compound is added in sections to the shortened borders of the resin tray; then the compound is heated with the flame from an alcohol air torch, tempered, and molded in the mouth to a form that will be in harmony with the physiologic action of the lim-

iting anatomic structures. The tray is carefully removed from the mouth, and the modeling compound border is chilled in ice water. The border molding is accomplished in the anterior region when the upper lip is elevated and extended out, downward, and inward (Fig. 8-11, *A* and *B*). In the region of the buccal frenum the cheek is elevated and then pulled outward, downward, and inward and moved backward and forward to simulate movement of the upper buccal frenum. Posteriorly the buccal flange is border molded when the cheek is extended outward, downward, and inward (Fig. 8-11, *C* to *E*).

The posterior palatal seal is formed through

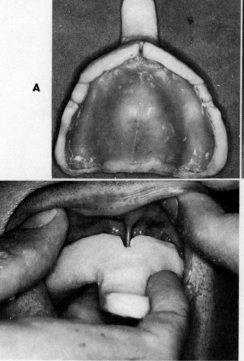

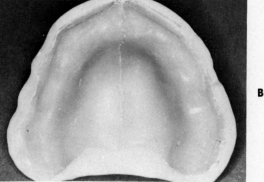

Fig. 8-10   A, The final impression tray covers the entire basal seat area. Its borders have not been molded in harmony with the limiting oral structures and must be corrected. A wax spacer has been left inside the tray to allow the tray to be properly positioned in the mouth during border molding. **B,** The borders of the tray are reduced so modeling compound can be added for border molding. **C,** Notice that space has been created between the borders of the tray and the reflection.

both hamular (pterygomaxillary) notches and across the palate over the vibrating line. The vibrating line is observed in the patient's mouth as the patient says a series of short "ahs," and the hamular notches are palpated. The posterior border of the impression tray is marked with indelible pencil, the palatal tissues are dried quickly, the tray is placed in the mouth, and the patient is again asked to say "ah." The tray is removed from the mouth, and the mark that has been transferred from the tray to the mouth is compared with the vibrating line and the hamular notches (Fig. 8-12, *A* and *B*). The tray must contain both hamular notches and must extend approximately 2 mm posterior to the vibrating line. If it is underextended, the length is corrected by the addition of modeling compound. A strip of low-fusing compound is traced on the impression over the vibrating line and through the hamular

notches. The compound is chilled and then heated with the alcohol torch, tempered, and seated in the mouth under pressure. The added material will spread out on both sides of the vibrating line and form a raised strip across the distal end of the impression (Fig. 8-12, *C*). This will enhance the posterior or palatal seal, which has the three functions: (1) it slightly displaces the soft tissues at the distal end of the denture to enhance the posterior border seal; (2) it serves as a guide for positioning the tray properly for the final impression; and (3) it prevents excess impression material from running down the patient's throat (Fig. 8-12, *C*).

After border molding is completed, the modeling compound forming the labial and buccal borders of the tray is reduced approximately 1 mm to make space for the final impression material. The spacer wax is removed from inside the tray for the same reason. Space must be

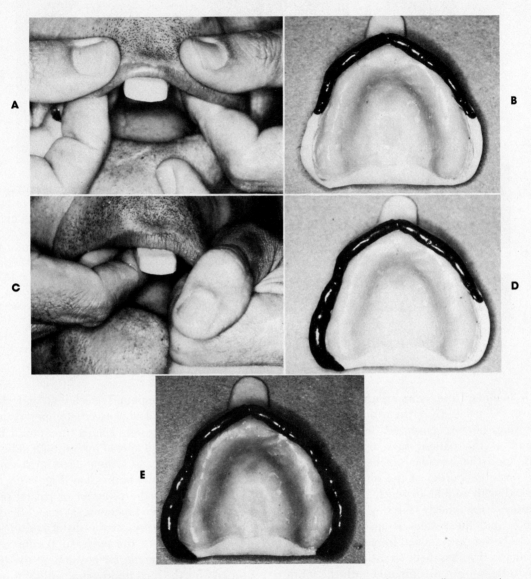

Fig. 8-11 A, Border molding in the anterior region by moving the upper lip outward, downward, and inward. **B,** Modeling compound border molded anteriorly. **C,** The buccal flange is border molded by moving the cheek outward, downward, inward, and backward/forward. **D,** Properly molded border of the left buccal flange. **E,** Completed labial and buccal borders. Notice that the wax spacer has remained inside the tray during the border-molding procedure.

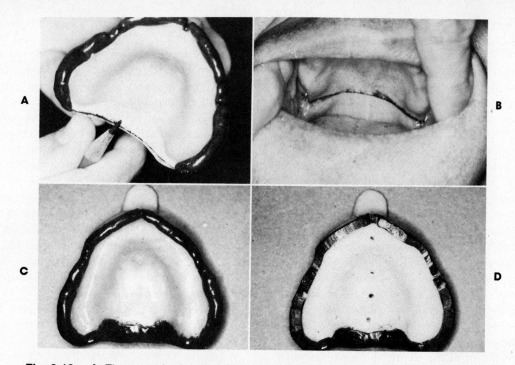

Fig. 8-12   A, The posterior border of the impression tray is marked with indelible pencil to denote its extent over the soft palate in the patient's mouth. **B,** The line has been transferred to the patient's mouth and indicates that the tray includes the vibrating line and both hamular notches posteriorly. **C,** Modeling compound has been added to the posterior border of the final impression tray; it will enhance the posterior palatal seal. The wax spacer is still in place in the tray. **D,** The labial and buccal borders of the tray have been reduced approximately 1 mm for the final impression material. The wax spacer has been removed, and holes have been drilled in the tray to selectively relieve pressure during making of the final impression. The posterior palatal seal remains intact.

provided within the tray for the final impression material. If this is not done, pressure spots will form in the impression. Pressure spots are regions where the tray displaces the soft tissues to be recorded in the impression. These regions of extra pressure will tend to dislodge the denture when it is completed and may impair the health of the tissues with which they come into contact. Holes are placed in the palate of the impression tray with a no. 6 round bur to provide escapeways for the final impression material (Fig. 8-12, *D*). The holes furnish relief during the making of the final upper impres-

sion for the median palatal raphe and in the anterolateral and posterolateral regions of the hard palate.

Making the final upper impression. The soft tissues in the mouth must be rested and healthy before the final impression is made. To allow tissue recovery, the patient *must* leave the old dentures out of the mouth a minimum of 24 hours before the making of the final impression.

Positioning the tray properly in the patient's mouth for the final upper impression is essential to a successful result and can be a difficult procedure. The sequence of steps used requires practice by the dentist for each patient but will help ensure the proper placement of the tray. The practice procedures are performed step by step without final impression material in the tray. First, the dentist centers the tray as it is carried to position on the upper residual ridge by observing the labial frenum going into proper relation to the labial notch (Fig. 8-13, *A*). Then, when the frenum is within 1 to 2 mm of being in the notch, the index fingers of each hand are shifted to the first molar region, and with alternating pressure the tray is carried upward—without displacement of the front end of the tray downward—until the posterior palatal seal of the tray fits properly in the hamular notches and across the palate (Fig. 8-13, *B*). The tray is held in position with a finger placed in the palate immediately anterior to the posterior palatal seal (Fig. 8-13, *C*). The practice procedure with the empty tray is repeated until the dentist feels confident of the proper position of the tray in the mouth.

The final impression material is mixed according to manufacturer's directions and uniformly distributed within the tray. The amount of material used and the spatulation time should be as uniform as possible from mix to mix. This uniformity is essential if the dentist is to become familiar with the working properties of the materials. All borders must be covered. Excess impression material is allowed to run out the posterior border of the tray before the tray is placed in the mouth (Fig. 8-14, *A*). An additional, small, amount of impression material is placed in the central palatal area of the tray to help prevent air from being trapped in this part of the final impression (Fig. 8-14, *B*). The tray is positioned in the mouth in a manner similar to that used during the practice sessions (Fig. 8-14, *C* to *E*).

Border molding is performed in the posterior regions on both sides first and then in the anterior region (Fig. 8-15, *A* to *C*).

When the final impression material has completely set, the cheeks and upper lip are ele-

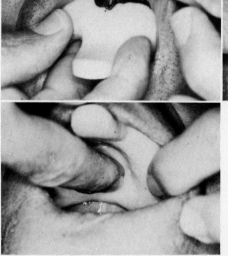

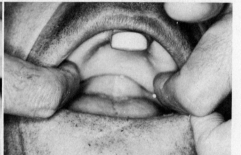

Fig. 8-13   **A,** During practice sessions the tray is centered in the mouth and the labial frenum is guided into the labial notch. **B,** The tray is carried upward and posteriorly until its posterior palatal seal can be seen and felt contacting the posterior palatal seal area in the patient's mouth. **C,** The tray is held in position with a finger placed immediately anterior to the posterior palatal seal.

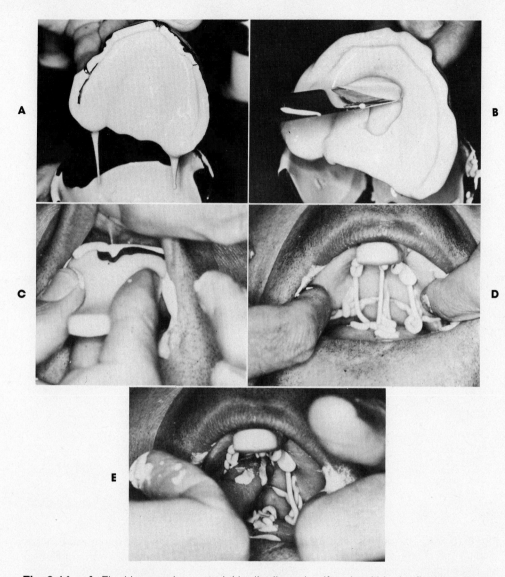

Fig. 8-14   A, Final impression material is distributed uniformly within the final impression tray. Excess is allowed to run out the posterior border of the tray. **B,** A small amount of impression material is added to the center of the tray to reduce the possibility of trapping air in this part of the impression. **C,** The final impression tray is positioned anteriorly by centering the labial notch in relation to the labial frenum. **D,** The posterior palatal seal is guided into position through the hamular notches in the region of the vibrating line by the placement of pressure alternately on each side with fingers in the first molar region of the tray. **E,** The final impression is held in position by a finger immediately anterior to the posterior palatal seal seal.

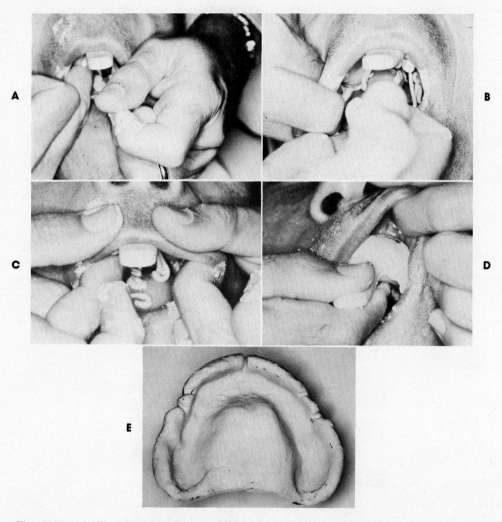

Fig. 8-15 **A,** The dentist molds the left posterior border of the final impression by extending the cheek outward, downward, and inward and moving it backward/forward in the region of the buccal frenum. **B,** The right posterior border of the impression is molded by the same procedures. The upper lip is properly supported by the tray during making of the final impression. **C,** The anterior border of the final impression is molded by moving the upper lip downward and inward with the thumbs. No side-to-side movement of the upper lip is desirable during this procedure. **D,** The upper lip is elevated, and the anterior wax handle is used to remove the final upper impression. **E,** Acceptable final upper impression. The borders are in harmony with the available space in the patient's mouth. There are no undesirable pressure spots. The impression shows that tissues forming the posterior palatal seal area have been placed to enhance the seal at the posterior border.

vated above the borders of the impression to introduce air between the soft tissue at the reflection and the border of the impression. While the lip is elevated, the dentist removes the impression from the mouth by grasping the handle of the tray and gently working the tray downward and forward in the direction of the labial inclination of the residual ridge (Fig. 8-15, *D*).

The impression is inspected for acceptability (Fig. 8-15, *E*). If it needs to be remade, and often this will be true, the impression material is removed, with particular care directed at the borders.

Remaking the final impression. Assuming that the tray was properly formed, faulty positioning is the most frequent reason that a final impression must be remade. A number of reasons for remaking final impressions are described in Chapter 10.

Pouring the cast. A technique for boxing the impression and pouring the cast is described in Chapter 10.

Second technique—one-step border-molded tray

A material that will allow simultaneous molding of all borders has two general advantages: first, the number of insertions of the tray for maxillary and mandibular border molding is reduced to two (a great time and motion saver); second, developing all borders simultaneously avoids propagation of errors caused by a mistake in one section affecting the border contours in another.

The requirements of a material to be used for simultaneous molding of all borders are that it should (1) have sufficient body to allow it to remain in position on the borders during loading of the tray, (2) allow some preshaping of the form of the borders without adhering to the fingers, (3) have a setting time of 3 to 5 minutes, (4) retain adequate flow while the tray is seated in the mouth, (5) allow finger placement of the material into deficient parts after the tray is seated, (6) not cause excessive displacement

of the tissues of the vestibule, and (7) be readily trimmed and shaped so excess material can be carved and the borders shaped before the final impression is made.

Hard acrylic resin and silicone materials have been used for this purpose, and both have serious deficiencies. Hard resins have a long setting time, do not attain proper consistency immediately after mixing (which requires a waiting time before insertion), and are difficult to trim. Also, if insertion is delayed too long, overextension will result. Heavy-bodied silicone materials do not allow preshaping or placement into deficient spaces with a finger after insertion, and they are difficult to trim after setting.

Polyether impression materials[*] meet all the requirements previously listed. They can be shaped with a moist finger in or outside the mouth and can be trimmed with a scalpel or a bur.

The following procedure utilizes polyether impression materials for border molding. It significantly reduces the time required for making impressions and also reduces the amount of motion used by the dentist, thus reducing the psychologic stresses of a busy practice.

Constructing the autopolymerizing acrylic resin impression tray

1. Make a preliminary upper impression, and pour the cast as described in the first technique (p. 177).
2. Construct an autopolymerizing acrylic resin final impression tray on the preliminary cast as in the first technique (p. 181).
3. Reduce the borders of the impression tray until they are 2 mm underextended and confirm the extension of the posterior palatal border (Fig. 8-12, *A* and *B*). Leave the relief wax in the impression tray (Fig. 8-16).

---

[*]Impregum, ESPE–Premier Sales Corporation, Norristown PA, 19401.

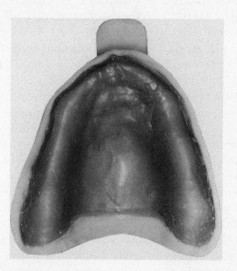

Fig. 8-16 The borders of the acrylic resin tray have been reduced. Relief wax remains inside the impression tray. Notice that it does not cover the borders or the posterior palatal seal area of the tray.

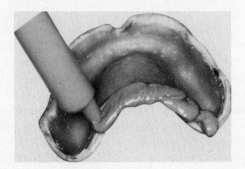

Fig. 8-17 Polyether material is placed across the posterior palatal seal area.

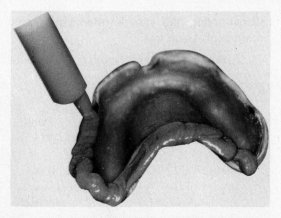

Fig. 8-18 The polyether material is continued around the borders of the impression tray until all have been covered.

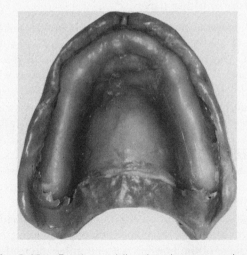

Fig. 8-19 Border molding has been completed, including the posterior palatal seal area. Notice that the relief wax is still in the impression tray.

Border molding the maxillary tray

1. Place adhesive for polyether impressions on the borders of the tray. Cover 6 mm inside the borders and 3 mm outside the borders.

2. Express a 3-inch strip of polyether material from the large tube onto a mixing pad. Next, express 2½ inches of catalyst from the small tube. The reason for using less catalyst than recommended is to provide sufficient working time to complete the border molding.

3. Thoroughly mix the material for 30 to 45 seconds using a metal spatula.

4. Position the polyether material on the borders, making certain that a minimum width of 6 mm exists on the inner portion (Figs. 8-17 and 8-18).

5. Quickly preshape the material to proper contours with fingers moistened in cold water.

6. Place the impression tray in the mouth as described in the first technique, making certain that the lips are sufficiently retracted to avoid scraping the material from the borders (Fig. 8-13).

7. Inspect all borders to be sure that impression material is present in the vestibule. If there is insufficient space, transfer some material from an adjacent site with a finger moistened in the patient's saliva.

8. Border mold as described in the first technique (Fig. 8-15).

9. Remove the tray when the impression material is set. The material is set when no permanent indentation results from a fingernail intruded into it.

10. Examine the border molding to determine that it is adequate (Fig. 8-19). The contour of the borders should be rounded. Any deficient sites can be corrected with a small mix of polyether or an addition of impression compound to adhere to the set polyether. Overexten-

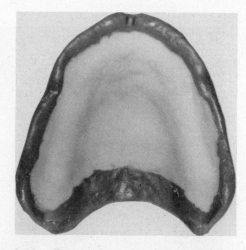

Fig. 8-20   The relief wax has been removed from the tray, and polyether material has been removed from the undercuts. The impression tray is now ready for the final impression.

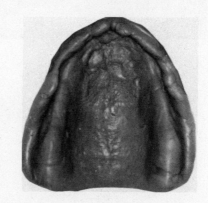

Fig. 8-21   The completed final impression with the one-step border-molded tray.

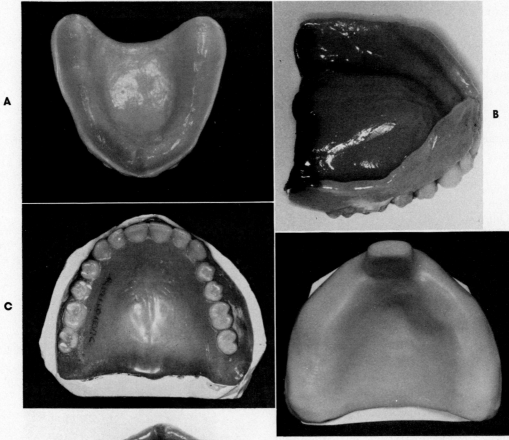

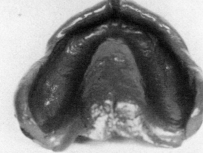

Fig. 8-22 The patient's original denture, **A,** is refitted with a treatment liner, **B,** and poured in laboratory stone, **C.** The optimized denture bearing surface is then covered with an autopolymerized tray, **D,** which is used for the final impression, **E.**

sions are readily detected because the tray will protrude through the polyether.

Preparing the maxillary tray to secure the final impression

1. Reduce the borders on the tray that protrude through the polyether. They indicate overextension or pressure spots. A denture bur can be used for their reduction.
2. Remove any material that extends internally within the tray more than 6 mm. A scalpel works best for this.
3. Remove the relief wax (Fig. 8-20). Heating the wax in warm water will make this easier.
4. Reduce the polyether where it extends into an undercut with a denture bur. This will allow the tray to go into place more easily.
5. Remove any excess material that has flowed onto the external portion of the tray.
6. Reduce the thickness of the labial flange to approximately 2.5 to 3 mm from one buccal frenum to the other.
7. Remove a small amount (about 0.25 mm) of material from borders that have not been previously adjusted. This includes the inner portion, the border, and the outer surface. It will create the necessary space for a thin film of impression material.
8. Make the final impression in silicone, metallic oxide paste, or rubber base (Fig. 8-21). An appropriate adhesive should be added on the impression surface of the tray when silicone material is being used.

Third technique—custom tray design based on the previously worn denture

Clinical experience has shown that a large number of edentulous patients seeking treatment with complete dentures are already wearing or possess complete dentures. Although these may need replacement for a number of reasons, they can usually be converted to adequate provisional prostheses by means of adjustments in their borders, refitting with a tissue conditioner or treatment liner, or improvement in their occlusal relationships. This approach is strongly recommended as a routine protocol to optimize supporting tissue health. It also, however, provides a prototype of the fitting surface of the denture. Logic and expediency suggest that these dentures can be regarded as a starting point for an accurate functional impression of the patient's denture-bearing surface. The denture is therefore treated like a standard impression, and a stone cast is poured. An acrylic resin tray is made on the cast over a wax spacer that is outlined just short of the borders of the impression (Fig. 8-22). The dentist can now presume that the tray reflects the border molding that was already developed on the originally resurfaced denture. The tray is tried in the mouth and checked for overextensions. The spacer is removed, relief holes are prepared, an adhesive is applied, and an impression is made in the preferred material. The final result will be indistinguishable from ones produced by the first and second techniques just described (Fig. 8-22).

The list at the end of Chapter 10 sums up the protocol that should be followed when making a complete maxillary impression.

BIBLIOGRAPHY

Fløystrand F: Vestibular and lingual muscular pressure on complete maxillary dentures, Acta Odontol Scand 44:71-75, 1986.

Fløystrand F, Karlsen K, Saxegaard E, Ørstavik JS: Effects on retention of reducing the palatal coverage of complete maxillary dentures, Acta Odontol Scand 44:77-83, 1986.

Minagi S, Sato Y, Akagawa Y, Tsuru H: Concept and technique for making an accurate final impression for complete dentures using a thixotropic impression material, Int J Prosthod 1:149-152, 1988.

Smith DE, Toolson LB, Bolender CL, Lord JL: One-step border molding of complete denture impressions using a polyether impression material, J Prosthet Dent 41:347, 1979.

CHAPTER 9

Biologic considerations for mandibular impressions

Biologic considerations for mandibular impressions are generally similar to those for maxillary impressions, and yet there are many differences. The basal seat of the mandible is different in size and form from the basal seat of the maxillae. The submucosa in some parts of the mandibular basal seat contains anatomic structures that are different from those found in the upper jaw. In addition, the nature of the supporting bone on the crest of the residual ridge usually differs between the two jaws. These variances are often sufficient to require major modifications in impression procedures for the mandible and the maxillae. The presence of the tongue and its individual size, form, and activity complicate the impression procedures for lower dentures and the patient's ability to learn to manage them. The clinical incorporation of the biologic principles of supporting and limiting structures will enable the dentist to unravel what is sometimes called the "mystery of the lower denture" and successfully provide prosthodontic treatment for edentulous patients.

The same fundamental principles are involved in the support of a mandibular denture as are involved in the support of a maxillary denture (Chapter 7). Both the support or stress-bearing area and the peripheral sealing area will be in contact with the denture's fitting or impression surface. The denture bases must extend as far as possible without interfering in the health or function of the tissues, whose support is derived from bone. The support for a mandibular denture comes from the body of the mandible. The peripheral retention seal is provided by the form of the denture's borders as determined by the macroscopic and microscopic anatomy of the limiting structures.

The total area of support from the mandible is significantly less than from the maxillae. The available denture-bearing area for an edentulous mandible is 14 cm² whereas for an edentulous maxilla it is 24 cm². This means that the mandible is less capable of resisting occlusal forces than the maxillae are and extra care must be taken if the available support is to be used to advantage.

SEQUELAE OF TOOTH LOSS

When the teeth are removed from the mandible, the alveolar tooth sockets tend to fill with new bone but the bone of the alveolar process starts resorbing. This means that the bony foundation for a mandibular denture becomes shorter vertically and narrower buccolingually. Thus the foundation for the basal seat is less favorable as a support for the denture. The bony crest of the residual ridge becomes narrower and sharper. Often, sharp bony spicules remain and can cause tenderness when pressure is applied by a denture.

The total width of the bony foundation (or the mandibular basal seat) becomes greater in the molar region as resorption continues. The reason is that the width of the inferior border of the mandible from side to side is greater than the width at the alveolar process from side to side (Figs. 9-1 and 9-2).

Other changes occur on the occlusal surface

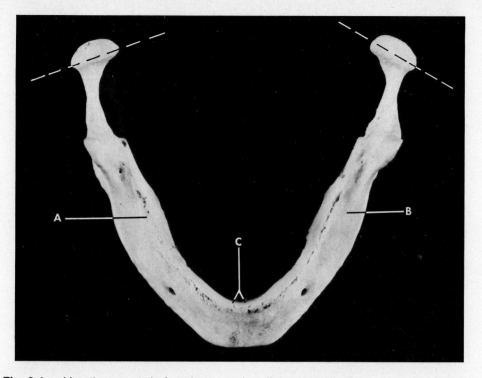

Fig. 9-1   After the removal of teeth, resorption of the alveolar process causes the bony support for a mandibular denture (the residual alveolar ridge) to become more narrow buccolingually and reduced in height. *A,* Crest of the residual ridge (cancellous bone); *B,* the buccal shelf (compact bone); *C,* the genial tubercles. Notice that if the buccolingual axes of the condyles of this mandible were extended posteriorly they would meet in the region of the foramen magnum.

of the bone. The shrinkage of the alveolar process in the anterior region moves the residual bony ridge lingually at first. Then, as resorption continues, this foundation moves progressively further forward (see Fig. 19-5). Bone loss frequently continues on the mandible below the level of the alveolar process.

With resorption of the alveolar process occlusal contours of residual ridges often develop that make them curved from a low level anteriorly to a high level posteriorly (Fig. 9-3). These conditions can cause severe problems of denture stability, which must be considered in impression making and in occlusion.

People who have these unfavorable conditions need dentures, however, and this means that the impressions must be made in such a way that maximum advantage is gained from each part of the basal seat.

MACROSCOPIC ANATOMY OF THE SUPPORTING STRUCTURES

Support for the lower denture is provided by the mandible (the bone) and the soft tissues overlying it. Some parts of the mandible are more favorable for this function than others, and pressures must be applied to the bone through the soft tissues according to the ability of the tissues and different parts of the bone to resist the stresses of occlusion.

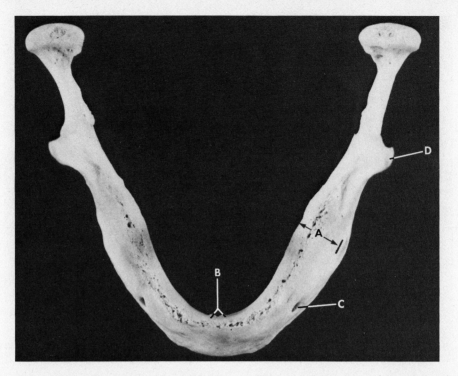

Fig. 9-2   Depending on the shape of the mandible and the nature of the resorption, when the alveolar ridge resorbs it often results in a mandibular basal seat *(A)* that becomes wider and larger. This change occurs because, as resorption moves the crest of the ridge more inferiorly, the width of the mandible becomes greater than that of the alveolar process at the time the teeth were removed. *A* denotes the width of the basal seat; *B,* the genial tubercules; *C,* the mental foramen; *D,* the coronoid process.

Crest of the residual ridge

The crest of the residual alveolar ridge is covered by fibrous connective tissue, but in many mouths the underlying bone is cancellous and without a good cortical bony plate covering it (Fig. 9-4). The fibrous connective tissue closely attached to the bone is favorable for resisting externally applied forces, such as those from a denture. However, if the underlying bone is cancellous, this advantage is mostly lost.

Buccal flange area and the buccal shelf

The area between the mandibular buccal frenum and the anterior edge of the masseter is known as the buccal shelf or buccal flange. It is bounded medially by the crest of the residual ridge, anteriorly by the buccal frenum, laterally by the external oblique line, and distally by the retromolar pad (Fig. 9-5). The buccal shelf may be very wide and is at right angles to the vertical occlusal forces. For this reason it offers excellent resistance to such forces. Some buccinator fibers are located under the buccal flange because the mandibular attachment of this muscle is close to the crest of the ridge in the molar region. This attachment is dissimilar to other muscle insertions insofar as the fibers run anteroposteriorly, paralleling the bone, and the denture does not resist the contracting

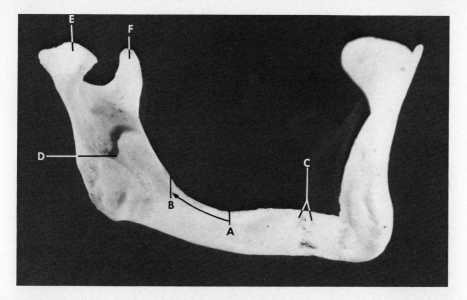

Fig. 9-3   Bony resorption has caused an anteroposterior curvature *(A to B)* in the bone of the basal seat as viewed from the side. Such an inclination of the residual alveolar ridge creates problems in maintaining the stability of a mandibular denture. Artificial teeth should not be placed over the line *B-A.* The genial tubercles, *C,* mandibular foramen, *D,* condyle, *E,* and coronoid process, *F,* are all indicated.

force of the muscle (Fig. 9-6). The inferior part of the buccinator is attached in the buccal shelf of the mandible, and thus contraction of the muscle does not lift the lower denture. The buccal shelf is the principal bearing surface of the mandibular denture, and it takes the occlusal load off the sharp narrow crest of the residual alveolar ridge that so many edentulous mandibles present (Fig. 9-6). It is covered with good smooth cortical bone, which is usually at right angles to the occlusal forces (Fig. 9-7).

These relative conditions vary from patient to patient, so a choice as to the best distribution of pressures on the mandibular basal seat must be made. If the residual bony ridge is unfavorable (that is, if it is sharp, spiny, or full of nutrient canals), masticatory pressures should be transferred to the buccal shelf. Otherwise, the residual ridge can help carry the load effectively. The accuracy of the diagnosis and the

skill with which the impressions are made will determine the effectiveness of the distribution of pressure to selected parts of the basal seat (Fig. 9-8). The requirements of mandibular impressions can be fulfilled by one of several selective pressure techniques.

Flat mandibular ridges

On the labial surface of the anterior region of the mandible several muscles are close to the crest of the ridge, especially in badly resorbed ridges. This proximity accounts for the short flanges necessary in this region. These muscles should not be impinged on, since their action is nearly at right angles to the flange. Many edentulous mandibles are extremely flat because of the loss of cortical bone (Fig. 9-7). The surface is weakened and changed in form by the more rapid resorption of the cancellous portion of the mandible. The bearing surface often becomes concave, allowing the attaching

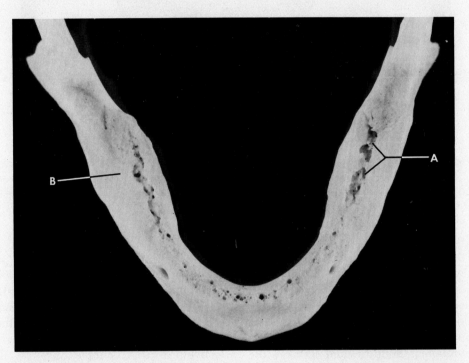

Fig. 9-4   The crest of the residual alveolar ridge consists of spongy or cancellous bone. Its porosity and roughness, particularly in the molar region, *A,* make it unsuitable as the primary stress-bearing area for a mandibular denture. Therefore the buccal shelf, *B,* is usually selected as the primary region for supporting a mandibular denture. (See Figs. 9-5 and 9-7.)

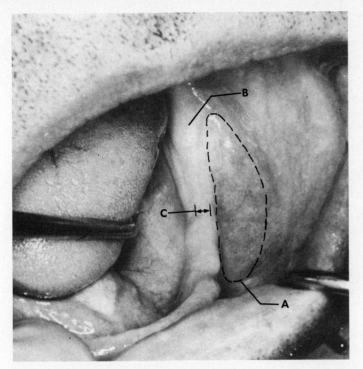

Fig. 9-5 The buccal shelf (within *dotted line*) in this patient's mouth extends posteriorly from the buccal frenum, *A,* to the retromolar pad, *B,* and from the external oblique line on the lateral to the crest of the residual alveolar ridge, *C,* medially.

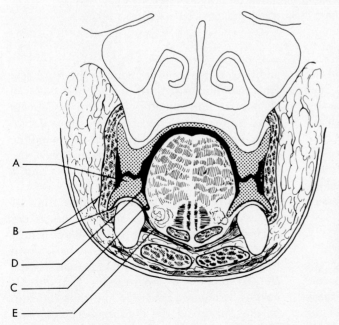

Fig. 9-6 Cross section showing a lower denture in place and its relation to the mandible, tongue, and cheeks. The polished contours of the denture, *A,* aid the muscles in pressing it to place. Notice that the attachment of the buccinator, *B,* goes under the buccal flange area to a point near the crest of the ridge. The lingual flange, *C,* extends away from the bony contour of the mandible and is under the tongue; this aids in seating the denture. *D,* The lingual polished surface contour provides space for the tongue and acts to place rather than displace the denture. The mylohyoid muscle, *E,* contracts during swallowing and should not be impinged on.

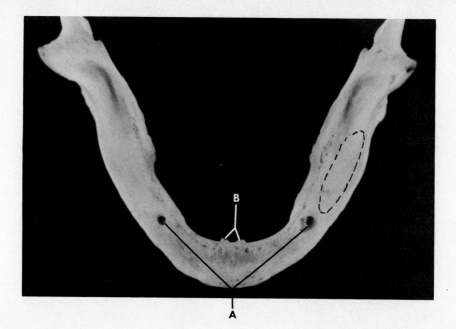

Fig. 9-7 The buccal shelf (outlined by the *dotted line*) consists of smooth compact bone. By both its nature and its position at right angles to the occlusal forces, it is well suited to provide support for a lower denture. The crest of the residual ridge should not be used as a primary stress-bearing area. Notice that the mental foramina, *A,* are on the crest of the ridge in this badly resorbed mandible. The mental vessels and nerves must be relieved of impingement by the denture base. Notice also the difference between the location of the mental foramina here and their more usual position in Figs. 9-1 and 9-2. *B* is the genial tubercles.

structures, especially on the lingual side of the ridge, to fall over onto the ridge surface. Such conditions require displacement of these tissues by the impression, which will gradually reestablish a suitable bearing surface. The crest of greatly resorbed ridges is often at the level of the mental foramina, and the nerves and blood vessels are easily compressed unless the area is palpated and relieved on the impression (Fig. 9-7).

Bone of the basal seat

The configuration of bone that forms the basal seat for a mandibular denture varies considerably among patients. Factors that influence the form of the supporting bone of the basal seat are listed in Chapter 7 (p. 151). In addition, important variations in the basal seat for a mandibular denture include the stages of change in the mandible, a sharp mylohyoid ridge, resorption in the area of the mental foramen, insufficient space between the mandible and the tuberosity, low mandibular ridges, the direction of resorption of the ridges, and a torus mandibularis.

Stages of change in the mandible. Fig. 9-9 portrays the mandible at various stages of development. The final illustration shows it fully formed, with loss of the alveolar process down to a point opposite the mental foramen. As the alveolar process is progressively lost, the attaching structures converge and thus the supporting surface of the denture becomes more and more limited.

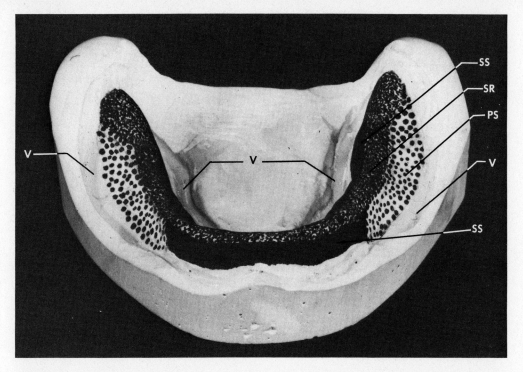

Fig. 9-8   Cast showing the distribution of forces in a selective pressure impression procedure. *PS*, Primary stress-bearing area (the buccal shelf); *SS*, secondary stress-bearing area (slopes of the residual ridge); *SR*, secondary relief area when the crest of the ridge is sharp and thin; *V*, peripheral seal area.

Mylohyoid ridge. Soft tissue usually hides the sharpness of the mylohyoid ridge, which can be found by palpation. The shape and inclination of the ridge vary greatly among edentulous patients.

In Fig. 9-10 are diagrams illustrating cross sections of the mandible to show the inclination of the mylohyoid ridge and the level of the mylohyoid muscle in the various parts of the mandible from the incisal to the third molar region. Note the various levels of attachment of the mylohyoid muscle as it extends posteriorly along the ridge from the symphysis mandibulae. Anteriorly the muscle attaches close to the inferior border of the mandible, and posteriorly it may be flush with the superior surface of the residual ridge. Fig. 9-11 depicts what would be

considered a desirable form of the mylohyoid ridge for an edentulous patient whereas in Fig. 9-12 the mylohyoid ridges are bulbous, irregular, and severely undercut. Extremely thin and sharp mylohyoid ridges are seen in Fig. 9-13, which illustrates another source of aggravation and soreness for edentulous patients.

Mental foramen area resorption. Severe resorption of bone near the mental foramina or the crest of the residual ridge results in compression of the mental nerves and blood vessels if relief is not provided in the denture base (Fig. 9-7). Pressure on the mental nerve can cause numbness of the lower lip.

Insufficient space between the mandible and the tuberosity. The maxillary sinus enlarges throughout life if it is not restricted by natural

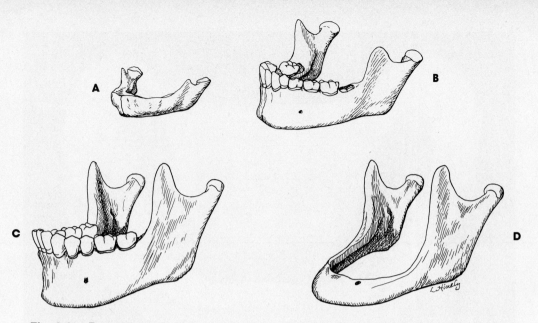

Fig. 9-9 Four stages of development of the mandible. **A,** At birth the condyles are not fully formed. **B,** At 8 years. **C,** Adulthood. **D,** Edentulism.

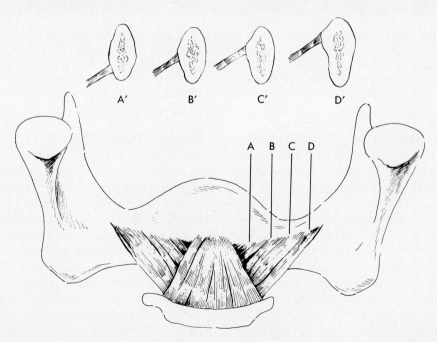

Fig. 9-10 Relationships of the mylohyoid muscle in various regions. The letters with prime signs denote cross sections of the designated areas: *A,* canine region; *B,* premolar region; *C,* first molar; *D,* third molar. In *D',* notice that the mylohyoid ridge approaches the level of the alveolar crest. The angle of the posterior lingual flange in the molar region is affected by this muscle; anteriorly, only the length of the flange is affected.

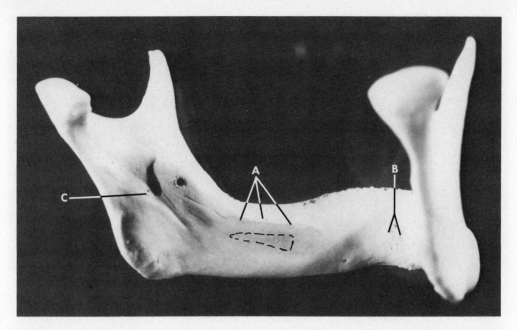

Fig. 9-11   An edentulous mandible with a moderate undercut beneath the mylohyoid ridge, *A*. The denture base cannot extend into this relatively slight undercut *(dotted line)* because the mylohyoid muscle, attaching to the ridge, moves outward and upward during contraction. Notice the location of the genial tubercles, *B*, midway between the superior and inferior borders of the mandible on its lingual surface. *C* is the mandibular foramen.

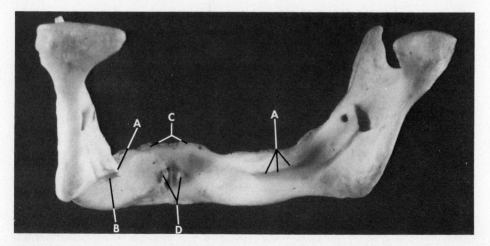

Fig. 9-12   An edentulous mandible with bulbous and irregular mylohyoid ridges, *A*, that are severely undercut, *B*, and cannot be used for retention. Notice the bony projection anteriorly on the crest of the alveolar ridge, *C*, and the genial tubercles, *D*.

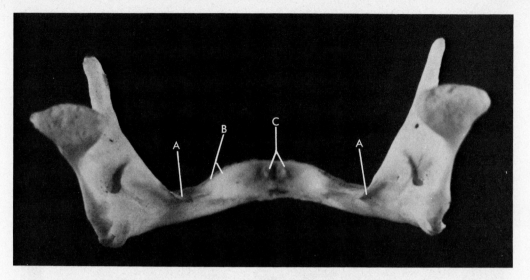

Fig. 9-13 An edentulous mandible with a flat residual alveolar ridge. The mylohyoid ridges, *A*, are knifelike and at the crest of the alveolar ridge. The spiny roughness of the alveolar ridge, *B*, cannot be detected when mucous membrane covers the ridge. The location of such roughness is usually indicated by a band of narrow fibrous tissue along the center of the ridge. Relief must be provided in the impression and the finished denture. Notice that the genial tubercles, *C*, are almost at the crest of the alveolar ridge anteriorly, an indication of the severe resorption that has occurred.

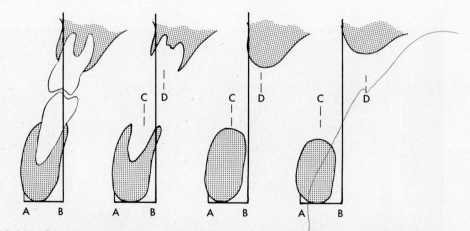

Fig. 9-14 Progressive resorption of the maxillary and mandibular ridges makes the maxilla narrower and the mandible wider. The lines *A-B* illustrate how this narrowing affects the bone. The lines *C* and *D* represent the centers of the ridges. Notice how the distance between them becomes greater as the mandible and maxillae resorb.

teeth or dentures, thus moving the tuberosity downward. The angle of the mandible is frequently made more obtuse by the early loss of posterior teeth with retention of the anterior teeth. Removal of this posterior support destroys the necessary counterbalance against muscle pull at the angle of the mandible. Such "straightening" of the mandible reduces the maxillomandibular space in the posterior region and is the cause of difficulty in obtaining sufficient space for the teeth and denture bases. The lack of space causes many denture failures.

Low mandibular ridges. Frequently the mandibular supporting area is depressed rather than elevated because of differences in the rate of resorption of cortical bone and cancellous bone. Lingually, on these greatly resorbed mandibles, the bone has shrunk down to the level of the attachments of the structures in the floor of the mouth. This makes the lingual flange of the denture more difficult to adapt.

Direction of ridge resorption. The maxillae resorb upward and inward to become progressively smaller because of the direction and inclination of the roots of the teeth and the alveolar process. Consequently, the longer the

maxillae have been edentulous, the smaller their bearing area is likely to be. The opposite is true of the mandible, which inclines outward and becomes progressively wider according to its edentulous age. This progressive change of the mandible and maxillae in the edentulous state makes many patients appear prognathic (Fig. 9-14).

Torus mandibularis. The torus mandibularis is a bony prominence usually found near the first and second premolars, midway between the soft tissue of the floor of the mouth and the crest of the alveolar process. In edentulous mouths where considerable resorption has taken place, the superior border of this prominence may be flush with the crest of the residual ridge on the lingual side. It varies in size from a pea to a hazelnut (Fig. 9-15). The cause for its occurrence is not known, but it is sometimes coincident with a bulbous torus palatinus. The torus mandibularis is covered by an extremely thin layer of mucous membrane and for this reason may be irritated by slight movements of the denture base. It should be removed surgically if relief cannot be provided for it inside the denture without breaking the border seal.

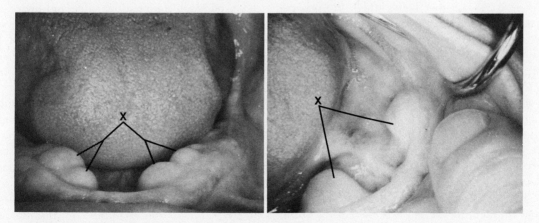

Fig. 9-15   Tori mandibulari, *X*. Surgical reduction of these will be necessary before a satisfactory seal can be developed by a mandibular denture.

MACROSCOPIC ANATOMY OF LIMITING STRUCTURES

Mandibular dentures should extend as far as possible within the limits of health and function of the tissues and structures that surround and support them. This is the same principle that governs the extent of maxillary dentures; but it is more difficult to apply to mandibular than to maxillary dentures, because the structures on the lingual side of the mandible must be considered as well as those around the labial and buccal surfaces of the denture. The structures on the lingual of the mandible are more complicated to control than those on the buccal and labial. The problem is the greater range of their movement and the speed of their actions.

Buccal and labial borders

The underlying structures around the border of a complete denture vary according to their location. This fact is overlooked constantly and is a reason why the best possible mandibular denture coverage is seldom attained. If a careful study is made and used, the size of the mandibular denture may be found larger than would be expected. Mandibular dentures should be wide back of the buccal frenum and narrow in the anterior labial region. The mandibular labial frenum contains a band of fibrous connective tissue that helps attach the orbicularis oris; therefore the frenum is quite sensitive and active and must be carefully fitted to maintain a seal without causing soreness (Fig. 9-16).

The part of the denture that extends between the labial frenum (labial notch) and the buccal frenum (buccal notch) is called the mandibular labial flange. This flange is limited in extension because the fibers of the orbicularis oris and the incisivus labii inferioris are fairly close to the crest of the ridge.

The buccal frenum connects as a continuous band through the modiolus at the corner of the mouth to the buccal frenum in the maxilla (see Fig. 19-6). These fibrous and muscular tissues pull actively across the denture borders, polished surfaces, and teeth. Therefore the denture should extend less in this region, and the impression must be functionally trimmed to have the maximum seal and yet not displace the denture when the lip is moved (Fig. 9-17).

The lower lip must be supported to an extent equal that provided by the natural teeth and their investing structures (Fig. 9-18). The length and thickness of the labial flange in the labial vestibules vary with the amount of tissue that has been lost. The tone of the skin of the lip and of the orbicularis oris depends on the thickness of the flange and the position of the teeth.

There is no muscle extending from the residual ridge to the lip between the two triangulari (depressors anguli oris), so the labial flange can be extended in length and thickness to supply the necessary support for the lip (Fig. 9-18).

Buccal vestibule. The buccal vestibule extends from the buccal frenum posteriorly to the outside back corner of the retromolar pad and from the crest of the residual alveolar ridge to the cheek (Fig. 9-18). The buccinator, in the cheek, extends from the modiolus (anteriorly) to the pterygomandibular raphe (posteriorly). Its lower side attaches in the molar region in the buccal shelf of the mandible (the part of the bone between the residual ridge and the external oblique line). The buccinator's action occurs in a horizontal direction, so it cannot lift the lower denture, even though the buccal flange of a properly extended denture will rest on its inferior attachment.

External oblique ridge and the buccal flange. The extension of the mandibular labial and buccal flanges is governed by the same general factors. The impression space in the labial vestibule between the labial and buccal frena is determined by the turn of the mucolabial fold (the line of flexure of the mucous membrane as it passes from the mandible to the lip and cheeks). The space is not extensive. The buccal flange area, which starts immediately posterior

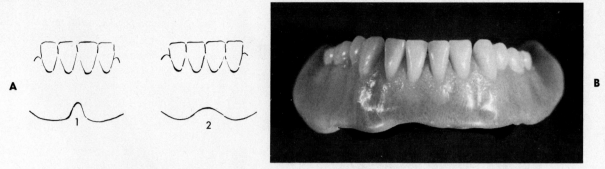

Fig. 9-16   The labial notch. In **A,** notice that it can be narrow or broad *(1 or 2)* depending on the width of the labial frenum. In **B,** the broadly contoured notch is correct for this patient. If it were too narrow for function of the labial frenum, soreness would result; if too broad, a loss of seal could occur.

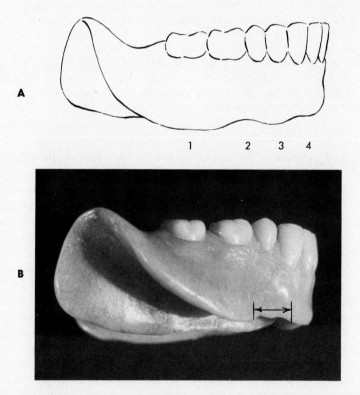

Fig. 9-17   **A,** Typical contours of the labial and buccal borders of a mandibular denture: *1,* Broad buccal flange; *2,* mandibular buccal notch for the buccal frenum; *3,* mandibular labial flange; *4,* labial notch for the labial frenum. **B,** Proper contour of the buccal notch *(arrow)* of a lower complete denture. The contours will vary somewhat for each patient.

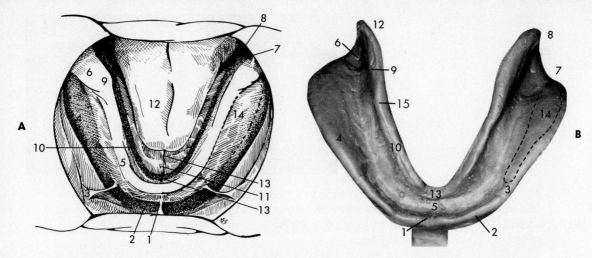

Fig. 9-18 Correlation of anatomic landmarks. **A,** In the mandibular arch: *1,* Labial frenum; *2,* labial vestibule; *3,* buccal frenum; *4,* buccal vestibule; *5,* residual alveolar ridge; *6,* retromolar pad; *7,* pterygomandibular raphe; *8,* retromylohyoid fossa; *9,* lingual tubercle; *10,* alveololingual sulcus; *11,* submaxillary caruncles; *12,* tongue; *13,* lingual frenum; *14,* buccal shelf and premylohyoid eminence. **B,** In the mandibular final impression: *1,* Labial notch; *2,* labial flange; *3,* buccal notch; *4,* buccal flange; *5,* alveolar groove; *6,* retromolar fossa; *7,* pterygomandibular notch; *8,* retromylohyoid eminence; *9,* lingual tubercular fossa; *10,* lingual flange; *12,* inclined plane for the tongue; *13,* lingual notch; *14,* buccal flange that fits on the buccal shelf; *15,* premylohyoid eminence.

to the buccal frenum and extends to the anterior portion of the masseter, swings wide into the cheek and is nearly at right angles to the biting force, thus providing the lower denture with its greatest surface for resistance to vertical occlusal forces (Fig. 9-19).

The external oblique ridge does not govern the extension of the buccal flange because the resistance or lack of resistance encountered in this region varies widely. The buccal flange may extend to the external oblique ridge, or up onto it, or even over it, depending on the location of the mucobuccal fold. However, palpation of the external oblique ridge is a valuable aid or landmark in helping to ascertain the relative amount of resistance or lack of resistance of the border tissues in this region.

The buccal shelf is successfully utilized, despite the fact that the buccinator fibers attach close to the crest of the ridge and the denture rests directly on a considerable portion of this muscle. The bearing of the denture on muscle fibers would not be possible except for the fact that the fibers of the buccinator and its pull when in function are parallel to the border and not at right angles to it, as the masseter fibers are; hence its displacing action is slight. More resistance is encountered in this region when the denture is first inserted than is manifested a few weeks after the patient has worn the completed dentures. Thus it is possible to stretch and displace these tissues and create this area, invaluable for biting resistance and stability, that is so sorely needed when the residual ridge is sharp or narrow.

Masseter muscle region. The distobuccal borders of the mandibular denture must converge rapidly to avoid displacement because of

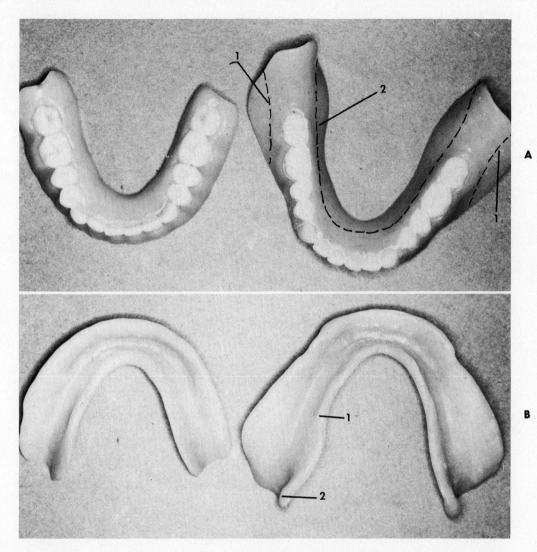

Fig. 9-19   A, The external form of a new denture *(right)* should permit the cheek, *1,* and tongue, *2,* to rest on the buccal and lingual flanges to help hold the denture in place. **B,** Here the lingual flange of the new denture slopes toward the tongue (from *1* to *2*) so it will accommodate the action of the mylohyoid muscle. It thus takes advantage of all the available basal seat to increase its retention, stability, and support. Immediately posterior to the buccal notch the buccal flange extends outward toward the cheek and provides the greatest surface area for resisting vertical occlusal forces.

contracting pressure of the masseter muscle, whose anterior fibers pass outside the buccinator in this region (Fig. 9-20).

When the masseter contracts, it alters the shape and size of the distobuccal end of the lower buccal vestibule. It pushes inward against the buccinator muscle and suctorial pad of the cheek.

The distobuccal border of the mandibular impression encounters the action of the masseter to a greater or lesser degree depending on the shape of the mandible and the origin of the muscle. If the ramus of the mandible has a perpendicular surface and the origin of the muscle on the zygomatic arch is medialward, the muscle pulls more directly across the distobuccal denture border; therefore it forces the buccinator and tissues inward, reducing the space in this region. If the opposite is true, greater extension is allowed on the distobuccal portion of the mandibular impression. One can register this masseter pull on the impression by softening the compound with an alcohol flame along the distobuccal border, tempering the compound in warm water, and, after seating the impression in the patient's mouth, exerting

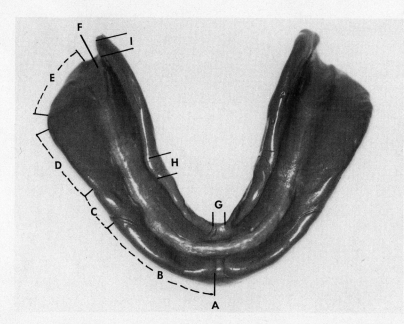

Fig. 9-20   Finished rubber base impression with border outline landmarks: *A,* Mandibular labial notch; *B,* mandibular labial flange; *C,* mandibular buccal notch; *D,* buccal flange; *E,* area influenced by the masseter; *F,* retromolar pad area; *G,* lingual notch; *H,* premylohyoid eminence; *I,* retromylohyoid eminence. Notice the *S* curve of the lingual flanges and also that, in the molar region, the flanges slope toward the tongue and extend below the attachment of the mylohyoid muscles on the mylohyoid ridges. The slope of the lingual flanges allows the mylohyoid muscles to contract and raise the floor of the mouth without displacing the lower denture. The length of the lingual flange in the molar region allows it to reach the mucolingual fold of tissue in the floor of the mouth to maintain the seal of the lower denture. The posterior end of the lingual flange bends laterally toward the mandible to fit into the retromylohyoid fossa. This part of the denture guides the tongue onto the top of the lingual flange.

a downward pressure by placing the index fingers on the impression in the second premolar region. While this downward pressure is being exerted on the impression by the dentist, the patient is instructed to exert a closing force. These opposing forces will cause the masseter to contract and trim the compound in that area since the relation of the mandible and maxillae causes the masseter to affect the distobuccal border directly. The relative size of the masseter will influence its action on the buccinator: a masseter that is of smaller diameter will have less influence (perhaps none) on the border.

Distal extension of the mandibular impression

The distal extent of the mandibular impression is limited by the ramus of the mandible, by the buccinator fibers that cross from the buccal to the lingual as they attach to the pterygomandibular raphe and the superior constrictor, and by the sharpness of the lateral bony boundaries of the retromolar fossa (which is formed by a continuation of the internal and external oblique ridges ascending the ramus). If the impression extends onto the ramus, the buccinator and adjacent tissues will be compressed between the hard denture border and the sharp external oblique ridge. This will not only cause soreness but also limit the function of the buccinator, which is part of the kinetic chain of swallowing.

The desirable distal extension is slightly to the lingual of these bony prominences and includes the pear-shaped retromolar pad, which forms a splendid soft tissue seal of the type that is so valuable in carrying out the principles involved in impression sealing.

Retromolar region and pad. The distal end of the mandibular denture region is bounded by the anterior border of the ramus. Thus the denture includes the retromolar pad posteriorly, which defines its posterior limit (Fig. 9-21). The retromolar pad (a triangular soft pad of tissue at the distal end of the lower ridge) must be covered by the denture to perfect the bor-

der seal in this region. It contains some glandular tissue and some fibers of the temporalis tendon, but it also has active structures working through it (see Fig. 9-35). Buccinator fibers enter it from the buccal side, and fibers of the superior pharyngeal constrictor enter it from the lingual; the pterygomandibular raphe enters the pad at its superoposterior inside corner. The actions of these structures limit the extent of the denture and prevent placement of extra pressure on the retromolar pad during impression procedures or when reducing the posterior borders of the pad on the cast.

Lingual borders

The lingual extension on mandibular impressions has been the most abused and misunderstood border region in complete denture construction. This misunderstanding is caused by the peculiarities of the tissue under the tongue, which has less direct resistance than the labial and buccal borders do and thus will not tolerate overextension of the lingual flange. Because of their peculiar lack of immediate resistance, these tissues are easily distorted when the impression is being made. Such extension over a long time will cause tissue soreness or dislodgment of the denture by tongue movement. The lingual border of the mandibular impression is

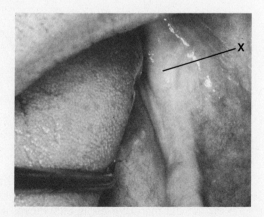

Fig. 9-21 The retromolar pad, *X*, is the posterior landmark for a mandibular denture.

easily carried down along the bony surface of the mandible into the undercut below the mylohyoid ridge, since the mylohyoid muscle is a thin sheet of fibers that in a relaxed state will not resist the impression. However, extension of the lingual flange under the mylohyoid ridge cannot be tolerated in function because it will displace the denture, causing soreness and limiting function, unless the flange is made to parallel the mylohyoid muscle when it is contracted. Although such a mechanical lock might seem desirable to secure additional retention, it cannot be tolerated because of physiologic factors. Therefore the border tissues in this area must be treated in a distinctly different manner from one involving the usual methods and materials (Figs. 9-10 to 9-12).

Influence and action of the floor of the mouth. An acceptable lingual border that will result in a stable denture can be secured with a proper understanding of the anatomy and function of the floor of the mouth. The mylohyoid muscle arises from the whole length of the mylohyoid line, extending from about 1 cm back of the distal end of the mylohyoid ridge to the lingual anterior portion of the mandible at the symphysis. Medially the fibers join those from the mylohyoid muscle of the opposite side, and posteriorly they continue to the hyoid bone. The muscle lies deep to the sublingual gland and other structures about the region of the second premolar, and so does not affect denture borders in this region except indirectly. However, the posterior part of the mylohyoid muscle in the molar region affects the lingual impression border in swallowing and moving the tongue. Fortunately, the posterior extension of the impression can go beyond the muscle's attachment line, since the mucolingual fold is not in this area. Thus the impression

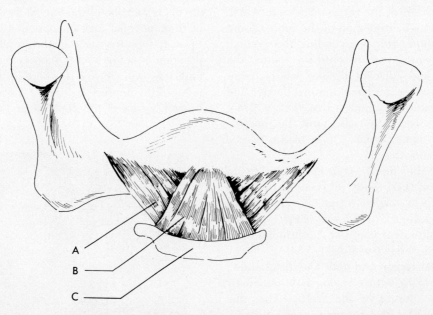

Fig. 9-22 Muscles of the floor of the mouth, posterior view. *A,* The mylohyoid; *B,* the geniohyoid; *C,* hyoid bone. Notice that the mylohyoid muscle is positioned more superiorly on the mandible as its attachment extends posteriorly on the mylohyoid ridge. For this reason, action of the mylohyoid affects the slope of the lingual flange of the impression in the molar region and causes the flange to slope toward the tongue.

may depart from a stress-bearing area of the lingual surface of the ridge and be suspended under the tongue in soft tissue on both sides of the mouth, thereby reaching the mucolingual fold of soft tissue for a seal. The distance that these lingual borders can be away from the bony areas will depend on the functional movements of the floor of the mouth and the amount that the residual ridge has resorbed (Figs. 9-6, 9-22, and 9-27).

Mylohyoid muscle and mylohyoid ridge. An extension of the lingual flange well beyond the palpable portion of the mylohyoid ridge, but not into the undercut, has other advantages. One is that the lack of direct pressure on this sharp edge of bone will eliminate a possible source of discomfort. If the impression is made with pressure on or slightly over this ridge, displacement of the denture and soreness are sure to result from lateral and vertical stresses. On the other hand, if the border stops above the ridge, vertical forces will still cause soreness, and the seal will be broken easily. If the flange is properly shaped and extended, it will com-

plete the lingual border seal in the retromylohyoid fossa and guide the tongue on top of the flange (Fig. 9-20).

Sublingual gland region. In the premolar region on the lingual side of ridge, the sublingual gland rests above the mylohyoid muscle. When the floor of the mouth is raised, this gland comes quite close to the crest of the ridge and reduces the vertical space available for flange extension in the anterior part of the mouth (Fig. 9-23).

The lingual frenum area is likewise rather shallow, sensitive, and resistant. It should be registered in function because at rest the height of its attachment is deceptive. In function, it often comes quite close to the crest of the ridge, although at rest it is much lower (Figs. 9-25 and 9-28).

Direction of the lingual flange. The extension of the lingual flange under the tongue is a concept vastly different from one that has it ending at the mylohyoid ridges. The lower border of the lingual flange runs parallel to the lower edge of the mandible from the lingual frenum

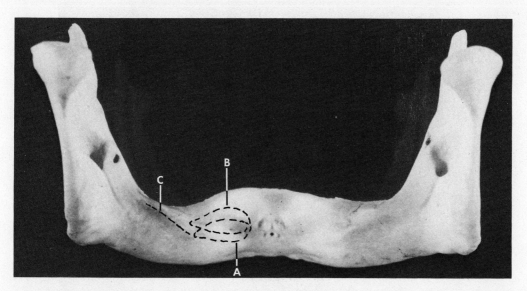

Fig. 9-23   Lingual side of the mandible showing the positions of the sublingual gland relative to the mylohyoid muscle, *A,* at rest and, *B,* in a contracted state. The mylohyoid line is denoted by *C.*

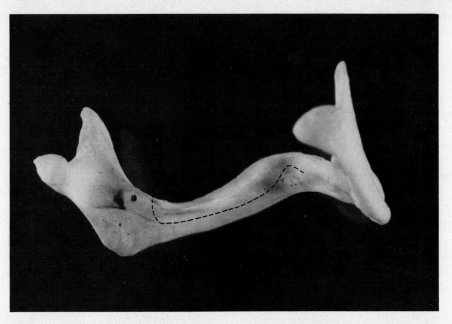

Fig. 9-24 *Dotted line* marks the lower border of the lingual flange on the left side. Notice that the flange roughly parallels the lower border of the mandible.

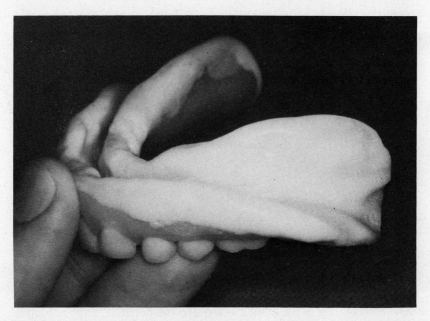

Fig. 9-25 A lower impression made in a lower denture with tissue-conditioning material. Notice that the lingual flange is shorter in the anterior than in the posterior region.

to the posterior end of the denture (Fig. 9-24). This makes the flange short in the anterior region and long in the posterior region because the crest of the ridge of the mandible turns up rather sharply as it approaches the ramus (Fig. 9-25). The posterior extension is bounded partially by the action of the glossopalatine muscle, which usually is no farther back than the distal extent of the retromolar pad.

Alveololingual sulcus

The alveololingual sulcus (the space between the residual ridge and the tongue) extends posteriorly from the lingual frenum to the retromylohyoid curtain. Part of it is available for the lingual flange of the denture.

The alveololingual sulcus can be considered in three regions.

1. The anterior region

    This extends from the lingual frenum to where the mylohyoid ridge curves down below the level of the sulcus. Here a depression (the premylohyoid fossa) can be palpated and a corresponding prominence (the premylohyoid eminence, Fig. 9-20, *H*) can be seen on impressions. The premylohyoid fossa results from the concavity of the mandible (as viewed from above) joining the convexity of the mylohyoid ridge (also from above) (Fig. 9-18). The lingual border of the impression in this anterior region should extend down to make definite contact with the mucous membrane floor of the mouth when the tip of the tongue touches the upper incisors.

2. The middle region

    This part of the alveololingual sulcus extends from the premylohyoid fossa to the distal end of the mylohyoid ridge (Fig. 9-18), curving medially from the body of the mandible. The curvature is caused by the prominence of the mylohyoid ridge. When the mylohyoid muscle and the tongue are relaxed, the muscle drapes back under the mylohyoid ridge.

If an impression is made under these conditions, the muscle and other tissues in this region will be trapped under the ridge and buccal to their functioning position when the tongue is placed against the upper incisors. The sublingual gland and submaxillary duct may be pushed down and laterally out of position by resistant impression material. This can be avoided by shaping this part of the lingual flange of the tray to slope inward toward the tongue and making the final impression with a very soft impression material.

When the middle of the lingual flange is made to slope toward the tongue, it can extend below the level of the mylohyoid ridge. Otherwise, it must end at the level of the mylohyoid ridge. If the flange slopes toward the tongue and extends below the mylohyoid ridge, the tongue can rest on top of the flange and aid in stabilizing the lower denture on the residual ridge. In addition, the slope of the lingual flange in the molar region provides space for the floor of the mouth to be raised during function (tongue movements and swallowing) without displacing the lower denture. The seal of the lower denture is maintained during these movements of the floor of the mouth because the lingual flange remains in contact with the mucolingual fold in the alveololingual sulcus (Figs. 9-26 and 9-27).

3. The posterior region

    This part of the alveololingual sulcus is the retromylohyoid space or fossa. It extends from the end of the mylohyoid ridge to the retromylohyoid curtain—being bounded on the lingual by the anterior tonsillar pillar (at the distal end by the retromylohyoid curtain and superior constrictor) and on the buccal by the mylohyoid muscle, mandibular ramus, and retromolar pad. The superior support for the retromylohyoid curtain is provided by part of the superior pharyngeal constric-

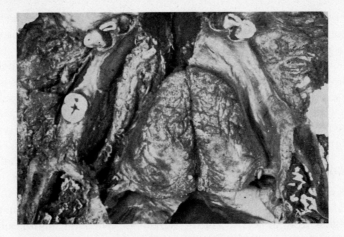

Fig. 9-26 The alveololingual sulcus has an *S* shape, starting at the midline. Notice that the *S* results from the contour of the residual ridge and the prominence of the mylohyoid ridge. This characteristic form is equally apparent on the dissected *(left)* and undissected *(right)* sides.

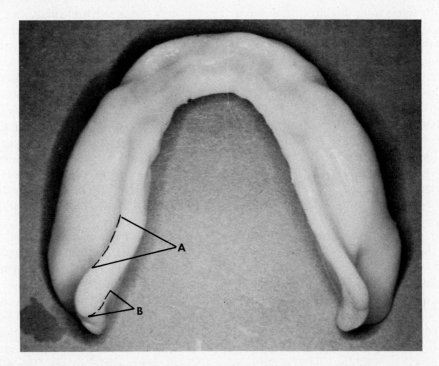

Fig. 9-27 A tissue-conditioning impression illustrates the typical *S* curve of the lingual flange. This type of contour permits tissues of the floor of the mouth to function normally. *A*, The slope of the lingual flange toward the tongue in the molar region allows the mylohyoid muscle to contract and raise the floor of the mouth without displacing the denture. *B*, The distal end of the lingual flange turns buccally to fill the retromylohyoid fossa. This part of the flange guides the tongue on top of the lingual flange of the denture.

tor. The actions of this muscle and of the tongue (and their effects on the alveololingual sulcus) determine the posterior extent of the lingual flange. The denture border should extend posteriorly to contact the retromylohyoid curtain (the posterior limit of the alveololingual sulcus) when the tip of the tongue is placed against the front part of the upper residual ridge.

The attachment of the mylohyoid muscle extends about 1 cm distal to the end of the mylohyoid ridge, which prevents the denture from locking against the bone in this region (Fig. 9-26). However, two objectives are accomplished when the lingual flange extends into this area. First, the border seal is made continuous from the retromolar pad to the middle of the alveololingual sulcus. Second, this part of the flange is so shaped that it guides the tongue on top of the lingual flange of the denture. Such a contour helps the patient control the denture without interfering in the functions of the soft tissues. When the lingual flange is developed in this manner, the border of the flange has a typical **S** curve as viewed from the impression surface (Fig. 9-27).

Lingual frenum and lingual notch. The lingual frenum (that is, the anterior attachment of the tongue) is extremely resistant and active and often wide (Fig. 9-18, *A, 13*). It forms the lingual notch in the lower impression. The denture border needs complete functional trimming so movements of the lingual frenum will not displace the denture or create soreness of this sensitive band of tissue (Fig. 9-28).

Lingual flange. The lingual flange of the denture occupies the alveololingual sulcus (the space between the residual alveolar ridge and the tongue). The distal end of the alveololingual sulcus ends at the retromylohyoid curtain. This curtain of mucous membrane is supported above by the superior constrictor and is pulled forward when the tongue is thrust out.

The distal extent of the lingual flange is partly limited by the glossopalatine arch, which is formed by the glossopalatine muscle and the lingual extension of the superior constrictor. Moving anteriorly, the lingual flange in the molar region is influenced by the mylohyoid muscle, which attaches to the mylohyoid ridge. The flange extends below and medialward from the mylohyoid ridge to occupy the alveololingual sulcus as limited by the mucolingual fold

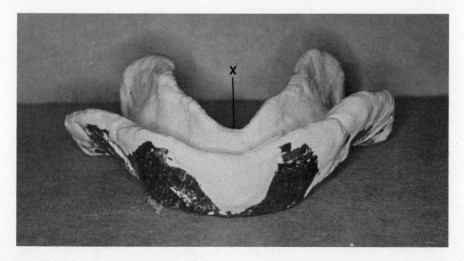

Fig. 9-28   *X* denotes the lingual notch in a completed impression. The lingual notch is usually broad and often is close to the crest of the ridge.

(the line of flexure of the mucous membrane as it passes from the tongue to the floor of the mouth). This means that the buccal surface of the flange rests not on mucous membrane in contact with bone but on soft tissue. The flange leaves the bony attachment at the mylohyoid ridge and slopes inward under the tongue to fill the alveololingual sulcus. Thus there is a space between the flange and the mucous membrane when the mylohyoid muscle is relaxed, but there is contact between the flange and the mucous membrane when the tongue is raised or thrust out (Fig. 9-29). This mucolingual fold is extremely flexible and mobile because of the type of tissue it is and because of the mobility of the entire floor of the mouth. The border tissue on the lingual side of the residual ridge is unlike the border tissue in any other part of the mouth as regards function and resistance in border molding (Fig. 9-6). It has so little resis-

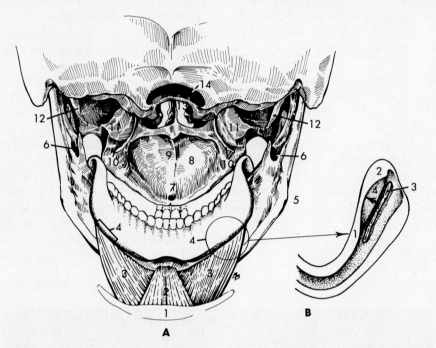

Fig. 9-29 **A,** Relationship of the mylohyoid muscle to the lingual flange of a denture, posterior view. Notice that the muscle attaches inferiorly to the flange from the middle of the mandible posteriorly through the premolar region. However, in the molar region, it attaches to the mylohyoid ridge superior to the border of the flange *(circle)* and its movement during contraction affects the shape of the lingual flange in the molar region. *1,* Hyoid bone; *2,* the geniohyoid muscle; *3,* the mylohyoid muscle; *4,* portion of the lingual flange *(circle)* covering the mylohyoid muscle; *5,* angle of the mandible; *6,* mandibular foramen; *7,* incisive fossa; *8,* hard palate; *9,* median palatine suture; *10,* pterygoid hamulus; *11,* lateral pterygoid plate; *12,* styloid process; *13,* nasal septum; *14,* foramen magnum. **B,** Lower denture, inferior view. *1,* Premylohyoid eminence; *2,* retromylohyoid eminence; *3,* the mylohyoid muscle (cut section covered by the lingual flange of the denture in the molar region); *4,* space in the denture for the mylohyoid muscle. *Arrow* denotes the direction that the mylohyoid muscle moves during contraction. Space in the lingual flange allows movement of the muscle and overlying floor of the mouth without displacement of the lower denture or creation of soreness in the floor of the mouth.

tance that it is easily distorted and for this reason needs a special type of technique and impression material to record its correct turn.

The anterior part of the lingual flange over the sublingual gland is usually shallow because of the mobility of the tissues that are controlled indirectly by the mylohyoid muscle. The mylohyoid muscle in this region extends nearly to the inferior border of the mandible, and yet the glandular and other tissues move above it in such a way that only a relatively short flange is usable (Figs. 9-22 and 9-23). The combination of a typical arch form of the lingual side of the mandible, the projection of the mylohyoid ridge toward the tongue, and the existence of a retromylohyoid fossa at the distal end of the alveololingual sulcus causes the border of the lingual flange to assume its typical S shape when viewed from the impression surface (Fig. 9-20). Starting at the midline, the flange curves outward, following the lingually concave residual ridge. At the premylohyoid fossa, which is located at the front end of the mylohyoid ridge, a premylohyoid eminence forms in the flange. At this point the border of the lingual flange curves away from the body of the mandible to accommodate the mylohyoid muscle when it is contracted or when the tongue is raised. At the distal end of the mylohyoid ridge, the lingual flange turns laterally toward the ramus to fill the retromylohyoid fossa and complete the typical S form. The distal end of the lingual flange is called the retromylohyoid eminence. Its most prominent contour lies medial, posterior, and below the level of the retromolar pad.

MICROSCOPIC ANATOMY*

In Chapter 7 the importance of microscopic anatomy to maxillary impression making, the histologic nature of the soft tissue and bone of the oral cavity, a classification of the oral mucosa, and clinical considerations of oral micro-

scopic anatomy have been discussed. A review of this part of Chapter 7 will be helpful at this point because the material is applicable also to considerations for mandibular impressions.

Supporting tissues

The microscopic anatomy of the supporting tissues of the lower impression will be described for the crest of the residual ridge and the buccal shelf.

Crest of the residual ridge. The mucous membrane covering the crest of the lower residual ridge is similar to that of the upper ridge insofar as, in the healthy mouth, it is covered by a keratinized layer and is firmly attached by its submucosa to the periosteum of the mandible. The extent of the attachment to the bone varies considerably. In some patients the submucosa is loosely attached to the bone over the entire crest of the residual ridge, and the soft tissue covering is quite movable. In a relatively few patients the submucosa is relatively firmly attached to the bone on both the crest and the slopes of the lower residual ridge. When the soft tissue is movable, it must be carefully registered in its resting position in the final impression. Occasionally surgical procedures are indicated to increase the amount of the "residual attached gingivae." When these tissues become inflamed, the submucosa is edematous, with infiltration by numerous inflammatory cells. Obviously, the tissue must be healthy at the time the final impression is made.

The mucous membrane of the crest of the lower residual ridge when securely attached to the underlying bone is histologically capable of providing proper soft tissue support for the lower denture. However, the underlying bone of the crest of the lower residual ridge is cancellous, being made up of spongy trabeculae (Fig. 9-30). Therefore the crest of the lower residual ridge may not be favorable as the primary stress-bearing area for a lower denture. The method of incorporating space in the final impression tray before the final impression is

*We wish to acknowledge the assistance of Dr. Steve Kolas, Professor, Department of Oral Pathology, Medical College of Georgia School of Dentistry, Augusta.

made ensures that proper relief will be provided for the crest of the lower residual ridge during making of the final impression.

Buccal shelf. Anatomically, the buccal shelf is defined as that part of the basal seat located posterior to the buccal frenum and extending from the crest of the lower residual ridge to the external oblique ridge (see Fig. 9-5). The mucous membrane covering the buccal shelf is more loosely attached and less keratinized than the mucous membrane covering the crest of the lower residual ridge, and it contains a thicker submucosal layer. Histologically, fibers of the buccinator are found running horizontally in the submucosa immediately overlying the bone.

The mucous membrane overlying the buccal shelf may not be as suitable histologically to provide primary support for the lower denture as the mucous membrane overlying the crest of the lower residual ridge. However, the bone of the buccal shelf is covered by a layer of compact bone (with its haversian systems) (Fig. 9-31). The nature of this bone, plus the horizontal supporting surface provided by the buccal shelf, makes it the most suitable primary stress-bearing area for a lower denture. The horizontal direction of the fibers of the buccinator allows the denture to rest on this part of the muscle without damage to the muscle or displacement of the denture.

The method of forming the lower final impression tray allows additional load to be placed on the buccal shelf during the making of the final impression (Fig. 9-32). The tray comes into direct contact with the mucosa of the buccal shelf, and the soft tissue is slightly displaced as the final impression is made.

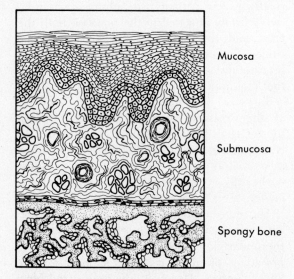

Fig. 9-30 Histology of the crest of the lower residual ridge. The submucosal layer of mucous membrane covering the crest may be of adequate thickness and firmly attached to the residual ridge. However, the bone that forms the crest of the lower ridge is cancellous or spongy; therefore this part of the ridge is generally not used for primary support of a lower denture.

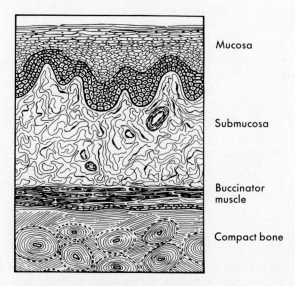

Fig. 9-31 Histology of the buccal shelf of the mandible. Bone forming the buccal shelf is compact, in contrast to the spongy bone that forms the crest of the lower ridge (Fig. 9-30). The nature of compact bone makes the buccal shelf suitable as the primary stress-bearing area for a lower denture.

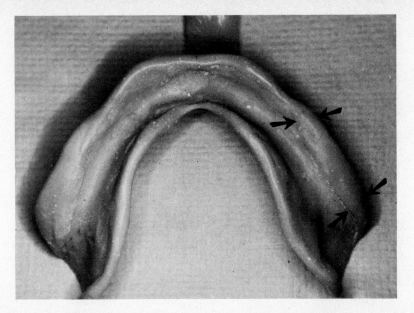

Fig. 9-32 Buccal flanges of the final impression tray in the region of the buccal shelf *(arrows)* are left in direct contact with the cast on both sides when the tray is made. This part of the tray directly contacts the mucosa of the buccal shelf during making of the final impression and places an additional load on the supporting tissues in this region. The rest of the tray has been relieved from the cast by a wax spacer.

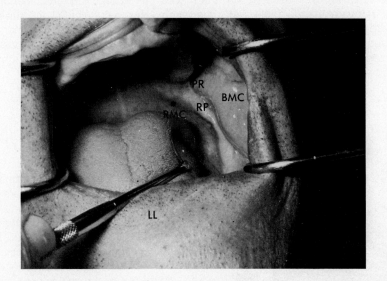

Fig. 9-33 Mucous membrane lining the retromylohyoid fossa, soft palate, retromolar pad, and cheek. *LL,* Lower lip; *RMC,* retromylohyoid curtain (formed by the mucous membrane covering the superior constrictor); *RP,* retromolar pad; *PR,* pterygomandibular raphe; *BMC,* buccal mucosa of the cheek. The retromylohyoid curtain lies at the posterior end of the alveololingual sulcus and is the posterior boundary of the retromylohyoid fossa. *Asterisk* denotes the location of the histologic section in Fig. 9-34, *A.*

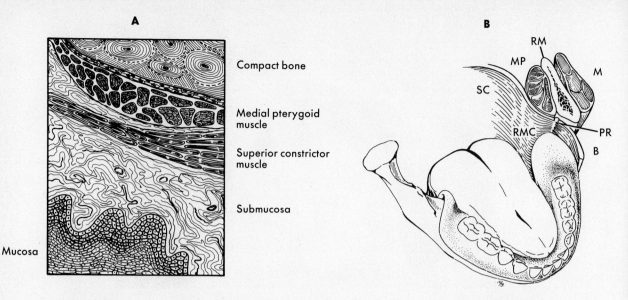

A

Compact bone

Medial pterygoid muscle

Superior constrictor muscle

Submucosa

Mucosa

B

RM

MP

M

SC

RMC

PR

B

Fig. 9-34   A, Histology of the retromylohyoid curtain at the site of the asterisk in Fig. 9-33. Notice the superior constrictor muscle and, posterior to it, the medial pterygoid muscle. Contraction of the medial pterygoid limits the space available for the posterior part of the lingual flange in the retromylohyoid fossa. **B,** Relationship of the medial pterygoid to the superior constrictor. When the medial pterygoid contracts, it forces the superior constrictor anteriorly, thus limiting the length of the lingual flange in this region. *B* is the buccinator; *M,* the masseter; *MP,* the medial pterygoid; *PR,* pterygomandibular raphe; *RM,* ramus of the mandible; *RMC,* the retromylohyoid curtain; *SC,* the superior constrictor. Contraction of the medial pterygoid, which lies posterior to the superior constrictor, causes the retromylohyoid curtain (mucosal covering of the superior constrictor) to move anteriorly, thus limiting the space in the retromylohyoid fossa for the retromylohyoid eminence at the posterior end of the lingual flange of a denture.

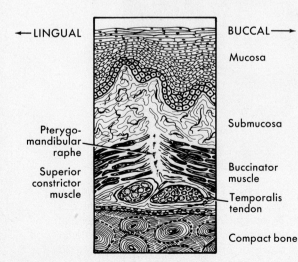

←— LINGUAL

BUCCAL —→

Mucosa

Submucosa

Pterygo-
mandibular
raphe

Superior
constrictor
muscle

Buccinator
muscle

Temporalis
tendon

Compact bone

Fig. 9-35   Histology of the posterior part of the retromolar pad. Notice the fibers of the buccinator laterally and of the superior constrictor medially. These join to form the pterygomandibular raphe. Fibers of the temporalis tendon lie deep to these structures. Because of the histologic makeup of the retromolar pad, it should not be displaced during making of the final impression.

Limiting tissues

The microscopic anatomy of the limiting tissues is described for the vestibular spaces, the alveololingual sulcus, and the retromolar pad.

The mucous membrane lining the vestibular spaces and alveololingual sulcus of the lower jaw is quite similar to that lining the vestibular spaces of the upper jaw. The epithelium is thin and nonkeratinized, and the submucosa is formed of loosely arranged connective tissue fibers mixed with elastic fibers. Thus the mucous membrane lining the vestibules and the alveololingual sulcus is freely movable, which allows for the necessary movements of the lips, cheeks, and tongue. Anteriorly the submucosa of the mucous membrane lining the alveololingual sulcus contains components of the sublingual gland and is attached to the genioglossal muscle. In the molar region the submucosa attaches to the mylohyoid muscle, and the mucous membrane covering of the retromylohyoid curtain is attached by its submucosa to the superior constrictor. Posterior to the superior constrictor fibers, which run in a horizontal direction, is found the medial pterygoid muscle running in a vertical direction (Figs. 9-33 and 9-34). The length and form of the lingual flange of the lower final impression tray must reflect the physiologic activity of these structures lest their normal movement be restricted or they tend to dislodge the lower denture.

The retromolar pad lies at the posterior end of the crest of the lower residual ridge. Histologically, its mucosa is composed of a thin, nonkeratinized epithelium; and, in addition to loose areolar tissue, its submucosa contains glandular tissue, fibers of the buccinator and superior constrictor, the pterygomandibular raphe, and the terminal part of the tendon of the temporalis (Fig. 9-35). Because of its histologic nature, the retromolar pad should be registered in a resting position in the final lower impression.

Cross sections of the mandible

Cross sections of the mandible reveal the proximity of muscle attachments and the lack of a broad bearing surface. The bony contour naturally is much narrower and sharper than the soft tissue contour. This fact often deceives the dentist as to the width and contour of the bearing surface.

CHAPTER 10

Mandibular impression procedures

A survey of dentists who include prosthodontic treatment in their practice would indicate that most of them believe making good mandibular impressions for edentulous patients is far more difficult than making good maxillary impressions. Why should this be true? The difficulty most likely stems from the lack of a true understanding of the functional anatomy of structures that determine the length and form of the mandibular lingual flange. These limiting structures are directly related to the tongue and the floor of the mouth and their combined movements, which are among the most complex in the body. An understanding of the role that they play can come only from continued study of their physiology and its clinical application. Both require a concerted effort. The lingual borders of properly molded mandibular impressions are as definite in length and form as are the buccal and labial borders of maxillary and mandibular impressions. Properly formed lingual borders of mandibular impressions do not happen by chance. They require cooperation of the patient to make the proper tongue and jaw movements that will create the desirable action of the floor of the mouth for border-molding purposes. They also require time, effort, patience, and a willingness on the part of the dentist to repeat difficult parts of the impression procedure as many times as necessary to obtain the desired result. The techniques for making mandibular impressions described in this chapter are based on the clinical application of the tolerances of the supporting structures and the function of the border tissues that make up the basal seat.

CLASSIFICATION OF MANDIBULAR IMPRESSIONS

Mandibular impressions for complete dentures are made in many kinds of materials and by many different techniques. The technique to use for each patient should be selected on the basis of the diagnosis of the basal seat and border tissues.

Impression techniques may be classified as (1) selective pressure and (2) pressureless. The choice is based on the objectives for the patient.

Selective pressure impressions. These are made in trays that have more space in them for the final impression material in some places than in others. The places that have less space or relief will transmit more pressure from the denture in function to favorable parts of the bone (such as the buccal shelf) and less pressure to unfavorable parts (such as a sharp ridge crest or bony spicule). We shall describe three selective pressure techniques for mandibular impressions, since they are ones that we routinely use with our patients.

Pressureless impressions. These are made with the least possible displacement of soft tissues covering the residual alveolar bone. They incorporate a large amount of space between the tray and the soft tissues of the basal seat and consequently require a very fluid type of impression material. Pressureless impression techniques are not described in this text.

CONSTRUCTION PROCEDURES

The same principles of construction are used for lower final impressions as for upper impressions (Chapter 8), even though particular techniques may vary.

First technique—selective pressure mandibular impression—border-molded special tray

Making the preliminary impression. The dentist should study the space available in the mouth for the lower impression to determine the general form, size, and health of the basal seat. Then an edentulous metal stock tray is selected that will provide for approximately ¼-inch (6 mm) bulk of impression material over the entire basal seat area. The patient is asked to raise his tongue slightly as the tray is placed in the mouth and to position the tongue in the tongue space of the tray (Fig. 10-1, *A*). Posteriorly the retromolar pads should be covered by the tray, and anteriorly the lingual surface of the labial flange should provide space for the necessary ¼ inch of impression material. The labial and buccal borders of the tray are observed in relation to the limiting anatomic

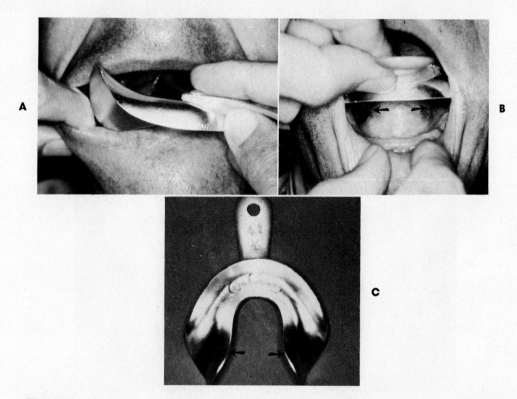

Fig. 10-1 Preliminary impression making. **A,** A lower stock metal tray is placed in the mouth by extension of one corner of the mouth with the index finger or a mouth mirror. The side of the tray is placed in the opposite corner, and the tray is rotated to position. **B,** The tray is raised anteriorly for observation of whether there is adequate space between the lingual flanges *(arrows)* and the lingual slope of the lower residual ridge to accommodate sufficient bulk of impression material. **C,** The lingual flanges of the tray slope toward the tongue in the molar region *(arrows)* so the mylohyoid muscle can contract as it raises the floor of the mouth. Notice the *S* shape of the lingual flange.

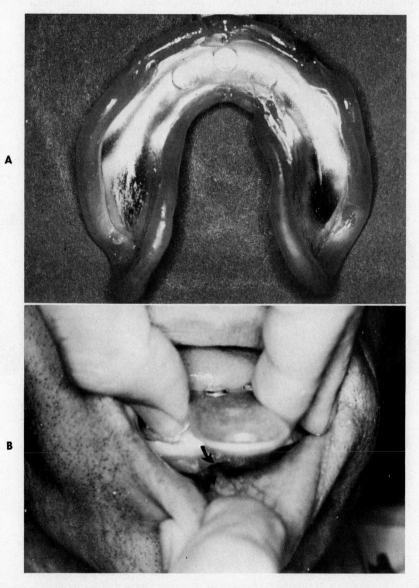

Fig. 10-2 Preliminary impression making. **A,** A rim of wax helps conform the borders of the tray to the mouth and confines the impression material in the tray. **B,** Space is provided in the boxing wax for the lower labial frenum. *Upper arrow* indicates the labial notch formed in wax; *lower arrow,* the lower labial frenum.

structures. The tray is raised anteriorly for observation of the relation between the lingual flanges and the lingual slope of the lower residual ridge (Fig. 10-1, *B*). The metal lingual flanges are reshaped by bending to allow for the action of the mylohyoid muscle (Fig. 10-1, *C*).

The borders of the tray are lined with a soft boxing wax so a rim is created within the tray to help confine the alginate (irreversible hydrocolloid) impression material that will be used for the preliminary impression (Fig. 10-2, *A*). The tray is again positioned in the mouth, with the patient's tongue raised slightly, and the borders of the tray are observed in relation to the limiting structures (Fig. 10-2, *B*). The entire basal seat area should be included within

the impression surface of the tray; all supporting tissues for the completed denture must be included in the overextended preliminary impression.

The tissue surface and borders of the metal tray, including the rim of wax, are painted with an adhesive material to ensure that the irreversible hydrocolloid adheres to the tray. The irreversible hydrocolloid is mixed according to directions of the manufacturer. The impression material is loaded into the lower stock tray from the lingual surface and evenly distributed to fill the tray to the level of the borders (Fig. 10-3, *A* and *B*). The tray is centered over the residual ridge, with the tongue raised slightly so it will be in the tongue space. As the tray is gently seated (by alternating pressure from an

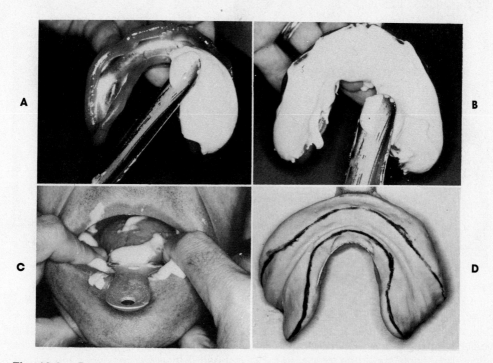

Fig. 10-3   Preliminary impression making. **A,** Irreversible hydrocolloid is placed in the tray so it moves the material ahead of it from one end of the tray to the other, eliminating any trapped air. **B,** The hydrocolloid is confined in the tray by a rim of molding wax and is evenly distributed. The impression is held in the mouth by an index finger from either hand placed on top of the tray in the region of the first molar. Notice the position of the tongue. **D,** The impression includes a negative record of all the basal seat area.

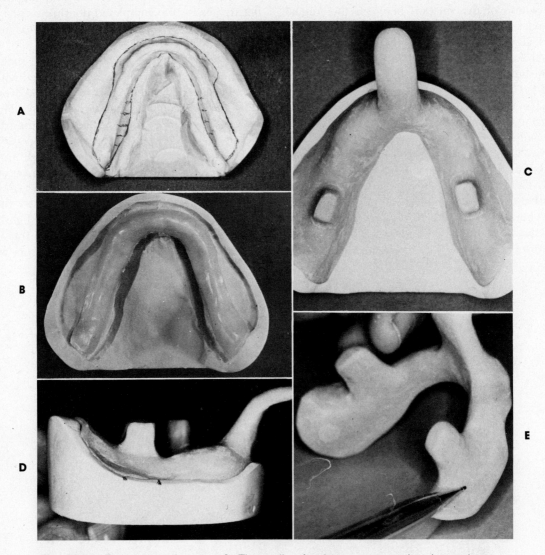

Fig. 10-4 Final impression tray. **A,** The outline for the wax spacer has been drawn on the preliminary cast. Notice that the buccal shelf on each side is not included. **B,** Wax has been adapted to the cast. The retromylohyoid fossae, buccal shelves, and borders are not covered by the wax. **C,** The lower final impression tray is formed on the cast of self-curing acrylic resin. **D,** The position of the handle is indicated by pencil marks on the cast. The handle should be located at the lowest part of the lower residual ridge, usually in the first molar region. **E,** The external surface of the lower impression tray should be similar in form to the completed denture.

index finger on either side of the tray in the first molar region), the patient is asked to let his tongue relax. The tray is held steadily in position for 1 minute after the initial set of the irreversible hydrocolloid (Fig. 10-3, *C*). Then the impression is removed from the mouth in one motion and inspected to ascertain that all the basal seat area is included (Fig. 10-3, *D*). Here, as was the case when this technique was discussed for the maxillary impression, the tray outline may be identified with an indelible marker on the impression or else later after the cast is poured (p. 183, Chapter 8).

Making the final impression tray. The cast is made of artificial stone poured into the irreversible hydrocolloid impression. The outline for a wax spacer, which will provide space in the tray for the final impression material, is drawn in pencil on the cast (Fig. 10-4, *A*). A wax spacer about 1 mm thick is placed over the crest and slopes of the residual ridge. The buccal shelf on each side and the retromylohyoid spaces on the cast are left uncovered (Fig. 10-4, *B*). Thus the completed final impression tray will contact the mucosa in the region of the buccal shelves and thereby help to position the tray correctly in the mouth and to place additional pressure in this primary stress-bearing area when the final impression is made. Extra wax can be placed over the lingual slopes of the cast below the level of the mylohyoid ridge to provide additional space for the action of the mylohyoid muscles when the final impression is made.

Self-curing (cold-curing or autopolymerizing) acrylic resin tray material is mixed and uniformly distributed over the cast so the final impression tray will be approximately 2 to 3 mm thick. An anterior resin handle is centered over the labial flange in the approximate position of the anterior teeth and shaped so as not to interfere with the position of the lip (Fig. 10-4, *C* and *D*). Two additional handles, one on each side, are placed in the first molar region. These handles are centered over the crest of the re-

sidual ridge at its lowest point and are approximately ¾ inch (19 mm) in height. The anterior handle is used to carry the final impression tray into the mouth and position it over the residual ridge. The posterior handles are used as finger rests to complete the placement of the tray on the residual ridge and to stabilize the tray in the correct position with minimal distortion of soft tissues while the final impression material sets. The flanges of the tray should be contoured like the flanges of the completed denture. Thus, while the impression is made, the limiting border tissues will be in a position similar to the one they should be in when the denture is in the mouth (Fig. 10-4, *E*).

Preparing the final impression tray. When the acrylic resin tray is removed from the lower preliminary cast, the wax spacer is left inside the tray (Fig. 10-5, *A*). Retaining the spacer allows the tray to be properly positioned on the lower residual ridge for border-molding procedures.

The available space for the impression is again observed in the patient's mouth and compared (length and width) to the flanges of the final impression tray. The buccal and lingual flanges of the tray are marked in pencil and reduced until the borders are short of the limiting anatomic structures (Fig. 10-5, *B*). When possible, observations are made with the modified tray in the mouth to ensure that space will be available for the addition of modeling compound.

Border molding the labial and buccal flanges. Stick modeling compound is added in sections to the borders of the resin tray, beginning with the labial flange, then the buccal flanges, and finally the lingual flanges. Each section of modeling compound is heated and border molded before the next section is added.

Border molding is accomplished for the labial flange when the lower lip is lifted outward, upward, and inward (Fig. 10-6, *A* and *B*). In the region of the buccal frenum the cheek is lifted outward, upward, inward, backward, and

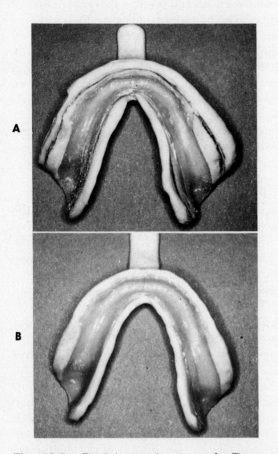

Fig. 10-5 Final impression tray. **A,** The wax spacer is maintained in the lower impression tray until border molding has been completed. A pencil mark indicates the approximate amount of tray shortening that will be needed before border molding. Notice that part of the right buccal flange has already been shortened. **B,** The flanges of the final lower impression tray have been reduced so they will be short of the limiting anatomic structures when the tray is placed in the patient's mouth.

forward to simulate movement of the lower buccal frenum. Posteriorly the buccal flange is border molded when the cheek is moved outward, upward, and inward (Fig. 10-6, *C* to *E*).

Border molding the lingual flanges. The lingual flanges are border molded in five steps:

1. With the tray in the mouth the length and thickness of the flange in the anterior region are observed relative to the available space in the alveololingual sulcus as limited by the lingual frenum, sublingual folds, and submaxillary caruncles. If space can be seen between the lingual border of the tray and these limiting anatomic structures with the tongue slightly raised, more modeling compound is added in this region. If the tray encroaches on the limiting structures, the lingual border is reduced before the border is molded.

   When the tray appears to fill the available space in the lingual anterior region, the labial surface of the lingual flange and border of the modeling compound between the premylohyoid eminences are heated and tempered. The tray is placed in the patient's mouth, and the patient is instructed to protrude the tongue (Fig. 10-7, *A*). This movement creates functional activity of the anterior part of the floor of the mouth, including the lingual frenum, and determines the length of the lingual flange of the tray in this region. Both premylohyoid eminences on the tray are usually visible after this procedure, and the lengths of the lingual flange on each side of the lingual notch will frequently be symmetric. This procedure often must be repeated while close observation is maintained on the flange and the space in the mouth.

2. The compound on the lingual surface of the flange is softened in the anterior region (from premolar to premolar) to a depth of 1 to 2 mm. The tray is placed in the mouth and the patient is asked to push the tongue forcefully against the

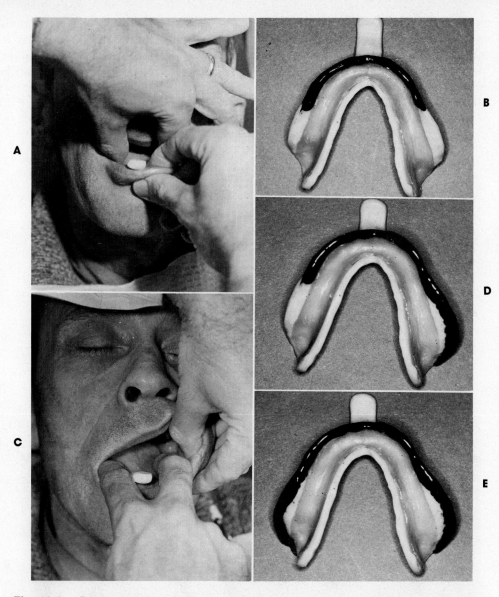

Fig. 10-6   Border molding. **A,** The procedure is accomplished in the lower anterior region by extension of the lower lip outward, upward, and inward. No side-to-side movement of the lip is necessary in this region since the lower labial frenum does not move from side to side during function. **B,** The labial flange of the lower final impression tray has been properly border molded in modeling compound. **C,** The posterior flange of the tray is molded by extending the cheek outward, upward, and inward as well as moving it backward/forward in the region of the buccal frenum. The tray is held in position by the posterior handles. **D,** The left buccal flange has been properly border molded. **E,** Both flanges molded; wax spacer is still in the tray.

front part of the palate (Fig. 10-7, *B*). This action causes the base of the tongue to spread out and develops the thickness of the anterior part of the lingual flange (Fig. 10-7, *C*).

The lingual flange will be shorter ante- riorly than posteriorly. At the premylohy- oid fossa in the canine-premolar region, the flange becomes longer and extends below the level of the mylohyoid line. It must slope toward the tongue more or less parallel to the direction of the fibers

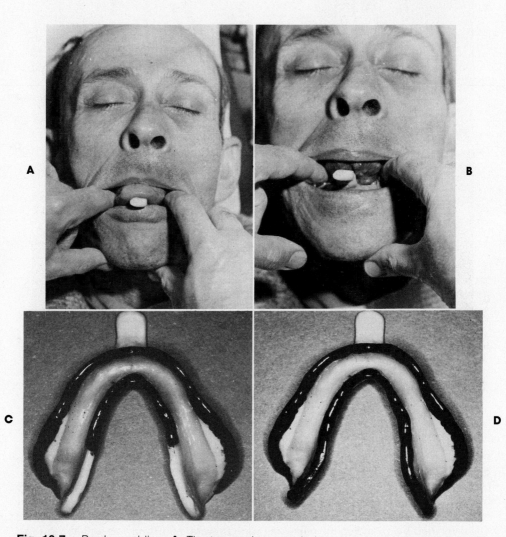

Fig. 10-7 Border molding. **A,** The tongue is protruded to regulate the length of the lin- gual flange. **B,** It is then pushed against the anterior part of the palate to regulate the thickness of the anterior lingual flange. **C,** The anterior part of the flange has been prop- erly border molded. **D,** Border molding for the lower tray complete. Notice that the bor- ders of the lingual flange are as definitely formed as the borders of the labial and buccal flanges. Wax is still in the tray.

of the mylohyoid muscle in the molar region.

3. Modeling compound is added to the lingual borders in the molar regions on both sides of the tray between the premylohyoid and postmylohyoid eminences. The compound is heated and tempered. Then the tray is placed in the patient's mouth, and the patient is asked to protrude the tongue. This develops the slope of the lingual flange in the molar region to allow for the action of the mylohyoid muscle. In some instances it will be necessary to thicken the flange by adding modeling compound to its lingual surface so its buccal surface can be cut away and sloped toward the tongue. If modeling compound builds up inside the lingual flange in this region because of the border-molding process, the excess should be removed. This will permit the mylohyoid muscle to function normally and will prevent pressure from being applied on the sharp mylohyoid ridge. It is better to have the tray contoured with too much slope toward the tongue in the molar region than with too little, since the final impression material will fill the excess space.

4. The compound on the border of the flange on both sides in the molar region is heated to a depth of 1 to 2 mm. The tray is placed in the mouth, and the patient again protrudes his tongue. The action of the mylohyoid muscle, which raises the floor of the mouth during this movement, determines the length of the flange in the molar region (Fig. 10-7, *D*).

The distal end of the lingual flange should extend about 1 cm distal to the end of the mylohyoid ridge. If this part of the preliminary impression lacks sufficient length, modeling compound is added to it. The flange should be so shaped that it turns laterally toward the ramus below the level of the retromolar pad and mylohyoid ridge.

5. Compound on the distal end of the flange

is heated, and the tray is placed in the mouth. The patient is instructed to protrude his tongue to activate the superior constrictor (which supports the retromylohyoid curtain). Then he is asked to close as the dentist applies downward force on the impression tray. The resulting contraction of the medial pterygoid muscle, acting posteriorly on the retromylohyoid curtain, can limit the space available for the border of the impression in the retromylohyoid fossa. Often compound must be added to the retromylohyoid eminence on the impression tray so the eminence will fill the retromylohyoid fossa properly during function of the limiting structures (Fig. 10-7, *D*).

The length and form of the lingual flange should be in harmony with the limiting anatomic structures on completion of the border molding for the distal corner of the flange. With the lower final impression tray in place in the mouth the patient should be able to wipe the tip of his tongue across the vermilion border of the upper lip without noticeable displacement of the lower tray.

The compound forming the posterior part of the retromolar fossa is heated, the tray is placed in the mouth, and the patient is asked to open wide. If the tray is too long, a notch will be formed at the posteromedial border of the retromolar fossa, indicating encroachment of the tray on the pterygomandibular raphe. The tray is adjusted accordingly (Fig. 10-7, *D*).

The final tray should be so formed that it can support the cheeks and lips in the same manner as the finished denture is to do. The lingual flange is shaped to facilitate making the final impression and guiding the tongue into the position it is to occupy relative to the finished denture. The lingual surface of the flange of the tray should guide the tongue into the same position it will occupy in relation to the finished denture.

The wax spacer is removed from the inside of the tray (Fig. 10-8, *A*). Several holes about ½ inch (12.5 mm) apart are marked in the center of the alveolar groove and the retromolar fossae of the tray and are cut in the tray with a no. 6 round bur (Fig. 10-8, *B*). They will provide escapeways for the final impression material and relieve pressure over the crest of the residual ridge and the retromolar pads when the final impression is made. The modeling compound borders of the lower final impression tray are shortened approximately 0.5 to 1 mm to make space for the final impression material (Fig. 10-8, *C*).

Making the final lower impression. Existing dentures must be left out of the mouth for a minimum of 24 hours before the lower final impression is made to allow the tissues of the basal seat to return to health and undistorted form. With proper education, the patient will understand the value of providing this period of rest for the supporting tissues and be willing to comply with this important requirement.

A good final impression cannot be made unless a properly fitting tray is in the correct position on the residual ridge. Therefore the dentist should practice proper positioning of the tray before making the final impression.

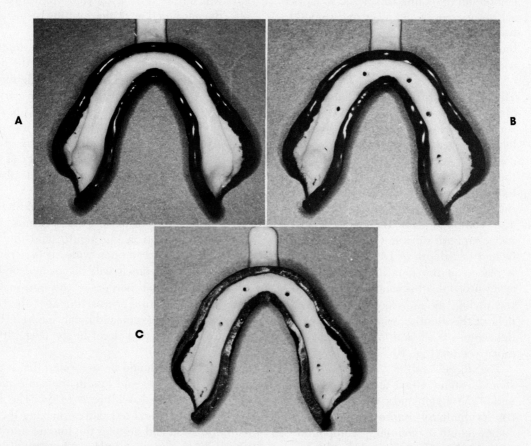

Fig. 10-8 Border molding. **A,** On completion of the procedure, the wax spacer is removed from the tray. **B,** Holes in the alveolar groove will provide an escapeway for the final impression material when this impression is made. **C,** Modeling compound borders have been shortened to provide space for the final impression material.

Practicing tray placement. In the practice procedure the empty lower final impression tray is inserted into the mouth by means of the anterior handle. With the mouth half open, the anterior part of the tray (next to the anterior handle) is placed against the left cheek while the right cheek is pulled laterally by the index finger of the left hand or a mouth mirror. Then the tray is rotated in the horizontal plane until it is over the residual ridge.*

At this time the patient is asked to raise his tongue slightly. The retromylohyoid eminences are alternately moved past the crest of the ridge. It may be necessary to adjust the tray posteriorly in the mouth beyond its correct position to initiate this procedure. Then the tray is moved forward and centered and moved downward toward its final position.

The index fingers are placed on top of the posterior handles, and by the alternate application of gentle pressure on each side, the tray is seated until the buccal flanges come into contact with the mucosa covering the buccal shelf. The amount of pressure used will determine the amount of displacement of the soft tissues on the buccal shelf. Heavier pressure will displace the soft tissue more and thus will provide more relief of the tissues over the crest of the ridge. Minimal tissue displacement, and therefore the minimal pressure, should be the objective unless the crest of the ridge is unfavorable for the support of the denture.

With the tray held steadily and not moving on the residual ridge, the patient is instructed to place his tongue under his upper lip in front of the upper anterior teeth, as if they were present. This will activate the floor of the mouth and border-mold the lingual flange of the impression. The dentist then carefully elevates the lower lip and corners of the mouth to complete the border-molding procedure (Fig.

*Left-handed dentists will use the opposite hands for each of these operations.

10-9). The fingers must be held in position on the posterior handles until the impression material has set.

Preparing the patient. The patient's clothing should be protected by a plastic apron. The face is lubricated with petroleum jelly, and a roll of gauze is placed under the tongue to help keep the mouth dry.

The final impression. An adhesive is painted on the basal surface of the tray. The final impression material is mixed in proper quantities according to manufacturer's directions and evenly distributed within the tray, care being taken that all borders are covered (Fig. 10-9, *A* and *B*). The gauze is quickly removed from under the patient's tongue. The final impression tray, carrying the final impression material, is positioned in the mouth and border molded as practiced (Fig. 10-9, *C* to *E*). It is held steadily for the time specified until the impression material has set. Then the completed impression is removed from the mouth and inspected for acceptability (Fig. 10-9, *F*).

Remaking final impressions. Impression making is not easy if it is done correctly. It requires great attention to details and a thorough understanding of the anatomy and physiology of oral tissues. The extra time that may be spent in making impressions, however, not only means the difference between success and failure but also will lead to the expenditure of less time in making adjustments to finished dentures.

Patients should be told that it is often necessary to make more than one impression to correct the tray before a final impression is acceptable. Many impressions must be remade. If the tray was correctly positioned in the mouth, errors in the impression indicate modifications of the tray that are necessary before another impression is made. The tray should *not* be modified unless it was correctly positioned when the impression was made. Errors in one impression must be corrected before the next one is made.

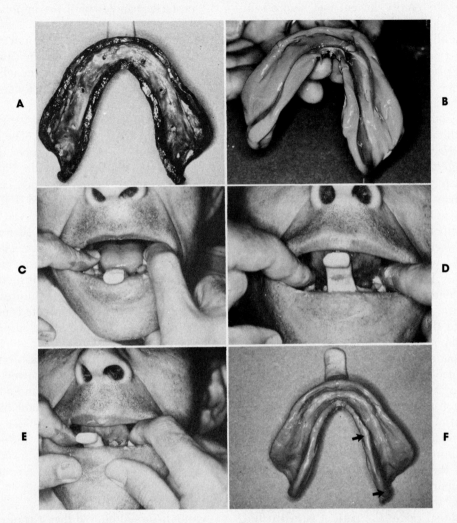

Fig. 10-9 Final impression making. **A,** Adhesive painted in the base of the tray ensures that the impression material will stick to the tray. **B,** The material must cover all the basal surface of the tray, including the borders. **C,** Then the impression is positioned correctly on the lower residual ridge by alternate pressure applications on each side of the tray until the buccal flanges contact the mucosa covering the buccal shelf. **D,** The tongue positioned under the upper lip will border mold the lingual flange of the final impression. **E,** The lower lip and corners of the mouth are elevated to complete the border-molding procedure in this region. **F,** The final impression shows that the tray was properly positioned on the lower residual ridge and that border molding was properly carried out. Notice that the lingual flange of the impression slopes toward the tongue between the premylohyoid and postmylohyoid eminences *(arrows).*

Following are some of the imperfections in an impression that will indicate it must be remade:

1. Incorrect tray position in the mouth
   a. A thick buccal border on one side with a thin border on the opposite side (This indicates that the tray was out of position in the direction of the thick border.)
   b. A thick lingual border on one side with a thin border on the opposite side (This implies that the tray moved toward the thin border.)
   c. Pressure spots on the inside surface of the labial flange (This may indicate that the anterior part of the tray was not completely seated on the residual ridge.)
   d. Pressure spots on the anterior part of the lingual flange (This suggests that the lower tray was too far forward in relation to the residual ridge [possibly as a result of anterior movement of the tray when the tongue was extended for border molding].)
   e. Excess thickness of final impression material in the alveolar groove of the tray or excess length of final impression material on the flange of the tray (This may indicate that the tray was not sufficiently seated on that part of the residual ridge.)
2. Pressure spots on secondary stress-bearing areas (such as on the alveolar groove of the lower tray or in the rugae of the upper tray)
3. Voids or discrepancies that are too large to be accurately corrected
4. Incorrect border formation as a result of incorrect border length of the tray
5. Incorrect consistency of the final impression material when the tray was positioned in the mouth
6. Movement of the tray while the final impression material was setting
7. Improper pressure by the posterior palatal seal

Boxing impressions and making the casts. A wax form can be developed around most preliminary and final impressions for complete dentures to give the proper form and simplify making casts. The procedure for developing this form is called boxing.

Boxing procedures cannot usually be used on impressions made in hydrocolloid materials because the material will not adhere to the impression or because the impression will be distorted.

A strip of boxing wax is attached all the way around the outside of the impression approximately 1 to 2 mm below the border and sealed to it with a spatula. The strip must be maintained at its full width, particularly at the distal ends of the impressions, to hold the vertical walls of the boxing away from the impressions and provide space for adequate thickness of the cast in these regions (Fig. 10-10, *A* and *B*). The vertical walls of the boxing are made of sheets of beeswax.

The tongue space in the lower impression is filled with a sheet of beeswax that is fitted and attached on the superior surface of the boxing wax. The beeswax tongue space filler is sealed to the boxing wax. The lingual borders of the impression must not be obliterated or disturbed by the beeswax filler or the boxing wax. The beeswax filler should be located just below the lingual border (Fig. 10-10, *C*).

A thin sheet of wax is used for making the vertical walls of the boxing. This may be special boxing wax, or a half sheet of beeswax may be cut lengthwise and used as boxing wax. It is attached around the outside of the boxing strip so as not to alter the borders of the impression. It should extend ⅜ to ⅝ inch (9 to 15 mm) above the impression so the base of the cast at its narrowest point will be of this thickness (Fig. 10-11, *A* and *B*). The impression should be supported in a level position by the boxing. The sheet of boxing wax should extend completely around the impression and be sealed to the boxing wax strip to prevent the escape of artificial stone when this is poured into the impression. The seal between the boxing wax and the impression can be tested by holding the impression toward the light to reveal any openings. Sufficient space must be available posteriorly between the impression and the boxing to provide for adequate thickness of casts distal to the impression.

If a modified plaster is used as the final impression material, a separating medium must

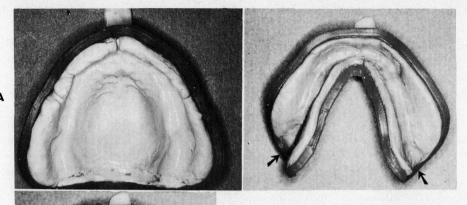

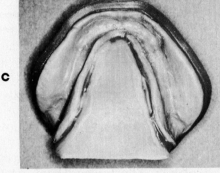

Fig. 10-10 Boxing the impression. **A,** Boxing wax has been attached just below the borders of the final upper impression. **B,** It extends for the full width at the posterior ends of the impression *(arrows)* to hold the vertical walls of the boxing in proper position. **C,** Beeswax tongue-space filler is securely attached to the wax.

be applied to it and allowed to penetrate into the plaster. Then the impression is soaked in water until all air has been eliminated from the plaster. Just before the cast is to be poured, all excess separating medium is rinsed from the impression and the excess water is shaken out.

Artificial stone is mixed according to manufacturer's directions. Sufficient stone is poured into the boxed impression that the base of the cast will be ⅜ to ⅝ inch (9 to 15 mm) thick. The artificial stone is allowed to harden for at least 30 minutes before separation.

After the final impression is separated from the cast, the borders of the cast are trimmed to leave a ledge of about ⅛ inch (3 mm) posteriorly and little or none anteriorly. The cast must be shaped to maintain the form of the borders of the impression and yet be easily accessible for adaptation of the materials used in making the occlusion rims (Fig. 10-11, *C* and *D*).

Second technique—selective pressure mandibular impression—one-step border-molded tray

Constructing autopolymerizing acrylic resin impression trays

1. Make a preliminary lower impression and pour the cast as described in the first technique (p. 225).
2. Construct an autopolymerizing acrylic resin final impression tray on the relieved preliminary lower cast as in the first technique (p. 229). Leave the relief wax in the tray (Fig. 10-12).
3. Reduce the borders of the tray until they are 2 mm underextended.

Border molding the mandibular tray

1. Prepare the mandibular tray for border molding in a similar manner as described for the maxillary tray (p. 189).

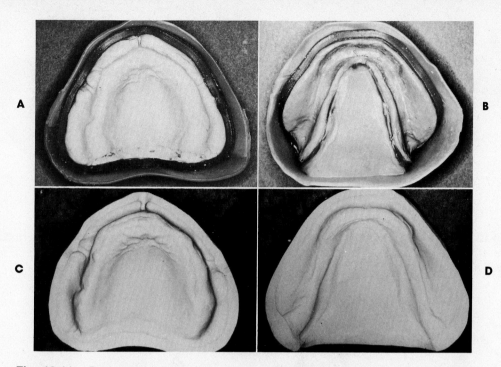

Fig. 10-11 Boxing the impression. **A,** The vertical wall of the boxing is securely attached to the boxing strip. The height of the wall will allow the base of the cast to be from ⅜ to ⅝ inch (9 to 15 mm) thick. **B,** This wall of the boxing is securely attached to a strip of boxing wax and to the posterior extent of the tongue-space filler. Notice that there is adequate space between the posterior ends of the impression and the vertical boxing. **C,** The final upper cast provides an accurate positive record of the basal seat and reflections. The thickness and form of the cast will permit easy adaptation of the materials used in making the occlusion rims. **D,** The lower final cast is formed so the posterior ends of the residual ridges are well supported, with artificial stone providing the needed strength in these regions.

2. Carefully evaluate the extensions of the tray intraorally.
3. Place adhesive over the borders of the tray.
4. Express a 4-inch strip of polyether material from the large tube and 3½ inches of catalyst from the small tube onto the mixing pad.
5. Thoroughly mix the material for 30 to 45 seconds using a metal spatula.
6. Position the polyether material on the borders. A minimum width of 6 mm must ex-

ist on the inner portion (Fig. 10-13). Since approximately twice the length of borders on the lower is involved as on the upper tray, loading must be done with minimal delay.
7. Place the impression tray in the mouth, making certain to retract the lips sufficiently to avoid scraping the polyether material from the borders.
8. Instruct the patient to elevate his tongue as the tray is seated.
9. Hold the lower lip out so the excess material can flow labially.

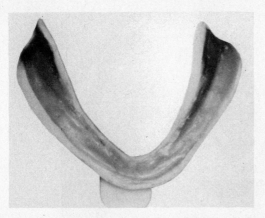

Fig. 10-12 One-step border-molded tray. The borders of the acrylic resin have been reduced; relief wax remains in the tray.

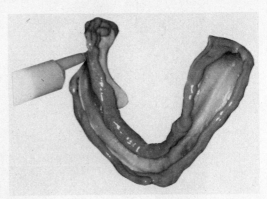

Fig. 10-13 Border molding the tray. Notice the polyether impression material extending around the tray borders, until all are covered.

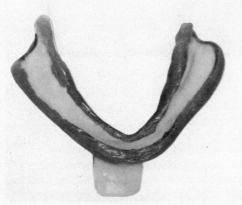

Fig. 10-14 Border molding the tray. The procedure has been completed; relief wax is no longer in the tray.

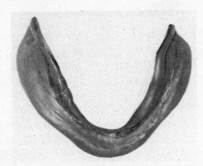

Fig. 10-15 The completed final impression with a one-step border-molded tray.

10. Have the patient drop his tongue until the tip contacts just behind the handle of the tray.
11. Quickly pull both cheeks buccally to make certain that the cheek mucosa is not trapped under the buccal flanges.
12. Complete the border-molding procedures as described in the first technique (Fig. 10-9, *C* to *E*).

13. Examine the borders for adequacy after the material has set (Fig. 10-14). The borders should be rounded.
14. Prepare the tray as described for the maxillary impression (p. 193).
15. Make the final impression in silicone, metallic oxide paste, or rubber base material (Fig. 10-15). Apply appropriate adhesive on the impression surface of the tray when using silicone.

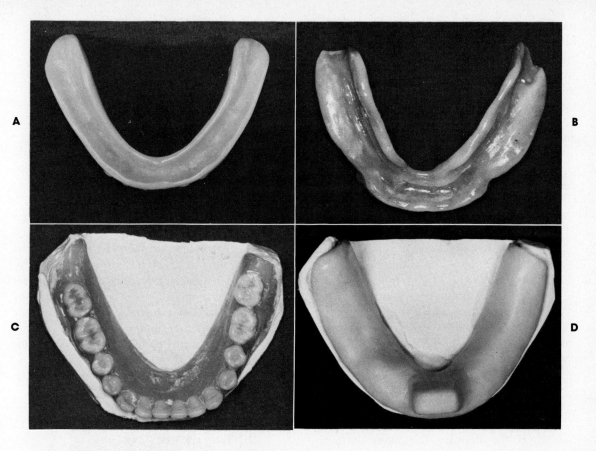

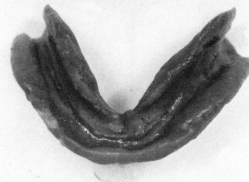

Fig. 10-16. The patient's original denture, **A,** is refitted with a treatment liner, **B,** and poured in laboratory stone, **C.** The optimized denture bearing surface area is then covered with an autopolymerized tray, **D,** which is used for the final impression, **E.**

Third technique—selective pressure mandibular impression—custom tray design based on the previously worn denture

This technique is similar to the one described for maxillary impressions in Chapter 8 and is illustrated in Fig. 10-16. The optimized fitting surface of the denture or the denture bearing (tissue-contacting) area is reproduced in stone. A wax spacer is placed to cover the entire cast, 3 to 4 mm short of the borders. A custom tray is fabricated over the spacer, and a final impression is made in the tray. Clinical experience suggests that any of these three techniques will produce an impression that fulfills biomechanical objectives. However, when advanced residual ridge resorption in the anterior mandible is present, and particularly if it is accompanied by high unfavorable soft tissue attachments (which minimize the amount of gingiva available for direct stress bearing), the first and third techniques are easier to apply.

Following is a summary of the events and considerations involved in making a mandibular impression:

1. Ensuring the health of tissues that comprise the denture-bearing surfaces
   a. Leave denture(s) out of the mouth.
   b. Optimize the patient's present denture(s) (tissue conditioning, occlusal adjustments).
   c. Prescribe preprosthetic surgery.
2. Preliminary impression(s)
   a. Use a stock tray with a wax strip border and irreversible hydrocolloid impression material.
   b. Identify the preferred peripheral outline of the custom tray. Mark a line between the attached and unattached mucosa. Make a laboratory stone cast.
   c. If the denture has been optimized (that is, functionally border molded) with a tissue conditioner, regard it as the preliminary impression. Make a laboratory stone cast.
3. Custom tray fabrication
   a. Outline the stress-bearing surface for the denture and cover it with a wax spacer.
   b. Make an acrylic resin tray that extends just past the identified junction of the attached/unattached mucosa.
4. Final impression
   a. Try the tray in the mouth and correct for any overextension(s).
   b. Develop a periphery for the tray in an effort to seal the denture's borders by using an incremental technique with a thermoplastic material (technique 1) or a one step technique with a rubber material (technique 2).
   c. If the third technique is used, border molding is not required.
   d. Use the preferred final impression material.
5. Working cast preparation
   a. Box and pour the final impression.
   b. Trim the cast.

CHAPTER 11

Biologic considerations in jaw relations and jaw movements

When the mandible moves as it does in carrying out the functions of mastication and speech, the various movements it makes and the relationships it assumes defy any simple description because of their complexity. However, when the mandible is motionless, definite relationships to the cranium or the maxillae can be established. Thus one needs to study certain static relationships to understand the motions made by the mandible in function. If we know the potential limits of the motions of the mandible, we will know the confines of the envelope of motion within which it can move.

To understand jaw motions, it is necessary to understand the factors involved in jaw relations.

ANATOMIC FACTORS

The mandibular bone has specific relationships to the bones of the cranium. The mandible is connected to the cranium at the two temporomandibular joints by the temporomandibular and capsular ligaments. The sphenomandibular and stylomandibular ligaments also connect the bones in such a way as to limit some motions of the mandible. The masseter, temporal, and medial pterygoid muscles supply the power for pulling the mandible against the maxillae, and the lateral pterygoid muscles connect the mandible to the lateral pterygoid plate in such a way as to act as a steering mech-

anism and protrude or move it laterally. (See Fig. 11-2.)

The other connection between the upper and lower jaws is through the *occlusal surfaces* of the teeth. For this reason the occlusion must be in harmony with jaw relations when the teeth are in contact.

TEMPOROMANDIBULAR ARTICULATION

Good prosthodontic treatment bears a direct relation to the structures of the TM articulation, since occlusion is one of the most important parts of treatment of patients with complete dentures. The TMJs affect dentures, and likewise dentures affect the health and function of the TMJs. Therefore a knowledge of the interrelationships of bony structures, tissue resiliency, muscle function, movements of the lips and of facial and masticatory muscles, and the occlusion, along with TMJ performance and overriding mental attitudes, seems indispensable to enabling the treatment of edentulous patients to qualify as a true health service. The relevant roles of these issues in complete denture treatment have been mentioned in various parts of this book. For a more thorough review of the anatomy and pathology of the TMJs, the reader is referred to relevant texts and articles.

Muscles

Muscles provide moving forces for all actions in the body. In dentistry, mandibular movements are the main focus since the participating muscles are involved in all functions of the masticatory system. Muscle force is necessary in chewing and in activities such as swallowing, smiling, talking, singing, etc. The mandibular musculature is also involved in grinding and clenching of the teeth and in other oral parafunctions that can lead to clinical problems. These muscular activities, likewise, take place in the complete denture wearer. Edentulous patients, furthermore, employ other muscle activities that are related to the retentive control and stability of a removable denture. The anatomy and physiology of the masticatory musculature are therefore most relevant to the rehabilitation of edentulous patients. Although an overview of the main muscles involved in mandibular movements follows, the reader should consult relevant texts for a more detailed description.

Muscles of mastication. The muscles of mas-

tication include the temporal, masseter, and medial and lateral pterygoids. The first three of these are closing muscles; the fourth is a guiding muscle that participates in jaw opening.

Temporalis. The temporal muscle arises on the side of the head from the whole of the temporal fossa and attaches to the tip and the inner and anterior surfaces of the coronoid process of the mandible (see Fig. 11-16). Its anterior fibers go down the anterior surface of the coronoid process of the mandible and down the anterior surface of the ramus, with some fibers extending into the retromolar pad and nearly as far forward as the third molar. The function of the posterior part of this muscle is to retrude the mandible and brace the condyle during lateral mandibular excursions to the same side. The function of the middle parts is to elevate the mandible into centric position. The temporal muscle does not participate in biting force when the mandible is in protrusion. Therefore

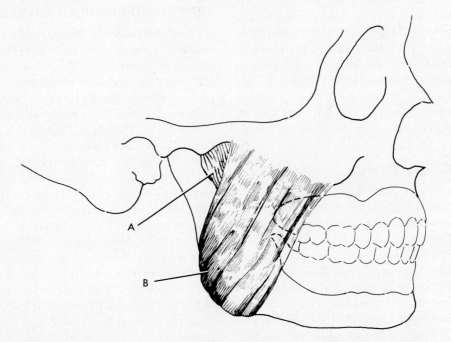

Fig. 11-1   The masseter. The buccal flange contour of the mandibular impression is influenced by the anterior fibers of this muscle. *A* is the deep portion; *B,* the superficial portion.

the action of this muscle is sometimes used as a test to determine whether the patient is closing in centric relation. When the mandible is in protrusion, no bulging can be felt with the fingers on the side of the head in the region of the temples.

Masseter. The masseter is a thick muscle consisting of two portions, the superficial and the deep. Arising from the zygomatic process of the maxilla and from the zygomatic arch of the zygomatic bone, it inserts on the outer surface of the ramus and the lateral surface of the coronoid process of the mandible. Its action is almost entirely that of an elevator of the mandible. The deep fibers aid in retruding the mandible from a forward position. The masseter muscle affects the border of the mandibular denture on the distobuccal corner of the buccal flange. Its action pushes the buccinator fibers against the denture border; for this reason the borders must converge rapidly toward

the retromolar pad. At the time the preliminary impression is made, while the compound on the border of the impression tray in this region is still soft, considerable downward force should be exerted on the lower jaw by the dentist so that the patient, in attempting to counteract this downward pressure, will cause the masseter muscle to contract, therefore forcing the softened compound away from impingement in this region (Fig. 11-1).

Pterygoideus medialis. The first portion of the medial pterygoid muscle arises from the medial surface of the lateral pterygoid plate and the palatine bone. The second portion arises from the pyramidal process of the palatine bone and the posterior end of the maxilla. The medial pterygoid inserts into the lower and posterior surfaces of the ramus and into the medial side of the angle of the mandible (Fig. 11-2). The action of this muscle is mostly that of an elevator, although it does assist in the lat-

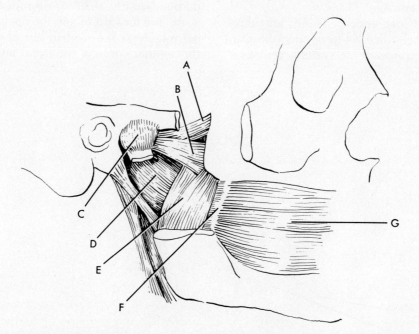

Fig. 11-2 Notice the difference in direction of the fibers of the medial (internal) and lateral (external) pterygoid muscles. *A,* Superior head of the lateral pterygoid; *B,* inferior head; *C,* capsule of the temporomandibular joint; *D,* the superior constrictor; *E,* the medial pterygoid; *F,* pterygomandibular raphe; *G,* the buccinator.

eral and protrusive movements of the mandible.

Pterygoideus lateralis. The lateral pterygoid muscle arises from two heads, the superior belly from the greater wing of the sphenoid bone and the inferior belly from the lateral pterygoid plate. Its fibers run horizontally backward and laterally. The superior belly attaches mostly to the disk and to the neck of the condyle, the inferior belly only to the neck of the condyle (Fig. 11-2). The principal action of the lateral pterygoid is protrusion of one or both condyles. With this activity the mandible is depressed or protruded. When only one condyle is protruded, the mandible moves laterally to the opposite side. The lateral pterygoids also guide the mandible into lateral or protrusive positions so food can be engaged by the teeth. The superior belly is active in a stabilizing capacity or in fixing the condyle and disk in a specific position during elevation of the mandible. However, it is *not* a muscle that elevates the mandible.

Muscles of depression. There are three groups of muscles that act to depress the mandible. The *suprahyoids* (digastricus, geniohyoideus, mylohyoideus, and stylohyoideus) and the *platysma* act as a group and are the primary movers in opening the mandible. The *infrahyoids* (extending from the hyoid bone to the sternum) act to stabilize the hyoid bone so the suprahyoid group can be effective. The third group (the *lateral pterygoids*) pull the condyles forward or medialward as the other groups act.

The mylohyoideus is the only one of these muscles that affects denture borders. Some of the salient factors regarding it are discussed here (Fig. 11-3). The mylohyoid muscle arises from the inner surface of the mandible on a line extending posteriorly from the symphysis mandibulae to the distal aspect of the third molar. The area of origin of the muscle on the mandible is known as the mylohyoid ridge. It is close to the crest of the alveolar process in the third molar region, but it gradually moves lower as it goes forward, until it is near the lower border of the mandible in the anterior portion (see Fig. 9-10). It runs medially, downward, and forward to join the opposite mylohyoid muscle at the median line and insert into the anterior cornu of the hyoid bone. The my-

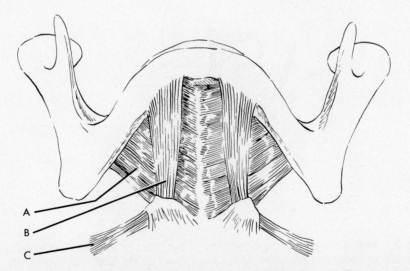

Fig. 11-3 Muscles of the floor of the mouth, anteroinferior view. *A,* The mylohyoid; *B,* anterior belly of the digastric; *C,* posterior belly of the digastric.

lohyoid muscle, together with the geniohyoid, forms the muscular floor of the mouth upon which the tongue and other structures rest (see Fig. 9-22). Although it aids in opening the mandible, its principal action is assisting in swallowing by raising the tongue and the floor of the mouth and elevating the hyoid bone. Consideration of the act of swallowing is extremely important for establishing the stability of a mandibular complete denture. When the mylohyoid muscle is in a tense state, it is pulled away from the mandible; therefore the lingual flange of the denture cannot impinge on this muscle without the denture's being displaced during swallowing or raising the tongue.

When the mylohyoid muscle is relaxed, it settles along the lingual surface of the mandible in the molar region. For this reason the impression material can follow incorrectly along the lingual contour of the mandible into the undercut below the mylohyoid ridge. If the lingual flange of a denture extends into the undercut, it will bind the muscle so the muscle is restricted in movement; otherwise, the muscle will cause displacement of the denture when contracted. Resorption of the alveolar process causes a sharpening of the mylohyoid ridge, and the resulting edge with the muscle attaching to it is a source of much discomfort because the hard surface of the denture irritates the end fibers of the muscle (see Fig. 9-13).

CLASSIFICATION OF JAW RELATIONS

Jaw relations are classified into three groups to make them more easily understood: (1) orientation, (2) vertical, and (3) horizontal relations. Considered in this manner, the relation of the mandible to the maxillae (or cranium) can be accurately determined in three dimensions. *Orientation* relations establish the references in the cranium. *Vertical* relations establish the amount of jaw separation allowable for dentures. *Horizontal* relations establish the front-to-back and side-to-side relationships of one jaw to the other. Thus, with specific distances designated, the mandible can be accurately located relative to the maxillae.

Orientation relations

When the mandible is kept in its most posterior position, it can rotate in the sagittal plane around an imaginary transverse axis passing through or near the condyles. The axis can be located when the mandible is in its most posterior position by means of a kinematic face-bow or hinge-bow, or it can be approximated by use of an arbitrary type of face-bow.*

Face-bow. The face-bow is a caliper-like device that is used to record the relationship of the jaws to the temporomandibular joints or the opening axis of the jaws and to orient the casts in this same relationship to the opening axis of the articulator. It is also a convenient instrument for supporting the casts while they are being attached to the articulator. It consists of a U-shaped frame or assembly that is large enough to extend from the region of the TMJs to a position 2 to 3 inches (5 to 7.5 cm) in front of the face and wide enough to avoid contact with the sides of the face. The parts that contact the skin over the TMJs are the condyle rods, and the part that attaches to the occlusion rims is the fork. The fork attaches to the face-bow by means of a locking device, which serves also to support the face-bow, the occlusion rims, and the casts while the casts are being attached to the articulator.

There are two basic types of face-bows: the arbitrary and the kinematic (or hinge-bow). The arbitrary face-bow is placed on the face with the condyle rods located approximately over the condyles. The kinematic face-bow is so designed that the opening axis of the mandible can be located more accurately (see Fig. 11-9, *B*).

The arbitrary face-bow is the one most used in complete denture techniques and is considered adequate for this purpose. The condyle rods of one particular model are positioned on a line extending from the outer canthus to the top of the tragus and approximately 13 mm in

---

*It is also possible to simulate mandibular orientation by an arbitrary "average" technique without using a face-bow (p. 327).

front of the external auditory meatus. This placement generally locates the rods within 5 mm of the true center of the opening axis of the jaws. The rods of another commonly used model are designed to fit into the external auditory meatuses. On the articulator the location of these rods approximately compensates for the distance that the meatuses are posterior to the transverse opening axis of the mandible.

The fork of arbitrary face-bows is attached to the maxillary occlusion rim so the record is a simple measurement from the jaws to the approximate axis of the jaws.

The fork of kinematic face-bows is attached to the mandibular occlusion rim. Then, as the patient retrudes the mandible and opens and closes the jaws, the dentist observes the movement of the points of the condyle rods. The condyle rods of kinematic face-bows have sharp points, so their motion can be observed more accurately. When the points rotate only and do not translate, they are on the opening axis of the jaw. At this position the mandible is as far back as it will go and can be considered in centric relation for the occlusal vertical dimension that has been established.

Since face-bows are used to orient casts on an articulator in the same relation to the opening axis of the articulator as the jaws are to the opening axis of the jaws, the face-bow record is not a maxillomandibular relation record. Rather, it is a record made for the orientation of the cast to the instrument. However, use of a kinematic face-bow can aid in recording centric relation.

The posterior terminal hinge axis of the mandible can be located only when the mandible is in its most posterior position (that is, centric relation, provided of course the vertical dimension of the jaws has been established). The difficulty of attaching the lower occlusion rim to an edentulous mandible so it will not move in relation to the bone prevents its more extensive use for edentulous patients. The inevitable movement of the recording base on the jaw makes determining the exact center of the opening axis quite difficult.

Value of the face-bow. Failure to use the face-bow may lead to errors in occlusion of the denture. It is true that the errors may be small if the error in orientation of the casts is small. Likewise, the errors produced by failure to use the face-bow would be negligible if all the interocclusal records were made precisely at the occlusal vertical dimension at which the occlusion was to be established and if teeth with zero degrees of inclination were used. However, if cusped teeth are used or interocclusal records are made with the teeth out of contact so the vertical separation of the casts or dentures must be reduced *on the articulator,* the face-bow record is essential. The face-bow transfer allows a more accurate arc of closure on the articulator when the interocclusal records are removed and the articulator is closed. It requires little time, and the convenience it provides in cast mounting saves that time.

Fig. 11-4 is a schematic of a comparative study of mounting dentures with and without a face-bow.

Fig. 11-5 shows the variations that can occur in registration of condylar guidance on the articulator when the casts are mounted at various heights—the highest mounting at *A*, the intermediate-height mounting at *B*, and the lowest mounting at *C*. Note that the cast-condylar angle remains 135 degrees regardless of the height of mounting.

Use of the face-bow. The use of a face-bow (Hanau Model C or any other) is predicated on an arbitrary location of the opening axis of the mandible. However, the condyle is not a point whereas its hinge axis or kinematic center is an exact point. To palpate for the center of the condyle or to set it by arbitrary lines is to use an approximation. Nevertheless, this method is better than not using a face-bow at all. The approximation works well in complete denture construction, but it produces inaccuracies when wax or plaster is interposed for maxillomandibular records or when fixed or partial dentures are constructed for vertical dimension increase. This difficulty can be removed by use

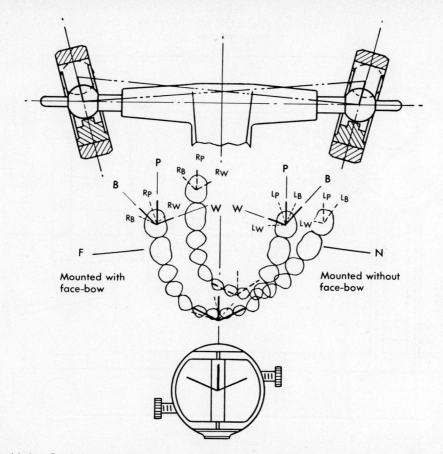

Fig. 11-4 Occlusion and the occlusal aspect with and without a face-bow mounting on the articulator. *B, P,* and *W* are balancing, protrusive, and working contacts. *F,* Denture mounted with a face-bow. Notice the direction of the balancing, protrusive, and working strokes for needle-point tracings in the anterior and molar regions. This mounting will coincide with movements in the mouth, and the tracings will reflect the directions of these movements. *N,* Denture mounted without a face-bow. The tracings will reflect movements of the articulator only, and the denture will thus occlude properly only on the articulator. When denture *N* is superimposed on denture *F,* the tracings of the two *(dotted lines)* will not coincide. Notice that the needle-point tracings of *N* are at an incorrect angle and therefore will not duplicate mandibular movements. The clinical importance of this failure is not known, however.

of a kinematic face-bow, which aids in finding the kinematic center of jaw opening, or by recording the appropriate vertical dimension clinically and not changing it on the articulator.

The Hanau Model C face-bow and most other arbitrary face-bows are adjusted to a point on the face. The point is marked 13 mm

forward from the external auditory meatus, on a line from the top of the tragus to the corner of the eye (outer canthus). Without clamping the condyle rods, the dentist centers the device so equal readings are obtained on both sides, and the wing nut of the clamp is tightened to hold the face-bow in place on the oc-

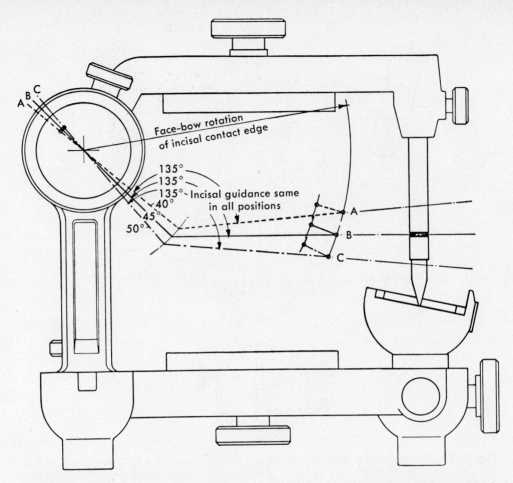

Fig. 11-5 Variance of condyle registrations on the articulator (40, 45, and 50 degrees), the result of mounting casts with a face-bow at various heights (A, B, and C). However, the cast-condylar angle remains the same in all positions, which is 135 degrees. Therefore movement of the cast in relation to condylar inclination is the same in all three positions, which fact makes the height of mounting immaterial.

clusal fork (see Figs. 15-6 and 15-7).

The Whip Mix is also an arbitrary face-bow (see Fig. 15-17). The ends of the bow are placed in the external auditory meatuses instead of over the condyles. However, when the instrument is attached to the articulator, the transverse axis of the articulator is ⅝ inch (15 mm) anterior to the position of the ends of the face-bow. This distance compensates for the distance between the external auditory meatus and the condyle. Thus the effective result is approximately the same as with other arbitrary face-bows.

Studies performed to compare the effectiveness of different types of face-bows have failed to demonstrate any significant differences. The face-bow registrations showed no great variation in repeated recordings. Numerous studies have also investigated the precision of various registration methods; but, regrettably, the question as to whether different methods of complete denture construction can produce significant differences in the end result has yet to be compellingly addressed in well-designed clinical studies.

The kinematic face-bow (see Fig. 11-9, *B*) is first fastened to the mandibular occlusion rim, and the patient is asked to make simple opening and closing movements with the mandible in its most retruded position (centric relation). These movements show whether the condyle rods are on the rotational center. If they are not, the points are adjusted during the opening movements until they rotate without any concentric arcing. When the hinge axis center has been determined, it is marked on the face with an indelible pencil. The face-bow is removed from the face-bow fork, and the condyle rods are straightened and made parallel. The face-bow is now used in the regular manner by being fastened into place over the previously determined rotational points. This type of transfer will be exact in the positional relation of the casts and, in addition, will permit a recording medium (wax, zinc oxide–eugenol, plaster) for interocclusal records to be interposed without the usual inaccuracy being produced. This fact is of great advantage in complete dentures, especially when the interarch distance is to be increased or decreased.

It should be remembered, however, that these theoretical advantages to the use of a face-bow may not necessarily produce a better clinical end result. One of the few systematic studies made to compare patient response to variations in denture technique failed to show any significant differences between a "complex" technique involving hinge axis location for a face-bow transfer to the articulator and a "standard" technique without face-bow and with an arbitrary mounting. Similar clinical results with dentures constructed by the two techniques have been found in both short- and long-term recall assessments. The registration included dentists' evaluations of occlusion, denture stability, retention, and conditions of denture-bearing tissues, together with patient satisfaction and adaptation. The results indicated that the success of denture treatment involves many factors and the use of a face-bow is not an essential one. Such documentation and extensive clinical experience have caused many practicing dentists to stop using a face-bow. This is, of course, no excuse for abandoning impeccable technique and sound principles of denture construction. It also is clear that imperfections may exist with both "complex" and "standard" techniques, which means that scrupulous clinical control and the acceptance of a need for adjustments are necessary with any method.

Vertical relations

The vertical jaw relations are those established by the amount of separation of the maxillae and mandible under specified conditions. They are classified as the vertical relations (or more properly the vertical dimensions) of (1) occlusion, (2) rest, and (3) other positions. Vertical relations are discussed further in Chapter 12.

The vertical dimension of *occlusion* is established by the natural teeth when they are present and in occlusion. In people who have lost their natural teeth and must wear dentures it is established by the vertical height of the two dentures when the teeth are in contact. Thus the vertical dimension of occlusion must be established for edentulous people so their denture teeth will be properly related to each other. Although it has been referred to as the vertical "relation" of occlusion, this term is now hardly ever used.

The vertical dimension of *rest* (or physiologic rest position of the mandible) is established by muscles and gravity. It is a postural relationship of the mandible to the maxillae, and the teeth do *not* determine it. The mandible is in its physiologic rest position when all the muscles that close the jaws and all those that open the jaws are in a state of minimal tonic contraction sufficient only to maintain posture. Since gravity exerts a force on the mandible, this force is added to the force from muscles applied to the mandible, and therefore the position of the head is important when observations of the vertical dimension of rest position are made. Specifically, the head must be held in an upright position by the patient and not supported by a headrest when these observations are made.

The value of the vertical dimension of rest position in denture construction lies in its use as a guide to the lost vertical dimension of occlusion. This is possible because the difference between the occlusal vertical dimension and the rest vertical dimension is the interocclusal distance. The interocclusal distance (formerly referred to as the "free-way space") is the distance or gap existing between the upper and lower teeth when the mandible is in the physiologic rest position. It usually is 2 to 4 mm when observed at the position of the first premolars. However, the clinically recorded rest position is not the same as the electromyographically determined one. A range of reduced muscle tension up to an interocclusal distance of about 10 mm has been reported.

An interocclusal distance is essential for the health of the periodontal tissues when natural teeth are present. It also is absolutely essential for complete denture patients. Failure to provide for it will cause "clicking" of the dentures during speech, soreness of the tissues of the basal seat, and rapid destruction of the residual alveolar ridges. When denture teeth are in contact without rest for the supporting tissues (except when the mouth is open for speech or eating), the bones of the mandible and maxillae will resorb in an effort to achieve that needed rest.

On the basis of these facts, it can be seen that if the correct vertical dimension of rest position is determined the vertical dimension of the occlusion rims or dentures can be easily adjusted to provide the necessary interocclusal distance. Then the occlusion may be tentatively established at this reduced distance to establish the vertical dimension of occlusion.

The vertical dimensions of *other* positions (for instance, when the mouth is half open or wide open) are of no significance in the construction of dentures.

Horizontal relations

The horizontal jaw relations are those in a horizontal plane of reference. The basic horizontal relationship is centric relation—*when the mandible is in its most retruded position at the established vertical dimension.* It is a reference relationship that must be recognized in any prosthodontic treatment. Horizontal jaw relations are discussed further in Chapter 13. Other horizontal jaw relations are deviations occurring in the horizontal plane: protrusion(s), right and left lateral excursions, and all intermediate positions. They are grouped together as eccentric relations.

All eccentric relationships (excursions) are in the same horizontal plane as centric relation, except that the articulating eminences push the mandibular condyles downward as the mandible is moved forward or laterally. Although they are essentially in the horizontal plane, concurrent changes are seen in the vertical dimensions between the posterior upper and lower residual alveolar ridges. These changes must be recorded if articulators are to be properly adjusted. They are known as the Christiansen phenomenon, and they result in the development of spaces between the upper and lower occlusal surfaces at the distal of the occlusion rims or dentures with downward/forward movement of the condyles.

Some dentists maintain that if the occlusion of the dentures is to be balanced so there is uniform contact between upper and lower teeth throughout the functional range of jaw movement the amount of this space must be determined. This can be done by means of interocclusal records, with the articulator adjusted accordingly. However, the value of such registrations is not supported by convincing documentation; and we therefore do not regard them as necessary for achieving clinically acceptable results.

MOVEMENTS OF THE MANDIBLE*

Mandibular movements are complex in nature and vary greatly among persons and within each person. Many different mandibular movements occur during mastication, speech, swallowing, respiration, and facial expression. Also, parafunctional movements (bruxism and clenching) may eventually cause pain and pathosis in the structures related to movement of the jaw. The dentist is the *scientist* who must understand the factors that regulate motion of the jaws. These include contacts of opposing teeth, the anatomy and physiology of the TMJs, the axes around which the mandible rotates, the actions of the muscles and ligaments, and the neuromuscular integration of all these factors. The dentist is also the *health clinician* who must relate an understanding of mandibular movements to their useful clinical application in the treatment of patients, particularly those who are edentulous.

Practical significance of understanding mandibular movements

A knowledge of mandibular movements is essential to developing tooth forms for dental restorations, understanding occlusion, arranging artificial teeth, treating TMJ disturbances, preserving periodontal health, and the designing, selection, and adjustment of articulators.

When dental operations involve more than single restorations, most dentists find that restorative procedures can be developed more accurately, conveniently, and quickly on the articulator than in the patient's mouth. The articulator, then, must closely simulate jaw

movements within the range of contacts between opposing teeth so the occlusion planned on the instrument will function properly in the patient's mouth. The degree of success in doing this depends on evoking the desired functional jaw movements in the patient, on accurately recording and transferring these to the instrument, and on the capabilities of the articulator. Many differences can be expected between the manner in which opposing tooth surfaces contact on a simple nonadjustable articulator and the manner in which they contact in the patient's mouth (Fig. 11-6, *A*). Fewer differences will be expected during movements of a more fully adjustable articulator (Fig. 11-6, *B*). The decision whether most adjustments of occlusion in eccentric jaw relations for finished restorations should be made on the articulator or in the patient's mouth will determine the selection of an appropriate articulator for restorative procedures. Nevertheless, regardless of the method chosen, careful refinement and control of the occlusion as determined intraorally will be necessary.

Methods of studying mandibular movement

Mandibular, and particularly condylar, activity has been studied for many years by a variety of methods, ranging from direct clinical observations to sophisticated electronic instrumentation. In 1889 Luce photographed the reflection of sunlight from beads placed opposite the condyles. Walker, in 1896, used a facial clinometer to measure condylar movements. Bennett, in 1908, traced the pathway of a light positioned opposite the condyle. Hildebrand recorded condylar movements by roentgen fluoroscopy in 1931. Studies have been conducted using mechanical and cinematographic techniques, cineradiography, and more recently photoelectric and electromagnetic techniques. Several of these techniques have been coupled with computer analysis to provide valuable information relative to the nature of the mandib-

*We wish to acknowledge the assistance of Jackie G. Weatherred, D.D.S., Ph.D., Coordinator of Physiology for Dentistry, Medical College of Georgia School of Dentistry, Augusta.

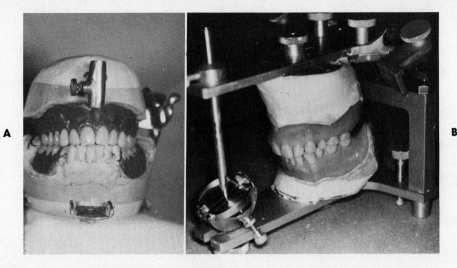

Fig. 11-6   A, This articulator is adjusted by an interocclusal centric relation record and is accurate only for the position at which the record was made. **B,** This articulator is adjusted by a face-bow record, an interocclusal centric relation record, and interocclusal protrusive and lateral records. An occlusion developed on this instrument will function in the patient's mouth with fewer discrepancies than will an occlusion developed on the articulator in **A.** However, in both cases subsequent intraoral occlusal refinement may still be required.

ular movements. Motion pictures of markers attached to the teeth and others positioned adjacent to the condyles have been made in single planes and with a prism beam splitter. Three-dimensional motion picture photography has depicted movement of markers attached to the teeth and to a pin inserted directly into the condyle (Fig. 11-7). Light-emitting diodes, computer-monitored radionuclide tracking, and optical pantography have been used to study mandibular movements. In addition, electronic instruments (including a Gnathic Replicator, a Dynamic Duplicator, an ultrasonic probe, and other sensing devices) have been computerized and programmed to cause casts of the patient's mouth to move in the same manner as the patient's mandible.

The studies have included the effects of tooth contact on condylar movements, the movement of working and balancing condyles during lateral mandibular excursions, and the presence or absence of opposing tooth contacts during mastication. Mandibular movements also have been studied during mastication, during movement from centric relation to centric occlusion, and during movement from the vertical relation of rest to the vertical relation of occlusion.

Studies of mandibular movements have revealed important information regarding factors that regulate jaw motion, which in turn have clinical implications in all aspects of occlusion. Through continued research dentists will learn new methods of developing harmony among the factors regulating jaw motion that will enable them to provide improved dental care for their patients.

Factors that regulate jaw motion

When opposing teeth are in contact and mandibular movements are made, the direction of the movement is controlled by the neuromuscular system as limited by the movement of the two condyles and the guiding influences

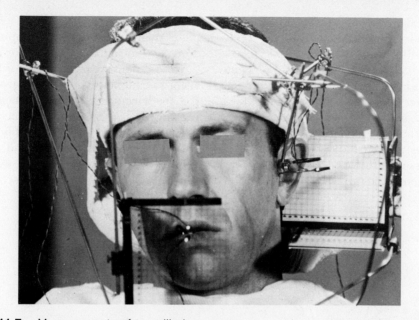

Fig. 11-7   Measurements of mandibular movements can be made when the pathways of small lights recorded by three motion picture cameras simultaneously in the frontal, sagittal, and horizontal planes are plotted. Grids give an indication of the amount of movement of the lights. The light at the end of a pin inserted into the condyle shows the direction of movement of the condyle, and the light facing forward shows the amount of rotation of the condyle during mandibular movements.

of the contacting teeth. When the opposing teeth are not in contact and mandibular movements occur, the direction of movement is controlled by the mandibular musculature as limited by condylar movement alone. The condyles and teeth modify only mandibular movements initiated by the neuromuscular system.

Any mandibular movement is the result of the interaction of a number of biologic factors. These include contacts of opposing teeth, the anatomy and physiology of the TMJs, the rotational axes of the mandible, and the actions of the controlling and moving muscles as directed by the associated neurophysiologic activities. For clarity, the manner in which each of these factors relates to jaw motion will be described individually.

Influence of opposing tooth contacts. An important aspect of many jaw movements includes the contacts of opposing teeth. The manner in which the teeth occlude is related not only to the occlusal surfaces of the teeth themselves but also to the muscles, TMJs, and neurophysiologic components including the patient's mental well-being.

When patients wearing complete dentures bring their teeth together in centric or eccentric positions within the functional range of mandibular movements, the occlusal surfaces of the teeth should meet evenly on both sides. In this manner the mandible is not deflected from its normal path of closure nor are the dentures displaced from the residual ridges. In addition, when mandibular movements are made with the opposing teeth of complete dentures in contact, the inclined planes of the teeth should pass over one another smoothly and not disrupt the influences of the condylar guidance posteriorly and the incisal guidance anteriorly.

Research has shown that condylar movement is limited not solely by the anatomy of the TMJs but also by the contacts of opposing teeth. Variations in condylar movement have been observed concomitantly as deflective occlusal contacts or steep incisal guidance from opposing canines change the pathway of mandibular movement. Thus the inclined planes of artificial teeth must be so positioned that they will be in harmony with the other factors that regulate jaw motion. A failure to develop this kind

of occlusion can disturb the stability of complete dentures and cause denture bases to move on the soft tissues of the residual ridges.

Several dentists have observed that patients adapt to complete dentures by avoiding eccentric tooth contacts during mastication and by chewing on both sides at the same time. Such a chewing pattern will presumably reduce the risk of denture dislodgment and may explain why patients appear to function well with dentures even when a balanced occlusion is no

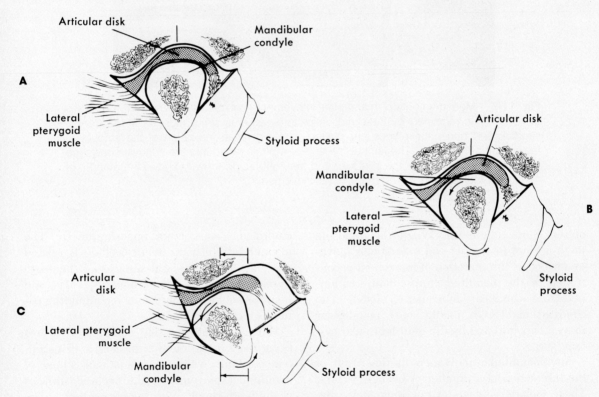

Fig. 11-8 The temporomandibular joint is divided by the articular disk into a superior and an inferior compartment. **A,** When the condyle is most retruded, notice its relation to the disk. Fibers of the lateral pterygoid are attached to both the neck of the condyle and (through the capsular ligament) the anterior part of the disk. **B,** With the jaws open and the mandible retruded, notice that a rotational movement *(arrows)* causes no condylar translation. **C,** With the mandible moving forward accompanied by slight opening, a rotational movement causes forward translation of the disk on the articular eminence (notice stretching of the fibrous capsule). All mandibular translatory movements affect the disk and eminence.

longer present. This occlusal change has been reported to occur in patients within a year or two following denture insertion.

Influence of the temporomandibular joints. Each TMJ is divided into a superior and an inferior compartment by the articular disk, in effect making two joints within each temporomandibular articulation (Fig. 11-8, *A*). However, the basic type of mandibular movement in the two compartments is different. In the upper compartment it is primarily translation, and in the lower compartment primarily rotation. This difference is related to the anatomic attachments of the articular disk to the lateral surfaces of the condyle and to the lateral pterygoid muscle.

All mandibular motion is either rotation or translation (or more commonly a combination of these). A rotational movement is one in which all points within a body describe concentric circles around a common axis. A translatory movement is one in which all points within a body are moving at the same velocity and in the same direction. Rotational movements of the mandible take place in the lower compartment of the TMJ between the superior surface of the condyle and the inferior surface of the articular disk (Fig. 11-8, *B*). Translatory, or gliding, movements of the mandible take place in the upper compartment of the TMJ between the superior surface of the articular disk as it moves with the condyle and the inferior surface of the glenoid fossa. The condyle can translate anteroposteriorly approximately ¾ inch (18 mm). Mandibular movements, except opening and closing with the mandible held by the patient or dentist in its most posterior position (posterior terminal hinge movement), are combinations of rotation and translation (Fig. 11-8, *C*).

Axes of mandibular rotation. Rotational movements of the mandible are made around three axes (transverse, vertical, and sagittal) that move constantly during normal jaw function.

During opening and closing, the mandible moves in the sagittal plane around a *transverse* axis that passes through or near both condyles (Fig. 11-9, *A*). The transverse axis can be located when opening and closing occur with the mandible in its most posterior position (Fig. 11-9, *B*). This axis is used to orient the maxillary cast properly on the articulator. The transverse axis moves with the mandible in lateral, protrusive, or lateroprotrusive movements. Thus, if the mandible is in a forward position and opening or closing occurs, the rotation will still take place about the same transverse axis in the lower compartment of the TMJ. However, since the mandible cannot be fixed in space in the forward position, the transverse axis will be instantaneous for any given location and will move and tilt with the mandible. (An instantaneous axis is one that operates while the mandible is translating to a series of different positions.)

In a lateral excursion the mandible rotates around a *vertical* axis passing through or near the condyle on the working side (the side toward which the mandible is moved) as the condyle on the opposite (balancing) side moves forward and medially (Fig. 11-9, *C*). Since it is physiologically impossible to make a lateral mandibular movement with no translation of the condyle on the working side, again the vertical axis is moving and tilting along with the mandible.

During a lateral mandibular movement, the condyle on the balancing side that is moving forward and medially also moves downward because of the slope of the articular eminence. This downward movement of the condyle on the balancing side causes the mandible to rotate around a *sagittal* axis passing through or near the condyle on the working side (Fig. 11-9, *D*). As the condyle on the working side rotates around the vertical axis and translates, the sagittal axis moves in a corresponding manner.

During these same mandibular excursions, in addition to rotating, the condyle on the

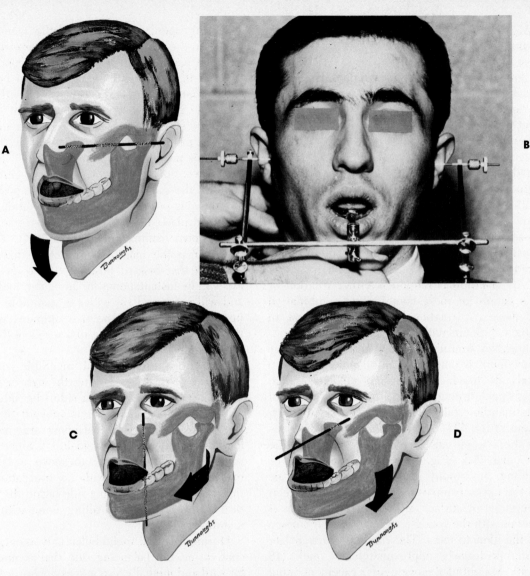

Fig. 11-9 **A,** When the jaws are opened or closed, the mandible rotates around a transverse axis that passes through both condyles. No matter the location of the condyles within the temporomandibular joint, the mandible rotates around a transverse axis during opening and closing movements. **B,** The patient makes a series of opening and closing movements with the mandible in its most posterior position relative to the maxillae. The condyle-locating pins are adjusted until they rotate with no arcing component during the retruded opening and closing movements. Thus they indicate the location of the transverse hinge axis around which the mandible is rotating. **C,** When the mandible is moved to the right, the left (balancing) condyle moves downward, forward, and inward, with rotation occurring around a vertical axis through the working condyle. **D,** In a right lateral mandibular excursion, there is a downward component of the balancing condyle. During this downward movement, the working condyle rotates around a sagittal axis. (**B** from Hickey JC, et al: J Prosthet Dent **13:**72-92, 1963.)

working side may also move laterally, anteriorly, posteriorly, upward, or downward. The exact nature of this translatory movement during lateral mandibular excursions is dependent on the movement itself and the anatomic form of the glenoid fossa, condyle, and articular disk.

One other important mandibular translatory movement, the direct lateral side shift that occurs simultaneously with a lateral excursion, was first described by Dr. Norman Bennett in 1908 and is called the *Bennett shift*. The amount of medial movement of the condyle on the balancing side during a lateral excursion governs the magnitude of the direct lateral slide of the mandible, which can be observed and measured by the movement of the condyle on the working side (Fig. 11-10).

The Bennett shift is an important component of lateral jaw movements for most patients, although its amount and timing vary among persons. Its precise incorporation is more significant in restoring the occlusion of dentulous than of edentulous patients.

The location of the axes of rotation, the establishment of the horizontal and lateral condylar guidances, and the provision for direct lateral shift of the mandible must be closely approximated on the articulator if they are to be adequately simulated. This transfer of information from the patient to the articulator requires an understanding of the capabilities and limitations of the articulator and is accomplished by means of accurate interocclusal records or pantographic tracings (Fig. 11-11). In either instance, for edentulous patients, the occlusion of the artificial teeth can be perfected better on the articulator than in the mouth because of the movement of the dentures on the basal seat tissues of the residual ridges.

Muscular involvement in jaw motion. The muscles responsible for mandibular motion generally show increased activity during any jaw movement. This increase in activity may be associated with movement of the mandible, fixation in a given position, or stabilization so

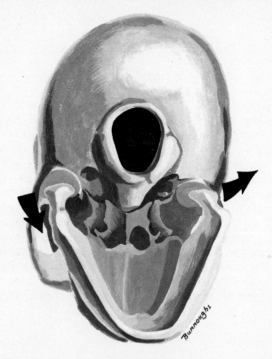

Fig. 11-10   The skull from the inferior aspect. During a right lateral excursion the mandible shifts bodily in a lateral direction. This direct lateral movement (Bennett shift) is the result of a mesial (inward) movement of the balancing condyle *(left arrow)* with a corresponding lateral (outward) movement of the working condyle *(right arrow).*

movement will be smooth and coordinated from one position to another. The activity and interaction of the muscles for a series of jaw movements have been determined by electromyography (Fig. 11-12).

Certain muscles are primarily involved in mandibular movements of particular clinical significance in establishing jaw relations. The role that these muscles play in regulating these mandibular movements are described as follows:

The *temporal muscles* have broad fan-shaped origins on the skull (Fig. 11-13). The fibers that form the posterior part of each muscle run more horizontally than those in the

Fig. 11-11 **A,** The most posterior relation of the mandible to the maxillae can be transferred from the patient to the articulator by means of an interocclusal centric relation record. Here a plaster interocclusal CR record is made between the occlusion rims. **B,** The relation of the mandible to the skull during selected mandibular movements can be transferred to the articulator with a pantographic tracing. Such tracings are made by fixed needle points that scribe lines on moving tracing tables attached by a clutch to the mandible. This complicated registration procedure is not considered necessary in complete denture construction.

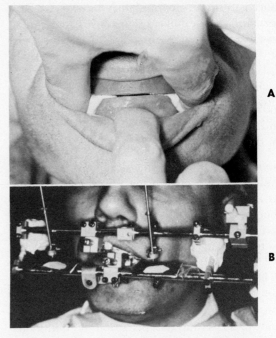

Fig. 11-12 Relative amount of activity in the muscles of mastication. The muscles listed at the top of the charts were measured electromyographically for their activity during various jaw movements. Each bar denotes the mean of 50 mandibular movements. **A,** The temporal muscles. Notice the relatively large amount of activity of the middle and posterior parts during hinge openings and retrusions of the mandible and the reduced activity when mandibular opening was uncontrolled. The posterior parts of the temporal muscles brace the mandible during lateral excursions to the same side. **B,** Left masseter, left lateral pterygoid (externus), and left digastric. Notice that the external pterygoid plays a major role in uncontrolled openings of the mandible but has little involvement in hinge openings. On the other hand, the digastrics are extremely active in uncontrolled opening, retrusion, and hinge-opening movements. (From Woelfel JB, et al: J Prosthet Dent **10:**688-697, 1960.)

LEFT ANTERIOR TEMPORAL MUSCLE
0 1 2 3 4 5 6 7 8 9 10 11 12

CLENCH
CLENCH LEFT
CLENCH RIGHT
CLENCH PROTRUDED
SLIDE LEFT
RETRUDE
HINGE OPEN
PROTRUDED LEFT
LEFT LATERAL EXCURSION
PROTRUDED RIGHT
PROTRUSION
OPEN UNCONTROLLED
SLIDE PROTRUDED
RIGHT LATERAL EXCURSION
SLIDE RIGHT

LEFT MIDDLE TEMPORAL MUSCLE
0 1 2 3 4 5 6 7 8 9 10 11 12

CLENCH
CLENCH LEFT
SLIDE LEFT
HINGE OPEN
RETRUDE
PROTRUDED LEFT
CLENCH RIGHT
LEFT LATERAL EXCURSION
CLENCH PROTRUDED
OPEN UNCONTROLLED
PROTRUDED RIGHT
RIGHT LATERAL EXCURSION
PROTRUSION
SLIDE PROTRUDED
SLIDE RIGHT

LEFT POSTERIOR TEMPORAL MUSCLE
0 1 2 3 4 5 6 7 8 9 10 11 12

CLENCH LEFT
CLENCH
SLIDE LEFT
HINGE OPEN
RETRUDE
LEFT LATERAL EXCURSION
PROTRUDED LEFT
CLENCH RIGHT
OPEN UNCONTROLLED
PROTRUDE
CLENCH PROTRUDED
PROTRUDED RIGHT
RIGHT LATERAL EXCURSION
SLIDE PROTRUDED
SLIDE RIGHT

RIGHT POSTERIOR TEMPORAL MUSCLE
0 1 2 3 4 5 6 7 8 9 10 11 12

CLENCH
CLENCH RIGHT
RETRUDE
HINGE OPEN
RIGHT LATERAL EXCURSION
PROTRUDED RIGHT
SLIDE RIGHT
PROTRUDED LEFT
LEFT LATERAL EXCURSION
PROTRUDE
OPEN UNCONTROLLED
CLENCH LEFT
CLENCH PROTRUDED
SLIDE LEFT
SLIDE PROTRUDED

A

LEFT MASSETER MUSCLE
0 1 2 3 4 5 6 7 8 9 10 11 12

CLENCH
CLENCH RIGHT
CLENCH PROTRUDED
PROTRUDED LEFT
PROTRUSION
RETRUDE
CLENCH LEFT
PROTRUDED RIGHT
RIGHT LATERAL EXCURSION
OPEN UNCONTROLLED
LEFT LATERAL EXCURSION
HINGE OPEN
SLIDE FORWARD
SLIDE RIGHT
SLIDE LEFT

LEFT EXTERNAL PTERYGOID MUSCLE
0 1 2 3 4 5 6 7 8 9 10 11 12

RIGHT LATERAL EXCURSION
PROTRUDED RIGHT
PROTRUSION
OPEN UNCONTROLLED
CLENCH PROTRUDED
CLENCH RIGHT
CLENCH
SLIDE FORWARD
SLIDE RIGHT
PROTRUDED LEFT
RETRUDE
CLENCH LEFT
HINGE OPEN
SLIDE LEFT
LEFT LATERAL EXCURSION

LEFT DIGASTRIC MUSCLE
0 1 2 3 4 5 6 7 8 9 10 11 12

OPEN UNCONTROLLED
RETRUDE
HINGE OPEN
PROTRUDED LEFT
PROTRUSION
CLENCH
PROTRUDED RIGHT
CLENCH PROTRUDED
CLENCH RIGHT
RIGHT LATERAL EXCURSION
LEFT LATERAL EXCURSION
CLENCH LEFT
SLIDE RIGHT
SLIDE FORWARD
SLIDE LEFT

RIGHT DIGASTRIC MUSCLE
0 1 2 3 4 5 6 7 8 9 10 11 12

OPEN UNCONTROLLED
RETRUDE
HINGE OPEN
PROTRUDED LEFT
PROTRUSION
PROTRUDED RIGHT
RIGHT LATERAL EXCURSION
CLENCH RIGHT
CLENCH PROTRUDED
CLENCH
LEFT LATERAL EXCURSION
CLENCH LEFT
SLIDE RIGHT
SLIDE FORWARD
SLIDE LEFT

B

Fig. 11-12   For legend see opposite page.

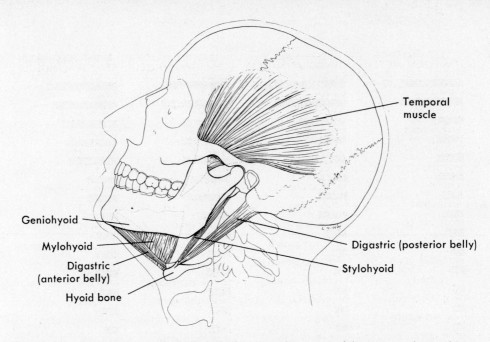

Labels on figure: Temporal muscle; Geniohyoid; Mylohyoid; Digastric (anterior belly); Hyoid bone; Digastric (posterior belly); Stylohyoid

Fig. 11-13   The middle, and particularly the posterior, parts of the temporal muscle contract isotonically (fibers actually shorten during contraction and cause movement of a part) and, in combination with the suprahyoid muscles, *position* the mandible in centric relation. Then these same muscles contract isometrically (fibers maintain their length during contraction and fix or hold a part in a particular position) to *maintain* the mandible in centric relation during making of an interocclusal CR record.

anterior and middle parts. When the posterior fibers contract, they tend to move the mandible posteriorly into centric relation or to hold it in its most posterior position during terminal hinge movement. Thus, when a patient is instructed to "pull your lower jaw back and close on your back teeth" to make a centric relation record or to locate the posterior terminal hinge axis, the temporal muscles and the inframandibular muscles retrude the mandible and maintain it in this most posterior position.

The *lateral pterygoids* move the mandible forward, if acting jointly, or to the opposite side, if acting individually (Fig. 11-14, *A*). During the conscious effort required in mandibular terminal hinge opening move-

ments, the lateral pterygoids remain relatively inactive. Meanwhile, the suprahyoids produce rotary jaw movement around a stationary transverse mandibular hinge axis (Fig. 11-14, *B*). During uncontrolled opening movements the lateral pterygoids are responsible for the forward movement of the condyles and the mandible. They also are responsible for the lateral and protrusive movements necessary to making an eccentric interocclusal record or pantographic tracing when adjusting the horizontal condylar guidances and lateral condylar guidances (Bennett shift) on the articulator.

The superior belly of each lateral pterygoid acts to fix or stabilize the condyle and disk during elevation of the mandible.

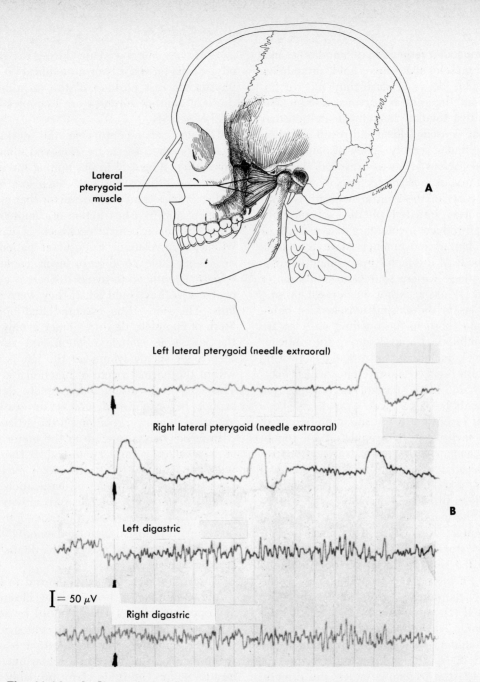

Fig. 11-14 **A,** Shortening of fibers of the lateral pterygoid moves the condyle on the same side forward. The muscle also holds or braces the condyle and disk in a forward position along the articular eminence in certain phases of mastication. Without this action, the condyle on the balancing side would drop back into the fossa as a result of the forces developed by the closing muscles of mastication. **B,** This electromyogram was made during a mandibular hinge or retruded opening movement. *Arrows* show the beginning of opening. Notice that the lateral pterygoids maintain their resting pattern while the digastrics, which are responsible for the opening movement, show increased electrical activity. (**B** modified slightly from Fig. 8 in Woelfel JB, et al: J Prosthet Dent **7:**361-367, 1957.)

Neuromuscular regulation of mandibular motion. The muscles that move, hold, or stabilize the mandible do so because they receive impulses from the central nervous system. The impulses that regulate mandibular motion may arise at the conscious level and result in voluntary mandibular activity. They also may arise from subconscious levels as a result of the stimulation of oral or muscle receptors or of activity in other parts of the central nervous system. The impulses initiated at the subconscious level can produce involuntary movements or modify voluntary movements. At any one time the cell body of the motor nerve may be influenced by these various sources to inhibition or excitation. When a closing movement occurs, the neurons to the closing muscles are being excited and those to the opening muscles are being inhibited. Impulses from the subconscious level, including the reticular activating system, also regulate muscle tone, which plays a primary role in the physiologic rest position of the mandible.

Certain receptors in mucous membranes of the oral cavity can be stimulated by touch, thermal changes, pain, or pressure. Other receptors located principally in the periodontal ligaments, mandibular muscles, and mandibular ligaments provide information as to the location of the mandible in space and are called proprioceptors (Fig. 11-15). The impulses generated by stimulation of these oral receptors travel to the sensory nuclei of the trigeminal nerve or, in the case of proprioceptors, to the mesencephalic nuclei. From there they are transmitted (1) by way of the thalamus to the sensorimotor cortex (conscious level) to produce a voluntary change in the position of the mandible, (2) by way of a reflex arc to the motor nuclei of the trigeminal nerve and directly back to the mandibular muscles to cause an involuntary movement of the mandible, or (3) by a combination of these two under the influence of subcortical areas such as the hypothalmus, basal ganglia, or reticular formation (Fig. 11-15). Involuntary movements of the mandible away from a source of pain during the making of jaw relation records or a modification of the physiologic rest position of the mandible because of denture soreness are examples of this kind of activity.

The loss of receptors in the periodontal ligaments when teeth are removed eliminates this source of control in positioning the mandible for edentulous patients. Such loss of control is an important biologic factor that must be compensated by construction of complete dentures that have centric occlusion in harmony with centric relation. Edentulous patients are no longer able to discern even contacts of opposing teeth or to avoid deflective occlusal contacts as they could when they were dentulous. Therefore it is essential that opposing teeth of complete dentures meet evenly when the jaw is in centric relation and also that they meet evenly whenever the jaw is closed within the normal range of functional activity. This kind of occlusion for complete dentures cannot be established unless the casts are mounted in centric relation on the articulator.

Impulses may also arise in the motor cortex as a result of voluntary thought. These impulses are transmitted to the motor nuclei and from there to the muscles of mastication so the mandible performs the desired activity (Fig. 11-15). Thus patients can be trained to make posterior terminal hinge movements of the mandible that may be used by the dentist to locate the transverse hinge axis.

Mastication was formerly believed to be the result of interaction between jaw closing and jaw opening reflexes as influenced by sensory input and conscious control. Recent evidence, however, indicates that mastication is a programmed event residing in a "chewing center" located within the brain stem (probably in the reticular formation of the pons) (Fig. 11-15). The cyclic nature of mastication (jaw opening and closure, tongue protrusion and retrusion) is the result of the action of this central pattern generator. Conscious effort may either induce or terminate chewing, but it is not required for

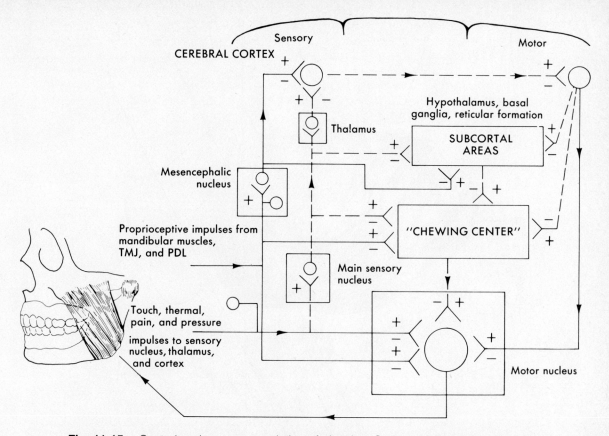

Fig. 11-15   Central and sensory regulation of chewing. Some peripheral sites influence motoneurons (+, facilitate; −, inhibit) relatively directly, by acting on the "chewing center" itself; others do so indirectly, by affecting the ascending projections to one or more of the higher centers (such as the sensorimotor cerebral cortex) that regulate motoneuron output via the chewing center. *Broken lines* denote less direct central pathways. (Based on Sessle BJ: In Roth GI, Calmes R, editors: Oral biology, St Louis, 1981, The CV Mosby Co.)

the continuation of chewing. In a similar manner sensory impulses from the orofacial region may modify the basic cyclic pattern of the chewing center to achieve optimal function (Fig. 11-15). The alteration of chewing characteristics (rate, force, duration) as related to the consistency of a bolus of food is an example of this type of influence. Finally, central influences from areas of the brain associated with other patterned or "learned" behavior, emo-

tion, and stress may inhibit or excite the chewing center.

The cerebellum does not initiate mandibular movement. Rather, it compares information from the motor cortex and other higher centers (signifying the appropriate or intended movement) to sensory information received from the periphery (signifying actual position and rate of movement). Acting as a feedback control mechanism, it sends appropriate signals back to the

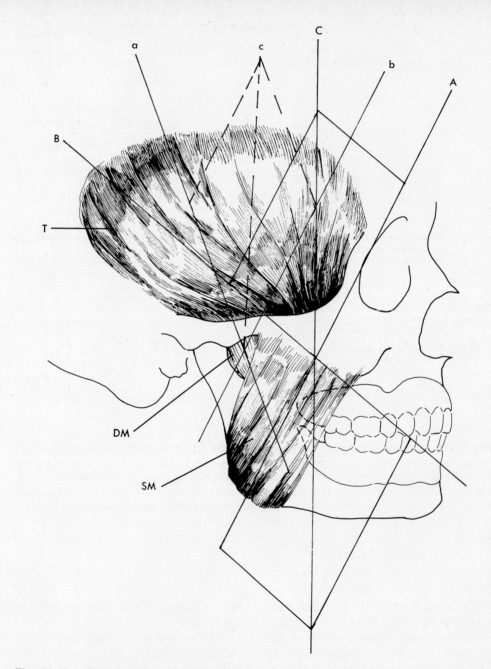

Fig. 11-16 Parallelograms of forces exerted by the muscles of mastication. *A*, Superficial portion of the masseter and the medial pterygoid; *a*, deep portion of the masseter. *B*, Posterior portion of the temporalis; *b*, anterior portion of the temporalis. *C* and *c*, Direction of the resultant forces; note that it follows the diagonals of the parallelograms and is in line with the long axes of the teeth. *T*, The temporal muscle; *DM*, deep portion of the masseter; *SM*, superficial portion of the masseter.

motor cortex to inhibit agonist muscles and excite antagonist muscles. In this way movement is terminated at the exact point of intention, ensuring a coordinated response from the muscles that are responsible for mandibular function.

The relatively continuous flow of impulses through specific pathways from oral receptors to the central nervous system and back to the regulating musculature establishes memory patterns for the individual. Thus persons with natural teeth may subconsciously develop mandibular closing patterns that bypass deflective occlusal contacts so the teeth meet evenly in centric occlusion. However, when memory patterns are disrupted by removal of teeth or placement of new restorations with an occlusion that is not in harmony with the existing mandibular movement pattern, mandibular movements may be significantly altered, causing pain, pathosis, and mental stress.

Clinical understanding of mandibular movement

Parallelogram of forces. From the standpoint of the prosthodontist, the skull presents some interesting facts that need to be taken into consideration. The factor of muscle pull in relation to the direction and strength of each muscle used in positioning the mandible after the loss of teeth is an important consideration (Fig. 11-16). The parallelogram of forces can be studied only in relation to the entire skull. The direction of these forces has much to do with the seating or unseating of dentures. The occlusal vertical dimension affects this direction of forces, a fact that makes positioning of the mandible after the loss of teeth so important. The relation of the ridges can be understood by studying the teeth in natural occlusion to observe the inclination of their roots and alveolar processes.

Envelope of motion in the sagittal plane. In an explanation of the clinical implications of mandibular movements, it is helpful to define the limits of possible motion and certain man-

dibular reference positions. Fig. 11-17 shows one method that may be used to record and study mandibular movements. Recent tests indicate that edentulous patients can make reproducible lateral border movements when stabilized baseplates are used to support the pantograph.

Fig. 11-18 shows an envelope of motion (maximum border movements) in the sagittal plane as scribed by a dentate subject. The trac-

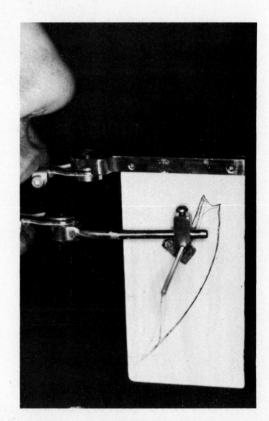

Fig. 11-17 A marker attached by means of a clutch to the lower teeth scribes a tracing on a plate attached by another clutch to the upper teeth. The tracing on the plate indicates the pathway of the mandible in the sagittal plane. An envelope of motion is thus portrayed indicating the extreme limits of mandibular movement in this plane for this particular patient.

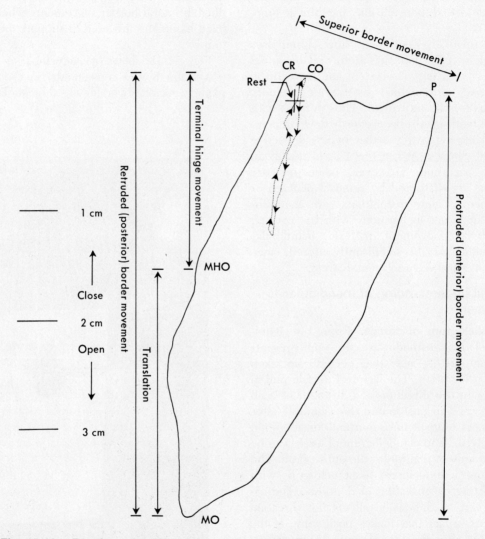

Fig. 11-18 Envelope of motion in the sagittal plane. *P,* Most protruded position of the mandible with the teeth in contact; *CO,* centric occlusion; *CR,* centric relation; *MHO,* maximum hinge-opening position; *MO,* point of maximum opening of the jaws; *Rest,* mandibular rest position.

ing was made from motion picture film when the pathway of a bead attached to a lower central incisor was plotted. The tracing starts at *P*, which represents the most protruded position of the mandible with the teeth in contact. As the mandible is moved posteriorly while tooth contact is maintained, a dip in the top line of the tracing occurs as the incisal edges of the upper and lower anterior teeth pass across one another. *CO* (centric occlusion) is reached when the opposing posterior teeth are maximally intercuspated. When the mandible is further retruded, as most people with natural teeth can do, the most posterior relation of the mandible to the maxillae is depicted by *CR* (centric relation). Centric relation and the mandibular position where centric occlusion occurs are two reference positions that are of extreme importance in constructing dental restorations. Single restorations are generally constructed to be in harmony with centric occlusion (that is, with the mandible positioned at *CO*). Multiple restorations, and certainly complete dentures, are so constructed that their occlusion will be in harmony with centric relation (i.e., with the mandible positioned at *CR*).

As the teeth separate, the mandible moves to its most retruded position from *CR* (Fig. 11-18) and the patient can continue to open in this retruded position, with no apparent condylar translation, to approximately *MHO* (maximum hinge-opening position). Any opening beyond *MHO* will force the condyles to move forward and downward from their most posterior position. *CR-MHO* represents the posterior terminal hinge movement. This movement is used clinically to locate the transverse hinge axis for mounting casts on the articulator. The posterior terminal hinge movement and centric relation at the vertical level of tooth contact coincide at *CR*. This terminal hinge movement can be made only by a conscious effort.

At approximately *MHO* (Fig. 11-18) the patient can no longer retain the mandible in the most retruded position; and as further opening occurs the mandible begins to move forward,

with translation of the condyles in a forward direction. Obviously, different muscles and impulses come into play. At *MO* (maximum opening) the jaws are separated as far as possible and the condyles are in or near their most anterior position relative to the mandibular fossae. The most forward line on the tracing, running from *MO* to *P*, represents the pathway of the mandible as it is moved from its most open position upward to its most protruded position until the teeth contact at *P*, which was the starting point for tracing the envelope of motion.

Any mandibular movement observed from the side will fall within this envelope of motion since it represents all extreme positions into which the mandible can be moved. However, few normal mandibular movements follow the border tracings; normal mandibular movements occur somewhere in front of the terminal hinge movement line, *CR-MHO*.

The dotted line beginning with the teeth in centric occlusion (at *CO*) and extending downward and then upward anterior to the path of the posterior terminal hinge movement line (*CR-MHO*) is a tracing of the masticatory cycle viewed in the sagittal plane and superimposed on the envelope of motion (Fig. 11-18). The arrows pointing downward indicate the pathway of the bead attached to the lower central incisor during the opening part of the chewing cycle, and the arrows pointing upward indicate the pathway during the closing part of the cycle. Note that the pathways occur anterior to the line representing the terminal hinge movement. This holds true for most persons with natural teeth. However, if restorations are so constructed that centric occlusion and centric relation coincide at *CR*, many of the chewing cycles will terminate at *CR*. This applies also to people whose occlusions have been equilibrated for centric relation. The important point to remember is that for edentulous patients the teeth should contact evenly throughout the normal range of function.

When the patient is relaxed and the jaw is in

the resting position, obviously the teeth are not in contact. Mandibular rest position normally occurs somewhere downward and slightly forward of *CR*, as indicated by *Rest* in Fig. 11-18. This is defined as the habitual postural position of the mandible when the patient is at ease and upright. The only muscle activity required is the minimal tonic contraction necessary to support the mandible against the force of gravity. The rest position is an important reference in prosthodontics, particularly for complete den-

ture patients, since it is a guide to reestablishing the proper vertical dimension of occlusion.

Envelope of motion in the frontal plane. The envelope of motion as seen in the frontal plane roughly resembles a shield. Fig. 11-19 shows such an envelope whose tracing was made from a motion picture film when the pathway of a bead attached to the lower central incisor was plotted. The tracing begins with the teeth in centric occlusion (at *CO*). As the mandible is moved to the right with the opposing teeth

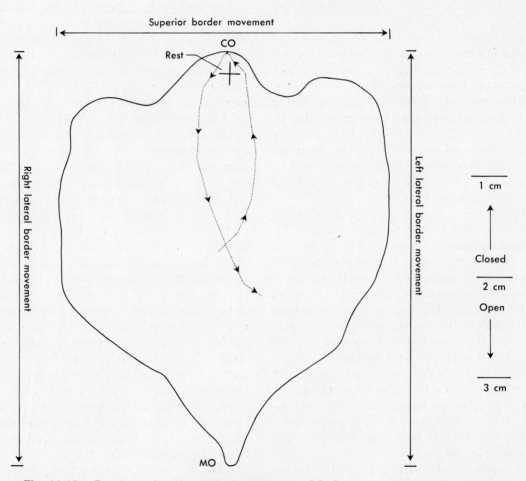

Fig. 11-19 Envelope of motion in the frontal plane. *CO*, Centric occlusion; *MO*, point of maximum opening of the jaws; *Rest*, mandibular rest position.

maintaining contact, a dip in the upper line of the tracing is created as the upper and lower canines pass edge to edge. The mandibular movement is continued as far to the right as possible. Then the opening movement is started and continued with the mandible in the extreme right lateral position until maximum opening occurs (at *MO*).

From *MO* (the position of maximum opening) the mandible is moved in an extreme left lateral excursion as it is closed until the opposing teeth make contact (Fig. 11-19). Then, with the opposing teeth maintaining contact, the mandible is moved from the extreme left lateral position back to where the opposing teeth again contact in centric occlusion, *CO*. The dip in the left side of the superior border movement is made when the upper and lower left canines pass edge to edge.

The dotted line beginning at approximately the middle of the tracing and extending upward (indicated by the upward-pointing arrows) represents the upward component of the masticatory cycle as the subject chews a bolus of food on the left side (Fig. 11-19). Note that the dotted line contacts the superior border of the envelope at *CO*, indicating that the opposing teeth have penetrated the bolus and come into contact with one another. The masticatory cycle moves to the right when the subject opens from centric occlusion as indicated by the downward dotted line (downward-pointing arrows). In the frontal view the rest position is located slightly downward and to the left for this individual, as indicated by *Rest* in Fig. 11-19.

BIBLIOGRAPHY

Celenza FV: An analysis of articulators, Dent Clin North Am **23**:305-326, 1979.

Ellinger CW, Somes GW, Nicol BR, Unger KW, Wesley RC: Patient response to variations in denture technique. III, Five-year subjective evaluation, J Prosthet Dent **42**:127-130, 1979.

Garnick JJ, Ramfjord SP: Rest position, J Prosthet Dent **12**:895-911, 1962.

Glantz PO, Stafford D, Sundberg H, Harrison A: A survey of dental prosthetic technology in some commercial laboratories in Sweden, Swed Dent J **3**:229-236, 1979.

Jemt T: Masticatory mandibular movements. Analysis of a recording method and influence of the state of the occlusion, Swed Dent J Suppl **23**:1-52, 1984.

Lundeen HC: Mandibular movement recordings and articulator adjustments simplified, Dent Clin North Am **23**(2):231-241, 1979.

Manns A, Miralles R, Guerrero F: The changes in electrical activity of the postural muscles of the mandible upon varying the vertical dimension, J Prosthet Dent **45**:438-445, 1981.

Michler L, Bakke M, Møller E: Graphic assessment of natural mandibular movements, J Craniomandib Disord **1**:97-114, 1987.

Mohamed SE, Schmidt JR, Harrison JD: Articulators in dental education and practice, J Prosthet Dent **36**:319-325, 1976.

Rugh JD, Johnson RW: Mandibular movements. In Mohl ND, Zarb GA, Carlsson GE, Rugh JD, editors: A textbook of occlusion, Chicago, 1988, Quintessence Publishing Co Inc.

Rugh JD, Smith BR: Mastication. In Mohl ND, Zarb GA, Carlsson GE, Rugh JD, editors: A textbook of occlusion, Chicago, 1988, Quintessence Publishing Co Inc.

Sessle BJ: Mastication, swallowing, and related activities. In Roth GI, Calmes R, editors: Oral biology, St Louis, 1981, The CV Mosby Co.

Tangerud T, Silness J: Kjeveregistrering ved behandling med helproteser. Nordisk klinisk odontologi, Copenhagen, 1987, Forlaget for Faglitteratur, vol 21A-IV, pp 1-23.

Winstanley RB: The hinge-axis: a review of the literature, J Oral Rehabil **12**:135-159, 1985.

Zarb GA: Oral motor patterns and their relation to oral prostheses, J Prosthet Dent **47**:472-478, 1982.

CHAPTER 12

Biologic considerations in vertical jaw relations

ANATOMY AND PHYSIOLOGY OF VERTICAL JAW RELATIONS

The vertical relation of the mandible to the maxillae is established by two factors: the mandibular musculature and the occlusal stops from the teeth or occlusion rims.

In infants and edentulous adults the vertical jaw relations are established by the *mandibular musculature*. This type of relation is known as the vertical relation (or dimension) of rest. There have been two main hypotheses about the postural rest position of the mandible. One involves an active, and the other a passive, mechanism. According to the first hypothesis this position is assumed only when the muscles that close the jaws and those that open the jaws are in a state of minimal contraction to maintain the posture of the mandible. The second hypothesis holds that the elastic elements of the jaw musculature, and not any muscle activity, balances the influence of gravity. However, numerous studies have shown evidence of electromyographic (EMG) activity at postural rest position. It is also well known that the jaw drops when one falls asleep and muscle tension is reduced further. The clinically recorded rest position—usually 2 to 3 mm below the intercuspal position—does not correspond to recorded minimal EMG activity. The mandible in the EMG rest position is usually several millimeters lower than in the clinical rest position. It is therefore more accurate to refer to a "range of posture" rather than to a single rest position.

The physiologic rest position is a postural position controlled by the muscles that open, close, protrude, and retrude the mandible. It is also controlled by the position of the head. This can be verified by declining and inclining the head: when declining, notice that the distance between the teeth is less than when holding the head in a normal alert position; when inclining, the distance is greater. Therefore the patient's head should be upright and unsupported when observations of physiologic rest position are being made.

The other factor establishing the vertical relation of the mandible to the maxillae is the *occlusal stop* provided by the teeth or occlusion rims. This is what is known as the vertical dimension of occlusion. The natural teeth establish the occlusal vertical dimension while they are developing and in place. When a child is young and the teeth are developing, many transient factors are active. These are involved with the relative length of the closing and opening mandibular musculature and with the eruptive force of developing teeth.

In the course of a lifetime many things happen to the natural teeth. Some are lost, some are so abraded that they lose their clinical crown length, some are attacked by dental caries, and in some a restoration fails to maintain their full clinical crown length. Consequently, even patients who have retained their natural teeth may have a reduced occlusal vertical dimension. The preextraction vertical measurement may not reliably indicate the dimension to be incorporated in complete dentures. Information about the occlusal vertical dimension with natural teeth should not be ignored, however. Instead, modifications from it should be made as indicated when the information is available.

As stated in Chapter 11, the masseter, medial pterygoid, and temporalis are the closing muscles involved in establishing vertical jaw relations. The opening muscles are the inframandibulars (mainly the platysma) and the suprahyoids (mylohyoideus, geniohyoideus, digastricus, and stylohyoideus). These muscles, plus gravity, help control the tonic balance that maintains the physiologic rest position.

The health of the periodontal ligaments that support the natural teeth and the health of the mucosa of the basal seat for dentures depend on rest from occlusal forces. An interocclusal distance or space between the maxillary and mandibular teeth is thus essential for the closing muscles, opening muscles, and gravity to be in balance when the muscles are in a state of minimal tonic contraction. The physiologic rest position allows the supporting tissues and structures to be relieved of occlusal stress. If this interocclusal distance is encroached on, symptoms of muscular fatigue may occur. In denture wearers the clinical consequence is irritation to denture-bearing area(s).

ESTABLISHMENT OF THE VERTICAL MAXILLOMANDIBULAR RELATIONS FOR COMPLETE DENTURES

The establishment of vertical maxillomandibular relations is a phase of prosthodontic treatment for edentulous patients in which it is difficult to arrive at definite conclusions from a practical viewpoint. The subject has been discussed as the "establishment of a vertical dimension," and this is the concept that we will be using in the present consideration. The relationships involved are those in a vertical direction as opposed to those in a horizontal direction (such as centric relation). Studies of growth and development have shown that the rest position of the mandible tends to remain relatively constant for reasonable lengths of time. However, several short- and long-term intraoral and general factors can influence the postural rest position. Dentists must keep this in mind when using the rest position as a guide for establishing vertical maxillomandibular relations. Unfortunately, there is no measure that tells the exact interarch distance; thus there is no proof for a "correct" vertical dimension at which the occlusion should be established. Nevertheless, most patients will adapt to a vertical dimension that is established by means of a combination of esthetic, functional, and patient-reported comfort considerations, together with information derived from studying the patient's rest position.

Compromises between comfort, esthetics, and function are often advisable and may be necessary to reduce the known vertical dimension of occlusion that has been obtained from preextraction records. Dentures may have favorable esthetics but still not be comfortable because of excessive leverage from the great amount of maxillomandibular space.

Nature reduces the interarch distance with gradual wear of the natural teeth, usually without damage to the structures concerned. The dentist attempting to restore youth by restoring the youthful vertical dimension of the face with dentures is likely to encounter great difficulty. The skin, hair, joints, eyes, ears, and all organs of the body undergo degenerative changes that are natural and occur with the passing of years. Therefore a sacrifice in comfort is often necessary to restoring a youthful appearance for the sake of esthetics. Much pressure is brought to bear by many patients trying to stave off old age; and if the dentist succumbs to this pressure, the prognosis will not be favorable.

The greatest danger in this phase of denture construction is an excessive interarch distance, because premature striking of teeth causes recurring trauma to the tissues and longer leverage, making the dentures more awkward to manipulate and more easily displaced. The interceptive occlusal contacts may result in clicking of the denture teeth. Extrusion of natural teeth caused by a loss of opposing teeth may bring the alveolar process with it, and closure of part of the interarch space in that region occurs. For full coverage of the denture bases, an abnormal amount of interarch space is needed to accommodate the artificial teeth. To bring the vertical dimension of the face back to normal requires surgery, controlled pressure molding of the maxillary tuberosities, retromolar pads, and soft tissue irregularities, or reduced denture base coverage. These factors should be studied by mounted diagnostic casts, radiographs, and digital examination before the treatment phase of constructing dentures is started.

Natural teeth provide the occlusal stop that determines the vertical dimension of occlusion. When the natural teeth have been lost, there should be adequate space for artificial teeth of the same size. The problem is simplified when the size of the lost natural tooth is known. If there is insufficient space for the denture teeth, they may be larger than the natural teeth or the newly established vertical separation of the jaws may not be great enough.

When an excessive amount of bone has been lost from various causes (such as periodontal disease, ill-fitting dentures that have been worn for many years, or partially edentulous mouths, especially with all the mandibular posterior teeth gone), it is possible to reduce the denture space an undesirable amount.

Reduced interarch distance lessens the biting force and consequently reduces soreness; therefore it often is used to this end. Narrow knife-edged ridges that cannot be made comfortable in any other manner may be treated by reducing the occlusal vertical dimension to decrease trauma and soreness. However, a reduced interarch distance results in a facial expression that is not desirable; and the vertical dimension of the face should be increased to a point that will be satisfactory and comfortable. With a reduced interarch distance, the lower

third of the face is changed because the chin has the appearance of being too close to the nose and too far forward. The lips lose their fullness, and the vermilion borders are reduced to approximate a line. The corners of the mouth turn down because the orbicularis oris and its attachments are pushed too close to their origin. The reduced vertical dimension of occlusion decreases the action of the muscles, with a resultant loss of muscle tone. This gives the face an appearance of flabbiness instead of firmness. A reduced interarch distance often causes a crease to form at the corners of the mouth, and may be associated with angular cheilitis. (See Chapter 2.)

The reduced interarch distance leads to a loss of the cubicle space of the oral cavity. Normally the tongue at rest completely fills the oral cavity, and a reduced interarch distance has a tendency to push the tongue toward the throat, with the result that adjacent tissues are displaced and encroached on. Such encroachment may mean obstruction of the opening of the eustachian tubes, which will interfere with ear function. This can be the cause of much discomfort. It has been claimed that impaired hearing may be due to a reduced vertical dimension of the face. However, these claims are difficult to support. One should nevertheless use caution whenever there is a large interarch distance by experimenting with a temporary splint over the teeth to test for improved hearing or increased discomfort before the final restorations are made.

Trauma in the region of the TM fossa may be attributed to a reduced interarch distance of the occlusion or to occlusal disturbances that accompany the inevitable aging changes in denture-bearing tissues. The symptoms of joint involvement often are obscure pain and discomfort, clicking sounds, headaches, and neuralgia.

If it is suspected that these various pathologic conditions are attributable to a reduced interarch distance, the dentures should be constructed as treatment dentures. The vertical dimension of occlusion should be built up gradually (for example, by adding acrylic on the occlusal surfaces of a lower denture). Complete restoration of the original occlusal vertical dimension in one set of dentures will likely result in failure because the patient is unable to accommodate to this great change in so short a time.

Methods of determining the vertical dimension

The methods for determining vertical maxillomandibular relations can be grouped roughly into two categories. The *mechanical* methods include use of preextraction records and measurements, ridge parallelism, and others. The *physiologic* methods include use of the physiologic rest position, the swallowing phenomenon, and phonetics as a means for determining the facial dimension at which occlusion should be established. The use of esthetics and patient-reported comfort adds to the mechanical and physiologic approaches to the problem.

All determinations of the vertical dimension must be considered tentative until the teeth are arranged on their trial bases. At tryin, observations of phonetics and esthetics can be used as a check against the vertical relations established by mechanical or physiologic means.

Mechanical methods
1. Ridge relation
   a. Distance from the incisive papilla to the mandibular incisors
   b. Parallelism of the ridges
2. Measurement of the former dentures
3. Preextraction records
   a. Profile radiographs
   b. Casts of the teeth in occlusion
   c. Facial measurements

Physiologic methods
1. Physiologic rest position
2. Phonetics and esthetics
3. Swallowing threshold
4. Tactile sense
5. Patient-reported perception of comfort

Mechanical methods
Ridge relation
Incisive papilla to mandibular incisors. The incisive papilla is used to measure the patient's vertical dimension. It is a stable landmark that changes comparatively little with resorption of the alveolar ridge. The distance of the papilla from the incisal edges of the mandibular anterior teeth on diagnostic casts averages approximately 4 mm in the natural dentition. The incisal edges of the maxillary central incisors are an average 6 mm below the incisive papilla. Therefore the usual vertical overlap of the opposing central incisors is about 2 mm (Fig. 12-1). Remember: These are average measurements; they should be used with caution, and they do not appear to be relevant in patients with severe resorption.

Ridge parallelism. Paralleling of the maxillary and mandibular ridges, plus a 5-degree opening in the posterior region, often gives a clue as to the correct amount of jaw separation. This paralleling is natural, because the teeth in normal occlusion leave the residual ridges in the posterior region parallel to each other, provided there has been no abnormal change in the alveolar process (Fig. 12-2).

Since the clinical crowns of the anterior and posterior natural teeth have nearly the same length, their removal tends to leave the residual alveolar ridges nearly parallel to each other. This would be ideal from a mechanical point of view, because the dentures would not tend to slide anteriorly or posteriorly; however, in most people the teeth are lost at different times, and when a person finally becomes edentulous the residual ridges are no longer parallel. If a person has lost teeth at irregular intervals or has suffered a great amount of bone loss because of periodontal disease or resorption, the lines of the ridges will naturally not be parallel; in addition, the edentulous ridges of the mandible and maxillae will become progressively more discrepant from the standpoint of width (Fig. 12-3).

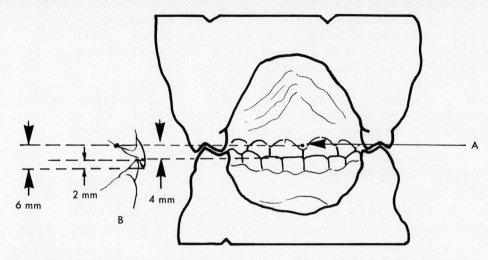

Fig. 12-1 Sectioned casts, posterior view. When the teeth are in centric occlusion, the incisal edges of the mandibular central incisors are 4 mm from the incisive papilla, *A*. A sagittal view of the central incisors, *B,* shows the vertical overlap to be about 2 mm.

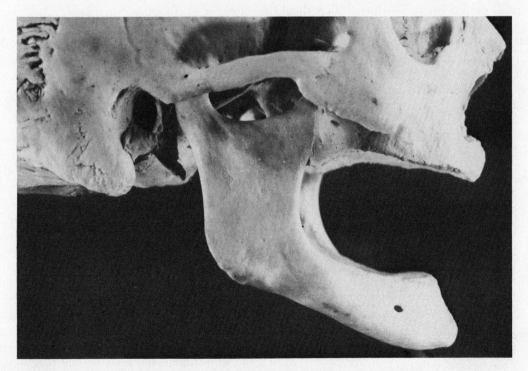

Fig. 12-2 The crest of the lower residual alveolar ridge will be approximately parallel to the crest of the upper ridge when the jaws are positioned at the vertical dimension of occlusion. This relationship is ideal for the stability of dentures.

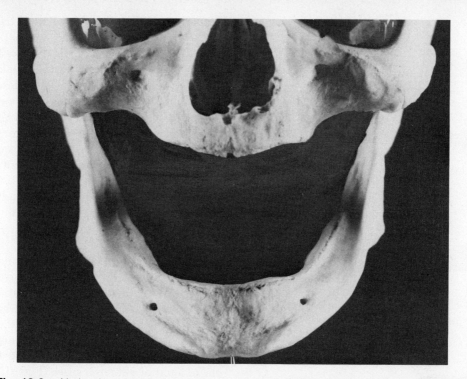

Fig. 12-3   Notice how in this edentulous skull the mandible has become progressively wider and the maxillae progressively narrower as resorption continued.

Measurement of the former dentures. Dentures that the patient has been wearing can be measured, and the measurements can be correlated with observations of the patient's face to determine the amount of change required. These measurements are made between the borders of the maxillary and mandibular dentures by means of a Boley gauge. Then, if the observations of the patient's face indicate that this distance is too short, a corresponding change can be made in the new dentures.

Preextraction records

Profile radiographs. Profile radiographs of the face may be used, but the problems of establishing a vertical dimension of rest and enlarging the image cause some inaccuracies.

Casts of teeth in occlusion. A simple method of recording the vertical overlap relation and the size and shape of the teeth is to use diagnostic casts mounted on an articulator. The casts give an indication of the amount of space required between the ridges for teeth of this size.

Facial measurements. Various devices for making facial measurements have been used in many different forms. Devices have been made to record the relation of the head to the central incisors vertically and anteroposteriorly by placement of a face-bow with auditory meatus plugs in position and with spectacle suspension. Another method is to record the distance from the chin to the base of the nose by means of a pair of calipers or dividers before the teeth are extracted.

Physiologic methods

Physiologic rest position. Registration of the jaw in physiologic rest position gives an indication as to the relatively correct vertical dimension. This may not be an exact guide; however, when used with other methods, it will aid in

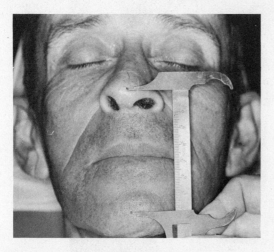

Fig. 12-4 A measurement is made between two points on the face when the jaws are at the vertical relation of physiologic rest position.

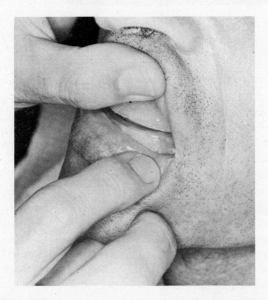

Fig. 12-5 With occlusion rims in the mouth and the jaws at the vertical dimension of rest position, the interocclusal distance seems satisfactory. Notice the space between the occlusion rims.

determining the vertical relation of the mandible to the maxillae. A suggested method is to have the patient relaxed when the wax occlusion rims are in place, with the trunk upright and the head unsupported. After insertion of the occlusion rims into the patient's mouth, the patient swallows and lets the jaw relax. When relaxation is obvious, the lips are carefully parted to reveal how much space is present between the occlusion rims. The patient must allow the dentist to separate the lips without help or without moving the jaws or lips. This interocclusal distance at the rest position should be between 2 and 4 mm when viewed in the premolar region.

The interarch space and rest position can be measured by indelible dots or adhesive tape on the face. If the difference is greater than 4 mm, the occlusal vertical dimension may be considered too small; if less than 2 mm, the dimension is probably too great. The occlusion rims are adjusted until the dentist is satisfied with the amount of interarch space (Figs. 12-4 to 12-6). It is essential that an adequate interocclusal distance exist when the mandible is in its physiologic resting position.

Phonetics and esthetics. Phonetic tests of the vertical dimension consist more of listening to speech sound production than of observing the relationships of teeth during speech. The production of *ch, s,* and *j* sounds brings the anterior teeth close together. When correctly placed, the lower incisors should move forward to a position nearly directly under and almost touching the upper central incisors. If the distance is too large, it means that too small a vertical dimension of occlusion may have been established. If the anterior teeth touch when these sounds are made, the vertical dimension is probably too great. Likewise, if the teeth click together during speech the vertical dimension is probably too great.

Esthetics, also, is affected by the vertical relation of the mandible to the maxillae. A study of the skin of the lips compared to the skin

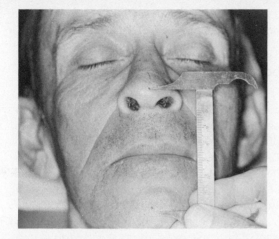

Fig. 12-6 With the occlusion rims in contact, the distance between the points on the face is 3 to 4 mm less than when the jaws are in the physiologic rest position. (See Fig. 12-4.)

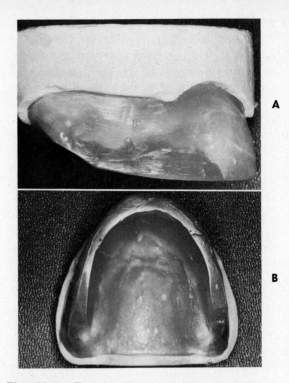

Fig. 12-7 The maxillary occlusion rim is contoured so its labial surface will be similar to that of the finished denture base and the artificial teeth. **A,** Side and, **B,** occlusal views show the contour and dimensions of the neutral zone, which have been approximated in this occlusion rim. Identical principles are employed in contouring mandibular occlusion rims.

over other parts of the face can be used as a guide. Normally the tone of the skin should be the same throughout. However, it must be realized that the relative anteroposterior positions of the teeth are at least equally involved in the vertical relations of the jaws as in the restoration of skin tone.

The contour of the lips depends on their intrinsic structure and the support behind them. Therefore the dentist must initially contour the labial surfaces of the occlusion rims so they closely simulate the anteroposterior tooth positions and the contour of the base of the denture, which, in turn, must replace or restore the tissue support provided by the natural structures (Fig. 12-7).

If the lips are not correctly supported anteriorly, they will be more nearly vertical than when supported by the natural tissues. In such a situation the tendency is to increase the vertical dimension of occlusion to provide support for the lips, and this can be disastrous.

The esthetic guide to the correct vertical maxillomandibular relation is, first, to select

teeth that are the same size as the natural teeth and, second, to estimate accurately the amount of tissue lost from the alveolar ridges. The amount of tissue lost can be judged from the dental history and the length of time the teeth have been missing.

Swallowing threshold. The position of the mandible at the beginning of the swallowing act has been used as a guide to the vertical dimension of occlusion. The theory is that, when a person swallows, the teeth come together with a very light contact at the beginning of the swallowing cycle. If denture occlusion is continually missing during swallowing, the vertical dimension of occlusion may be insufficient (too far closed). On this basis, a record of the relation of the two jaws at this point in the swallowing cycle is used as the vertical dimension of occlusion. The technique involves building a cone of soft wax on the lower denture base in such a way that it contacts the upper occlusion rim when the jaws are too wide open (see Fig. 13-11). Then the flow of saliva is stimulated by a piece of candy or otherwise. The repeated action of swallowing the saliva will gradually reduce the height of the wax cone to allow the mandible to reach the level of the vertical dimension of occlusion. The length of time this action is carried out and the relative softness of the wax cone will affect the results. We have not found consistency in the final vertical positioning of the mandible by this method, however.

Tactile sense and patient-perceived comfort. The patient's tactile sense is used as a guide to the determination of the correct occlusal vertical dimension. An adjustable central bearing screw is attached in the palate of the maxillary denture or occlusion rim, and a central bearing plate is attached to the mandibular occlusion rim or trial denture base (see Fig. 13-8). The central bearing screw is adjusted first so it is obviously too long. Then, in progressive steps, the screw is adjusted downward until the patient indicates that the jaws are closing too far. The procedure is repeated in the opposite direction until the patient indicates that the teeth feel too long. The screw then is adjusted downward until the patient indicates that the length is about right, and the adjustments are reversed alternately until the height of the contact feels right. The problem with this method relates to the presence of foreign objects in the palate and the tongue space. The final determination must be made at the tryin after the teeth are in position. Patient participation in the decision to establish a vertical dimension record should also be considered, since there are both physiologic and psychologic advantages to this approach.

Tests of vertical jaw relations with the occlusion rims

The vertical separation of the jaws that is established in the mouth with the occlusion rims and mounted on the articulator is the vertical dimension of occlusion. This preliminary relationship is established and maintained by the occlusion rims. It precedes the determination of the horizontal jaw relationship and the eventual preliminary centric relation record.

Following are some of the tests that aid the dentist in confirming the correct vertical relation of occlusion with the occlusion rims:

1. Judgment of the overall facial support
2. Visual observation of the amount of space between the rims when the jaws are at rest
3. Measurements between dots on the face when the jaws are at rest and the occlusion rims in contact
4. Observations made when sibilant-containing words are pronounced, to ensure that the occlusion rims come close together but do not contact
5. The patient's opinion on perceived comfort with the established occlusion rim height

The use of these tests enables the dentist to make preliminary and tentative determinations of the vertical dimension of occlusion. The final determination, however, cannot be made by any method until the teeth are set in the wax trial dentures and the vertical dimension is verified in the mouth.

BIBLIOGRAPHY

Brill N, Fujii H, Stoltze K, Tryde G, Kato, H, Møller E: Dynamic and static recordings of the comfortable zone, J Oral Rehabil 5:145-150, 1978.

Broekhhuijsen ML, van Willigen JD, Wright SM: Relationship of the preferred vertical dimension of occlusion to the height of the complete dentures in use, J Oral Rehabil 11:129-138, 1984.

Fay EF, Eslami A: Determination of occlusal vertical dimension: a literature review, J Prosthet Dent 59:321-323, 1988.

Heath MR, Boutros MM: The influence of prostheses on mandibular posture in edentulous patients, J Prosthet Dent **51**:602-604, 1984.

L'Estrange PR, Vig PS: A comparative study of the occlusal plane in dentulous and edentulous subjects, J Prosthet Dent **33**:495-503, 1975.

Manns A, Miralles R, Santander H, Valdivia J: Influence of the vertical dimension in the treatment of myofascial pain-dysfunction syndrome, J Prosthet Dent **50**:700-709, 1983.

Mohl ND, Zarb GA, Carlsson GE, Rugh JD, editors: A textbook of occlusion, Chicago, 1988, Quintessence Publishing Co Inc.

Rugh JD, Drago CJ: Vertical dimension: a study of clinical rest position and jaw muscle activity, J Prosthet Dent **45**:670-675, 1981.

Silverman MM: The comparative accuracy of the closest-speaking-space and the freeway space in measuring vertical dimension, J Acad Gen Dent **22**:34-36, 1974.

Tallgren A: The continuing reduction of the residual alveolar ridges in complete denture wearers: a mixed-longitudinal study covering 25 years, J Prosthet Dent **27**:120-132, 1972.

Toolson LB, Smith DE: Clinical measurement and evaluation of vertical dimension, J Prosthet Dent **47**:236-241, 1982.

Tryde G, McMillan DR, Christensen J, Brill N: The fallacy of facial measurements of occlusal height in edentulous subjects, J Oral Rehabil **3**:353-358, 1976.

Yemm R, El-Sharkawy M, Stephens CD: Measurement of lip posture and interaction between lip posture and resting face height, J Oral Rehabil **5**:391-402, 1978.

CHAPTER 13

Biologic considerations in horizontal jaw relations

The principles of good occlusion apply to both dentulous and edentulous patients. However, different requirements are necessary in the occlusion for complete dentures because artificial teeth are not attached to the bone in the same manner as natural teeth. Thus an occlusion that is physiologically acceptable or desirable for the preservation of the attachment apparatus of natural teeth may not be applicable for complete dentures. To maintain stability of complete dentures, the opposing teeth must meet evenly on both sides of the dental arch when the teeth contact anywhere within the normal functional range of mandibular movement. An occlusion for complete dentures that provides these even contacts can be developed only when centric occlusion is in harmony with centric relation.

The most posterior position of the mandible relative to the maxillae at the established vertical dimension (centric relation) is a bone-to-bone relationship that is classed as horizontal because variations from it (eccentric relations) occur in the horizontal plane. Eccentric excursions may be either anterior or lateral; those that occur anteriorly are known as protrusions. Centric relation is a reference relationship that is constant for each patient, provided the osseous and soft tissue structures in the TMJs are healthy. Inflammation or swelling and osseous changes can alter it, but for clinical purposes it is considered constant in the healthy patient. Therefore it is the reference against which the desired occlusal condition should be coordinated.

CONFUSION IN TERMINOLOGY AND CONCEPTS

The term *centric relation* is given a number of different meanings in its application to the development of dental restorations. However, the use of a single definition is essential to improving communications throughout dentistry.

Centric relation has been defined as (1) the mandibular position that coincides with the median occlusal position, (2) a mandibular position determined by the neuromuscular reflex learned when the primary teeth are in occlusion, (3) the mandibular position that exists when the centers of vertical and lateral motion are in their posterior terminal hinge position, (4) the relationship of the mandible to the maxillae when the mandible is braced during swallowing, (5) a mandibular position synonymous with the physiologic rest position, and (6) a mandibular position synonymous with the position of the mandible during swallowing. The confusion in terminology has been aggravated by controversy over the connection between centric relation and the intercuspal position. Some authors have argued in favor of the "muscular position" on grounds that it is the one most frequently used in function; it has been defined as the position reached after a relaxed mandibular closure from the rest position, and it usually coincides with the intercuspal (or tooth) position in the natural dentition. However, research has shown that the muscular position is extremely variable and is not recordable with the same predictability as the retruded position is.

This confusion can be eliminated by accepting one definition: *Centric relation is the most posterior position of the mandible relative to the maxillae at the established vertical dimension.* All other horizontal mandibular positions are eccentric and can apply to centric relation without changing or confusing its meaning. The apparent competition between the centric relation/retruded contact position and the muscular position used in recording maxillomandibular horizontal relationships seems to have been won by the first concept (at any rate, according to the prosthodontic literature).

MUSCLE INVOLVEMENT IN CENTRIC RELATION

Centric relation is not a resting or postural position of the mandible. Contraction of muscles is necessary to move and fix the mandible in it. However, this neuromuscular activity does not affect the validity of its definition.

The anatomic attachments of the posterior and middle parts of the temporal and the suprahyoid muscles (primarily the geniohyoideus and the digastricus), together with EMG studies, indicate that these muscles move and fix the mandible in its most retruded position relative to the maxillae. The temporal, masseter, and medial pterygoid muscles elevate the mandible to a particular vertical relation with the maxillae. The lateral pterygoids show little activity when the mandible is in centric relation (Fig. 13-1).

HARMONY BETWEEN CENTRIC RELATION AND CENTRIC OCCLUSION

The understanding of CR (centric relation) is complicated by failure to distinguish between centric relation and centric occlusion. This has come about by the incorrect usage of the word *centric* to mean either centric relation or centric occlusion. "Centric" is an adjective and must be used with either *relation* or *occlusion* to be specific and meaningful. Centric relation is a bone-to-bone relationship whereas centric occlusion is a relationship of upper and lower

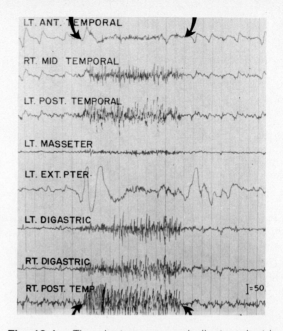

Fig. 13-1 The electromyogram indicates electrical activity of the muscles labeled when the mandible was moved from the resting position into centric relation and from CR back to the resting position. An increase in both frequency and amplitude of activity *(arrows)* denotes the time during which the mandible was in CR. Notice the striking increase from the middle and posterior parts of the temporal and digastric muscles, because these are responsible for positioning and holding the mandible in CR. Notice also that the anterior parts of the temporalis, masseter, and external (lateral) pterygoid show little increase above resting activity when the mandible is in CR.

teeth to each other (Fig. 13-2). Once CR is established, CO can be built to coincide with it or to provide a broad area of tooth contact in this position (a so-called "freedom in centric").

Confusion also results from the fact that in many people, CO of the natural teeth does not coincide with CR of the jaws. In the natural dentition CO is usually located anterior to CR, the average distance being 0.5 to 1 mm. In edentulous subjects the lack of teeth, and consequently of any centric occlu-

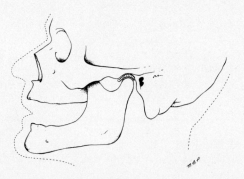

Fig. 13-2 Centric relation is a bone-to-bone relationship. The mandible is in its most retruded position relative to the maxillae. Centric occlusion should be established in harmony with this position.

sion, makes it necessary to use CR as a reference position. A more controversial issue is whether or not these positions should coincide.

Natural tooth interferences in CR initiate impulses and responses that direct the mandible away from deflective occlusal contacts into CO. Impulses created by closure of the teeth into CO establish memory patterns that permit the mandible to return to this position, usually without tooth interferences.

When natural teeth are removed, many receptors that initiate impulses resulting in positioning of the mandible are lost or destroyed. Therefore the edentulous patient cannot control mandibular movements or avoid deflective occlusal contacts in CR in the same manner as the dentulous patient can. Deflective occlusal contacts in CR cause movement of denture bases and displacement of the supporting tis-

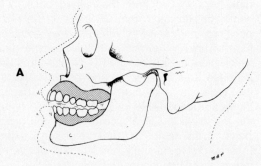

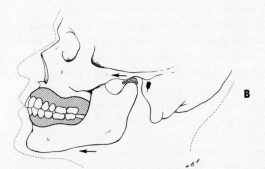

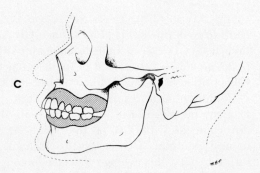

Fig. 13-3 **A,** Centric occlusion is not in harmony with centric relation. When the mandible is in CR, the opposing teeth do not contact evenly. **B,** Centric occlusion not in harmony with centric relation. For the opposing teeth to meet evenly as they do in CO, the mandible must be moved away from CR. Notice that the condyle has moved forward in the glenoid fossa to permit the opposing teeth to contact evenly. This is not a desirable situation for edentulous patients. **C,** Centric occlusion is in harmony with centric relation. Opposing teeth contact evenly when the mandible is in its most retruded position relative to the maxillae. This is the desirable situation for all edentulous patients.

sues or direct the mandible away from this relation. Therefore CR must be recorded for edentulous patients to enable CO to be established in harmony with it (Fig. 13-3). This can usually be achieved with CO and CR coinciding. However, in some patients a broader area of stable contacts near CR is necessary, the so-called "freedom in centric" or "long centric."

ORIENTING CENTRIC RELATION TO THE HINGE AXIS

The upper cast can be accurately oriented to the opening axis of the articulator by the location of a physiologic transverse hinge axis and a face-bow transfer. The physiologic transverse hinge axis is located by a series of controlled opening and closing movements of the jaws when the mandible is held in its most retruded position relative to the maxillae. These mandibular movements are called terminal hinge movements and are the part of the posterior border movement that occurs without translation (Fig. 13-4).

As in the determination of the physiologic transverse hinge axis, when a centric relation record is made the mandible is in its most retruded position to the maxillae. However, the centric relation record is made at an established vertical distance of the jaws corresponding to a specific vertical position of the terminal hinge movement. Therefore, when the upper cast is correctly oriented to the hinge axis of the articulator by an accurate face-bow transfer, the lower cast will also be correctly oriented to the opening axis of the instrument when it is mounted with an accurate CR record. This is true because the mandible was in its most retruded position relative to the maxillae both for locating the transverse hinge axis and for recording CR.

ORIENTING CENTRIC AND VERTICAL RELATIONS

Many vertical relations are possible between the mandible and the maxillae. However, there is a most retruded position of the mandible for each vertical relation and there is a change in the horizontal mandibular position for each change in the vertical dimension. Such changes occur even though the condyles are maintained in their most retruded position. This most retruded position is centric relation for that specific vertical measurement. A vertical dimension of occlusion must be established between the jaws of an edentulous patient to provide adequate interocclusal distance and allow the mandibular muscles to function at their optimal physiologic length.

The CR record must be made at the established vertical dimension of occlusion when an

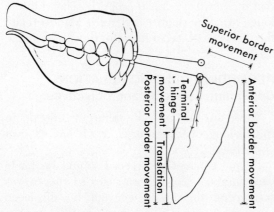

Fig. 13-4 This tracing depicts an envelope of motion scribed in the sagittal plane. Having the patient open and close with the mandible in its most retruded position relative to the maxillae (terminal hinge movement) is the method used for locating the transverse hinge axis. Centric relation is the most retruded position of the mandible at a specific vertical distance along the pathway of terminal hinge movement. Thus the mandible is in CR for both locating the posterior transverse hinge axis and establishing CR. Notice that the masticatory cycle *(arrows pointing upward and downward)* terminates with the teeth in contact when the mandible is in CR. (From Hickey JC: Dent Clin North Am, pp 587-600, November 1964.)

arbitrary face-bow transfer is used to orient the casts to the opening axis of the articulator. This is necessary because the opening and closing (transverse) axes of rotation of the articulator will be the same as those of the patient only when the casts are mounted with a correctly located physiologic transverse hinge axis. When an arbitrary hinge axis is used, the amount of error introduced by opening or closing the vertical dimension of occlusion on the articulator will depend on the interrelationship between the arbitrary location to the true hinge axis and the vertical opening of the articulator. Thus, when the CR record is made at or very close to the desired vertical dimension of occlusion, little or no change (opening or closing) will be necessary on the articulator and the likelihood of errors from this source will be greatly reduced.*

SIGNIFICANCE OF CENTRIC RELATION

Correct registration of CR is essential in the construction of complete dentures. Many dentures fail because the occlusion is not planned or developed in harmony with this position. The maxillomandibular musculature is so arranged that a patient can easily move his mandible into centric relation. Thus CR serves as a reference relationship for establishing an occlusion. When the CR and CO of artificial teeth do not coincide or a "freedom in centric" is not present, the stability of the denture bases is in jeopardy and the edentulous patient is subjected to unnecessary pain or discomfort.

The irregular loss of teeth often creates deflective occlusal contacts that guide the mandible into a slightly protrusive or lateral position, or both. The muscles, bones, ligaments, teeth, and all related structures grow into a coordinated center for muscular activity. The stability of natural teeth is jeopardized when the mandible is deflected away from CR. To change this center for muscular activity is to imperil the

stability of dentures. The edentulous patient does not have the same level of neuromuscular sensitivity as the dentulous patient and cannot learn to avoid the deflective contacts on opposing teeth of complete dentures.

CR is the horizontal reference position of the mandible that can be routinely assumed by edentulous patients under the direction of the dentist. This makes it possible for dentists to verify the relationship of casts on the articulator when they are mounted in CR. However, patients cannot routinely close their teeth into CR when it is established on the articulator somewhere else. Thus errors in mounting casts on the articulator may result from incorrect positioning of the occlusion rims in the mouth, unequal pressures on opposite sides of the jaws during the making of interocclusal records, and errors in the mounting procedures. These errors can go undetected when CR is not used as the horizontal reference position.

Edentulous patients use CR closures in mastication and in other mandibular activities, such as swallowing. Therefore the casts must be mounted on the articulator in this position so the opposing teeth on complete dentures will meet evenly when the patient closes in CR.

An accurate CR record will properly orient the lower cast to the opening axis of the articulator and orient CR to the hinge axis of both the articulator and the mandible. Assuming that the maxillary cast is properly related to the hinge axis, the dentist is thereby able to relate the lower cast accurately to the same hinge axis.

RECORDING CENTRIC RELATION
Conflicting concepts and objectives

There are two basically different concepts in the making of CR records. Each has its own objectives.

In one concept the record should be made with minimal closing pressures so the tissues supporting the bases will not be displaced

---

*This is particularly important if a face-bow is not used.

while the record is being made. The objective of this concept is for the opposing teeth to touch uniformly and simultaneously at their first contact. The uniform contact of the teeth will not stimulate the patient to clench and relax the closing muscles in periods between mastication.

The second concept is that the records should be made under heavy closing pressure so the tissues under the recording bases will be displaced while the record is being made. The objective of this concept is to produce the same displacement of the soft tissues as would exist when heavy closing pressures were applied on the dentures. Thus the occlusal forces will be evenly distributed over the supporting residual ridges when the dentures are under heavy occlusal loads. If the distribution of the soft tissues is uneven, however, the teeth will contact unevenly when they first touch. This uneven contact tends to stimulate nervous patients to clench and relax their closing muscles, which may cause soreness under the denture bases and changes in the residual ridges.

There is some logic in both concepts, and the dentist must decide which will be best for each patient. Regardless of the method selected, the recording technique and the procedures used for testing the occlusion must be based on the objective of the concept chosen. If the minimal closing pressure method is used, the occlusion should be tested at the first contact of the teeth. If the heavy closing pressure method is used, the occlusion should be tested under heavy closing pressure. If centric relation records are made with heavy pressure, it is illogical to expect the teeth to occlude evenly at their first contact.

Although little research evidence is available to support one or the other of these proposed concepts for recording CR, clinical experience and empirical data do seem to endorse the use of a technique based on minimal closing pressure to produce the desired information on the patient.

Complications in recording centric relation

CR has been defined as the most retruded unstrained position of the condyles in the glenoid fossae at a given degree of opening. This definition is often misunderstood because the word *unstrained* is taken to mean an absence of anteroposterior strain whereas it should also include an absence of superoinferior strain. This definition is also impossible to use in a practical sense. The condyles are not available for visual observation. The definition given earlier in this chapter (p. 283) is more accurate and usable. The structure of the TMJs is such that one joint can be displaced downward by uneven pressure when records are made and yet the condyles will still be in their most retruded position. This situation cannot occur on the articulator, and thus a deflective occlusal contact may be the source of instability, soreness, and resorption despite the correctness of the other relations. If the jaws operated as a hinge, the maxillomandibular relation would then be automatically registered correctly; but the condyles are not hinges, and they can be easily malpositioned, with resultant difficulties. The basal seats for denture bases made from the best impressions will not withstand the ravages of an incorrect CR from any cause.

Centric registrations are complicated further by the fact that soft tissues are of varying density. Hanau referred to tissue resiliency as *real-eff*, an acronym for "phase *r*esiliency *a*nd *l*ike *eff*ect." This resiliency is present in both the mucosa and the TMJs. Thus, undue pressure in securing the relation must be avoided, lest excessive displacement of the soft tissues result.

Even though a balanced and equalized registration has been made, it often is lost in the cast-mounting procedure and processing of dentures. Some of these changes are unavoidable because of changes in denture base materials during processing. For this reason, it is necessary to reestablish a carefully equalized CR after the dentures have been completed.

The theoretical ideal of an equalized occlusal relationship is a centric registration made with the same soft tissue placement that existed when the impressions were made. The objective is difficult to accomplish with present knowledge, however. Attempts to record CR with minimal closing pressure have included the use of soft plaster of Paris, zinc oxide–eugenol paste, and carefully softened wax. Maxillomandibular records made in these materials that harden in the mouth are reasonably effective.

Retruding the mandible to centric relation

One of the most difficult and most important tasks is retruding the mandible to its centric relation. Some of the difficulties encountered are biologic, some psychologic, and some mechanical. The methods used to attain retrusion can be divided into passive and active. With passive methods, the patient is as relaxed as possible and the dentist guides the mandible in a terminal hinge axis movement, or gently pushes the chin backward into a retruded position. With active methods, the patient responds to instruction by actively retruding the mandible.

The *biologic* difficulties arise from a lack of coordination in groups of opposing muscles when the patient is requested to close in the retruded position. This lack of synchronization between the protruding and retruding muscles may be due to the habitual eccentric jaw positions adopted by the patient to accommodate a malocclusion. For example, a patient having only anterior teeth will have a habit of protruding the jaw and, when asked to retrude it, may find it difficult to do so. In securing this retruded position, what may seem like awkwardness of the patient is in fact difficulty performing consciously what has been unconsciously avoided for so long.

The *psychologic* difficulties involve both the dentist and the patient. The more the dentist tries to overcome the apparent inability of the patient to retrude the mandible, the more confused the patient may become and the less likely he is to respond to the directions provided by the dentist. The dentist must be prepared to spend adequate time securing the CR record. This is always one of the most important steps in the construction of complete dentures. Most complete dentures constructed without an accurate CR record are doomed to failure. Several methods should be available as aids for the patient to retrude the mandible. One patient may respond to one method and another to another. A central bearing point and plate supported by the recording bases are excellent for exercising a forward and backward jaw movement. They provide a sliding surface against which the patient can rest his jaws while exercising the mandibular musculature. However, a particular disadvantage of such contraptions is that they restrict the available tongue space, which may in turn produce recording errors. Another effective method involves the use of stretch-relax exercises. The patient is instructed to open wide and relax, to move the jaw right and relax, to move the jaw left and relax, and to move the jaw forward and relax four times in each of four sessions a day. The results to be expected are that the patient will be able to follow the dentist's directions in moving the jaw to CR and to the desired eccentric positions.

The *mechanical* difficulties encountered in securing CR records are due to poorly fitting baseplates. It is essential that the bases on which CR records are made fit perfectly and not interfere with each other (Fig. 13-5). The amount of pressure that the patient exerts at the time of registering CR is difficult to control. Minimal pressure should be exerted during the registration, to avoid displacement of the soft tissues as much as possible. This is obviously difficult to do. If minimal pressure is exerted at the time of this registration, the jaw relation will be recorded with minimal tissue displacement and the denture will have a uniform occlusal contact when the teeth first touch. Whereas one side of the mouth might

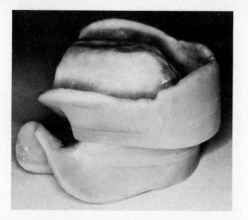

Fig. 13-5 Acrylic resin–lined occlusion rims provide accurately fitting bases for jaw relation records. These records cannot be made accurately and transferred to the articulator when the bases do not properly fit on the residual ridges.

have a thicker layer of soft tissue than the other side and this would not change the moment of first contact of the teeth, under functional loads the pressures would be unequal as a result of unequal displacement of the soft tissue. Patients compensate for this difference by selective placement of food in their mouth. Interocclusal plaster or wax registrations give a better impression of the displacement of soft tissues in all parts of the mouth than is possible with a record made by a central bearing point. This is especially true if the tissue depth is uneven and the opposing ridge relation or size is not normal.

Methods for assisting the patient to retrude the mandible. A number of methods are used to assist the patient in retruding his mandible:

1. Instruct the patient by saying, "Let your jaw relax, pull it back, and close slowly and easily on your back teeth."
2. Instruct the patient by saying, "Get the feeling of pushing your upper jaw out and closing your back teeth together."
3. Instruct the patient to protrude and retrude the mandible repeatedly while he holds his fingers lightly against his chin.

4. Instruct the patient to turn the tongue backward toward the posterior border of the upper denture.
5. Instruct the patient to tap the occlusion rims or back teeth together repeatedly.
6. Tilt the patient's head back while the various exercises just listed are carried out.
7. Palpate the temporal and masseter muscles to relax them.

The simplest, easiest, and often most effective way of causing a retrusion of the mandible to CR is by verbal instruction to the patient. "Let your lower jaw relax, pull it back, close on your back teeth." These instructions must be given in a calm and confident manner. When the patient is responding properly, the dentist should say so. In this manner, the patient's awareness of the desired position is reinforced.

Many patients do not realize the jaw movements they can make. By getting the feeling of pushing their upper jaw forward, they automatically pull their lower jaw back. Once they have achieved this, it is easy for them to repeat the desired motion.

When the mandible is protruded and retruded with a relaxation each time, movements into the desired position can be felt by the patient with his own fingers on the chin. The dentist can then aid by a slight pressure on the point of the chin. The patient may get an idea of the movement by feeling the dentist's or the dental assistant's chin. This protruding and retruding of the mandible is done repeatedly until the patient is trained in the movement and the dentist can feel the patient's mandible reach its retruded position.

The series of stretch-relax movements mentioned earlier can also be helpful. These exercises will help to get the mandible into the position of CR. The dentist soon develops a sense of touch as to when the mandible is back to the desired position.

When the patient's tongue attempts to reach for the posterior border of the upper denture, retrusion of the mandible will make the denture border easier to reach. Thus the desired retrusion can be achieved. The problem with this method is the likelihood of displacing the mandibular denture or recording base by the action of the tongue.

Tapping the occlusion rims or back teeth together rapidly and repeatedly is used to help the patient retrude the mandible, since it is believed that the center of muscle pull will gradually work the mandible back. However, it is difficult to record these positions, and a patient can easily tap in a slightly protrusive or lateral position. The results should be checked by other tests:

Tilting the head backward
This will place tension on the inframandibular muscles and tend to pull the mandible to a retruded position. However, it is extremely difficult to obtain registrations with the head in this position because of the awkwardness of insertion and removal of the recording medium and occlusion rims from the mouth when the head is so tilted. Having the patient recline may overcome some of these problems, as well as provide the physiologic advantage of making it easier to retrude the mandible.
Massaging the jaw muscles
The temporal muscle shows reduced function when the mandible is in a protruded position. For this reason its contraction can be felt when the mandible is in or near its retrusive position and the patient is asked to open and close. Massage or palpation of the masseter and temporal muscles will help the patient relax.
Having the patient swallow
Swallowing may bring the mandible to a retruded position and may be an aid in retruding the mandible to CR. However, a person can swallow when the mandible is not completely retruded so this method must be verified by another technique.

Research has shown that the most reproducible recording of a retruded mandibular position in dentate subjects is achieved by gently guiding the mandible backward with the subject relaxing his jaws. This can also be effective in helping record CR in edentulous patients.

Methods of recording centric relation

The various methods used for recording centric relation may be classified as static or functional, and each of these may be extraoral or intraoral techniques.

The *static* methods are those that involve first placing the mandible in CR with the maxillae and then making a record of the relationship of the two occlusion rims to each other. This method has the advantage of causing minimal displacement of the recording bases in relation to the supporting bone. Intraoral records in the static class are made with wax or plaster, with or without a central bearing point and with or without intraoral or extraoral tracing devices to indicate the relative position of the two jaws.

The *functional* methods are those that involve functional activity or movement of the mandible at the time the record is made. These methods have the disadvantage of causing lateral and anteroposterior displacement of the recording bases in relation to the supporting bone while the record is being made. The records in the functional class include the various chew-in techniques suggested by Needles, House, and Essig and Paterson. They also include methods that make use of swallowing for positioning and recording the relative position of the jaws.

Accurate records of CR have been made by all the methods in both classes although incorrect records also have been made by the methods in both classes. This means that, irrespective of the method used, subsequent clinical checking and rechecking must be done throughout the denture construction phase.

Extraoral tracings and devices. A needle point tracing made on a tracing table coated with carbon or wax can be used to indicate the relative position of the upper and lower jaws in the horizontal plane (Fig. 13-6, *A*). These tracings are shaped somewhat like a Gothic arch and thus are referred to as Gothic arch tracings. They may also be known as arrow point tracings.

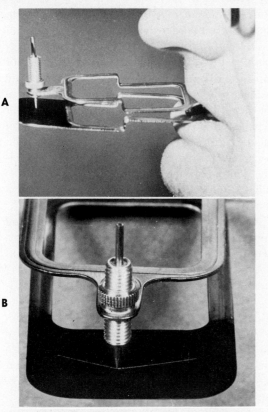

Fig. 13-6 A, A needle point tracing device attached to the upper occlusion rim remains fixed during mandibular movement. The lower tracing plate, attached to the lower occlusion rim, moves during mandibular movement. The tracing made on the lower plate provides an indication of the horizontal location of the mandible relative to the maxillae. **B,** The needle point tracer is in the apex of the tracing, indicating that the mandible is in its most retruded position relative to the maxillae.

To make an arrow-point or needle-point tracing, one condyle moves forward and inward during a lateral mandibular movement followed by a movement in the opposite direction with rotation around the opposite condyle. The movements are approximate rotations alternately around the two condyles. They cut lines extending to a point representing the most retruded position of both condyles. Therefore,

when both condyles are resting in their most retruded positions, the needle point of the tracer will be resting on the apex of the tracing thus created (Fig. 13-6, *B*). A needle point tracing is fundamentally a single representation of the position of the mandible and its movement in the horizontal plane.

Many needle-point tracings are not indicative of an exact centric relation because of the roundness of the apex. The lateral movements should be made until the apex is sharp to indicate the true retruded position of the mandible. A dull or rounded apex on a tracing may be caused when the condyles do not reach their most posterior position in the TMJ or when the recording bases move on their basal seats. A rounded apex can be corrected only by repeated manipulation of the mandible from side to side and in a protruded relation to the maxillae. The central–bearing point tracing device affords a sliding table that permits the patient to protrude and retrude the mandible easily while the tracing is made.

A double needle-point tracing, one anterior to the other, also can be made by increasing or decreasing the vertical dimension at which the tracing is scribed. With a central bearing point the height of the screw is increased or decreased. These two tracings afford an excellent illustration of how the centric position varies at different levels of the occlusal vertical dimension. The extraoral tracing should be extended a reasonable distance from the recording bases so the tracing may be enlarged to a size that can be properly evaluated. Tracings made inside the mouth or close to the occlusion rims are often small, and it is difficult to be certain that the apex of the tracing is sharp. Some needle point tracing devices combine the central bearing point and the needle point tracer into one by having the bearing point cut the tracing on the opposite plate.

Tracing devices that make use of the central bearing point are placed on and fastened to the baseplates, care being taken to center them laterally and anteroposteriorly so pressure will be

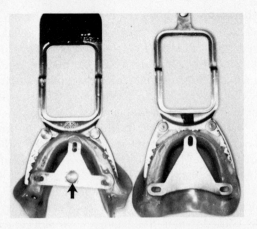

Fig. 13-7 *Right,* Central bearing plate centered and attached on the occlusal surface of the upper occlusion rim. *Left,* Central bearing plate containing the central bearing point *(arrow)* centered and attached to the lower occlusion rim. The vertical space between the jaws when the occlusion rims and tracing devices are in the mouth can be adjusted by raising or lowering the central bearing point.

equally distributed laterally and anteroposteriorly (Fig. 13-7). This is predicated on the assumption that the center of the mandibular occlusion rim and the center of the maxillary occlusion rim coincide. However, there is a certain latitude; thus the equalization of pressure is fairly well achieved when the two centers are close to the same point. For this reason it is a mistake to use a central bearing point device when the ridge relations are not normal or when there is an excess of soft tissue on the ridges. Likewise, an uneven distribution of soft tissue in different parts of the basal seat can cause errors in a vertical direction even though the mandible itself is in the correct horizontal position of CR.

It is important not to accept any part of the tracing except the apex as an indication of CR. When patients chew lightly, they may often close their jaws in eccentric positions.

Extraoral tracings may be used in combination with wax or modeling compound occlusion rims on temporary bases or in combination with a central bearing point. Extraoral tracings made without a central bearing point are not considered satisfactory because, although they indicate the correct anteroposterior position of the mandible, they may not record the correct maxillomandibular (superoinferior) relation of the jaws. It is extremely difficult to maintain equalized pressure on blocks of wax or modeling compound, so there is not much to be gained by securing a tracing without using a central bearing point.

Intraoral tracing devices. Intraoral tracing devices combine a central bearing point with a needle point tracing made inside the mouth. The bearing point is sharp and makes a tracing on the opposing central bearing plate (Fig. 13-8). A hole may be drilled in the plate at the apex of the intraoral tracing, or a plastic disk with a hole in it may be placed over the apex of the tracing. The hole or depression is used to ensure that the patient's jaw is in the retruded position while the registration is being recorded with plaster or some such material.

Interocclusal centric relation records. Interocclusal records are made with a recording medium between the occlusion rims, the trial denture bases, or the completed dentures. Materials that are commonly used include plaster, wax, zinc oxide–eugenol (ZOE) paste, and cold-curing acrylic resins. The patient closes into the recording medium with the lower jaw in its most retruded position and stops the closure at a predetermined vertical relation. Interocclusal records are relatively easy to make, but their success depends on the clinical judgment of the dentist and the cooperation between dentist and patient. This method is simple because mechanical devices are not used in the patient's mouth and are not attached to the occlusion rims.

Interocclusal registrations are, in some respects, preferred to registrations using mechanical aids. The earliest registrations of CR generally were made with a large mass of wax.

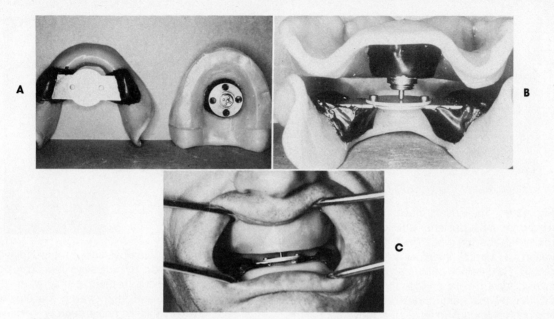

Fig. 13-8   The Coble intraoral tracing device. **A,** On the *right,* the adjustable central bearing point is attached in the palate of the upper occlusion rim. On the *left,* the tracing plate is centered in the first molar region of the lower occlusion rim. **B,** Tracing point in contact with the central bearing plate as viewed from the posterior aspect of the occlusion rims. **C,** The patient is making an intraoral needle point tracing by moving his mandible from side to side. The apex of the tracing will indicate the position of centric relation.

This resulted in many incorrect and inaccurate records. The difficulties in handling wax interocclusal records involved uneven softening and uneven thickness of the recording material and the possible distortion of the record after it was made. Impression plaster, ZOE paste, acrylic resin, polyether, and silicone offer little resistance when closure is made into them; their resistance is uniform throughout, and they set hard enough that the interocclusal records will not be distorted after they set. By adding a small amount of alcohol to the ZOE paste the setting time can be reduced. This may be an advantage in patients in whom the denture bases are difficult to keep immobile.

The technique for making plaster interocclusal records is quite simple. The patient is comfortably seated upright in the dental chair with his feet flat on the footrest. His head is supported by the headrest to control its movement as well as any movements of the occlusion rims and recording medium.

The thumb and index or middle finger of the dentist's hand are placed between the opposing teeth or occlusion rims. The hand is inverted to cover the patient's eyes and help prevent anxiety if the patient should see the dentist's concern when instructions are not followed properly. The forefinger of the dentist's other hand is placed on the labial surface of the lower anterior teeth or rim to help retain the denture base on the residual ridge and to feel the anteroposterior movement of the mandible. As the patient closes in CR, the dentist moves the thumb and finger out of the way, allowing the patient's closing force to maintain both denture

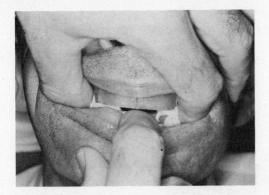

Fig. 13-9   The patient closes into soft plaster to record the most posterior position of the mandible relative to the maxillae. This kind of recording is called a direct interocclusal centric relation record. The position of the hands when making an interocclusal record permits the dentist to ascertain that the trial denture bases are in proper position on the residual ridges, to feel movement of the mandible as the patient closes his jaws together, to help guide the mandible during closure, and to cover the patient's eyes.

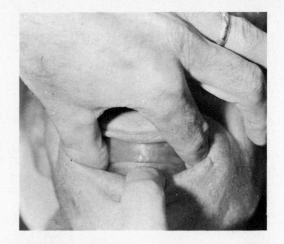

Fig. 13-10   An interocclusal centric relation record can be made by adjusting the occlusion rims until they appear to meet evenly when the mandible is in CR and then sealing the rims together. However, this is unsatisfactory because displacement of the soft tissues of the basal seat is unequal and movement of the occlusion rims cannot be avoided.

bases in position on the residual ridges (Fig. 13-9).

An alternative but similar placement of the dentist's hands is as follows: One hand keeps the upper denture base in position while the other controls the lower jaw. The thumb and forefinger of this hand are placed on the lower base in the region of the left and right first molars and the center of this hand pushes gently backward on the chin. The other fingers can be used to check the relaxation of muscles in the floor of the mouth.

Sufficient trial closures are made to allow both the dentist and the patient to become familiar with the procedure. The relationship of the opposing anterior teeth or occlusion rims when the mandible is in CR at the desired vertical dimension during the trial closure is the dentist's guide to the proper amount of jaw closure when the interocclusal record is made. Most incorrect CR records can be recognized at the time they are made, but further checks and tests must be used to detect small errors.

This can be done by setting the posterior teeth in centric occlusion on the articulator and observing their occlusion in the mouth.

Other methods of recording centric relation. Several other methods of recording CR have had mixed results.

Some have been made by adjustment of the occlusion rims until they contact fairly evenly in the mouth at the desired vertical relationship. Strips of Celluloid or paper placed between the rims are held tight while under closing pressure. If a strip pulls out easily, it indicates less pressure on this side than on the other. The height of the occlusion rims is reduced at the location of excess pressure, or built up at the location of reduced pressure. Such a procedure is most often unsatisfactory.

Another method of obtaining records with wax occlusion rims is to heat the surface of one of the rims and have the patient close into this softened surface to make a new maxillomandibular relation impression (Fig. 13-10). This procedure does not remove the errors of unequal pressure.

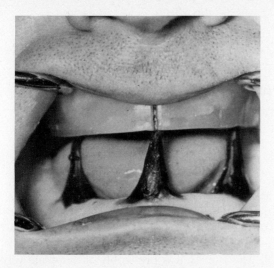

Fig. 13-11 Soft cones of wax attached to the mandibular base form an interocclusal record as they are forced against the upper occlusion rim when the patient swallows. Swallowing should establish the proper horizontal and vertical relations of the mandible to the maxillae.

A great improvement in the method of softening wax rims is deep heating posterior portions of the mandibular wax rim and leaving the anterior portion cool to maintain the predetermined vertical dimension of occlusion. Deep heating sometimes is referred to as *pooling*. Deep pooling is accomplished by insertion of a hot wax spatula down into the center of the lower occlusion rim, first on one side and then on the other, thus allowing time for the inner hot portion of the wax to soften the outer portion enough that the outer walls will collapse readily under closing pressure. The maxillary rim is not softened, and thus it will not be affected during its contact with the heated mandibular rim. After the wax has been chilled, the surplus is trimmed away, since it would guide the mandible back into the same relation during subsequent mandibular closures. In other words, the surplus wax would not permit a testing or verification of the centric relation record.

Still another method utilizes softened wax placed over the occlusal surfaces of the posterior mandibular teeth. The recording wax is not placed over the anterior teeth lest it tend to cause the patient to protrude his mandible. In this method the maxillary teeth close into wax instead of wax contacting wax as in other methods. The advantage of this method is that comparatively small surfaces are in contact rather than large flat wax surfaces. A disadvantage is that most often the record must be made at an increased vertical dimension of occlusion to prevent contact of opposing teeth.

Swallowing and chew-in records are included as physiologic techniques for recording CR. In one technique soft cones of wax are placed on the lower trial denture base. The wax cones contact the occlusal surface of the upper occlusion rim when the patient swallows. This provides a record of the horizontal relation of the mandible to the maxillae (Fig. 13-11). Unfortunately, the mandibular position recorded by this method is not necessarily consistent with CR and is not repeatable.

BIBLIOGRAPHY

Bergman ,B, Olsson CO: Zinkoxid-eugenolpasta som hjälpmedel vid käkregistrering, Sven Tandlak Tidskr **61:**169-226, 1968.

Brill N, Tryde G: Physiology of mandibular positions, Front Oral Physiol **1:**199-237, 1974.

Helkimo M, Ingervall B, Carlsson GE: Comparison of different methods in active and passive recording of the retruded position of the mandible, Scand J Dent Res **81:**265-271, 1973.

Langer A: The validity of maxillomandibular records made with trial and processed acrylic resin bases, J Prosthet Dent **45:**253-258, 1981.

Mohamed SE, Christensen LV: Mandibular reference positions, J Oral Rehabil **12:**355-367, 1985.

Mohl ND, Zarb GA, Carlsson GE, Rugh JD, editors: A textbook of occlusion, Chicago, 1988, Quintessence Publishing Co Inc.

Myers ML: Centric relation records—historical review, J Prosthet Dent **47:**141-145, 1982.

Steenks MH, Bosman F: Reference positions of the mandible, J Oral Rehabil **12:**537-538, 1985.

Winstanley RB: The hinge-axis: a review of the literature, J Oral Rehabil **12:**135-159, 1985.

Yurkstas AA, Kapur KK: Factors influencing centric relation records in edentulous mouths, J Prosthet Dent **14:**1054-1065, 1964.

CHAPTER 14

Recording and transferring bases and occlusion rims

Dentists should not be exclusively concerned with the vertical forces delivered through the occlusal surfaces of the teeth to the denture-bearing tissues. The horizontal forces exerted on the external surfaces of the dentures are also important and have to be taken into consideration in the making of complete dentures. Fish described a denture as having three surfaces: the impression, the occlusal, and the polished surface. All three are developed independently in complete denture prosthodontics; but they are integrated by the dentist to create a stable, functional, esthetic result. The polished surface of a denture consists of the nonarticulating parts of the teeth along with the labial, buccal, lingual, and palatal parts of the denture base material. The design and orientation of this surface are determined by its relationship to the functional role of the tongue, lips, and cheeks (Fig. 14-1, *A* to *C*). The polished surface occupies a position of equilibrium among these groups of muscles and is frequently referred to as the neutral zone (Fig. 14-1, *D*).

Occlusion rims are employed as provisional substitutes for the planned complete dentures and are used to record both the neutral zone and the maxillomandibular relations. They are made on the stone cast that represents the denture-supporting tissues and consist of a denture base and a wax rim (Fig. 14-2).

The denture base, or recording base, must be rigid, accurate, and stable. It is referred to as a trial denture base if it is made of wax or, preferably, autopolymerizing (cold-curing) acrylic resin. Such a denture base will be used at both the registration and the tryin appointments. On the other hand, the denture base can be made of processed acrylic resin, and eventually the selected teeth are processed to it. The rim itself is preferably of baseplate wax because that is easy to manage and convenient.

TRIAL DENTURE BASE, OR RECORDING BASE

Wax bases are frequently used (Figs. 14-3 and 14-4) and must be reinforced with wire. Sometimes they are lined with a zinc oxide–eugenol (ZOE) impression paste seated on the cast, to which a separating medium has been applied. These bases may be bulky and brittle, but dentists frequently find them easier to work with when setting up teeth, especially when a restricted interarch distance exists. Autopolymerizing resin trial denture bases are also extensively used. Undercuts first have to be blocked out on the cast to avoid possible damage, and the resin in its doughlike state is molded onto the cast. Alternatively, a wax template is lined with cold-curing resin (Fig. 14-5), though this is slightly more time-consuming; or an autopolymerizing resin base can be made by the "sprinkle-on" method (Fig. 14-6). In both cases the monomer and polymer are applied alternately until a relatively even thickness of resin base is achieved, and in both the casts are placed in hot water in a pressure cooker for 10 minutes under 30 pounds of pressure. This produces rapid polymerization, and excess monomer is eliminated. Both methods produce a base that is rigid, stable, and easily contoured

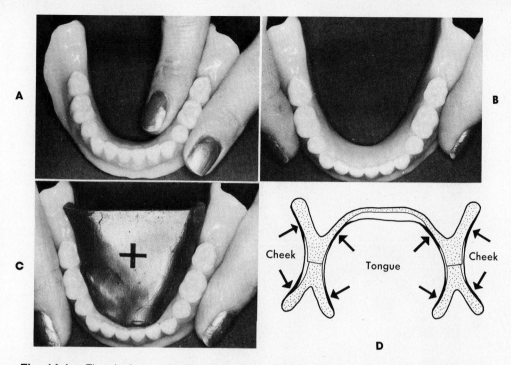

Fig. 14-1   The design and orientation of the denture's polished surface are influenced by functional activities of the tongue, cheeks, and lips. **A** to **C,** Relative positions of the groups of muscles making up the tongue, cheeks, and lips simulated by the fingers. The area marked + in **C** represents a "tongue" of wax. **D,** *Arrows* indicate the direction of muscular activity in a coronal plane through the molar region of the two occlusion rims. *Shaded areas* denote the neutral zone.

and polished. Acrylic resin baseplates are excellent for making maxillomandibular relation records. They fit accurately and are not easily distorted. Their only disadvantage is that they may take up space needed for setting the teeth, necessitating some grinding of the resin base in required areas. They may also be loose because of the necessary blockout of undercuts in the cast. A trial denture base and occlusion rim made of extra-hard baseplate wax are easiest for arranging the teeth (Figs. 14-3 and 14-4). The wax can be softened all the way through to the cast, so the teeth can be set directly against the cast if necessary. For many patients "hard" baseplate materials must be cut

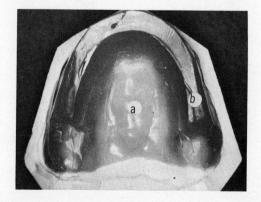

Fig. 14-2   Maxillary occlusion rim. The recording base, *a,* is usually made of hard baseplate wax or cold-curing resin. The rim, *b,* is wax.

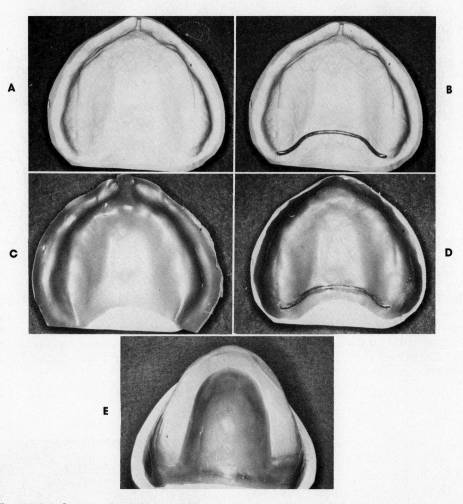

Fig. 14-3 Construction of an extra-hard wax occlusion rim. **A,** The maxillary cast is dusted with talcum powder as a separating medium. **B,** Ten-gauge reinforcement wire is adapted to the posterior palatal area to extend through the hamular notches, 2 mm in front of the vibrating line. **C** and **D,** A sheet of softened baseplate wax is pressed firmly against the cast to form the recording base. **E,** The roll of softened wax is sealed to this base and contoured to the desired arch form. The rim is built to a height slightly greater than the total length of the teeth and the amount of residual alveolar ridge shrinkage.

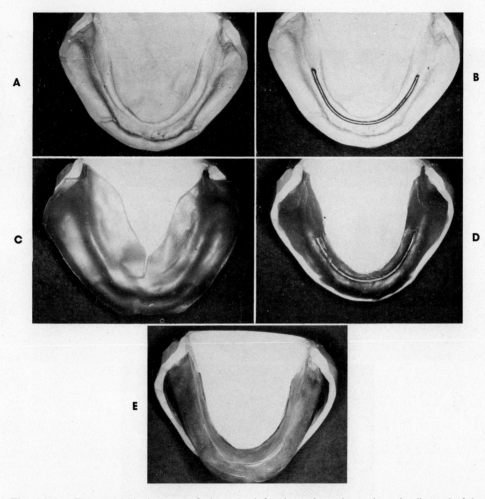

Fig. 14-4   This mandibular cast, **A,** has a reinforcing wire adapted on the lingual of the residual ridge. **B** to **D,** A sheet of softened baseplate wax is closely adapted to the potential denture-bearing area of the cast to form the recording base. **E,** The roll of softened wax is sealed to the base and contoured to the desired form.

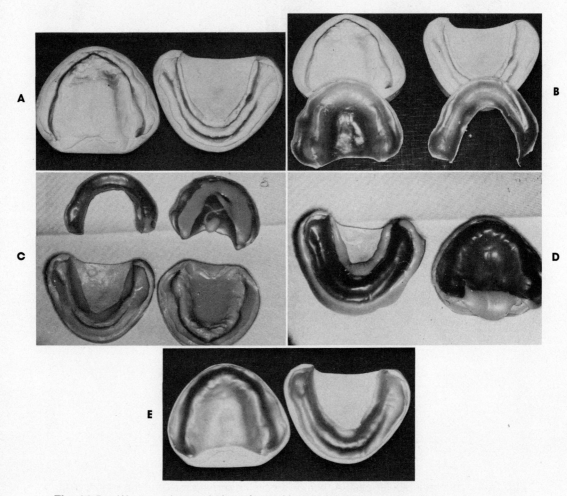

Fig. 14-5 Wax template technique for making a trial denture base. **A,** Master casts prepared by waxing out the undercuts and applying a separating medium. **B,** Wax templates are formed and, **C** and **D,** lined with autopolymerizing acrylic resin. In **E** the completed (well-fitting and stable) trial base is ready for the addition of occlusion rims.

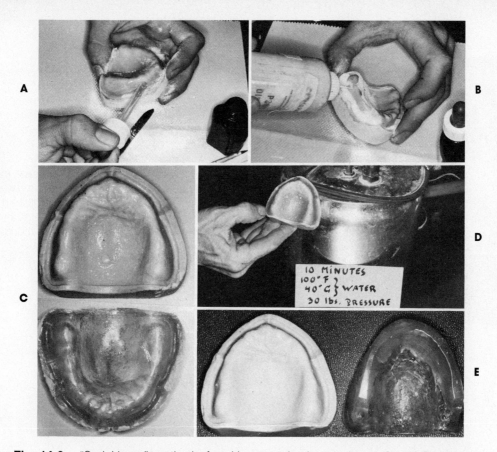

Fig. 14-6 "Sprinkle-on" method of making a resin denture base. **A** and **B,** Monomer and polymer are applied alternately until an evenly thick base is developed, **C.** The base and cast, **D,** are placed in a pressure cooker to complete polymerization. **E,** The denture base is trimmed and polished, and a wax rim is sealed onto it.

away to allow the teeth to be set in their proper places.

The denture base can be processed onto the final cast before the relations-registration appointment. This procedure offers the dentist the advantage of using the base or fitting surface of the completed denture throughout all the patient's clinical appointments. This base may be made of heat-curing, cold-curing, or one of the "pour"-type acrylic resins. After the maxillomandibular relations have been confirmed and the setup completed, the teeth are processed to this base.

OCCLUSION RIMS

The occlusion rims can be used to establish (1) the level of the occlusal plane, (2) the arch form (which is related to the activity of the lips, cheeks, and tongue), and (3) the preliminary jaw relation records, the vertical and horizontal jaw relationships (including tentative facial support), and an estimate of the interocclusal distance. Unfortunately, none of these determinations can be made in a precise scientific way and most of the knowledge concerning them is theoretical. However, there are several basic principles that have proved to be successful

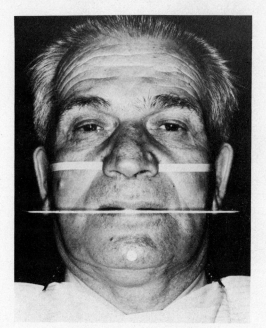

Fig. 14-7 For demonstration purposes, the ala-tragus line on this patient has been bilaterally taped on. The occlusal plane is established when the wax occlusion rim is made parallel to this line. A Fox plane-guide may be used for the paralleling.

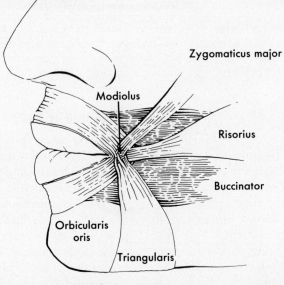

Fig. 14-8 The modiolus.

clinically, and these can be used to help achieve the objectives enumerated.

Level of the occlusal plane

Many dentists use a technique wherein the occlusal plane is established on the maxillary occlusion rim. The procedure entails developing the occlusion rim so the incisal plane is parallel to the interpupillary line and at a height that allows for the length of the natural tooth plus the amount of tissue resorption that has occurred. The upper lip can be a guide if it is of average length. The occlusal plane, posteriorly, is made to parallel the ala-tragus line on the basis of the position of most natural occlusal planes (Fig. 14-7). Then the lower occlusion rim is adjusted to meet evenly with the upper rim and reduced until sufficient interocclusal distance has been obtained. This procedure is adequate for many patients and usually results in satisfactory dentures. It certainly cannot be regarded as applicable to all patients, however.

There are other approaches to occlusal plane determination. One involves tongue function and its relation to the occlusal plane and mandibular denture stability. When this is related to Fish's description of the neutral zone and the activity of the modiolus muscles, a rational and clear guide for occlusal plane determination evolves. The food bolus is triturated while resting on the mandibular occlusal surfaces (occlusal table). This table is an area bounded by the cheek tissues buccally, the tongue lingually, the pterygomandibular raphe and its overlying tissues distally, and the contraction of the corner of the mouth mesially. The mesial boundary is a point where eight muscles meet at the corner of the mouth. The meeting place, called the *modiolus* (Latin, hub of a wheel), forms a distinct conical prominence at the corner of the mouth (Fig. 14-8). If the thumb is placed inside the corner of the mouth and the finger outside on the prominence and then the lip and cheek are contracted, the modiolus feels like a knot. The modiolus becomes fixed every time the buccinator contracts, which is a natural accompaniment of all chewing efforts.

The contraction of the modiolus presses the corner of the mouth against the premolars so the occlusal table is closed in front. Food is crushed by the premolars and molars and does not escape at the corner of the mouth unless seventh nerve damage has occurred (as in Bell's palsy).

The practical application of this approach lies in developing the polished surface of the denture in the occlusion rims and establishing the height of the occlusal plane. The corners of the mouth are marked on the occlusion rims to provide the dentist and technician with anterior landmarks for the height of the first premolars (Fig. 14-9, *A* to *C*). The retromolar pads are relatively stable posterior landmarks, even in patients with advanced ridge reduction. It has been shown that the mandibular first molar is usually at a level corresponding to two thirds of the way up the retromolar pad (Fig. 14-9, *D*). The retromolar pads are circled on the final casts. The land of the cast (edge) is marked at points two thirds the length of the pad from its anterior border. These points will aid in determining the height of the distal end of the occlusal plane. The anterior and posterior landmarks are joined when the wax is melted to this level with a hot spatula. It will be observed that the resultant occlusal plane is almost invariably parallel to the residual alveolar ridges and to the interpupillary line. Its height will conform to activities of the tongue, cheek, and corner of the mouth (Fig. 14-9, *E*), which tend to enhance mandibular denture stability. The maxillary occlusion rim is next adjusted to meet evenly with the mandibular rim and reduced until an adequate interocclusal distance is obtained.

The tests that aid the dentist in establishing the correct vertical dimension of occlusion by means of occlusion rims are reviewed in Chapter 13.

Following are the tests most frequently used:
1. Judgment of the overall facial support
2. Visual observation of the space between the rims when the jaws are at rest
3. Measurements between dots on the face

when the jaws are at rest and when the occlusion rims are in contact

4. Observations when the *s* sound is enunciated accurately and repeatedly—the average speaking space

This last ensures that the occlusion rims come close together but do not contact. It must be emphasized that the interocclusal (interrim), or speaking, space that exists between the posterior teeth when the patient is enunciating *s* sounds is not related to the interocclusal space of rest position. Clinical experience suggests that this space is about 1.5 to 3 mm for most patients. However, patients with a Class II occlusion tend to have a larger speaking space (3 to 6 mm), and Class III occlusion patients have a critically small space of about 1 mm.

Both tests 1 and 2 are particularly effective if

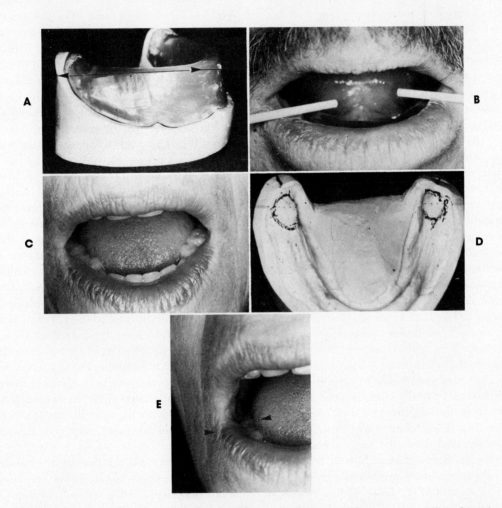

Fig. 14-9 A mandibular occlusion rim, **A,** is trimmed to conform to two pairs of landmarks: the right and left corners of the mouth, **B** and **C,** and a point two thirds the way up the retromolar pads, **D.** The wax rim is melted with a hot spatula to the level indicated by the *arrows* in **A.** Mandibular teeth set to this level, **E,** will conform to the tongue and cheeks and to activities of the corners of the mouth *(arrowheads).*

the patient's old dentures are used for comparison. Old dentures can be valuable for prognostic purposes, especially if they are used with treatment liners to recover an optimal vertical dimension of occlusion. Old dentures can also have their facial surfaces selectively augmented with a soft wax to assist the dentist in assessing the required cosmetic support from the dentures' polished surfaces. This is a useful step when the shape of the dental arch form is determined, as it should be, by the dentist.

It is now possible to proceed to the next clinical step and make a preliminary centric relation record. However, the dentist may elect to consider the development of arch forms at this appointment, using the patient's occlusion rims. This step will provide even more essential information regarding horizontal placement of the artificial teeth. Consequently, a discussion of dental arch form will precede the discussion on making centric relation records.

Arch form

Both the width of the occluding surfaces and the contour of the arch form of the occlusion rims should be individually established for each patient to simulate the desired arch form of the artificial teeth. Such an analogue of the missing teeth and their supporting tissues will enable the dentist or technician accurately to follow instructions for arranging the artificial teeth. This can serve to reduce the amount of time spent with the patient by the dentist at the tryin appointment and allow more time for perfecting the arrangement of the teeth.

Fish drew the profession's attention to the concept of a neutral zone in complete denture construction. He argued that the natural teeth occupy a zone of equilibrium, with each tooth assuming a position that is the resultant of all the various forces acting on it. This is usually a stable position unless actual changes in the dentition have occurred. When natural teeth are replaced by artificial teeth, it is logical to set the artificial teeth in a position as close as possible to the one previously occupied. The

same forces that stabilized the natural teeth can then be used to stabilize the dentures. In the treatment of partially edentulous patients, it is common to find that sufficient natural teeth remain to provide a guide for the positions of the artificial teeth. When the patient is edentulous, it is not always easy to determine where the natural teeth were in relation to the partially or totally resorbed alveolar ridges. Clinical judgment must be brought to bear in such situations, and this may be quite challenging.

Certain types of dentitions are accompanied by specific patterns of soft tissue behavior. Clinical observation of denture patients suggests that these characteristic types of soft tissue movements persist into old age and offer a clue to the location of the preexisting natural teeth. The best guide to determining and designing the arch form is to consider the pattern of bone resorption where the teeth are lost and the utilization of anatomic landmarks that are relatively stable in position.

Clinical experience and reports confirm that the denture space or neutral zone can be reproduced with only a limited variation that lies within the range of clinical acceptability.

Mandibular arch. The occlusion rim is designed to conform to the arch form that in the dentist's judgment the patient had before the natural teeth and alveolar bone were lost. In the lower jaw a larger proportion of bone loss occurs on the labial side of the anterior residual ridge. The loss occurs equally on the buccal and lingual of the residual ridge in the premolar region, but in the molar region it appears to be primarily from the lingual of the ridge because of the cross section shape of the mandible (which is wider at its inferior border than at the ridge crest). Thus the residual ridge almost invariably becomes more lingually placed in the anterior region and more buccally placed in the posterior region. The occlusion rim is contoured as a guide when artificial teeth are placed labial to the ridge in the anterior region, over the ridge in the premolar region, and slightly lingual to the ridge in the molar region.

The curvatures of the occlusion rims, which simulate the arch form of the posterior teeth, follow the curvature of the mandible itself when seen from above. Lines are drawn on the cast for accurately evaluating the arch form. One line is drawn from the lingual of the retromolar pad and extended anteriorly to a point just lingual to the crest of the ridge in the premolar region. This line aids in positioning the lingual surfaces of the posterior teeth, and it establishes the lingual extent of the occlusion rim (Fig. 14-10). This lingual line can be curved similar to the curvature of the body of

the mandible. The anterior part of the occlusion rim is contoured to compensate for the estimated bone loss in this region, and the corners of the mouth are used as guides for determining an approximate location for the canines and first premolars. The experienced dentist learns to visualize the artificial teeth (represented at this state by the contoured rim) as growing out of the alveolar bone and following the curvature of the bone. The end result is an arch form that is frequently not on the residual ridge. Several techniques using soft waxes, ZOE impression pastes, and tissue conditioners have been proposed as adjunctive efforts to establish a correct neutral zone for the arch form. When advanced anterior ridge reduction has been accompanied by migration of the mentalis muscle attachment to the crest of the ridge, a certain amount of compromise is essential and the rim is trimmed very thin and placed on, or lingual to, the ridge crest. If this sort of compromise creates an intolerable situation for the patient, surgical labial sulcus deepening in this area may be considered. Some dentists and technicians have subscribed to a tooth-on-the-ridge philosophy, which has seriously undermined efforts for denture stability and esthetics. The concept of a neutral zone in the context of a keen understanding of patterns of alveolar ridge resorption enables the dentist to determine the arch form for the patient receiving treatment (See Fig. 17-3.)

Maxillary arch. Bone reduction usually occurs on the labial and buccal areas of the maxillary residual ridge. Consequently the residual ridge is usually palatal to the original location of the natural teeth. The maxillary teeth should be labial and buccal to the residual ridge if they are to be placed in the neutral zone and occupy the position of their predecessors. Frequently this pattern of bony reduction is ignored, and the dentist finds a contracted maxillary arch form within the confines of the mandibular arch form. This oversight guarantees inadequate labial support. The incisive papilla appears to occupy a stable locale on the palate,

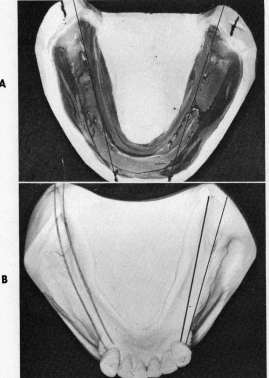

Fig. 14-10 **A,** A straight line drawn from lingual of the retromolar pad to a point just lingual to the crest of the ridge in the premolar region can act as a guide for positioning artificial posterior teeth. **B,** A partially edentulous cast with a straight line on the right and a curved line on the left showing the curvature of the body of the mandible.

unless it is modified surgically. Clinical experience indicates that the incisal edges of the maxillary central incisors are usually 8 to 10 mm anterior to the center of the incisive papilla. The tips of the canines are also related to the center of the papilla, and a high percentage of canines are ± 1 mm in front of the papilla (Fig. 14-11, *A*). The papilla is circled and used as a rough guide in locating the anteroposterior position of the maxillary anterior teeth (Fig. 14-11, *B*). It has also been shown that after the teeth are lost the canines should be located in a coronal plane passing through the posterior border of the papilla. A patient's old dentures, preextraction photographs, or diagnostic casts and photographs made before the dentition deteriorated may be employed to assist not only in selecting artificial teeth but also in establishing the optimal labial support for the patient.

If the patient has been wearing inadequate dentures, tooth loss will have a pronounced effect on the appearance of the lips and adjacent tissues. As a result of the loss of substance and the reduction in elastic properties, the connective tissue will not provide sufficient resistance to the activities of the orbicularis oris and associated muscles. Consequently the effect of the degenerative changes in the skin becomes exaggerated and the lips appear to have aged to a much greater extent than the surrounding parts. The skin becomes roughened, and deep vertical lines appear in the body and margins of the lips. There is a noticeable shortening/thinning of the lips because of a tendency for the lip margins to roll inward. The nasolabial fold changes direction to become almost continuous with the groove at the corner of the mouth, and the lips and cheeks are no longer distinctly separated (Fig. 14-12). Such a loss of well-defined demarcation tends to produce a generally disordered appearance of the lower half of the face. At this stage it may be difficult to visualize proper lip support in an attempt to counter the changes just described. However, the more experienced dentist will generally use the occlusion rim to achieve the best compromise be-

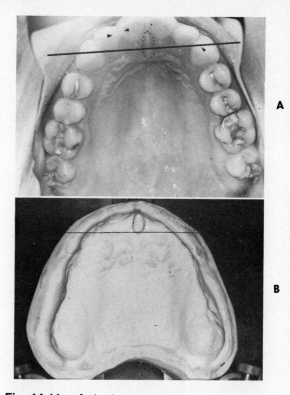

Fig. 14-11   **A,** In the natural dentition the tips of the maxillary canines are frequently ± 1 mm anterior to the center of the incisive papilla *(dotted circle).* **B,** On an edentulous cast the papilla is *circled* since it provides a rough guide to positioning the maxillary canines.

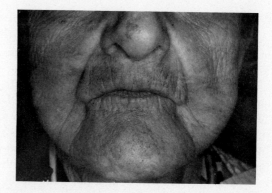

Fig. 14-12   Degenerative skin changes create virtual continuity between the nasolabial fold and the corner of the mouth.

tween neutral zone determination and harmonious labial support. Cheek support is probably not affected as much as lip support by altering labial support, since the buccinator is stretched between the pterygomandibular raphe and the modiolus muscles. It must be remembered that the longer the period of edentulism the greater will be the loss of the original muscle patterns and the less easily and completely will they be relearned when even the best dentures are provided. The more accurate the replacement and the sooner it occurs, the easier will be the task of relearning.

The anterior position of the maxillary occlusion rim is so modified that the lower lip gently caresses the rim during pronunciation of the letter *f*. The rim is usually parallel to the interpupillary line and at a height that accommodates the length of the natural tooth plus the amount of assessed bone reduction that has occurred. It is possible, though rather difficult to visualize, to simulate proper length and lip support by contouring the labial aspect of the maxillary occlusion rim. It would be preferable, and in fact easier, for the dentist to select the anterior teeth for the patient's denture at the examination appointment and set them for proper length and lip support in the occlusion rims. Further characterization of the anterior arrangement could then be done at the patient's next appointment.

Preliminary centric relation record

The preliminary centric relation record is made after the occlusion rims have been contoured, and it is designed to simulate the position that will be occupied by the artificial teeth and tissues of the complete dentures (Fig. 14-13). The occlusion rims are used to establish a preliminary centric relation record and to transfer it by means of a face-bow to a semiadjustable articulator. Once the anterior teeth have been placed in their final positions in the occlusion rim, a record is made of the jaw relation when the incisor teeth are in an edge-to-edge position. This record will enable the den-

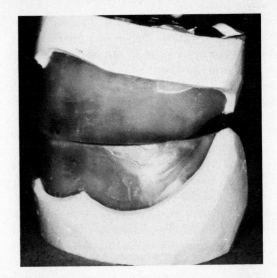

Fig. 14-13 Two occlusion rims have been contoured and adjusted and are now ready to be used for making the preliminary CR record.

tist to adjust the condylar guidances of the articulator.

An articulator is used in complete denture construction to simulate jaw movements, for convenience and because of the lack of a solid base in the patient's mouth. The use of a semiadjustable articulator requires that at least four jaw relations be transferred from the patient to the instrument: (1) the relation of the jaws to the opening axis (Chapter 15), (2) the vertical separation of the jaws, (3) the horizontal relation of the lower to the upper jaw in CR, and (4) the relation of the lower jaw to the upper jaw when the mandible is protruded (Chapter 20) so the incisor teeth will be edge to edge. Quite obviously, all these records must be made by the dentist.

The vertical and horizontal relations of the jaws are integral components of the CR position in edentulous patients. The provisional vertical dimension of occlusion is first established, and the horizontal jaw relation record is made at this level.

BIBLIOGRAPHY

Barrenäs L, Ödman P: Myodynamic and conventional construction of complete dentures. A comparative study of comfort and function, J Oral Rehabil. (In press, 1989.)

Beresin VE, Schiesser FJ: The neutral zone in complete and partial dentures, ed 2, St Louis, 1978, The CV Mosby Co.

Berry DC, Wilkie JK: An approach to dental prosthetics, vol 2, Pergamon series on dentistry, London, 1964, Pergamon Press.

Fish EW: An analysis of the stabilising factors in full denture construction, Br Dent J 52:559-570, 1931.

Fish, W: Principles of full denture prosthesis, ed 4, London, 1948, Staples Press Ltd.

Karlsson S, Hedegård B: Study of the reproducibility of the functional denture space with a dynamic impression technique, J Prosthet Dent 41:21-25, 1979.

Lee JH: Dental aesthetics, Bristol, 1962, John Wright & Sons Ltd.

Lott F, Levin B: Flange technique: an anatomic and physiologic approach to increased retention, function, comfort, and appearance of denture, J Prosthet Dent 16:394-413, 1966.

Nairn RI: The circumoral musculature: structure and function, Br Dent J 138:49-56, 1975.

Pound E: Controlling anomalies of vertical dimension and speech, J Prosthet Dent 36:124-135, 1976.

Watt DM, Likeman PR: Morphological changes in the denture bearing area following the extraction of maxillary teeth, Br Dent J 136:225-235, 1974.

Wright CR: Evaluation of the factors necessary to develop stability in mandibular dentures, J Prosthet Dent 16:414-430, 1966.

CHAPTER 15

Relating the patient to the articulator

The final test for success or failure of complete dentures is made in the patient's mouth. A demonstration of an excellently planned and executed occlusion on the articulator, though an important mechanical entity in itself, is meaningless unless that occlusion functions in the mouth in harmony with the biologic factors that regulate the mandibular activity of the patient.

If it were practical to do so, the patient's mouth would be the best articulator. However, it is mechanically impossible to perform intraorally many of the procedures involved in construction of complete dentures. Furthermore, the dentist must consider the movement of the trial dentures on supporting soft tissues in the mouth and the difficulties posed by the presence of saliva and the patient's ability to cooperate. The convenience for the dentist and dental laboratory technician dictates that an articulator be used.

ARTICULATORS

Articulators are a mechanical analogue for the TMJs and the upper and lower dental arches, a device to which maxillary and mandibular casts can be attached, with the intent of simulating the functional and parafunctional contact relationships of one arch to the other. They are used to hold casts in one or more positions in relation to each other for the purposes of diagnosis, arranging artificial teeth, and development of the occlusal surfaces of fixed restorations. They have been made in hundreds of different designs. The designs have been based on (1) theories of occlusion and (2) the types of records used for their adjustment. Some articulators are simple, with only one function—to hold the casts in centric relation with each other. Most of these consist of a simple hinged device. Other articulators are complex, and some of these require a complicated apparatus for transferring records of jaw relationships from the patient's mouth to the articulator. The necessary records may be simple or complex depending on the instrument being adjusted. It must be emphasized, however, that even the most sophisticated articulator fails to reproduce the complex movements of the masticatory system. Furthermore, the inherent rigidity of an articulator contrasts with the enormous modifications of movement

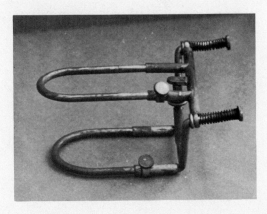

Fig. 15-1   The Bonwill articulator.

that a mandible performs throughout functional and parafunctional activities. Still, articulators are essential in prosthodontic treatment, and a brief review of their development is useful to understanding how the study of occlusion has evolved from anatomic and cadaver studies to neurophysiologic ones.

Articulators based on theories of occlusion

In the history of articulators, at least three theories of occlusion have been proposed as bases for the inventors' articulator designs. These will be briefly described.

The *Bonwill theory* of occlusion proposed that the teeth move in relation to each other as guided by the condylar controls and the incisal point. It was known as the theory of the equilateral triangle, in which there was a 4-inch (10 cm) distance between the condyles and between each condyle and the incisor point. The articulator designed by W.G.A. Bonwill is shown in Fig. 15-1. It allows lateral movement, but since the condylar guidances are not adjustable they permit movement of the mechanism only in the horizontal plane.

The *conical theory* of occlusion proposed that the lower teeth move over the surfaces of the upper teeth as over the surface of a cone, generating an angle of 45 degrees with the central axis of the cone tipped 45 degrees to the occlusal plane. The Hall Automatic articulator, designed by R.E. Hall (Fig. 15-2), conforms to the conical theory of occlusion. It should be noted that teeth having 45-degree cusps are necessary when dentures are made on this instrument.

The *spherical theory* of occlusion showed the lower teeth moving over the surface of the upper teeth as over the surface of a sphere with a diameter of 8 inches (20 cm). The center of the sphere was located in the region of the glabella, and the surface of the sphere passed through the glenoid fossae along or concentric with the articulating eminences. The theory was proposed by G.S. Monson in 1918, based on the observations of natural teeth and skulls made by von Spee, a German anatomist. The "maxillomandibular instrument" (Fig. 15-3), devised by Monson, operated on the spherical theory of occlusion. The Hagman Balancer and one phase of the Pankey-Mann occlusal reconstruction technique also had their bases in the spherical theory of occlusion.

The articulators that function on theories of occlusion have one common fault: they make

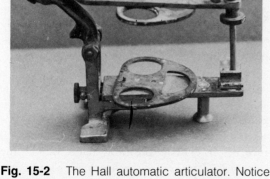

Fig. 15-2 The Hall automatic articulator. Notice its steep incisal guidance, which necessitates using teeth with high cusps.

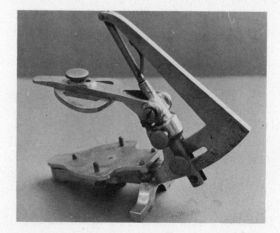

Fig. 15-3 The Monson maxillomandibular instrument.

no provision for variations from the theoretical relationships that occur in different persons. When the varying inclinations of condylar paths of the two sides of many patients are recognized, the need for modification becomes apparent. Also the wide variation in the paths of jaw movements among persons makes individually variable condylar guidances on articulators essential.

Articulators based on the type of record used for their adjustment

Three general classes of records are used for transferring maxillomandibular relationships from the patient to the articulator: interocclusal records, graphic records, and hinge-axis records. Some articulators are designed for use with only one type of record. Others use combinations of two or three types of records.

Interocclusal record adjustment. Most articulators in common use today for complete denture construction are adjusted by some kind of interocclusal records. These records may be made in wax, plaster of Paris, ZOE paste, or cold-curing acrylic resin. Each record is of only one positional relationship of the lower jaw to the upper jaw. Articulators may or may not have the capability of adjusting to all interocclusal records. It is at this point that differences in articulators become apparent. Some are adjustable to CR records only, and some to protrusive and centric relation records. Others are adjustable to lateral relation records as well.

The mechanical features that determine whether an articulator can be adjusted to accommodate interocclusal records include (1) individually adjustable horizontal condylar guidances, (2) variable controls for the Bennett (direct lateral) shift, (3) variable intercondylar distances, (4) split-axis condylar guidance controls (to allow the Bennett shift in the instrument to be upward, downward, forward, or backward, as the articulator is moved into lateral positions), and (5) adjustable incisal guidance controls.

The recorded and adjusted relationships and positions of the casts on the articulator are accurate only at the positions where the interocclusal records are made. All other relationships on the articulator are approximations.

Graphic record adjustment. Articulators designed for use with graphic records are generally more complicated than those designed for interocclusal records. Since graphic records consist of records of the extreme border positions of mandibular movements, the articulators must be capable of producing at least the equivalent of curved movements. The reason is that the border movements of the mandible are in curves.

These instruments and others similar to them are capable of reproducing, with reasonable accuracy, the border movements of the mandible, provided the graphic records themselves are accurate. Accurate graphic records for this purpose are not too difficult to make, as long as the complicated kinematic face-bow and "jaw writing" apparatus is firmly attached to the jaws. This is a simple procedure if natural teeth exist in both jaws, but it becomes more difficult, and the records even unreliable, when patients are edentulous. This is especially true when the basal seats for the dentures are unfavorable.

Hinge-axis location for adjusting articulators. All the instruments that can be adjusted to graphic records have one feature in common: the necessity for correct location of the opening axis of the mandible. A failure to locate the "hinge axis" of the patient's mandible correctly will make adjustment of these instruments impossible.

One instrument, the Transograph, depends entirely on the accurate location of the hinge axis for its adjustment. It is adapted from a kinematic face-bow assembly, and the tests for accuracy are made with wax interocclusal records of centric position made in varying thickness. The Transograph provides no opportunity for adjustment to protrusive or lateral jaw relations.

SELECTION OF AN ARTICULATOR FOR COMPLETE DENTURES

The large number of articulators available, and the wide range of adjustment possibilities in these articulators, can leave the dentist quite confused when one must be chosen. However, this need not be so. The choice of articulator is made on the basis of what is expected of it.

If occlusal contacts are to be perfected in centric occlusion only, a simple, sturdy, hinge-type articulator without provision for lateral or protrusive movements can be selected. This type of instrument has been called one-dimensional because only one interocclusal record is necessary for its adjustment and use.

If denture teeth are to have a cross-arch and cross-tooth balanced occlusion, the minimum requirement is a semiadjustable articulator. This may be an instrument with individually adjustable condylar guidances in both the vertical and the horizontal plane, such as the simple instruments in the Hanau University series, the Whip Mix articulator, or the Dentatus articulator.

If more control of the occlusion is desired, a completely adjustable three-dimensional articulator is of value. A three-dimensional articulator requires a CR record, at least two lateral records, and some means for controlling the height and inclinations of the cusps. The means for their adjustment may be interocclusal records or three-dimensional graphic tracings made by a kinematic face-bow apparatus.

The more complicated articulators pose some problems in making complete dentures because of the resiliency of the soft tissues of the basal seat on which the recording bases must rest. Because this resiliency permits some movement of the bases in relation to the bone, the records made are not necessarily records of the true path of movement of the bone. Therefore it becomes essential that the casts representing the patient's mandible and maxillae be oriented on the articulator similarly to the manner in which the jaws of the patient are oriented to one another and to the skull. To ac-complish this, certain measurements and records must be taken from the patient and transferred to the articulator to relate the patient to the articulator.

Several articulators have been employed in the fabrication of complete dentures. We recognize that excellent results can be obtained with a wide variety of articulating instruments; however, we believe that extensive clinical experience and testing justify the recommendation of at least three instruments used extensively in clinical practice—the Hanau model 130-28, the Whip Mix, and the Dentatus articulators.

Hanau articulator

The Hanau articulator is a semiadjustable arcon* type of instrument. It consists of an upper member containing the condylar guidance elements and a lower member to which the condylar spheres are attached. The upper and lower members are mechanically connected (Fig. 15-4).

The Hanau articulator is classed as a modified two-dimensional instrument. The upper cast is oriented to the upper member (which represents the skull) by either a kinematic or an arbitrary face-bow transfer record (Fig. 15-5). The arbitrary face-bow is routinely used for complete dentures. The Hanau face-bow consists of a U-shaped frame or assembly that is large enough to extend from the region of the TMJs to a position 2 to 3 inches (5 to 7.5 cm) in front of the face and wide enough to avoid contact with the sides of the face. The parts that contact the skin over the TMJs are the condyle rods, and the part that attaches to the occlusion rims is the fork. The condyle rods are positioned on a line extending from the outer canthus to the top of the tragus and approximately 13 mm in front of the external auditory meatus (Fig. 15-6). This placement of the rods will locate them within 2 mm of the true center of

---

*For *ar*ticulator and *con*dyle.

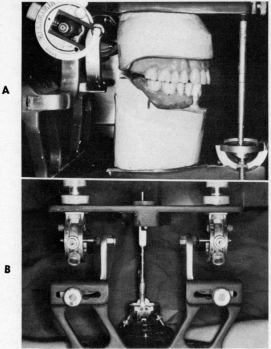

A

B

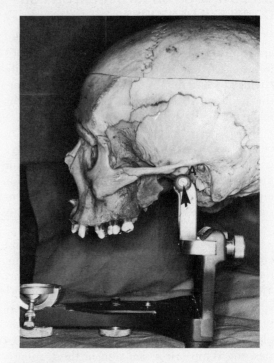

Fig. 15-4 The Hanau model 130-28 articulator, **A,** side and, **B,** rear views. Notice that the upper member of the articulator carries the "condylar housing" or simulated glenoid fossa. The mechanically connected lower member carries the condylar spheres, which are contained in the upper member's condylar housing.

Fig. 15-5 The upper member of this articulator has been replaced by a dry skull to simulate the relationship of the condylar housing, *A,* to the condylar sphere *(arrow).*

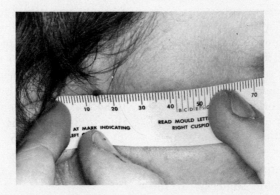

Fig. 15-6 Measuring 13 mm on a line extending from the top of the tragus to the outer canthus. This provides an arbitrary center for the opening axis of the mandible.

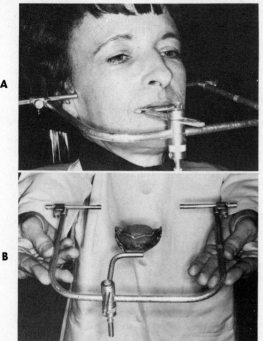

Fig. 15-7   **A,** The Hanau face-bow fork attached to the maxillary occlusion rim properly locates the face-bow on this patient's face. **B,** The completed face-bow record.

the opening axis of the jaws. The fork of the face-bow is attached to the maxillary occlusion rim, thus the record is a simple measurement from the jaws to the approximate axis of the jaws (Fig. 15-7).

Theoretical evidence indicates that articulator adjustments for patients' varying intercondylar widths may be of significance in fixed prosthodontic procedures. This is probably not the case in the treatment of complete denture patients and is considered an elective procedure. The Hanau articulator is machined to accept different intercondylar distances and can be adjusted to each patient's intercondylar width (Fig. 15-8). In this manner the location of the vertical axes of rotation of the patient's mandible can be approximated on either side of the articulator.

The lower cast is oriented to the lower member of the articulator, representing the mandible, by relating the lower to the upper cast through an interocclusal CR record (Fig. 15-9).

The horizontal condylar guidances are adjusted by an interocclusal protrusive record. The lateral condylar guidances may be set arbitrarily or may be adjusted by right and left lat-

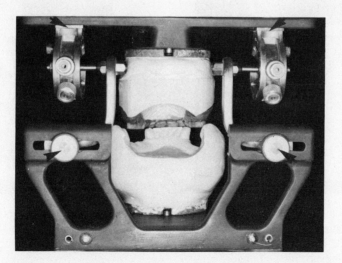

Fig. 15-8   Although the intercondylar width is adjustable on the Hanau *(arrows),* adjustments are rarely needed in complete denture construction.

eral interocclusal records. The lateral condylar guidances on this articulator do not allow upward, downward, forward, or backward movement of the working condylar sphere.

The articulator is provided with an adjustable incisal guide table that is routinely used for removable prosthodontic restorations. The angulation of the lateral plates of the table is calibrated in degrees, and the plates can be positioned at the desired lateral incisal guidance. The table is adjustable anteroposteriorly to provide the necessary guidance for protrusive movement.

The articulator has a straight incisal guide pin with a flat end, which permits movements

on the guide table. The pin on the Hanau articulator is adjustable and allows for vertical changes without changes in pin position relative to the middle of the incisal guide table (Fig. 15-10).

Whip Mix articulator

The Whip Mix articulator is a semiadjustable arcon type of instrument that consists of an upper member, containing the condylar guidances, and a lower member, to which are attached the condylar spheres (Fig. 15-11). The upper and lower members are not mechanically connected but can be held together when necessary by a rubber band.

The Whip Mix articulator is classed as a modified two-dimensional instrument. The up-

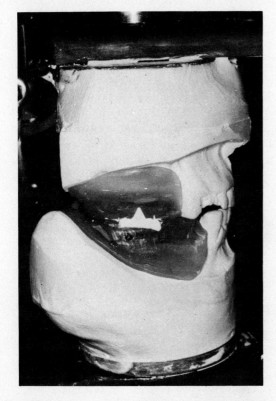

Fig. 15-9 The mandibular cast for an immediate denture patient is related on the Hanau by means of an interocclusal CR record. The maxillary cast is usually mounted first on the articulator. In another technique the mandibular and maxillary casts are mounted simultaneously.

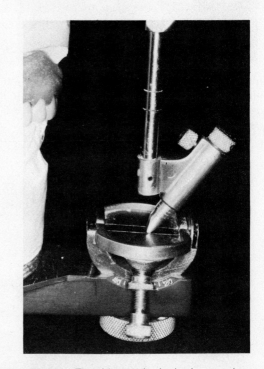

Fig. 15-10 The Hanau incisal pin can be adjusted vertically without moving away from the middle of the incisal guide table.

per cast is oriented to the upper member (which represents the skull) by either a kinematic or arbitrary face-bow transfer record. The arbitrary face-bow is routinely used for complete dentures. It is positioned posteriorly by ear posts that fit into the external auditory meatuses and anteriorly by a plastic nasion relator that fits into the concavity of the bridge of the nose. These three points establish an approximation of the axis-orbital plane on the patient that can be transferred to the articulator.

The distance between the condylar spheres (intercondylar distance) is semiadjustable in a lateral direction and can be regulated for small (88 mm), medium (100 mm), and large (112 mm) intercondylar widths of the patient as determined by an indicator on the face-bow (Fig. 15-12, *A* and *B*). Metal shims permit the distance between the condylar guidance elements on the upper member to be adjusted in harmony with the intercondylar widths on the lower member (Fig. 15-12, *C*). Thus the location of the vertical axes of rotation of the mandible can be approximated on the articulator.

The lower cast is oriented to the lower member of the articulator, representing the mandible, by relating it to the upper cast through an interocclusal CR record. The horizontal condylar guidances are adjusted by an interocclusal protrusive record, and the lateral condylar

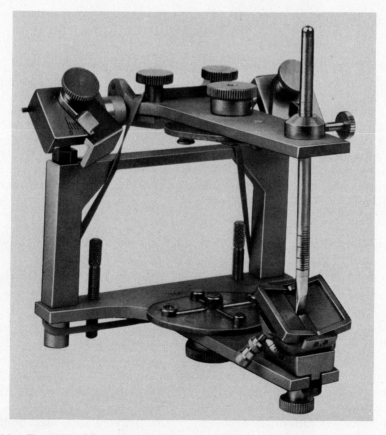

Fig. 15-11 The Whip Mix articulator is a two-piece instrument designed on the arcon principle. (Courtesy Whip Mix Corporation, Louisville Ky.)

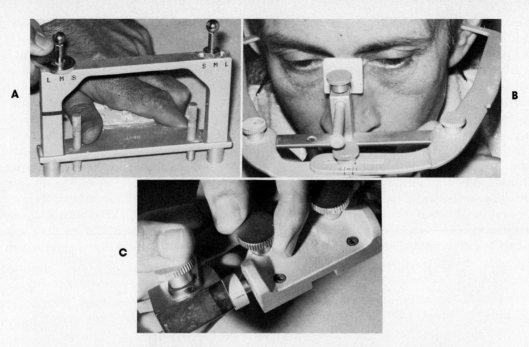

Fig. 15-12   **A,** The condylar spheres of the Whip Mix articulator removed from the frame of the lower member are adjusted for varying intercondylar distances according to the needs of the patient. Intercondylar distances are small, medium, and large, with an increment of 12 mm between gradations. **B,** The face-bow is properly oriented to the patient. The intercondylar width of the patient is indicated by a measuring gauge on the anterior part of the bow. The intercondylar width for this patient is *M* (medium). **C,** One metal spacer is added on each side for a medium intercondylar width. This will properly adjust the condylar housing on the upper member of the articulator to the condylar spheres when they are in medium position on the lower member. Two metal spacers are required on each side for a large intercondylar width.

guidances by right and left interocclusal lateral records. The lateral condylar guidances on the Whip Mix articulator do not allow upward, downward, forward, or backward movement of the working-side condylar sphere (Fig. 15-13).

The articulator has interchangeable fixed and adjustable incisal guide tables. The fixed table, made of plastic, can be individually modified by cold-curing acrylic resin. The adjustable table, made of metal, is used for removable prosthodontic restorations. The lateral plates of the adjustable incisal guide table can be positioned at the desired lateral incisal guidance, and the angulation of the plates calibrated in

degrees. The entire table is adjustable anteroposteriorly to provide the necessary guidance for the protrusive movement (Fig. 15-14).

The articulator has a straight incisal guide pin. One end of this pin is rounded to fit the concavity in the fixed incisal guide tables, and the other end is flat to permit movements on the guide table. Since the incisal guide pin is straight, its vertical position in the upper member of the articulator changes its relation to the middle of the guide table.

Orienting the upper cast on the Whip Mix articulator. The upper occlusion rim is placed in the patient's mouth. Adjustments are made so

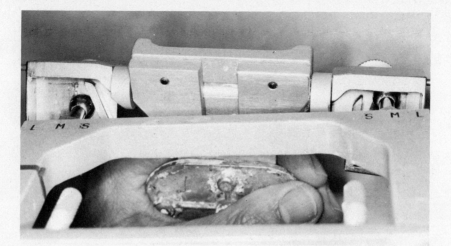

Fig. 15-13 The condylar housing and spheres of the Whip Mix articulator, seen from below. The balancing condylar sphere on the *left* has moved downward, forward, and inward as dictated by the condylar guidances on the left. Simultaneously the working condylar sphere on the *right* has moved laterally (Bennett shift); however, the condylar housing will not permit full freedom of the working sphere during this movement.

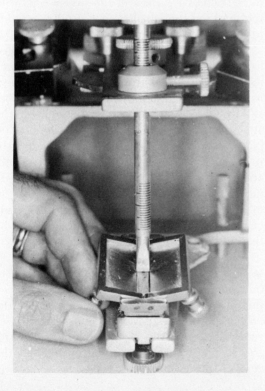

Fig. 15-14 The incisal guide table can be adjusted anteroposteriorly for protrusive movement, and the lateral plates can be raised or lowered for harmony with the lateral incisal guidance.

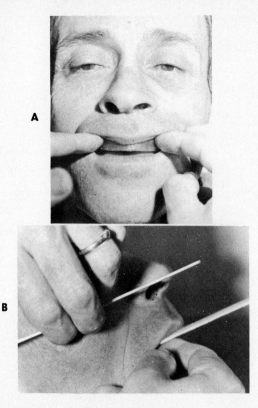

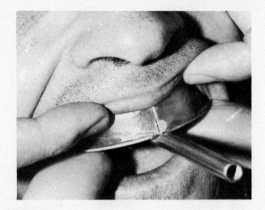

Fig. 15-16 The Whip Mix face-bow fork attached to the occlusal surface of the upper occlusion rim.

Fig. 15-15 **A,** The upper occlusion rim has been adjusted to represent the approximate length of the natural anterior teeth, with the incisal plane parallel to the interpupillary line. **B,** Occlusal plane of the upper occlusion rim roughly paralleling the ala-tragus line.

the occlusal surface of the rim anteriorly is in the approximate position formerly occupied by the natural teeth. The upper lip should be adequately supported, the incisal plane should parallel the interpupillary line, and the occlusal plane should roughly parallel a line from the ala to the tragus (Fig. 15-15). These modifications should be made quickly, since it is not necessary for the upper occlusion rim to be in its final form when orienting the upper cast on the articulator.

With the upper occlusion rim in the mouth, the face-bow fork is preliminarily positioned in line anteroposteriorly with the middle of the head and a mark is made on the labial surface of the occlusion rim to indicate this position. Then the face-bow fork is heated and attached to the occlusal surface of the upper rim, with the mark on the labial surface used as a guide to the proper position (Fig. 15-16).

The upper occlusion rim and the attached face-bow fork are placed in the patient's mouth. The patient is instructed to hold them in position with thumbs pressing against both sides of the bottom of the face-bow fork. The attachment mechanism for the face-bow is placed over the end of the fork, and the ear posts are guided into the external auditory meatuses until they fit snugly. The anterior locking device on the face-bow is tightened to maintain this position, and a notation is made of the estimated cranial width as indicated by the marker on the front of the face-bow.

The plastic nasion relator (nosepiece) is attached to the supporting crosspiece of the face-bow, and the face-bow is adjusted vertically so the nosepiece fits into the concavity of the bridge of the nose (nasion). The face-bow is securely locked to the fork in this position (Fig. 15-17). The nasion relator that determines the vertical position of the face-bow anteriorly

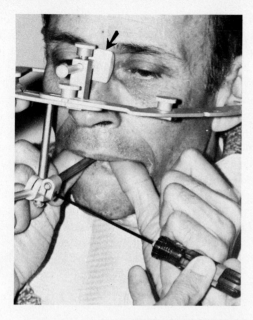

Fig. 15-17   The Whip Mix face-bow properly oriented to the patient's face with the nasion relator *(arrow)* and securely attached to the face-bow fork. The patient is holding the upper occlusion rim and attached face-bow fork securely in position on the residual ridge. Notice that the face-bow is aligned at the approximate level of the infraorbital notch when positioned by the plastic nasion relator.

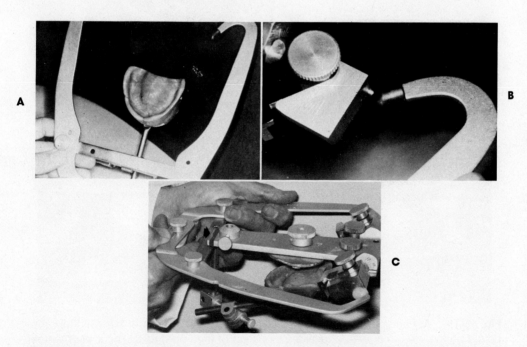

Fig. 15-18   A, The Whip Mix face-bow with attached fork and occlusion rim removed from the patient. Notice that the upper occlusion rim is lined with acrylic resin for an accurate fit on the cast and in the mouth. **B,** Ear posts of the face-bow are attached to small metal rods extending from the condylar housing. **C,** The forward end of the upper member of the articulator rests on the anterior crosspiece of the face-bow *(arrowhead).*

forms a third point of reference and, together with the ear posts posteriorly, establishes the axis-orbital plane of the patient, which will be transferred to the articulator. The nasion relator has been so designed that when it is positioned at nasion the face-bow will be located anteriorly in the approximate region of the infraorbital notch.

The ear posts are carefully disengaged from the auditory meatuses, and the face-bow and attached upper occlusion rim are removed from the patient (Fig. 15-18, *A*). The condylar posts on the lower member of the articulator and the condylar guidance mechanisms on the upper member are adjusted to correspond with the cranial width as indicated by the face-bow.

The face-bow, holding the upper occlusion rim, is attached posteriorly to the upper member of the articulator when the holes are fitted in the ear posts over small metal rods that extend laterally from each condylar housing (Fig. 15-18, *B*). The metal rods are located approximately 6 mm posteriorly from the actual transverse axis of the articulator to compensate for the location of the ear posts in the external auditory meatuses, which are roughly the same distance posteriorly from the mandibular transverse hinge axis of the patient. The forward end of the upper member of the articulator, with the incisal guide pin removed, rests on the anterior part of the face-bow (Fig. 15-18, *C*). Since the anterior part has been positioned at the approximate level of the infraorbital notch on the patient's face by the nasion rela-

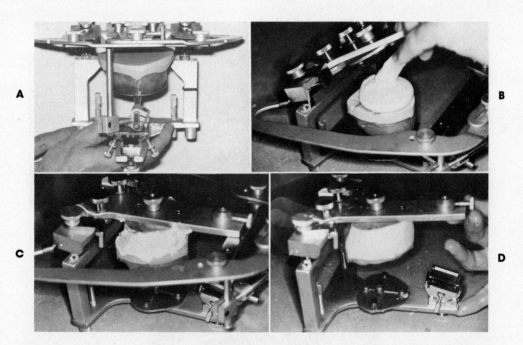

Fig. 15-19 **A,** Face-bow, occlusion rim, cast, and upper member of the Whip Mix supported on the lower member to facilitate mounting of the upper cast. The lower member of the articulator is used in this procedure for convenience only. **B,** With the upper member elevated, fast-setting plaster is distributed over the top of the upper cast. **C,** The upper member of the articulator has been closed back into position on the anterior part of the face-bow. **D,** Mounting of the upper cast on the articulator completed. Notice the neat appearance of the plaster that attaches the upper cast to the mounting ring.

tor, the upper cast will automatically be oriented on the articulator in the same relationship as the upper jaw of the patient is to the TMJs posteriorly and to the infraorbital notch anteriorly (the axis-orbital plane).

The upper member of the articulator and the attached face-bow, occlusion rim, and upper cast can be conveniently supported by the lower member of the articulator while the upper cast is attached to the upper member of the articulator with fast-setting artificial stone (Fig. 15-19). The upper cast is now oriented on the upper member of the articulator similarly to the way the upper jaw is oriented to the skull of the patient (Fig. 15-20).

Establishing preliminary vertical relations on the Whip Mix. After the upper occlusion rim has been adjusted for facial support, vertical height, and the angulation of the incisal and occlusal plane (with the face-bow used to orient the upper cast correctly on the articulator), refinements are made in the form of the upper

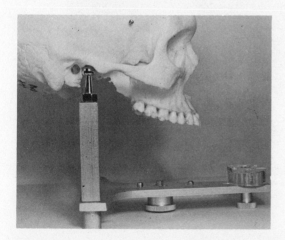

Fig. 15-20   A skull has been substituted for the upper member of the Whip Mix to show the manner in which the relationship of the upper cast to the articulator should simulate that of the upper jaw to the patient's head. (From Hickey JC, et al: J Prosthet Dent **18:**425-437, 1967.)

occlusion rim. Remember: The size and form of the rim represent the natural dental arch plus the part of the residual ridge that has been lost by resorption. The length of the upper residual ridge relative to the length of the upper lip can be helpful in developing the length of the occlusion rim anteriorly. If the upper lip is long compared to the residual ridge, the level of the occlusion rim may be slightly above the vermilion border of the lip. If the lip is short, the occlusion rim may extend several millimeters below the vermilion border.

The height of the lower occlusion rim is preliminarily adjusted (with the upper rim out of the mouth); thus anteriorly it will be at the level of the corner of the mouth and posteriorly at the level of the posterior third of the retromolar pad, approximating the height of the occlusal plane of the completed dentures. The lower rim is adjusted labially for proper support of the lower lip.

With both occlusion rims in the mouth, observations are made to determine what modifications may be needed to establish a preliminary vertical dimension of occlusion. These observations include (1) a determination of the interocclusal distance, (2) measurements of the facial height at mandibular rest position when the occlusion rims are not in the mouth as compared to measurements with the occlusion rims in the mouth, (3) the space between the rims during phonetic testing, and (4) the nature of the facial support of the patient. The occlusion rims are adjusted until an adequate interocclusal distance seems present (Fig. 15-21).

Making the preliminary centric relation record. After the vertical dimension between the jaws has been established with the occlusion rims in the mouth, the preliminary CR record is made. CR is *always* the horizontal relation for orienting the lower cast to the upper cast of edentulous patients.

With the occlusion rims in the mouth, sufficient trial closures in CR are practiced until

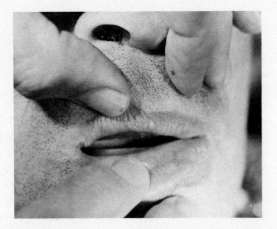

Fig. 15-21 Space between the upper and lower occlusion rims indicates that an adequate interocclusal distance has been established when the mandible is at the vertical dimension of rest.

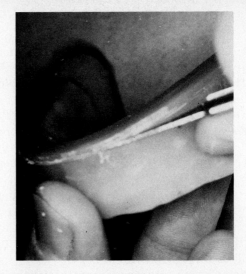

Fig. 15-22 The lower occlusion rim is reduced to make space for the recording medium; in this manner the CR record can be made as close to the desired vertical dimension of occlusion as possible.

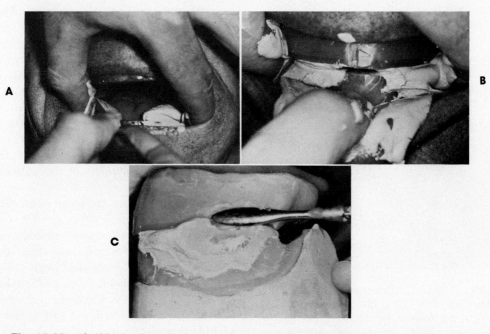

Fig. 15-23 **A,** With both occlusion rims in the mouth and supported, recording medium is added to the occlusal surface of the lower rim. **B,** The patient closes in CR as rehearsed previously. Closure is stopped at the predetermined vertical, with no contact between opposing occlusion rims. **C,** The occlusion rims are placed on the lower cast and securely sealed together before the lower cast is mounted on the articulator.

both the dentist and the patient become familiar with the position. The hand position used by the dentist and the instructions given the patient are similar to those described previously.

When the patient can consistently follow the instructions, approximately 2 mm of wax is removed from the occlusal surface of the lower occlusion rim to provide space for the recording medium (Fig. 15-22). The CR record must always be made at or as close as possible to the desired vertical dimension without contact of the opposing occlusion rims. The dentist observes the relationship of the occlusion rims when the mandible is in CR and stops the closure at the desired vertical dimension during additional trial closures. A space of approximately 2 mm should exist between the rims at the preliminary vertical dimension. Two V-shaped cross grooves are made on the occlusion rims in the molar region, one on each side. These serve as keys for the recording material should the interocclusal record and rims come apart.

The recording medium, a fast-setting plaster-like material (Impressotex), is placed on the lower occlusion rim on each side in the molar-premolar region. Under guidance of the dentist, the patient closes into the plaster with the mandible in CR. The same procedures are followed as used in the trial closures (that is, stopping when the occlusion rims reach the predetermined vertical distance) (Fig. 15-23, A and B). It is essential that both rims be correctly positioned on the residual ridges while the record is being made.

After the recording medium has set, the patient opens carefully and the occlusion rims and interocclusal record are removed (Fig. 15-23, C). They can often be taken out as one unit. There must be no contact of the opposing occlusion rims posteriorly or through the plaster. Such contacts will displace the tissues under the denture base, cause movement of the

occlusion rims on the basal seat, or shift the mandible away from CR. If contact between the rims occurs, a new interocclusal record must be made.

Some patients will have difficulty maintaining the mandible in a fixed position while the plaster interocclusal record sets. In these instances, wax instead of plaster is used as the recording medium.

Orienting the lower cast on the Whip Mix. The lower cast is seated on the lower occlusion rim. The upper member of the articulator is inverted on the laboratory bench with the incisal guide pin centered vertically so it will contact the middle of the incisal guide table. The lateral condylar guidances are set at zero, and the horizontal condylar guidances at 35 degrees to support the condylar spheres. The upper occlusion rim, with the lower rim and lower cast attached, is properly positioned on the upper cast (Fig. 15-24, A and B). Fast-setting plaster is distributed over the bottom of the lower cast and the mounting ring of the lower member of the articulator (Fig. 15-24, C).

The condylar spheres of the lower member of the articulator are placed in the condylar housing of the upper member, and the front part of the lower member is rotated downward until the incisal guide table contacts the incisal guide pin (Fig. 15-24, D). The condylar spheres must be in contact with the posterior part of the condylar housings. Additional plaster is added around the cast. The mounting must be neat (Fig. 15-25). Both casts are now oriented on the articulator as the jaws are oriented to the skull (Fig. 15-26).

Dentatus articulator

The Dentatus is similar to the other articulators just described. It is employed quite extensively in European dental schools, particularly the Scandinavian ones. It too is a semiadjustable instrument that, like the others, can be modified according to several patient variables.

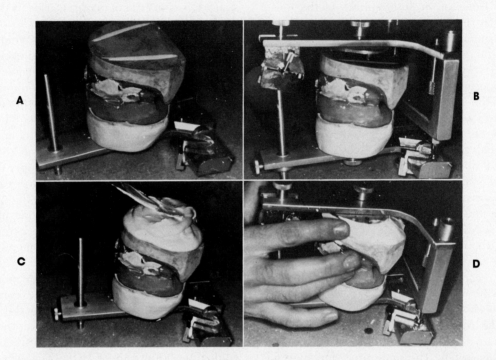

Fig. 15-24 **A,** The occlusion rims and lower cast are placed in position on the upper cast, which is attached to the upper member of the Whip Mix. **B,** The lower member of the articulator is positioned on the inverted upper member, leaving adequate space between the mounting ring on the lower member and the lower cast. **C,** With the lower member of the articulator removed, fast-setting plaster is distributed over the surface of the lower cast. **D,** The lower member is placed on the upper member. The condylar spheres must fit snugly against the posterior part of the condylar housings and the incisal guide table must contact the incisal guide pin. The lower cast is attached to the lower member of the articulator by fast-setting plaster.

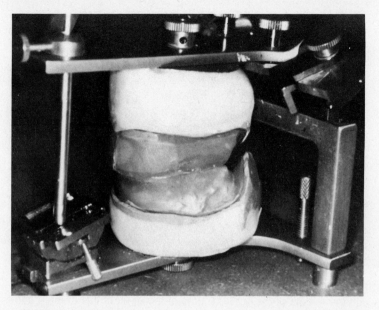

Fig. 15-25 The lower cast has been attached to the lower member of the Whip Mix in proper relation to the upper cast by means of an interocclusal CR record. Notice the neat appearance of the mountings.

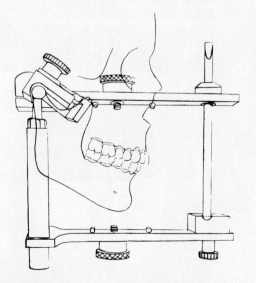

Fig. 15-26 Superimposition of a skull on the articulator to show how properly mounted casts should be oriented to the articulator as the jaws of the patient are oriented to the skull. (From Hickey JC, et al: J Prosthet Dent **18**:425-437, 1967.)

ARBITRARY OR AVERAGE CAST ORIENTATION TECHNIQUE

Practically all prosthodontic literature states that a face-bow transfer is essential for avoiding errors in the occlusion of finished dentures. It is also easy to acknowledge the theoretical advantages of using a face-bow to orient the maxillary cast on the articulator. However, the scientific documentation for the *clinical* necessity of using a face-bow is lacking. Any type of face-bow, and all articulators, suffer from errors and can only approximate conditions in the patient's masticatory system. Consequently, careful adjustments must be performed at insertion of most prostheses, especially dentures, regardless of the occlusal system or articulator used. Many dentists have recognized this fact and have abandoned the use of a face-bow, adopting instead a technique of mounting casts arbitrarily. (Some dentists may even have developed a bad conscience as a result.)

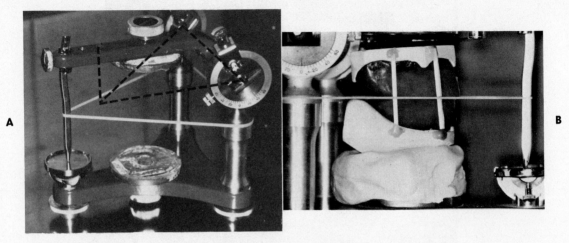

Fig. 15-27 A, The Bonwill triangle is indicated by *dotted lines.* **B,** The casts are mounted with the middle of the occlusal rims at the apex of this triangle and the occlusal plane horizontal.

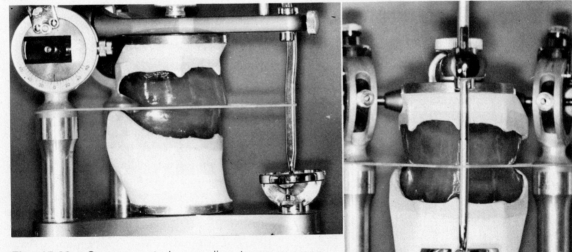

Fig. 15-28 Casts mounted according to an average-value technique. **A,** Lateral view; **B,** anterior view.

We hasten to affirm that following sound principles in other phases of denture construction is necessary for acceptable clinical results; but, in fact, a systematic study comparing a "complex" technique with a "standard" technique and no face-bow transfer showed *no significant* clinical differences between dentures made by the two methods. An arbitrary mounting of the maxillary cast can be easily accomplished on any semiadjustable articulator by aligning the occlusal plane of the wax occlusion rim horizontally with a rubber band placed halfway up the articulator's three vertical posts so the apex of the Bonwill triangle coincides with the middle point (Fig. 15-27). The lower cast is then mounted exactly as if a face-bow transfer had been utilized (Fig. 15-28).

BIBLIOGRAPHY

Beard CC, Clayton JA: Studies on the validity of the terminal hinge axis, J Prosthet Dent **46**:185-191, 1981.

Carlsson GE, Åstrand P: Registering av kondylbanelutningen medelst intraorala vaxindex hos patienter med totala plattproteser, Sven Tandlak Tidskr **57**:615-631, 1964.

Celenza FV: An analysis of articulators, Dent Clin North Am **36**:305-326, 1979.

Ellinger CW, Somes GW, Nicol BR, Unger JW, Wesley RC: Patient response to variations in denture technique. III, Five-year subjective evaluation, J Prosthet Dent **42**:127-130, 1979.

Ericson S, Ransjö K: Klinisk undersökning av några bettregistreringsmetoder, Sven Tandlak Tidskr **56**:1-7, 1963.

Kotwal KR: The need to use an arbitrary face-bow when remounting complete dentures with interocclusal records, J Prosthet Dent **42**:224-227, 1979.

Mohl ND, Zarb GA, Carlsson GE, Rugh JD, editors: A textbook of occlusion, Chicago, 1988, Quintessence Publishing Co Inc.

Tangerud T, Silness J: Kjeveregistrering ved behandling med helproteser. Nordisk klinisk odontologi, Copenhagen, 1987, Forlaget for Faglitteratur, vol 21A-IV, pp 1-23.

Thorp ER, Smith DE, Nicholls JI: Evaluation of the use of a face-bow in complete denture occlusion, J Prosthet Dent **39**:5-15, 1978.

Walker PM: Discrepancies between arbitrary and true hinge axes, J Prosthet Dent **43**:279-285, 1980.

Yanus M, Finger IM, Weinberg R: Comparison of a universal mounting jig to a face bow, J Prosthet Dent **49**:623-627, 1983.

CHAPTER 16

Selecting artificial teeth for the edentulous patient

The selection of artificial teeth for an edentulous patient requires knowledge and understanding of a number of physical and biologic factors that are directly related to the patient. The dentist must perform this phase of prosthodontic care for edentulous patients, since he is the only person who can accumulate, correlate, and evaluate the biomechanical information so the selection of artificial teeth will meet the individual esthetic and functional needs of the patient.

The selection of artificial teeth is a relatively simple non–time-consuming procedure, but it requires the development of experience and confidence. The dentist has many guides available to help in selecting both anterior and posterior artificial teeth.

ANTERIOR TOOTH SELECTION

The selection of anterior teeth for edentulous patients when all records of form, color, and size have been lost is a clinical procedure that can best be accomplished only by trial in the patient's mouth.

The selection of the most suitable teeth for each patient will have much to do with the eventual success or failure of complete denture service. Anterior teeth that are not in harmony with the patient's facial color, form, and size will cause problems in denture construction and in the reaction of the patient to the completed dentures. It is in this phase of denture service that the opportunity exists for an expression of the artistic ability of the dentist.

Much of the effectiveness of tooth selection depends on the ability of the dentist to interpret what is seen. The selection of teeth is not a mechanical exercise. Formulas, average values, and measurements can serve as a starting point; but they cannot take the place of good artistic judgment. Careful observation of the faces and teeth of people with natural teeth will develop in the dentist a sense of dentofacial harmony that is the objective of tooth selection and esthetics. There must be harmony of color, form, size, and arrangement of teeth if dentures are to defy detection.

Preextraction guides

Preextraction guides include photographs, diagnostic casts, radiographs, the teeth of close relatives, and extracted teeth.

Frequently, patients can supply photographs that show the natural anterior teeth or at least the incisal edges of some teeth (Fig. 16-1, *A*). Photographs will often provide general information about the width of the teeth and possibly their outline form that is more accurate than information from any other source. In addition, an algebraic proportion can be established from the photograph. The known factors are the interpupillary distance of the patient, the interpupillary distance on the photograph, and the width or length of the central incisor on the photograph. This information is helpful in assessing the patient's complaints about esthetics (Fig. 16-1, *B*) and achieving a pleasing result with new dentures (Fig. 16-1, *C*). The unknown factor is the precise width or length of the natural central incisor.

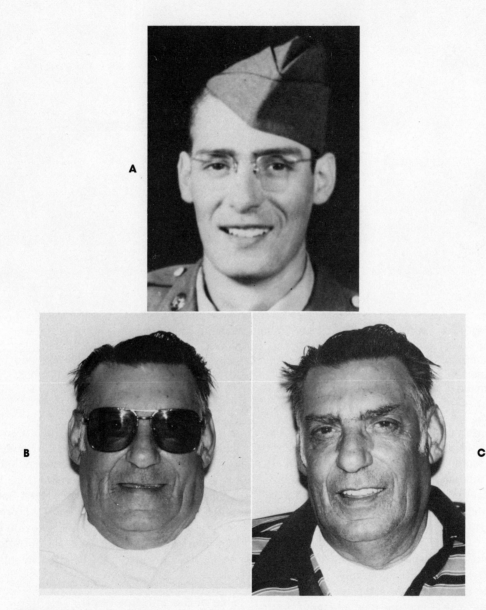

Fig. 16-1   **A,** The natural teeth at 20 years of age. **B,** Poor esthetics 45 years later with 15-year-old dentures. **C,** New dentures have restored the patient's appearance. The original photograph was helpful in achieving a result that pleased both the patient and his wife.

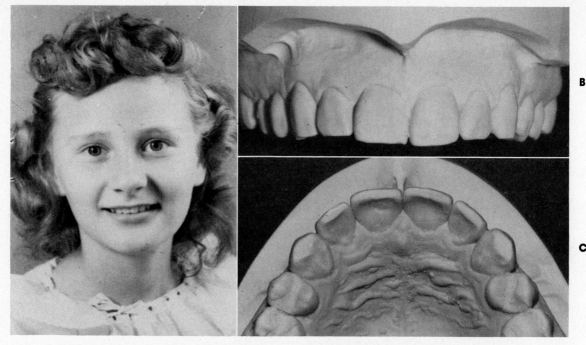

Fig. 16-2 **A,** This patient's childhood photograph provided assistance in selecting denture teeth for her at age 54. **B** and **C,** Diagnostic casts made of her 30-year-old daughter furnished additional assistance. The daughter's tooth shade (Vita A1 for the centrals and laterals, A2 for the canines) also substantiated her mother's request for a light tooth shade.

Diagnostic casts of the natural teeth are also reliable guides in both selecting and arranging anterior teeth. In most instances artificial teeth that are similar in appearance to the patient's natural teeth are desirable. The size and form of the anterior teeth can be determined on the diagnostic cast, and comparable artificial teeth selected.

Intraoral radiographs made before the natural teeth were lost can supply information about the size and form of the teeth to be replaced and can sometimes be obtained from the patient's previous dentist. However, radiographic images are always slightly enlarged and may be distorted because of the divergence of the x rays. Patients are grateful for the extra effort of the dentist in this important aspect of their appearance.

In the absence of other records, a son's or daughter's tooth size, color, and arrangement can be effectively used in selecting and arranging artificial teeth for their parents (Fig. 16-2).

Sometimes patients keep extracted anterior teeth or dental casts given them by a previous dentist. The extracted teeth will provide excellent information as to the size and form for the artificial teeth but cannot be used in selecting color.

Size of the anterior teeth

The size of the teeth should be in proportion to the size of the face and head (Fig. 16-3). Generally, larger persons have large teeth. However, there are variations in which a large person may have small teeth and spaces between the teeth, or a small person may have

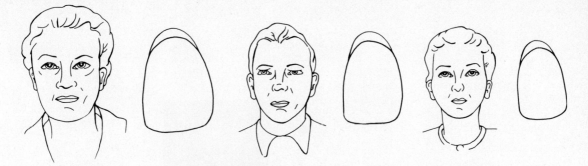

Fig. 16-3   The shapes of artificial teeth chosen to be in harmony with the size of the patient's face.

unduly large teeth and much irregularity in their alignment. Tactful questions asked of the patient and photographs can reveal this information.

Women's teeth are often smaller than men's. This is especially true of the lateral incisors, which normally should be more delicate in women than in men. A distinct difference between the sizes of the central and lateral incisors is desirable, particularly in women.

The growth of alveolar bone requires the presence and eruption of teeth. Thus the size of the casts has a relationship to the size of the anterior teeth. However, when attempts are made to determine the size of artificial teeth by measurement of edentulous casts, the results will be incorrect. The teeth will be too small because of resorption of the residual ridges. If the width of the anterior teeth is to be determined by measurements, the occlusion rims should be contoured for esthetics and the measurement should be made around the curve of the labial surface of the occlusion rim. The approximate location of the distal surfaces of the upper canines can be indicated by marks made on the upper rim at the corners of the mouth (Fig. 16-4, *A* and *B*). Then the distance between the marks is measured around the labial surface of the occlusion rim (Fig. 16-4, *C*), and anterior teeth of this width are arranged as indicated by the occlusion rim.

Other methods for selecting the size of anterior teeth. An estimation of the position of the apex of the upper natural canine can be found by extension of parallel lines from the lateral surfaces of the alae of the nose onto the labial surface of the upper occlusion rim (Fig. 16-5), but this is not sufficiently reliable for use as the means for the final selection. Measurements on the occlusion rim will provide an indication of the width of the upper anterior teeth.

Anthropometric measurements can be helpful in the selection of artificial teeth. Studies of 555 skulls indicated that the greatest bizygomatic width divided by 16 gives an approximation of the width of the upper central incisor (Fig. 16-6), and that dividing by 3.3 provides an estimation of the overall width of the upper six anterior teeth. A face-bow may be used to determine the bizygomatic width. The ratio of the cranial circumference to the width of the upper anterior teeth has been shown to be 10 to 1 in over 90% of 509 subjects studied (Kern, 1967). As a general guide, upper anterior teeth whose overall width as listed on tooth-selection charts is less than 48 mm are relatively small. Those listed as over 52 mm are relatively large.

Form of the anterior teeth

The forms of artificial anterior teeth should harmonize with the shape of the patient's face (Fig. 16-7). The outline form is considered

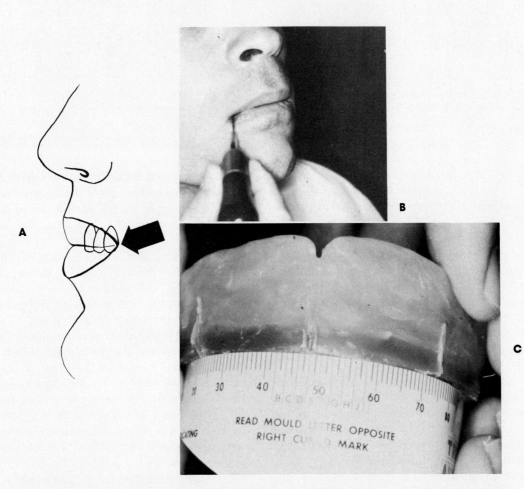

Fig. 16-4 **A,** The distal surface of the natural upper canine is usually located near the corner of the mouth. **B,** A mark is made on the properly contoured upper occlusion rim at the corners of the mouth on both sides. **C,** The distance between the marks at the corners of the mouth is measured around the labial surface of the occlusion rim to indicate the overall width of the upper six artificial anterior teeth.

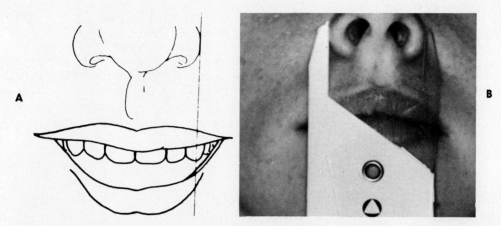

Fig. 16-5   A, A vertical line extending along the lateral surface of the ala often will pass through the middle of the natural upper canine. **B,** A plastic measuring caliper is available that provides a measurement of the interalar width and suggests possible molds of artificial anterior teeth that will be in harmony with this width.

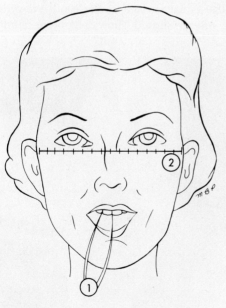

1:2 = 1:16

Fig. 16-6   Measurements on skulls indicate that the width of the natural central incisor, *1,* is approximately $\frac{1}{16}$ the bizygomatic width, *2.*

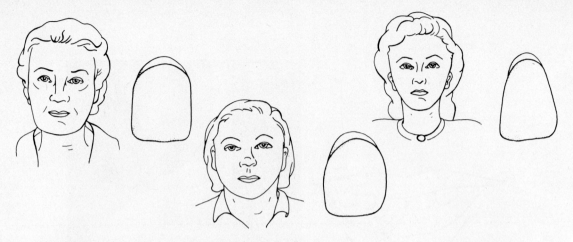

Fig. 16-7   Shapes of artificial teeth chosen to be in harmony with the outline of the patient's face.

from a front view of the patient and from the labial of the upper central incisor. The outlines of faces can be grouped into three basic classes: square, tapering, and ovoid. These are further subdivided on the basis of a combination of the characteristics of the three classes. Other variations arise in the proportions of the length and width of the faces.

The same types of variations in the forms of teeth have been provided by the manufacturers of artificial teeth. The problem is to select a tooth form that is in harmony with the form of the face of each individual patient. For this dentists should study faces of people and the forms of their natural teeth. Teeth that are in harmony with the outline form of the face will look good; teeth that are not in harmony will not look as good. This kind of study can help dentists recognize harmony or disharmony of form when they work with their patients.

The teeth selected must be "nice-looking" in themselves. Some molds of teeth have pleasing forms; others look mechanical. The nice-looking teeth are much more easily arranged into a pleasing composition than are teeth that have no esthetic value as individuals. The shape of the labial surface is probably more important than the outline form, which can be

changed when the incisal edges are ground (Fig. 16-8). This grinding should be done on almost all anterior teeth according to the age of the patient.

The labial surface of the tooth viewed from the mesial should show a contour similar to

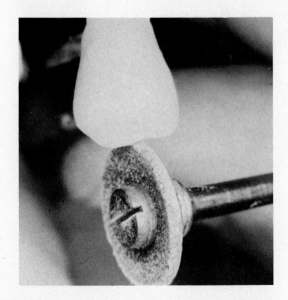

Fig. 16-8   The outline of an upper canine is modified to make it more natural in appearance and acceptable for the individual patient.

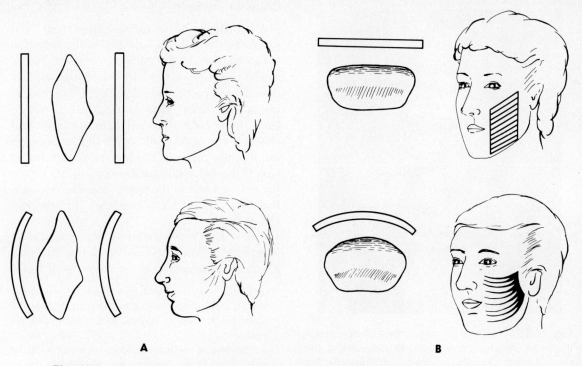

Fig. 16-9 **A,** Labial surfaces of artificial teeth chosen to be in harmony with the profile of the face. **B,** The labial surfaces of artificial teeth viewed from the incisal edge should be in harmony with the convexity or flatness of the face.

that when viewed in profile (Fig. 16-9, *A*). The three general types of profiles are convex, straight, and concave. The labial surface of the tooth viewed from the incisal should show a convexity or flatness similar to that seen when the face is viewed from under the chin or from the top of the head (Fig. 16-9, *B*).

The labial surface characteristics of anterior teeth should follow nature. For this, dentists must depend on the manufacturers. Curved and convex surfaces refract or reflect light and appear smaller than flat surfaces. The eye can measure a straight surface, but an optical illusion will be produced by a rounded surface. Tooth forms look more artificial when nature's curvatures are missing.

The curvatures of anterior teeth can be seen when observed from the mesial, distal, incisal, and labial surfaces. There may also be reverse curvatures, in the form of minute irregularities.

A study of natural teeth under slight magnification reveals no smooth glassy surfaces, so it is important that minute irregularities be reproduced in artificial teeth to give a natural effect.

The contact areas or surfaces of anterior teeth should show wear as occurs in natural teeth through life. Broadened contact areas look more natural because they seem compatible with elapsed years.

Labiolingually thick teeth can be rotated and spaced to give the three-dimensional depth so necessary for esthetics; therefore they should be selected preferentially.

The dentogenic concept in selecting artificial teeth

Tooth selection using the concepts of "dentogenics" is based on the age, sex, and personality of the patient (Frush and Fisher, 1955, 1956, 1957). It seems reasonable that a large

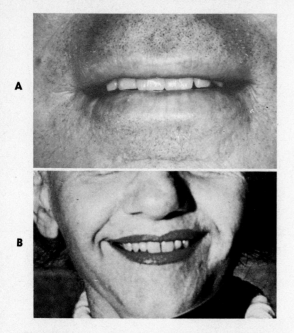

Fig. 16-10 Artificial teeth that are appropriate for this man, **A,** and this woman, **B,** because of the relative sizes, outlines, contours, and arrangement of the teeth. Teeth selected for the woman would be inappropriate for the man.

rugged man would have teeth of a size and form different from those of a delicate-appearing woman. The squareness of tooth form tends to portray masculinity whereas more rounded incisal and proximal contours connote femininity (Fig. 16-10). Lateral incisors that are smaller than the centrals tend to make the arrangement of teeth more feminine; on the other hand, central and lateral incisors that are more nearly the same size appear masculine. Dentogenic concepts provide information that can be used with other methods of selecting artificial teeth.

The selection of teeth under any concept is the dentist's responsibility. A work authorization order that merely indicates the age, sex, and personality of the patient does not fulfill professional requirements.

Color of the teeth

A knowledge of the physics, physiology, and psychology of color is valuable in the selection of tooth color.

The colors recognized by the human eye are the effect of certain wavelengths of light on the retina. The colors of faces and teeth therefore come from light reflected onto the rods and cones of the retina. Although the human eye can identify colors of the spectrum from red to violet, the color of most concern to dentists is the yellow band in the spectrum. The reason is that the colors of teeth and faces are primarily yellow.*

Color has four qualities: hue, saturation (chroma), brilliance (value), and translucency. All these are involved in the selection of teeth.

Hue is the specific color produced by a specific wavelength of light acting on the retina. It is the color itself, such as bluish, greenish, or reddish yellow.

The hue of teeth must be in harmony with the color (hue) of the patient's face. If the two are in harmony, the effect will be pleasant (as two harmonious notes on a piano). If the color of the teeth and that of the face are not in harmony, attention will be called to the teeth, just as a discord between two notes on a piano will be noticed (Fig. 16-11). Disharmony of light waves or sound waves attracts attention. Disharmony of the hue of the teeth with the basic hue of the face makes dentures look artificial.

Saturation (chroma) is the amount of color per unit area of an object. For example, some teeth appear more yellow than others. The hue could be the same (that is, the yellow in both teeth could be the same yellow), but there is more of it in some teeth than in others.

Brilliance (value) is the lightness or darkness of an object. Variations in brilliance are produced by dilution of the color (the hue) by white or black. When the yellow in teeth is diluted with white,

---

*Two color-order systems have been developed for use in matching artificial teeth with the patient's natural coloring: the Munsell and the Commission Intérnationale de l'Éclairage (CIE). Refer to Rosenstiel et al: *Contemporary Fixed Prosthodontics*, 1988, Mosby, pp 381-383.

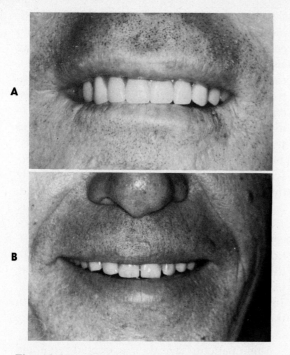

Fig. 16-11 **A,** Artificial teeth that do not harmonize with the face in color, size, and shape. **B,** The size and color of these teeth blend with the size and color of the patient's face.

the result is a light tooth; when the yellow is diluted with black, the result is a dark tooth. The relative amount of white or black in the teeth determines their lightness or darkness.

People with fair complexions generally have teeth with less color, and the colors are less saturated; thus the teeth are lighter and in harmony with the colors of the face. People with dark complexions generally have darker teeth that are in harmony with the coloring of the face. However, the lightness or darkness (brilliance) of the face (the frame for the teeth in the mouth) can alter the apparent brilliance of the teeth. Light teeth in the mouth of a patient with a very light complexion may appear dark. Likewise, dark teeth in the mouth of a patient with a very dark complexion may appear lighter than they are.

Translucency is the property of an object that permits the passage of light through it but does not give any distinguishable image. The light rays are so broken up and diffuse that they cannot pass directly through the object as they would if the object were transparent. Translucency of artificial teeth has the effect of mixing the various colors (hues) of the porcelain with the changing colors in the oral cavity. This results in teeth that look alive because of the changes in light and color reflected from them and passing through them with different light sources.

The apparent color of teeth is different when the lighting of the interior oral cavity is changed. When the mouth is nearly closed, the teeth will appear darker than when it is open wide and the interior well lighted. Also, when light is reflected through the teeth from the oral cavity, the teeth will appear lighter and more pink than in other light situations. The pink color of the interior of the mouth shows through the translucent material as it does through the enamel of natural teeth. For this reason, tooth manufacturers are striving to place translucent material in the same places in artificial teeth as nature has placed enamel in natural teeth.

The basic color of Caucasian faces is yellow. Blue is the complementary color of yellow. Thus, if the dentist stares at a blue card or cloth for 30 seconds before observing the color of teeth and faces, it will be possible to make a more accurate observation of the yellow color. The problem is to distinguish between the various gradations of yellow, from reddish yellow to greenish yellow. Preparing the retina beforehand to be more sensitive to yellow will simplify this.

The general classification of skin pigmentation ranges from sallow to ruddy to olive to swarthy. In hair there are black, brown, red, and blond. In eyes there are blue, gray, brown, and black. So many combinations of color exist, in fact, that it would be impractical to manufacture enough shades to match them all. The color of the hair has been used by some dentists as a guide, but this is unreliable and can be inaccurate because hair color changes more rapidly than tooth color. Also persons can change the color of their hair from week to week. The color of the eyes has been suggested as a guide to the color of the teeth, but likewise this is not sound since the iris is so small compared to the total face and the eyes are not close to the teeth.

The color of the face should be the basic guide to tooth color. The face is the frame into which the picture (the teeth) will fit. The hue of the teeth must harmonize with the colors in the patient's face. Saturation of color in the teeth must correspond to saturation of color in the face. Brilliance of the teeth must correspond to the lightness or darkness of the face. Teeth that are too light or too dark will be conspicuous, and denture teeth should not be conspicuous. Translucency, which is a characteristic of enamel, makes possible some variation in the effect of the color with different lip and mouth positions. This variation is essential to the illusion of naturalness.

Age and tooth color. For some persons the color of the natural teeth progressively darkens with age. In youth the pulp chambers are large and the red color of the pulp affects the total color of the tooth. Later the pulp chamber becomes smaller as a result of the deposition of

secondary dentin in it; this makes the tooth more opaque and reduces the effect of pulp color. As wear occurs on the teeth (from eating and toothbrushing and other abrasive forces), the tooth surface becomes smoother and more reflective. With wearing of the incisal edges, enamel is lost and its translucency begins to disappear. Also the dentin becomes exposed to and picks up stains from the oral fluids, foods, medicines, tobacco, and anything else the person may have had in his mouth. Consequently the teeth take on a somewhat brownish tinge, particularly the incisal edges of lower anteriors.

Although some persons' natural teeth become darker with age, there are many exceptions to this; it is therefore incorrect to establish a rule that prescribes light teeth for young patients and darker teeth for older ones (Fig. 16-12). Tooth color must be in harmony with the facial coloring at the time the dentures are made.

Some patients save their extracted teeth and ask the dentist to match this color. However, such a means of color selection will always lead to erroneous artificial tooth color because the

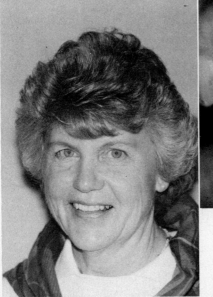

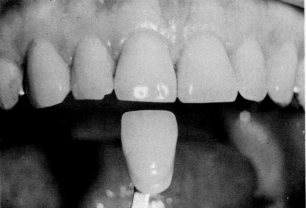

Fig. 16-12 A woman in her late 50s whose natural teeth match A2 on the Vita shade guide. If she were a denture patient, it would be inappropriate to insist that she have a darker tooth shade because of her age.

color of a tooth changes immediately when it is removed from the mouth and becomes nonvital; it blanches further as the tooth dries out. Thus, extracted teeth are valuable for size and form selection but should *not* be used for color selection.

Selecting the color of artificial teeth. Observations of the shade-guide teeth should be made in three positions: (1) outside the mouth along the side of the nose, (2) under the lips with only the incisal edge exposed, and (3) under the lips with only the cervical end covered and the mouth open (Fig. 16-13). The first step will establish the basic hue, brilliance, and saturation; the second will reveal the effect of the color of the teeth when the patient's mouth is relaxed; the third will simulate exposure of the teeth as in a smile.

Basic considerations are the harmony of tooth color with the color of the patient's face and the inconspicuousness of the teeth. The color selected should be so inconspicuous that it will not attract attention to the teeth. The color of the teeth should be observed on a bright day when possible, with the patient located close to natural light. The teeth should also be observed in artificial light, since denture patients are often seen in this environment.

The "squint test" may be helpful in evaluating colors of teeth with the complexion of the face. With the eyelids partially closed to re-

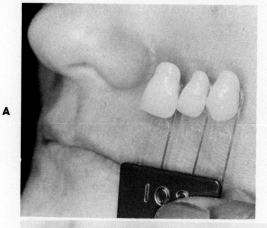

A

B

C

Fig. 16-13 Testing tooth color with shade-guide teeth. **A,** The color is matched with that of the skin of the cheek. **B,** The color is next observed under the upper lip with the incisal edges exposed. **C,** The color is then observed with the labial surfaces uncovered and the mouth open for the effect when light reflects from inside the mouth.

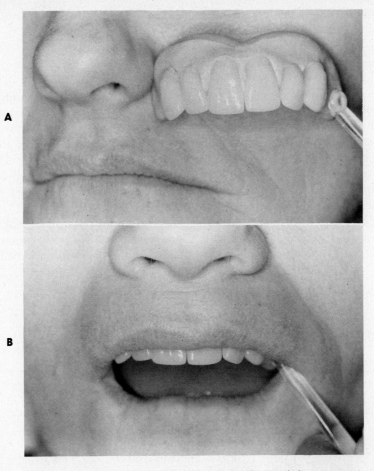

Fig. 16-14 The preliminary selection of artificial anterior teeth is set on a tooth selector, **A,** for quick observation in the patient's mouth, **B.**

duce light, the dentist compares prospective colors of artificial teeth held along the face of the patient. The color that fades from view first is the one that is least conspicuous in comparison to the color of the face.

Preliminary tryin of selected teeth

Molds of anterior teeth that seem suitable can be easily appraised when they are arranged on the upper occlusion rim or on a tooth selector (Fig. 16-14). Anterior teeth must be selected with sufficient width to fill the available space in the mouth and to provide for irregu-

larities in individual tooth position. The final decision regarding the selection of anterior teeth is made by observations of the trial (wax) dentures in the patient's mouth.

Because it is expensive and time consuming to replace all teeth with ones that are a different color or size, every effort must be made to select the correct teeth initially. A common error is to choose teeth that are too small and of a color that does not harmonize with the patient's facial coloring (Fig. 16-15). The dental assistant can play an active role in selecting both the shade and the mold of teeth to be

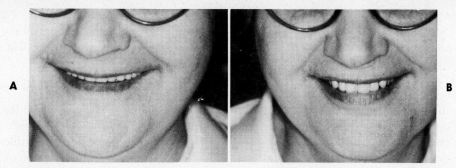

Fig. 16-15   A, Artificial teeth that are too small and too light colored. The seemingly endless row of teeth, together with improper support of the lips, creates what has been called the "denture look." **B,** Artificial teeth that are of proper size and in correct position to support the lips. The upper six anterior teeth fill the available space. Notice that in **A** eight to ten teeth occupy the space occupied by six or seven in **B.**

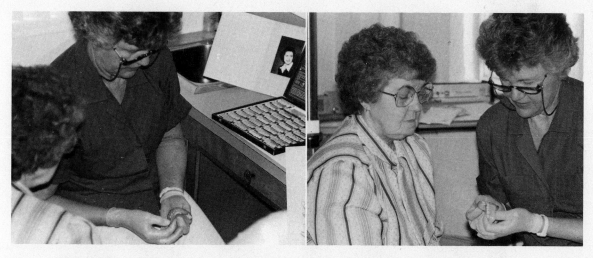

Fig. 16-16   An experienced dental assistant can help select the mold and shade of anterior teeth. Frequently the patient will communicate more openly with the assistant than with the dentist.

used (Fig. 16-16). Frequently the patient will feel more comfortable interacting with an assistant than with the dentist. The dentist must review any choice made, however.

POSTERIOR TOOTH SELECTION

The posterior teeth are selected for color, buccolingual width, total mesiodistal width, length, and type according to cuspal inclination and material. They should also be chosen in accord with the size and contour of the mandibular residual ridge.

All posterior teeth are not exact reproductions of natural teeth, which is as it should be. A complete denture needs anchorage and support different from those of natural teeth, and therefore the occlusal surfaces of artificial teeth should be modified. Masticating efficiency is only one consideration in the selection of posterior tooth forms. Comfort, esthetics, and preservation of the underlying bony and soft tissue structures are also important.

Posterior denture teeth are generally classified into two types: anatomic and nonanatomic. Strictly speaking, all denture teeth are designed geometrically, but the term *anatomic* is used for those artificial posterior teeth that more nearly resemble the teeth of a dentition. Manufactured artificial tooth forms can only be

a start in developing an occlusion. The dentist must modify the forms of the occlusal surfaces and arrange the teeth to fit the plan of occlusion.

Buccolingual width of posterior teeth

The buccolingual widths of artificial teeth should be greatly reduced from the widths of the natural teeth they replace. Artificial posterior teeth that are narrow in a buccolingual direction enhance the development of the correct form of the polished surfaces of the denture by allowing the buccal and lingual denture flanges

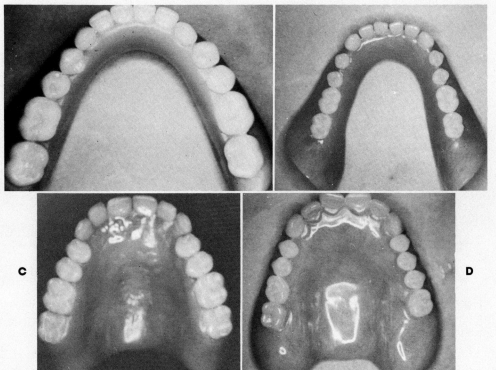

Fig. 16-17   A, Posterior teeth that are too wide in relation to the denture base. **B,** Posterior teeth of proper size in relation to the denture base. Notice that the buccal and lingual flanges slope away from the occlusal surfaces of the posterior teeth. This allows the cheeks and tongue to help maintain the lower denture in position on the residual ridge. **C,** Upper posterior teeth that are too large in relation to the denture base. **D,** Upper posterior teeth of proper size relative to the denture base. Notice the slope of the upper buccal flanges in relation to the occlusal surfaces of the posterior teeth. Forces created on the denture bases by the cheeks will help maintain the upper denture in position.

to slope away from the occlusal surfaces. This occlusal form permits forces from the cheeks and tongue to help maintain the dentures on their residual ridges (Fig. 16-17). Narrow occlusal surfaces with proper escapeways for food also reduce the amount of stress to the supporting tissues of the basal seat during mastication. On the other hand, the posterior teeth should have sufficient width to act as a table upon which to hold food during its trituration.

Mesiodistal length of posterior teeth

The length of the mandibular residual ridge from the distal of the canine to the beginning of the retromolar pad is usually available for artificial posterior teeth. Artificial posterior teeth are made by the manufacturer with varying overall mesiodistal widths (Fig. 16-18, A).

After the six anterior mandibular teeth have been placed in their final position, a point is marked on the crest of the mandibular ridge at the anterior border of the retromolar pad. This is the maximum extent posteriorly of any artificial tooth on the mandibular ridge. However, if the residual ridge anterior to this point slopes upward, smaller or fewer teeth must be used to avoid having a tooth over a pronounced incline at the distal end of the ridge. This shortened occlusal table will often prevent the lower denture from sliding forward when pressure is applied on the molars.

A ruler can be used to measure from the distal surface of the mandibular canine to the point that has been marked at the end of the available space (Fig. 16-18, B). The total mesiodistal width in millimeters of the four posterior teeth is often used as a mold number. For example, mold 32L of the Dentists' Supply Company signifies that the four posterior teeth have a total mesiodistal dimension of 32 mm and a long occlusocervical length.

The posterior teeth should not extend too close to the posterior border of the maxillary denture because of the danger of cheekbiting. However, if the posterior teeth do not extend far enough posteriorly, the forces of mastication will place a heavier load on the anterior part of the residual ridges. When the mandibular ridge slopes up sharply at its distal end, the posterior teeth must not be placed on this slope (Fig. 16-18, C). To do so will cause the lower denture to slide forward when forces are applied to the posterior teeth over the slope.

Posterior teeth are not arranged over the retromolar pad, because the pad is too soft and too easily displaced. Putting teeth over it will allow the denture to tip during mastication. Therefore only three posterior teeth should be used on each side of the denture in most patients (Fig. 16-18, D).

Vertical length of the buccal surfaces of posterior teeth

It is best to select posterior teeth corresponding to the interarch space and to the length of the anterior teeth. Artificial posterior teeth are made by manufacturers in varying occlusocervical lengths. The length of the maxillary first premolars should be comparable to that of the maxillary canines to have the proper esthetic effect (Fig. 16-19). If this is not done, the denture base material will appear unnatural distal to the canines. If the ridge laps are fairly thin and long, the posterior teeth can be readily positioned over full ridges without sacrificing leverage or esthetics. The form of the dental arch should copy as nearly as possible the arch form of the natural teeth they replace.

Commonly used materials

Both posterior and anterior teeth are currently available in vacuum-fired porcelain, acrylic resin, and a new hard acrylic resin (Fig. 16-20).

Porcelain teeth are most resistant to wear and staining. Unfortunately, they are also more likely to chip or fracture (Fig. 16-21). This problem has become much more troublesome since the vacuum-fired porcelains have been used (Fig. 16-22).

Acrylic resin teeth are the least resistant to wear, and they tend to collect stain more rap-

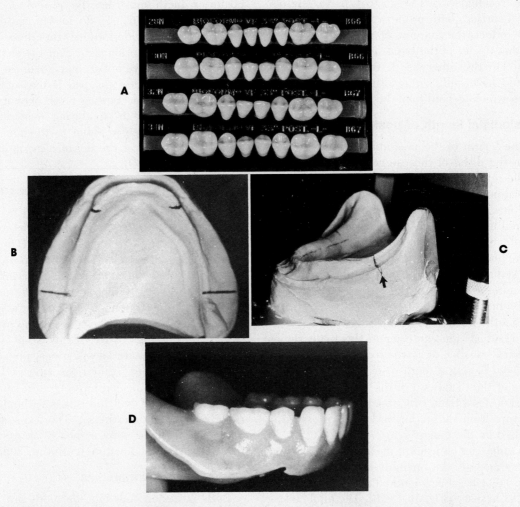

Fig. 16-18   A, Artificial posterior teeth are manufactured with varying mesiodistal widths. The four posterior teeth in mold *28M* have a total mesiodistal width of 28 mm whereas the four in mold *34M* have a total of 34 mm. **B,** Marks on the cast indicate the available space for artificial posterior teeth. **C,** This mark *(arrow)* indicates to the dentist or dental laboratory technician the distal extent of the posterior teeth. **D,** Three posterior teeth are used on each side of a lower denture because they adequately fill the space available between the distal surface of the lower canine and the retromolar pad (or the beginning of the steep incline at the distal of the mandibular ridge).

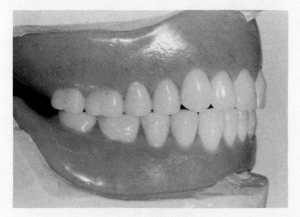

Fig. 16-19 The available interarch space be-tween residual ridges is a guide for the length of posterior teeth. The length of the premolar must be in harmony with that of the canine. This is an important factor when the patient is seen from the side.

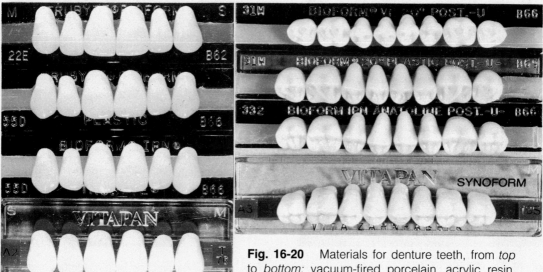

Fig. 16-20 Materials for denture teeth, from *top* to *bottom:* vacuum-fired porcelain, acrylic resin, hard-type acrylic resin (*third row* Dentsply IPN, *fourth row* Vitapan).

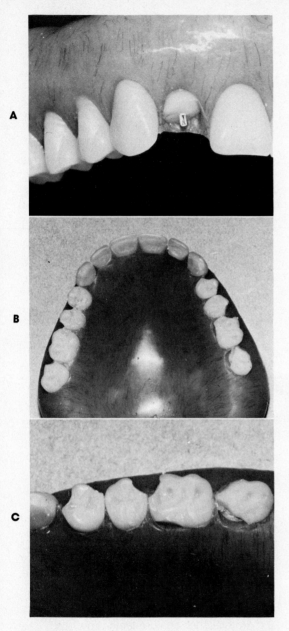

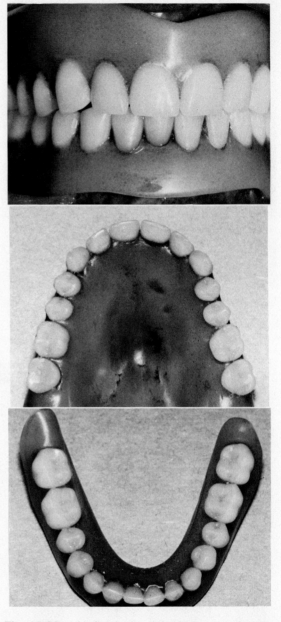

Fig. 16-21   Problems with vacuum-fired porcelain teeth. **A,** Fractured lateral incisor in a 3-year-old upper denture. **B** and **C,** Chipped and fractured upper posteriors in a 2-year-old denture worn opposing a complete lower denture by a bruxing and clenching 65-year-old man.

Fig. 16-22   Air-fired porcelain denture teeth worn by a 65-year-old woman for 43 years. Notice the lack of chipping and fracturing commonly seen with current vacuum-fired porcelain.

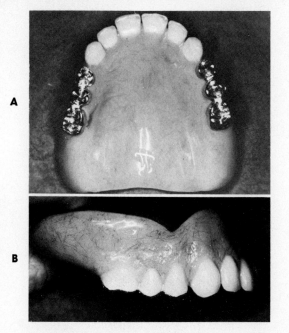

A

B

Fig. 16-23 **A,** The occlusal surfaces of these posterior teeth have been cast in gold. **B,** Notice that the gold is barely visible when the denture is viewed from the side.

idly than porcelain; they are the least likely to chip or fracture, however. A composite resin is available that is harder than the regular acrylic resin, but it tends to collect stain, which makes it unacceptable for many patients.

The new hard acrylic resin teeth are more wear resistant than regular acrylic resin teeth (Ogle, 1985), and they do not have the major staining problem noted with the composite resin.

Types of posterior teeth according to materials

The changing trend in tooth materials. For many years porcelain was the favorite tooth material, because of the rapid wear of acrylic resin. However, with the tendency for porcelain teeth to chip and fracture, acrylic resin gained in popularity. The new generation of

hard acrylic resin teeth has considerably lessened the use of porcelain during the past decade.

Acrylic resin posterior teeth are specifically called for when they oppose natural teeth or teeth whose occlusal surfaces have been restored with gold. They reduce the possibility that the artificial teeth will cause unnecessary abrasion and destruction of the natural or metallic occlusal surfaces of the opposing teeth. Gold occlusal surfaces can be developed for the artificial teeth and used in a similar manner (Fig. 16-23).

Acrylic resin is also desirable when the tooth must be excessively reduced in length because of a small interarch distance. The chemical bonding of the resin with the denture base prevents these teeth from breaking away from the denture base. In addition, it is desirable when a tooth must be shaped to fit a small space for esthetic purposes or be placed in contact with the retainer for a removable partial denture.

Acrylic resin posterior teeth must *not* be used with porcelain anterior teeth on complete dentures. The resin will wear more rapidly than the anterior porcelain and eventually create excessive and destructive occlusal forces in the anterior part of the mouth. The anterior basal seat is usually least able to withstand increased stresses.

Types of posterior teeth according to cusp inclines

The cuspal inclines for posterior teeth depend on the plan of occlusion selected by the dentist. For example, if a steep vertical overlap and low posterior tooth inclines are used, a spaced horizontal overlap of the anterior teeth must be selected. If a flat or nearly horizontal incisal guidance angle is chosen, shallow posterior tooth inclines should be selected, particularly if the condylar guidance also is shallow. In edentulous patients the incisal guidance angle is determined by the dentist; therefore the posterior tooth inclines are chosen at the time the horizontal overlap of the anterior teeth is set

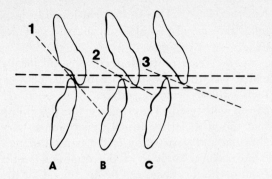

Fig. 16-24 **A,** No horizontal overlap, with the resultant incisal angle, *1.* **B,** Same vertical overlap but greater horizontal overlap, with less inclination of the incisal angle, *2.* **C,** Same vertical overlap but still greater horizontal overlap, with even less inclination of the incisal guide angle, *3.*

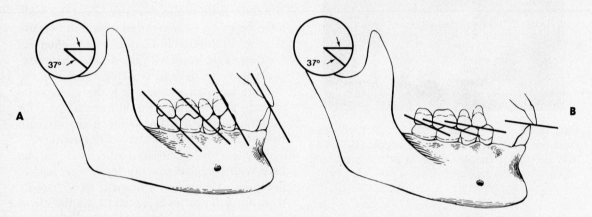

Fig. 16-25 Two figures with the same condylar inclination but different incisal guide inclinations. **A,** Steep vertical overlap, with resultant steep cusp inclines. **B,** Less steep incisal angle, with resultant flatter cusp inclines.

(Figs. 16-24 and 16-25). The influence of cusp inclines on denture stability is discussed in Chapter 21.

Posterior artificial teeth are manufactured with cusp inclines that vary from relatively steep to practically flat. Commonly used posterior cuspal inclinations are 33, 20, and 0 degrees (Fig. 16-26). The inclination is measured as the angle formed by the mesiobuccal cusp of the lower first molar with the horizontal plane.

Posterior teeth with 33 degrees of cuspal incline offer the maximum opportunity for a fully balanced occlusion. However, the final effective height of the cusp for a given patient depends on the way the teeth are tipped and on the interrelation of the other factors of occlusion (that is, the incisal guidance, condylar guidance, height of the occlusal plane, and compensating curve). Maintaining a shallow incisal guidance compatible with esthetics allows a balanced occlusion to be developed with as little cusp height on the posterior teeth as possible, thus reducing lateral forces on the residual ridges. Posteriors with 20 degrees of cuspal

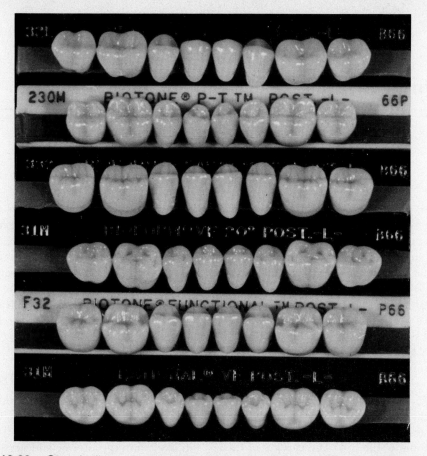

Fig. 16-26 Cusp inclines of molds for posterior teeth: *32L,* 33 degrees; *230M,* 30 degrees; *33L,* 30 degrees; *31M,* 20 degrees; *F32,* 10 degrees; *31M,* 0 degrees.

incline are semianatomic in form and wider buccolingually than the corresponding 33-degree teeth. They provide less cusp height with which to develop balancing contacts in eccentric jaw positions than 33-degree teeth do. Nonanatomic teeth, with 0 degrees of cuspal incline, are advisable when only a centric relation record is being transferred from the patient to the articulator and no effort is directed to establishing a cross-arch balanced occlusion. They are also effective when it is difficult or impossible to record centric jaw relations precisely from the patient or there are abnormal jaw relationships.

BIBLIOGRAPHY

Frush JP, Fisher RD: How dentogenic restorations interpret the sex factor, J Prosthet Dent 6:160-172, 1956.

Frush JP, Fisher RD: Age factor in dentogenics, J Prosthet Dent 7:5-13, 1957.

Frush JP, Fisher RD: The dynesthetic interpretation of the dentogenic concept, J Prosthet Dent 8:558-581, 1958.

Kern BK: Anthropometric parameter of tooth selection, J Prosthet Dent 17:431-437, 1967.

Ogle RE, David LJ, Ortman HR: Clinical wear study of a new tooth material. II, J Prosthet Dent 54:67-75, 1985.

CHAPTER 17

Preliminary arrangement of artificial teeth

Once the casts have been tentatively mounted on the articulator, the teeth are set in the occlusion rims so a more accurate observation can be made than was possible with the occlusion rims alone. The vertical jaw relations, established by adjustment of the occlusion rims, and the horizontal jaw relation (CR), established by a preliminary interocclusal record, are likely to be incorrect. These records must therefore be recognized as tentative and subject to correction when new information is available.

The profile contours of the occlusion rims may also be incorrect and are subject to change when teeth and wax, instead of wax alone, control the contours of the lips. The carving of the labial surfaces of the occlusion rims must therefore be considered tentative. The establishment of anterior tooth positions on the trial dentures is the dentist's responsibility and should preferably be carried out by the dentist or else be prescribed specifically to the dental technician.

Most dentists, however, prefer to carve the wax occlusion rims as accurately as they can for determining the desired amount of lip support and to have their assistant or technician make the preliminary arrangement of teeth as guided by the wax contours. Subsequently, these dentists make corrections in the tooth positions and even in the positions of the arches of anterior teeth when the wax trial dentures are observed in the mouth at the tryin appointment.

Other dentists will set the anterior teeth in the wax trial dentures themselves and thus reduce the time required for resetting the anterior teeth at the time that the wax dentures are tried in the mouth. These dentists use the information gained when the preliminary jaw relation records were made and other guides that might not be available to dental auxiliaries to assist them in the preliminary arrangement of teeth.

GUIDES FOR PRELIMINARILY ARRANGING ANTERIOR TEETH

The carved occlusion rims should provide reliable guides for placement of the anterior teeth in the wax occlusion rims. They indicate the likely anteroposterior and vertical positions of the incisor teeth on the basis of support obtained from the lips and mandible.

The length of time each jaw has been edentulous is in direct proportion to the amount of resorption that can be *expected.* The amount of resorption, in turn, can indicate the distance the teeth should be set from the residual ridge. If the patient's teeth have been out only 3 weeks, for example, the artificial teeth should be placed with the ridge lap of the tooth against the cast. However, even this is not always correct. It may be that the patient lost the teeth as a result of severe periodontal disease that destroyed much bone *before* the teeth were removed. Also the patient may have lost some bone from the anterior part of the jaws through surgery at the time the teeth were removed. The dentist can learn about these possibilities while making the diagnosis and can use the information when setting the central incisors in wax.

If the patient was edentulous for a long time or had natural teeth opposing a complete denture, much bone may have been lost from the residual ridge. In this situation the artificial teeth should *not* be placed against the ridge. As a general rule, the longer the natural teeth have been out the farther the artificial teeth should be from the residual ridge. This rule applies also when teeth are removed from the mouth at different times. Then shrinkage will be greater from one jaw than from the other. The teeth should be placed closer to the residual ridge when there is less shrinkage and farther from the ridge when there has been more resorption. The objective is to place the occlusal plane of the teeth in the same position it occupied when the natural teeth were in place.

Relationship to the incisive papilla

The incisive papilla is a guide to anterior tooth position because it has a constant relationship to the natural central incisors. It is found in the lingual embrasure between these incisors. Naturally, then, it should serve to position the midline of the upper dental arch or, more specifically, the central incisors in the dental arch.* However, the mesial surfaces of the central incisors of many people are not exactly in the center of their face or mouth. Therefore when information on the position of the central incisors is available, the positions of the artificial teeth should be made more like those of the natural teeth so the teeth will look more natural. Thus, at least until the teeth are in the mouth, a line marking the center of the incisive papilla on the cast can be extended forward onto the labial surface of the cast and then cut into the labial surface of the wax oc-

clusion rim (Fig. 17-1). The central incisors set on either side of this line will have positions quite similar to those of the natural teeth insofar as right and left orientations are concerned.

The incisive papilla is a guide also to the anteroposterior position of the teeth. The labial surfaces of the central incisors are usually 8 to 10 mm in front of it. This distance, for obvious reasons, will vary with the size of the teeth and the labiolingual thickness of the alveolar process carrying the natural teeth, so it is not an absolute relationship. Furthermore, as severe resorption of the residual ridge in a vertical direction occurs, the incisive papilla may move

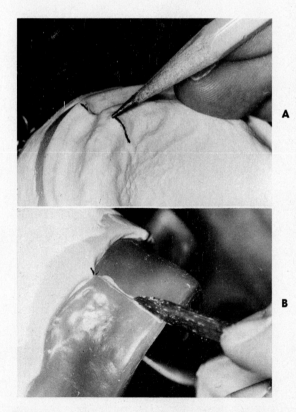

Fig. 17-1   The incisive papilla is used to help locate the midline of the dental arch. **A,** A mark is made on the cast through the center of the papilla. **B,** The mark is transferred to the occlusion rim as a guide to placement of the maxillary incisors.

---

*Although the incisive papilla is a useful guide for locating the midline, it is still advisable to locate and mark the midline on the wax rim when maxillomandibular registrations are made.

distally. Thus the distance from the papilla to the labial surface of the teeth may become greater when much bone has been lost from the maxillary residual ridge in a vertical direction.

Resorption of bone from the labial surface of the maxillary arch or surgical reduction of the labial plate of bone from the maxillae will cause the incisive papilla to *appear* to move forward. Obviously, this cannot happen, so an incisive papilla found on the labial occlusal surface of a cast indicates that the anterior teeth must be set in front of the residual ridge by a distance corresponding to the amount of change in the bone.

Relationship to the reflection

Another guide to positioning the central incisors is the relationship of the labial surfaces of these teeth to the reflection of soft tissues under the lip or as recorded in the impression and cast. Notice in Fig. 17-2 that the labial surfaces and incisal edges of the teeth are anterior to the tissues at the reflection, where the den-

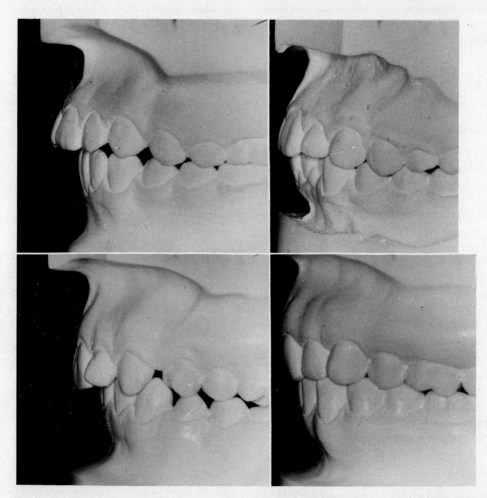

Fig. 17-2 Notice the relation of the labial surface of the central incisor to the line of inclination of the residual ridge.

ture borders would be placed.

There is an obtuse angle between the labial surface of the central incisor root and the labial surface of the clinical crown of the tooth. This fact must be kept in mind when placing an artificial incisor in the wax denture base (that is, the occlusion rim). The root of the natural tooth extends into the alveolar process, with a relatively thin layer of bone over it labially (Fig. 17-2). This means that the labial surface of the residual ridge can be used as a guide to determining the proper inclination of anterior teeth. *The accuracy of this guide decreases as resorption of the residual ridge progresses, however.* Nevertheless, the imaginary root of the artificial tooth must extend into the residual ridge (with allowance made for the loss of

bone). Clinical judgment is essential in the evaluation and application of these guides.

Factors governing the anteroposterior position of the dental arch

The anteroposterior position of the dental arch should be governed chiefly by consideration of the orbicularis oris and its attaching muscles and by the tone of the skin of the lips. Superficially, this means the position and expression of the lips. The orbicularis oris affects and is affected by the following seven muscles: the quadratus labii superioris, caninus, zygomaticus, quadratus labii inferioris, risorius, triangularis, and buccinator. These muscles control expression and reflect the personality and appearance of every person wearing complete

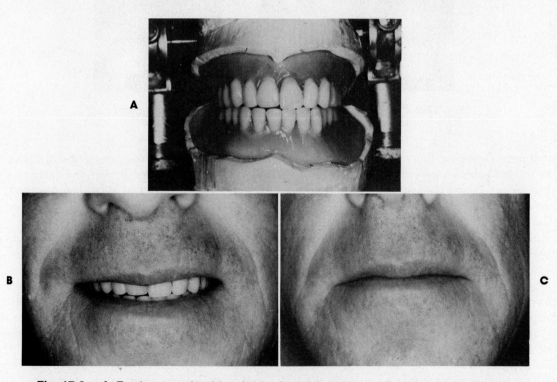

Fig. 17-3   A, Teeth set on the ridge *(patient's right)* and not on the ridge *(patient's left),* the latter to simulate their former natural position. **B** and **C,** Contrast this arrangement in the patient's mouth. The left side of the mouth is esthetically more pleasing. It must be emphasized, however, that such a tooth arrangement is not always feasible or desirable since it also depends on the patient's preference and any circumoral changes.

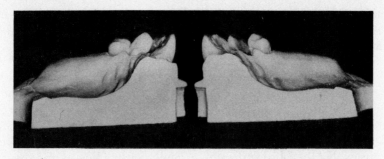

Fig. 17-4   Cast sawed in half to show the relative positions of teeth.

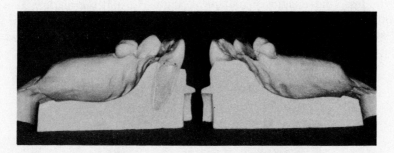

Fig. 17-5   Inclination of the central incisor root simulated on the cast.

dentures. Dropping the orbicularis oris backward throws this entire group of muscles closer to their origin and slackens them so they cannot be effective when stimulated to contract. The tone and action of these muscles depend on the anteroposterior support provided by the teeth and the denture base material.

Setting teeth over the maxillary anterior ridge is often carried to an extreme, which undermines the esthetic result. The greatest harm is done in setting the maxillary anterior teeth back to the ridge or under the ridge, regardless of the amount of resorption that has taken place. A study of the anterior alveolar process discloses that it is at an angle to the labial faces of the maxillary incisors. In other words, its direction is upward and backward (Fig. 17-2). Therefore the crest of the ridge is considerably more to the posterior in a re-

sorbed ridge than it is in a recent extraction. If the rule of setting teeth over the ridge is followed after the residual ridge has resorbed, a prematurely aged appearance will be the result (Fig. 17-3).

In Figs. 17-4 to 17-7 a cast has been sawed in two along the median suture for a study of the relative positions of an artificial tooth to a resorbing ridge. One side of the cast was left intact to show the relation of the former natural teeth to the maxilla. The central incisor was removed from the other side of the cast to show the evolution of an edentulous ridge, with the artificial tooth placed in relation to the ridge and to its former position (the untouched half of the cast). This depicts how far upward and backward the tooth could have been placed had it been set to follow the edentulous ridge. If all the artificial teeth had been placed to follow

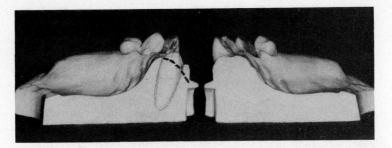

Fig. 17-6   The central incisor has been removed from the cast, and the anticipated bony reduction marked.

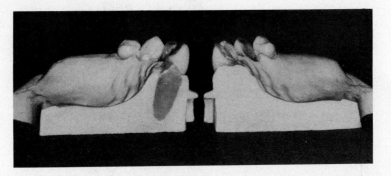

Fig. 17-7   An artificial tooth is waxed into place to reproduce the central incisor and restore both tooth position and gingival tissue contour.

this ridge, the orbicularis oris and its attaching muscles would have lost their correct anatomic relationship; an aged and expressionless appearance would have resulted.

SETTING MAXILLARY ANTERIOR TEETH IN WAX FOR THE TRYIN

The technique for setting anterior teeth in the wax occlusion rims is, at the same time, simple and exacting. If the occlusion rims have been accurately carved to support the lips and the maxillomandibular jaw relationship, they will act as a guide to the correct anteroposterior tooth position in the dental arch. If they have not been accurately carved, the dentist must decide what alterations in labial surface contour will be necessary when the teeth are set up. For example, if the lip needs more support when the occlusion rims are in the mouth, the incisors should be set in front of the labial surface of the wax rim. If the lips are too full at that time, more of the labial surface of the occlusion rims should be cut away before the teeth are set.

If the carving of the occlusion rims has been accurately done, cut away a small section of wax where a central incisor is to be placed. Then heat the wax where the occlusion rim is cut away until the wax pools (becomes molten) in that place. This will provide a "socket" for the artificial tooth.

Place the tooth in the molten wax and move it into the desired position with its mesial surface on the midline and its incisal edge just overlapping the occlusal surface of the lower occlusion rim.

Repeat this for the adjacent central incisor. (See Fig. 17-8.)

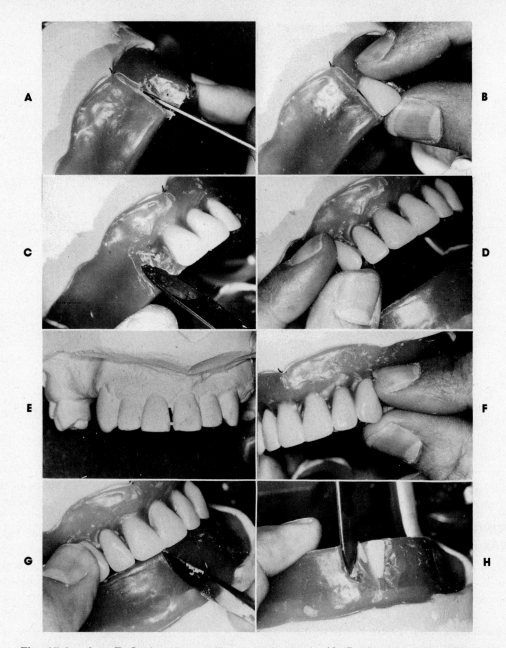

Fig. 17-8 **A** to **F,** Setting the maxillary anterior teeth. (**A,** Pooling the wax with a hot spatula to form a socket for the left central incisor; **B,** the end of this tooth is placed in the wax as indicated by preextraction records; **C,** preparing the socket for the lateral incisor; **D** and **E,** adjusting the right canine to match its position on the diagnostic cast; **F,** adjusting the left canine.) **G** and **H,** Setting the mandibular anterior teeth. (**G,** The midline is marked on the mandibular arch to correspond with that of the maxillary arch; **H,** the mandibular incisors are set in the same manner as the maxillary incisors.)

Then set the remaining upper anterior teeth in the wax, alternating their placement on the two sides of the dental arch. Be careful to follow the arch form indicated by preextraction casts or photographs if they are available. If these records are not available, use the residual ridge as a reference, keeping in mind the history of the residual ridge— whether the teeth have been out a long time or bone has been lost from it by pathosis or by surgery. Always, the imaginary roots of the artificial teeth must extend into the residual alveolar ridge (before resorption), even though the patient may wish it different.

When the occlusion rim is removed from the cast, observe the long axes of the teeth and visualize them as extending into the residual ridge. Be sure that the imaginary roots do not interfere with each other. This can best be seen by removing the occlusion rim from the cast and looking over the labial flange of the occlusion rim to visualize the imaginary roots extending into the alveolar groove of the trial denture base.

Importance of proper anteroposterior positioning of the anterior teeth

Fig. 17-9 is a series of drawings that shows the importance of the teeth and the labial flange of the denture base to the position and form of the lips. In Fig. 17-9, *A,* this inclination will maintain lip fullness and length in its natural form. To prevent the upper lip from thinning, lengthening, and losing the vermilion line contour, the incisors must be placed out to their former positions so the lip action will remain the same. In Fig. 17-9, *B,* the incisors are set with reduced vertical overlap. Notice the consequential turning in and lengthening of the lip. In Fig. 17-9, *C,* the incisor and border are inclined still more lingually, which produces a

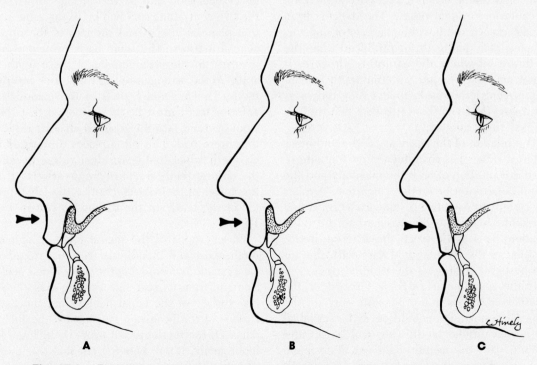

A **B** **C**

Fig. 17-9 Facial distortion caused by incorrect positions of the maxillary teeth. **A,** Favorable tooth and denture border position; **B,** less favorable; **C,** esthetically unfavorable.

thin and expressionless lip. This is attributable to the incline caused when the upper incisor is set back to contact the lower.

Anterior artificial teeth should almost invariably be placed in exactly the same positions as were previously occupied by the natural teeth, and the labial surface of the denture base material should duplicate as nearly as possible the contour and position of the mucous membrane covering the alveolar ridge. To change either will change the support for the lips as well as the tone and action of the muscles involved in appearance and facial expression. Any attempt to reduce the horizontal overlap of the anterior teeth will alter the support of the lips. Although this could be indicated in some situations (for example, patients with maxillary protrusion), such liberties should be taken only in unusual and exceptional circumstances.

When the horizontal overlap of natural teeth is reduced to develop contacts in centric occlusion, unfavorable occlusal forces are applied on the anterior residual ridges. The dangers from this far exceed the possible dangers of unfavorable leverage that might be produced when the teeth are set where the natural teeth were. It is not necessary for the anterior teeth to contact in centric occlusion unless they did so as natural teeth. Even then, it is best that they be set just out of contact.

The relation of the maxillary and mandibular anterior ridges has an influence on the anteroposterior position of both the maxillary and the mandibular anterior teeth. A common error is to attempt to establish a standard vertical and horizontal overlap without regard to the ridge relation. This is incorrect; the anteroposterior position of the teeth should vary with the anteroposterior relation of the residual ridges.

If the mandibular ridge is forward of the maxillary ridge (as in a prognathic person), the upper anterior teeth should never be set labial to the mandibular teeth. They can be set end to end, with the incisal edges cut at an angle that would have a seating action on the maxillary denture. When the prognathism is extreme, it is not possible to have tooth contact

in the incisor region because the maxillary incisors will then have to be too far anterior and too much leverage will result; also the tooth position will then put the upper lip under too much tension.

Extremely high ridges may seem to create a problem unless it is realized that natural teeth once came out of these ridges. Insufficient space between the residual ridges is an indication that either the artificial teeth are longer than the natural teeth or the vertical dimension of the face is too short. However, if only parts of the ridges are too close together, the cause may be an excess of fibrous tissue on the ridge. This occurs most frequently in the upper tuberosity region, and surgical removal of excess fibrous tissue is indicated.

SETTING MANDIBULAR ANTERIOR TEETH IN WAX FOR THE TRYIN

The lower anterior teeth should be set in the lower occlusion rim so the mesial surfaces of the two central incisors will be in the same sagittal plane as the mesial surfaces of the upper central incisors. The same basic principles are involved in the arrangement of these teeth as apply to the arrangement of the upper anterior teeth. The imaginary roots of the mandibular anterior teeth must be so positioned that they would extend into the residual alveolar ridge if they were real. This often places the mandibular teeth labial to the residual ridge, because the natural teeth are most frequently labial to the apices of their roots. (Notice the labial profile of the teeth on the diagnostic cast in Fig. 17-10.)

Observations of the incisal edge, imaginary tooth apex, and mandibular residual ridge are easily made by removing the mandibular occlusion rim from its cast and sighting over the labial surface of the labial flange from the basal surface of the occlusion rim toward the incisal edges. If the teeth are not properly inclined labiolingually, it will be apparent that the imaginary tooth roots cannot extend into the residual ridge.

Any difference in the arch form of the teeth

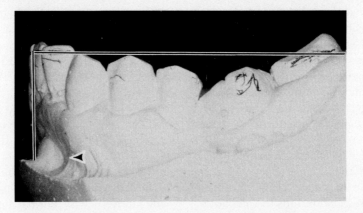

Fig. 17-10   The apices of imaginary roots of the lower anterior teeth *(arrowhead)* are lingual to the incisal edges and labial surfaces of the crowns of these teeth. When the residual alveolar ridge resorbs, artificial teeth must be placed labial (anterior) to the ridge; otherwise, the lip will not be properly supported.

and the arch form of the residual ridge can be easily detected by this same observation. It is important to recognize that the natural teeth erupted from the alveolar process and that the artificial teeth must be so placed that their imaginary roots also could have erupted from the alveolar process (with allowance made for bone lost through disease, surgery, accident, or resorption).

The height to which the lower anterior teeth are set is tentatively determined by the height to which the mandibular occlusion rim has been built. Normally, this will allow for a slight vertical overlap of the upper anterior teeth over them. Before the first tryin, this overlap will be about 1.5 mm, subject, of course, to change after the trial dentures are in the mouth.

Horizontal overlap

The horizontal overlap of the maxillary over the mandibular teeth should be fairly uniform from one side of the dental arch to the other. The amount of projection of the upper over the lower teeth in the horizontal plane will vary with the differences in size between the two jaws. If the upper jaw is much larger than the lower, the upper and lower teeth should be placed where the natural teeth were, without attempting to make them contact in the centric jaw position. The upper teeth should be related to the upper jaw and the lower teeth to the lower jaw, regardless of their relationships to each other. To change from this basic position invites problems and either supports part of the face too much or leaves another part unsupported.

Remember: This first tooth setup is only tentative. Changes in the vertical or horizontal jaw relationships indicate the need for changes in the tooth positions. If the teeth are correctly set labiolingually with respect to their residual ridges, the subsequent changes will be only in their relative heights and in the irregularities that need to be developed in their arrangement to make them appear more natural.

PRELIMINARY ARRANGEMENT OF POSTERIOR TEETH

The preliminary arrangement of posterior teeth involves the application of principles similar to those applied in the tentative arrangement of anterior teeth. The artificial posterior teeth should be placed as near as possible to where the natural teeth were placed. This, in fact, is easier said than done, however, since there are not as many guides or indicators to posterior tooth position as there are to anterior tooth position. Therefore the final position of the occlusal plane, the final arch form, and even the final length (posterior extent) of the occlusal plane cannot be determined until the jaw relations are tested and found correct.

The tests are essential, and the posterior teeth must be arranged in such a way that the tests can be made: This means that the height and orientation of the occlusal plane must be nearly correct, the opposing teeth must have specific and precise relationships to each other, and the lower dental arch must be properly formed.

Orientation of the occlusal plane

The orientation of the anterior occlusal plane is determined by esthetics. The position at which the incisal edges of the anterior teeth meet is the level of the anterior plane of occlusion. If these teeth are set in the same positions as were occupied by the natural teeth, the front of the occlusal plane will be correctly located.

The posterior (or distal) plane of occlusion should be so located that if it were extended it would be level with the junction between the middle and distal thirds of the retromolar pad. Stated another way, the distal occlusal plane should be at a level two thirds the way up the retromolar pad (as simulated in Fig. 17-11).

If the anterior teeth are correctly placed for esthetics, the location of the distal occlusal plane will place the plane at a level that is familiar to the tongue. If the plane is located higher or lower to gain leverage, the dentures will interfere with normal tongue action. This will be more dangerous to denture stability than unfavorable leverage will.

The height of the occlusal plane in the anterior region of dentures is influenced by the length of the lips, ridge fullness, ridge height, the amount of maxillomandibular space, and the incisal guide angle. The ridge height may be excessive in the mandibular anterior region and insufficient in the maxillary anterior region, or vice versa, or both the anterior and posterior ridges may be high or low. These factors will influence the location of the occlusal

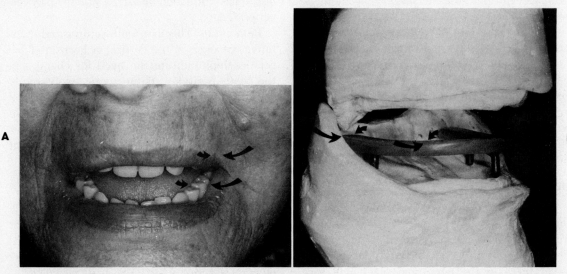

Fig. 17-11 *Arrows* in **A** and **B** suggest the relative orientation of the occlusal plane's anterior (corner of mouth) and posterior (two thirds up the retromolar pad) landmarks.

plane for some patients. The ideal is to locate the plane in the same position as it was when the natural teeth were present. The maxillomandibular space and the ridge height and fullness in the posterior regions often influence the positioning of the occlusal plane, even though they should not. Often the occlusal plane is marked out on the wax rims to follow an arbitrary line on the face, the ala-tragus line. However, this is not an accurate guide since it varies just as much as the shapes of ridges vary.

The inclination of the occlusal plane is important to the stability or instability of dentures. If the plane is too low in the anterior region or too high in the posterior region, the maxillary denture will tend to slide forward under pressure. If the reverse is true, the mandibular denture will tend to slide forward. Ideally the plane of occlusion should parallel both residual ridges.

The vertical orientation and inclination of the occlusal plane are not a simple matter of dividing the maxillomandibular denture space equally. This space is governed by the relative amount of bone lost from the two ridges; if more bone has been lost from the maxillae than from the mandible, the occlusal plane must be closer to the mandible than to the maxillae, and vice-versa. The occlusal plane must be placed as near as possible to the position of the occlusal plane of the natural teeth. It should *not* be at a level that would favor the weaker of the two ridges (basal seats). The most reliable guides are the height of the corners of the mouth and the height of the retromolar pads. At this point in the procedure, the height of the anterior teeth is tentative and will be modified as indicated by the observations made at tryin.

Tentative buccolingual position of the posterior teeth

The buccolingual position of the posterior teeth and the posterior arch form are determined anteriorly by the positions (or arch form) of the anterior teeth and posteriorly by the shape of the basal seat provided by the mandible. The curvature of the arch of anterior teeth should flow pleasingly toward the posterior teeth. The posterior teeth must continue this curvature in such a way that they are properly related to the bone that supports them and to the soft tissues that contact their buccal and lingual surfaces. In the final tooth arrangement the posterior form of the arch will be determined to a great extent by the "neutral zone" between the cheeks and tongue. This is the space resulting from the removal of the posterior teeth and the loss of bone from the residual ridges. The pressure of the cheeks and tongue against the buccal and lingual surfaces of the erupting natural teeth were strong enough to influence their alignment in the dental arch. These same forces are applied against dentures (Figs. 17-12 and 17-13). Therefore the final arrangement of the arch must be developed with respect for these external forces.

Leverage and posterior tooth positions. Posterior teeth will have their most favorable leverage if they are set close to the residual ridge and lingual to it. However, this is not practical, because of the disturbing influence it would have on other relationships (such as the vertical dimension of occlusion, face height, esthetics, and the space allotted for the tongue) (Figs. 17-14 and 17-15).

Posterior teeth placed buccal to the ridge can cause a denture to tip when pressure is applied to them in this bad-leverage position. The effect of such bad leverage is magnified as the occlusal plane is located further away from the ridge (the basal seat) (Fig. 17-15). The solution to the problem is to recognize the location of the occlusal surfaces of the natural teeth and to place the artificial teeth as near as possible to that position. However, this is not easily done when the upper jaw is wider or narrower than the lower jaw. These situations require special handling of the occlusal surfaces of the posterior teeth in their final arrangement into balanced occlusion.

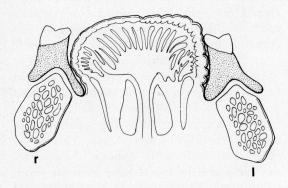

Fig. 17-12 Mandibular teeth positioned too far toward the buccal of the ridge *(r)* and too far toward the lingual *(l)*.

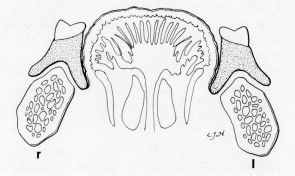

Fig. 17-13 Positions of the mandibular teeth corrected from those shown in Fig. 17-12.

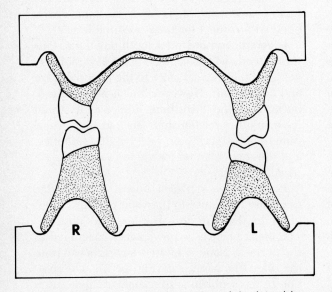

Fig. 17-14 *R,* Incorrect division of the interridge space; *L,* correct division.

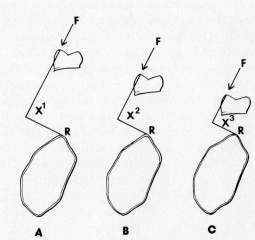

Fig. 17-15 The amount of leverage or torque (X^1, X^2, X^3) exerted on the occlusal plane is a function of the height of the plane above the ridge. It can be established by the following formula:
Torque = Force *(F)* × Distance from fulcrum *(R)*

Tentative arch form of the posterior teeth

The basic principle for the buccolingual positioning of posterior teeth is that they should conform to the shape of the residual ridge. In other words, the teeth should be in the position they would occupy if they had erupted from the residual ridge. The basic rule, then, is

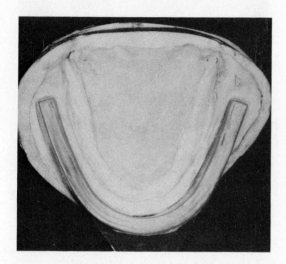

Fig. 17-16   Arch too wide.

that a perpendicular erected from the buccal side of the crest of the ridge should bisect the buccal cusp of the lower first molar. This principle and rule apply regardless of the differences in the widths of the upper and lower jaws. Therefore the arch form and buccolingual posterior tooth positions are keyed to the mandibular basal seat regardless of alterations that may be necessary if the upper jaw is wider or narrower than ideal. The form of each dental arch must be consistent with its foundation and harmonious within itself. The tentative arrangement of the posterior teeth can respect these guides.

This thought regarding placement of the arch and occlusal plane can best be conveyed by thinking of each arch as a piece of wire or strip of carding wax that may be moved up or down or backward or forward and may be bent wider or narrower.

Figs. 17-16 to 17-20 present a series of mandibular arch forms from the superior aspect showing some errors in position and width and the final favorable solution to these errors. They emphasize treating the arch as a unit before treating individual teeth in the final ar-

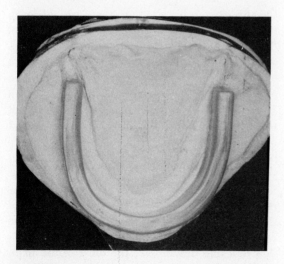

Fig. 17-17   Arch too wide in the premolar region, too narrow in the molar region.

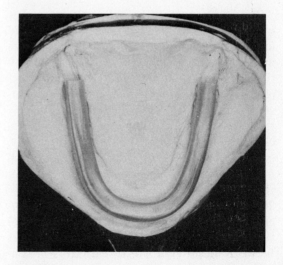

Fig. 17-18   Arch too narrow in the molar region.

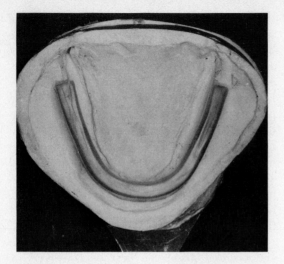

Fig. 17-19 Arch too far lingual in the anterior region.

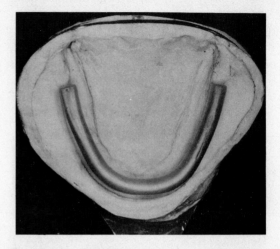

Fig. 17-20 Favorable arch form. The posterior part follows the curvature of the residual ridge.

rangement. Such a procedure saves time and aids obtaining the desired result.

Generally the posterior teeth will fall between two lines extending posteriorly from the distal surface of the canines to the buccal and lingual margins of the retromolar pad.

SETTING POSTERIOR TEETH FOR THE TRYIN

The posterior teeth are set in a tight centric occlusion. The mandibular teeth are positioned in the wax occlusion rim over the residual ridge in their ideal buccolingual relationship, with the maxillary teeth also in a tight centric occlusal arrangement regardless of their buccolingual positions. The objective here is to have the intercuspation of the posterior teeth so precise that any deviation in the mouth will be easily detected. Teeth with 30-degree cuspal inclinations are probably more effective for checking the accuracy of jaw relations than are 20-degree or 0-degree teeth. The 30-degree inclined cusps magnify horizontal errors in occlusion and make them easy to detect. Contacts between these teeth will reveal errors in centric occlusion in the mouth as the dentist instructs the patient to "pull the jaw back, close

just until any tooth touches, and then close tight." Any touch of the teeth and slide from that contact can be felt in the fingers. The touch and slide are an error that can be easily detected.

Guidelines for centric occlusion

There are three specifications for teeth in CO: (1) the upper teeth should overlap the lower teeth; (2) the long axis of each upper tooth should be distal to the long axis of the corresponding lower tooth; and (3) each tooth except the lower central incisor and the upper last molar should be opposed by two teeth. These are the specifications for tooth arrangement in testing the accuracy of CR records and mounting of casts. The teeth must be set in these relationships for the dentist to be able to make the necessary tests and observations.

There are two basic approaches to the arrangement of posterior teeth in centric occlusion. Both procedures are in current use. One involves setting the maxillary teeth first in relation to a line drawn over the crest of the mandibular ridge and then setting the mandibular teeth to the maxillary teeth. The other involves setting each mandibular tooth or all the teeth before the corresponding maxillary tooth or teeth are set. This second method permits the mandibular teeth to be set more accurately in relationship to the residual ridge than the first does. Most residual ridges are curved laterally between the position of the canine and the retromolar pad. The teeth should be set to follow this curve to provide the maximum tongue space and balance the pressure of the tongue with the pressure of the cheek. If the posterior part of the dental arch was curved when the natural teeth were present, this same relationship must be established if the support of the cheeks is to be restored.

Procedure for setting the posterior teeth into centric occlusion only

Arranging the posterior teeth for tryin is illustrated in Fig. 17-21. An alternative method of setting up nonanatomic posterior teeth is described in Chapter 21 and Figs. 21-34 and 21-39. *The latter method is very easy to carry out, since the occlusal surfaces of posterior teeth permit complete anteroposterior and buccolingual freedom of placement.*

Following is a description of our recommended techniques for setting cusped teeth:

Reduce the height of the posterior segments of the occlusion rim on one side, keeping the full height of the occlusion rims on the other side. This will make space for the teeth on one side and maintain the vertical dimension of the occlusion rims on the other side.

Pool enough wax distal to the maxillary canine to make a socket for the maxillary first premolar.

Place the cervical end of the premolar in the pooled wax so its long axis is parallel to the buccal surface of the canine.

Place the second maxillary premolar in the wax with a similar alignment and length.

Pool wax in the mandibular occlusion rim directly under the adjacent proximal surfaces of the upper premolars.

Place the cervical end of the lower second premolar in the pooled wax so it is too long. Then close the articulator to allow the upper teeth to force this tooth into the soft wax. Hold a finger against the cervical end of the tooth to keep its lingual cusp in contact with the upper two teeth.

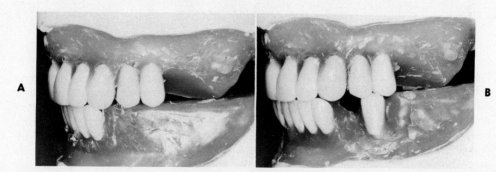

Fig. 17-21 Steps in arranging the posterior teeth for tryin. This procedure automatically intercuspates all posteriors into a tight centric occlusion. **A,** Maxillary first and second premolars set in alignment with the maxillary canine to continue the arch form established by the anterior teeth. The buccal premolar surfaces parallel the buccal canine surface. **B,** Mandibular second premolar set too high in pooled wax, and the articulator closed to push it down to its correct position. The wax remains soft enough that the tooth can be rotated or inclined as necessary. *Continued.*

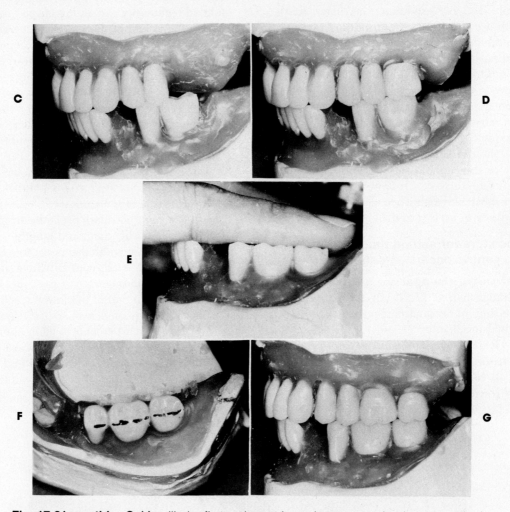

Fig. 17-21, cont'd   C, Mandibular first molar set in such a manner that it contacts both second premolars and its buccal cusps are bisected by a perpendicular erected on the buccal of the residual ridge. **D,** Maxillary first molar set in the pooled wax socket so it is slightly too long. The articulator is closed to force it into the soft wax socket. An index finger can be used to assist the tooth into its correct intercuspation and inclination by pressing against the cervical end while the articulator is being closed. **E,** Mandibular second molar set in a similar manner as the mandibular first molar **(C).** The finger acts as a template to ensure that all the mandibular cusps are harmoniously related to each other and that the occlusal plane aims at a level near the top of the retromolar pad. **F,** Alignment of the lower buccal cusps corresponding with the curvature of the residual ridge. **G,** Maxillary second molar set too long in its wax socket. It can be held by a finger placed against its cervical end while the articulator is closed.

Pool wax distal to the lower second premolar for the first molar tooth and push the cervical end of this tooth into the wax. Align it buccolingually in relation to the ridge crest as previously determined. Align the buccal and lingual cusps with those of the second premolar. Push the first molar down into the wax so its occlusal surface is aiming toward the top of the retromolar pad. Then close the articulator. This will bring the mesial inclines of the molar into contact with the distal inclines of the second premolar. The tooth contact should not disturb the position of the molar. If it does, push the molar further into the wax.

Pool wax for the upper first molar and position this tooth as the others. Place the cervical end of the tooth in the molten wax; then, holding the end, close the articulator to seat the occlusal surfaces together.

Pool wax for the lower second molar. Push this tooth into the wax in the desired buccolingual relationship, aligning the cusps with those of the first molar and aiming the occlusal surface toward the top of the retromolar pad. An index finger placed on the occlusal surfaces of the mandibular teeth at this time will reveal disharmonies in the height of the cusps and their alignment. Make the necessary adjustments.

Pool wax in the position of the upper second molar and place this tooth in position in the soft wax (but a millimeter or so too long). Then close the articulator while holding a finger against the cervical end of the upper tooth. This will occlude the teeth and position the molar in proper centric occlusion with the lower tooth.

Use a hot spatula to seal the wax around the cervical ends of all the teeth.

Repeat the procedure on the opposite side. Then after the wax is cooled, carve any excess from around the teeth and smooth the wax for tryin.

The occlusion will be adjusted only for CO at the tryin. The posterior teeth will have to be reset, to develop balanced occlusions in the other jaw positions after verification of the jaw relations and final arrangement of the anterior teeth for esthetics.

Setting posterior teeth is essentially a mechanical problem, and their anteroposterior position depends on the proper anteroposterior setting of the anterior teeth. A change in this position for esthetics will necessitate rearranging all the teeth. When the anterior setup is acceptable, the final anteroposterior position of the posterior teeth can be readily determined.

After the position of the anterior teeth has been determined in the mouth, it can act as an exact guide to the size of the posterior teeth. The posterior teeth may need to have their sizes changed, however. The distance between the distal surface of the mandibular canine and the mesial end of the retromolar pad is measured for the total anteroposterior space that may be covered by the teeth. The occlusocervical lengths of the posterior teeth are determined by the height and fullness of the ridges. The maxillae do not afford landmarks by which to measure whereas the mandible rises with an upward curvature that prevents setting the teeth too far posteriorly. The anterior teeth are in their final arrangement, and they establish the anterior limit of the posterior occlusion (Fig. 17-22). The distal extent of the posterior teeth is determined by the incline of the lower residual ridge. This may be as far forward as the normal position of the first molar in some mouths. If a tooth is placed on this incline, the denture will tend to slide forward when pressure is applied. It may be necessary to omit an upper and a lower premolar or molar from the dentures to avoid placing teeth on this incline. The buccolingual width of the posterior teeth should be less than the width of the natural teeth, to reduce biting pressure and increase tongue space. Remember that many tongues become abnormally wide because of reorganization of their intrinsic musculature when posterior teeth are lost and not replaced. The decreased buccolingual diameter of the teeth also

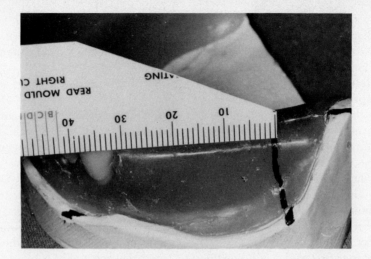

Fig. 17-22 Measuring the proper size of posterior teeth. *Vertical line* denotes the anterior edge of the retromolar pad. Posterior teeth should not be placed over the retromolar pad or the upward incline of the lower residual ridge.

contributes to a more favorable slope of the lingual surface of the lingual flange.

GENERAL CONSIDERATIONS

The ideal position of artificial teeth is precisely the same as of the natural teeth that they replace. When this objective is achieved, the soft tissues of the face will be supported as they were when the natural teeth were present. The pressures of the soft tissues against the artificial teeth will be the same as against the natural teeth when these were erupting. Such pressures were effective in aligning the natural teeth in the dental arch, and they can be effective in maintaining the dentures in place, provided of course the artificial teeth are aligned in dental arches that are in the same positions as the arches of the natural teeth. The situation has been described as follows: The cavity produced in a patient's mouth by the removal of teeth and the subsequent shrinkage of residual ridges is like a cavity in a tooth; it must be filled but not overfilled. The artificial teeth and the denture base material of the dentures should fill the usable space but not overfill it

and thus interfere with the action of oral or facial structures.

The anterior teeth play an important role in three basic oral functions: esthetics, incision, and phonetics. For *esthetics,* they must be of the same size and shape as the natural teeth and must occupy the same basic positions. Pre-extraction diagnostic casts and photographs can be invaluable for the placement of these teeth if they are available. If not available, the judgment and knowledge of the dentist concerning dental and oral anatomy must serve as a guide. The dentist's judgment is based on knowledge of the changes that occur in the residual ridges after the teeth are lost and of the tone of the skin around the mouth as compared to that in other parts of the face. For *incision,* certain mechanical considerations must be coordinated with the occlusion of the posterior teeth. These are discussed in Chapter 21. For *phonetics,* tooth position is closely associated with that for esthetics. In fact, phonetics can serve as a guide to esthetics and to the establishment of the vertical dimension of the jaws.

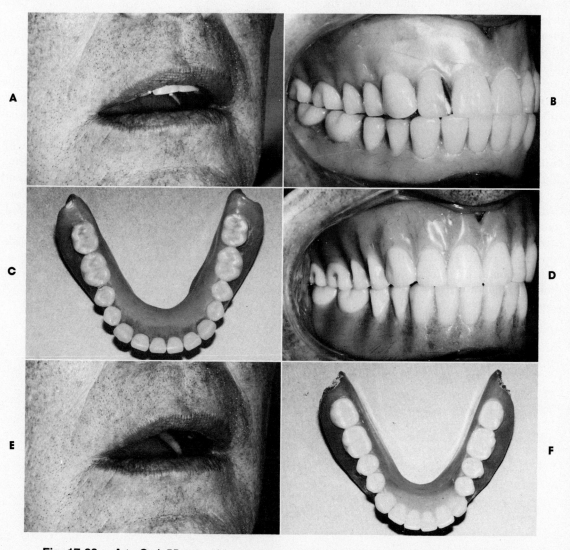

Fig. 17-23 **A** to **C,** A 55-year-old man who had successfully worn dentures for 15 years was given a new set with an elevated occlusal plane, **D.** This caused his anterior teeth to be invisible, **E.** The restricted tongue space, **F,** and elevated occlusal plane made it virtually impossible for him to manage the dentures, and he gave up attempting to wear them at the age of 56.

Esthetics and leverage

Frequently esthetics and leverage go hand in hand. An arch that is too broad in the premolar region will cause the patient to have the appearance of too many teeth; furthermore, the premolars will have improper tipping leverage. If the anterior teeth are set parallel to each other in every inclination and rotation, with perfect regularity and symmetry, they will have an unfavorable effect. Nature allows many apparent irregularities of anterior teeth, though usually not without a pattern that is more or less pleasing for an individual person. Irregularities can be used to great advantage by the dentist in making dentures appear natural. To be effective, however, irregularities must be correlated with the arch form and facial contour. Details must be worked out at the tryin. Any irregularities must be of a type that could appear in nature. For example, if two teeth are to be inclined or overlapped, their positions should be such that the roots (if they had roots) would not interfere with each other or with the teeth adjacent to them. It is still not possible to have two things occupy the same space at the same time, even if they are imaginary.

Common errors

Some of the common errors in arrangement of teeth include (1) setting the mandibular anterior teeth too far forward to meet the maxillary teeth, (2) failing to make the canines the turning point of the arch, (3) setting the mandibular first premolars to the buccal of the canines, (4) setting the maxillary posterior teeth over the ridge and then occluding them with the mandibular posterior teeth, thereby bringing them too far to the lingual in the second molar region and causing tongue interference and mandibular denture displacement, (5) failing to establish the occlusal plane at the proper level and inclination (Fig. 17-23), (6) establishing the occlusal plane by an arbitrary line on the face, and (7) not rotating the anterior teeth to give a narrower effect.

CHAPTER 18

Perfection and verification of jaw relation records

The vertical dimension and centric relation of edentulous jaws are tentatively established with the occlusion rims as described in Chapter 15. After the preliminary arrangement of the artificial teeth on the occlusion rims, it is essential that the accuracy of the jaw relation records made with the occlusion rims be tested, perfected if incorrect, and then verified to be correct. The dentist must assume that the preliminary jaw relation records were incorrect until they can be proved correct. This mental attitude of the dentist—attempting to prove that the jaw relation records are wrong—is essential in perfecting and verifying jaw relation records.

Patients should be advised to leave existing dentures out of the mouth for a minimum of 24 hours before the jaw relation records are perfected and verified at the time of the tryin appointment. Unfortunately, most patients will find this to be an unreasonable request. An acceptable alternative is to have the existing dentures relined with a soft temporary material. Whichever approach is taken, the soft tissues of the basal seat will be rested and in the same form as they were when the final impressions were made. If this procedure is not followed, the distorted condition of the soft tissue can prevent the registration of accurate interocclusal records.

It is almost impossible to overemphasize the importance of perfection and verification of jaw relation records. The appearance and comfort of the patient, occlusion of the teeth, and health of the supporting tissues are all directly related to the accuracy of jaw relation records.

VERIFYING THE VERTICAL DIMENSION

The mandibular trial denture is placed in the mouth, and then the maxillary trial denture is inserted. The patient is instructed to close lightly so the maxillary labial frenum remains absolutely free; this is necessary before the relation of the lip to the teeth can be observed. If the denture border causes binding of the frenum, the labial notch should be deepened.

Next, a tentative observation of the centric occlusion is made. The mandible is guided into CR by a thumb placed directly on the anteroinferior portion of the chin with instructions to "open and close until you feel the first feather touch of your back teeth." At first contact the patient opens and repeats this closure, only this time stopping the instant a tooth touch is felt, and then closing tight. The procedure will reveal errors in centric relation by the touch and slide of teeth on each other. Errors in CR can interfere with tests for vertical relations.

The vertical dimensions of occlusion and of rest must now be given careful consideration, because the final positions of the anterior and posterior teeth will depend to a great extent on the amount of space that is available vertically. Unfortunately, however, there is no precise scientific method of determining the correct occlusal vertical dimension. The acceptability of the dentures' vertical relations depends on the experience and judgment of the dentist. Nevertheless, the factors that govern final determination of this relation can be said to hang on careful consideration of

1. Preextraction records
2. The amount of interocclusal distance to

which the patient was accustomed, either before the loss of natural teeth or with old dentures

3. Phonetics and esthetics
4. The amount of interocclusal distance between the teeth when the mandible is in its rest position
5. A study of facial dimensions and facial expression
6. Lip length in relation to the teeth
7. The interarch distance and parallelism of the ridges as observed from the mounted casts
8. The condition and amount of shrinkage of the ridges

A combination of these factors and considerations may be used to aid in determining an acceptable vertical dimension. An elaboration on the various theories is given in Chapter 12.

It is obvious that verification of vertical maxillomandibular relationships is a challenge and requires assessment of many factors by the dentist.

VERIFYING CENTRIC RELATION

After the vertical dimension has been determined, CR is verified. This can be done by intraorally observing intercuspation or by an extraoral method on the articulator.

Intraoral observation of intercuspation

The test for accuracy of the preliminary CR record involves the observation of intercuspation when the mandible is pulled back by the patient as far as it will go and closure is stopped at the first tooth contact. The patient is guided into CR by a thumb placed on the anteroinferior portion of the chin and the index fingers bilaterally on the buccal flanges of the lower trial denture (Fig. 18-1). With the index fingers the dentist checks that the lower trial denture is seated in an inferoanterior direction. The patient pulls his lower jaw back as far as it will go and closes just until the back teeth make a "feather touch." As tooth contact approaches, the dentist's index fingers should rise off the buccal flanges. Pressure on the buccal

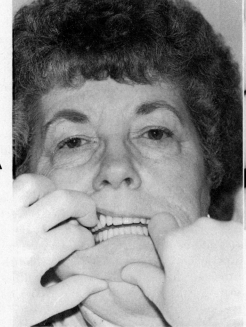

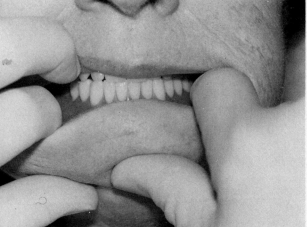

Fig. 18-1 **A,** Hand and finger positions for checking the accuracy of CR records. **B,** As tooth contact approaches, the index fingers are raised off the buccal flanges to avoid displacement of the lower denture.

flanges or stretching the lip with the index fingers will create the risk of posteriorly displacing the lower trial denture. Then the patient closes tightly. Any error in CR will be apparent when the teeth slide over each other, especially if anatomic teeth are used (Fig. 18-2). A second closure made with the same instructions and a stop at first tooth contact will permit visual observation of any error.

Errors in the mounting may prevent some teeth from intercuspating when the first contact is made. If the patient stops the closure at the instant the first teeth touch, an error will be indicated by the space between the lower tooth or teeth and the teeth they were supposed to touch. The amount of error observed in this manner will be magnified by the effect of the inclined plane contacts. All the teeth that occluded uniformly on the articulator must have equally uniform contacts in the mouth; if they do not, the touch and slide observation will prove the mounting incorrect.

Once it is determined that the mounting is incorrect, a preliminary observation of esthetics is made. If the anterior teeth are not placed to support the lip properly, their positions are corrected. Then vertical overlap of the anterior teeth is carefully noted. This is important be-

cause the amount of vertical overlap will be a guide to the amount of closure permitted when the next interocclusal record is made.

Because complete dentures rest on movable soft tissues, it is difficult to detect anything other than gross occlusal errors by visual observation of the occlusion. As a result one should not rely on visualization for the final determination of cast mounting accuracy.

Intraoral interocclusal records. The posterior teeth are removed from the lower occlusion rim, and both occlusion rims are placed in the mouth. Impression plaster, or an interocclusal registration paste, is mixed, and with the hands in the same position as for testing the previous record, the selected recording medium is placed on both sides of the lower occlusion rim in the molar and premolar regions. This may be done with a narrow plaster or cement spatula. Then the patient is instructed to pull the lower jaw back and close slowly until requested to stop and hold that position. The closure is stopped when the anterior teeth have the same vertical overlap as they had before the posterior teeth were removed. Thus the vertical relation of the two jaws will not have changed. When the plaster or registration paste is set, the new record is removed with the two occlusion rims and the lower cast is remounted on the articulator.

In an alternate technique an abbreviated beeswax occlusion rim is used to replace the removed posterior teeth. (The rim may replace all the posterior teeth, or else a "tripod" of beeswax stops can be used, Fig. 18-3.) The patient is guided into the most retruded mandibular position at the selected vertical dimension when the upper posterior teeth will indent the softened opposing wax rims. The lower cast is remounted on the articulator, and the lower posterior teeth are reset in CO.

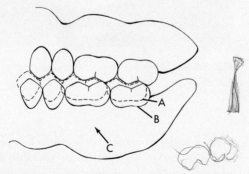

Fig. 18-2   An error in CO that is due to an error in CR mounting will produce contact of the inclined planes of the cusps, *B*. Further closure will allow the teeth to slide into CO, *A*. The path of closure is an arc, *C*, about the posterior terminal hinge axis.

The occlusion rims, with the teeth in good tight CO, are returned to the mouth, and the same tests are made as before. If the teeth occlude perfectly and uniformly when the lower jaw is drawn back as far as it will go, the CR

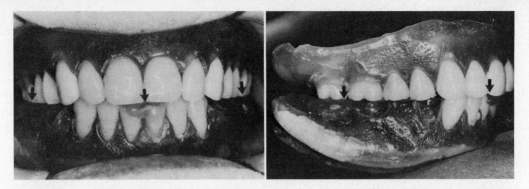

Fig. 18-3   A modified beeswax interocclusal record of CR is made to correct an error in the preliminary mounting of casts. The lower posterior teeth are removed so there will be no contact between upper and lower trial dentures. The vertical overlap of anterior teeth is a guide to the vertical dimension at which CR will be recorded. The beeswax tripod of stops is identified by *arrows*.

mounting may be assumed correct. There should be uniform simultaneous contact on both sides of the mouth, in the front and back and without any detectable touch and slide.

It is essential with this procedure that the dentist *try* to find an error in the previous record. The record must be assumed incorrect unless no touch and slide can be detected. The entire procedure is repeated until all doubt as to the correctness of the relationship of the casts is gone.

Extraoral articulator method

CR can be checked or verified by an extraoral method in which observations are made on the articulator rather than in the mouth. The technique is easy, and hence attractive, but its use depends on taking one or two liberties. A CR registration in soft wax is placed between the opposing teeth. The teeth do not contact through the wax; thus the record is made at a slightly increased vertical dimension. Although clinical experience endorses this technique, a purist might argue that such verification is likely to work correctly only if a kinematic hinge axis rather than an arbitrary facebow recording is used originally. Since conclusive research to support such an argument is

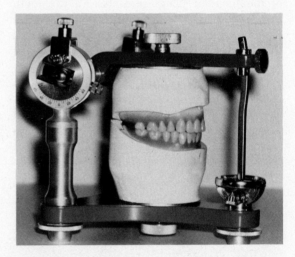

Fig. 18-4   Artificial teeth positioned on a Dentatus ARH articulator.

absent and since extensive clinical application of the technique has led to predictable and reproducible results, it deserves description.

Remember: The purpose of the extraoral method is to determine whether the position of the teeth on the articulator (Fig. 18-4) is the same as that in the patient's mouth (Fig. 18-5). As mentioned previously, it is difficult to de-

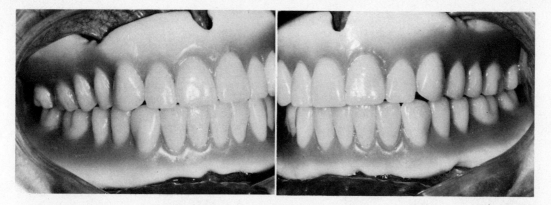

Fig. 18-5 The same trial dentures as shown in Fig. 18-4 being evaluated for proper occlusion. Clinical observation of tooth contacts is not as accurate as the extraoral method.

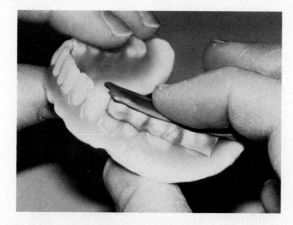

Fig. 18-6 A second layer of warmed Aluwax is applied to the first layer, which has been carefully adapted to the posterior teeth.

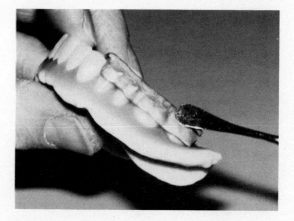

Fig. 18-7 The two layers of Aluwax are sealed with a warm spatula.

tect occlusal errors by clinical observation so wax, plaster, or a bite registration paste must be used as the recording medium in this technique.

Impression material (for example, two pieces of Aluwax) is placed over the posterior mandibular teeth (Fig. 18-6). A thickness is chosen that will eliminate the danger of making contact with the op-

posing teeth when biting pressure is exerted. No wax is placed on the anterior teeth because anterior tooth contact tends to cause the patient to protrude his lower jaw. The teeth must be completely dry and the wax pressed firmly on the teeth to eliminate voids between it and the teeth. The two thicknesses of wax are sealed with a warm spatula (Fig. 18-7). The chilled upper trial denture is placed in the patient's mouth. Next, just the wax portion is im-

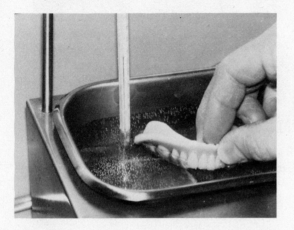

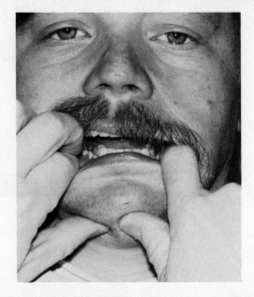

Fig. 18-8 Only the Aluwax is immersed, in 130° F (54° C) water for 30 seconds.

Fig. 18-9 The mandible is guided into CR with the thumb on the anteroinferior portion of the chin and the index fingers seating the lower trial denture in a downward and forward direction.

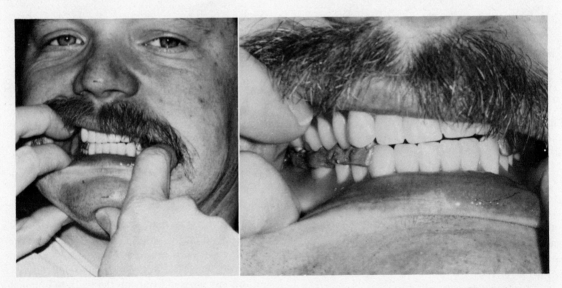

Fig. 18-10 The patient is instructed to close lightly into the softened wax. The index fingers should be slightly raised from the buccal flanges at this point.

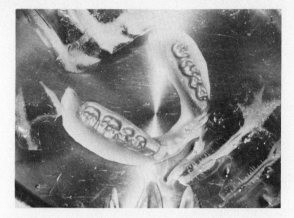

Fig. 18-11 The lower trial denture and attached Aluwax are chilled in ice water for several minutes.

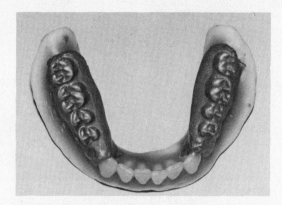

Fig. 18-12 The occlusal record should be approximately 1 mm deep and free of any penetration by the underlying teeth.

mersed in a water bath of 130° F (54° C) for 30 seconds (Fig. 18-8). Both the temperature and the time are critical in achieving a uniformly softened wax. (Aluwax retains heat longer than baseplate wax, which provides more working time for the next step.)

The mandibular trial denture is seated with the index fingers bilaterally positioned on the buccal flanges. The mandible is guided into CR by a thumb on the anteroinferior portion of the chin to direct some guidance toward the condyles. The thumb must be on the point of the chin, not under it; the patient is guided in a hinge movement, closing lightly into the wax (Fig. 18-9). As contact with the wax approaches, the index fingers are raised from the buccal flanges. The patient then closes into the wax until a good index is made (Fig. 18-10). Care must be taken that the patient does not penetrate the wax and make tooth contact. If one method of suggested retrusion does not work, another may. In any case a minimum amount of occlusal pressure should be exerted on the wax.

The lower trial denture is then carefully removed from the mouth and placed in ice water to chill the wax thoroughly (Fig. 18-11). Next the trial dentures are removed from the ice water and dried. It is important that the imprint of the opposing teeth be crisp and about 1 mm deep, with no penetration of the wax by a maxillary tooth (Fig. 18-12). If penetra-

tion occurs, it will likely deflect the occlusal contact as well as shift the bases or change the maxillomandibular relation horizontally and vertically. The chilled dentures are returned to the patient's mouth and the patient is guided into CR. The record is acceptable if there is no tilting or torquing of the trial dentures from initial contact to complete closure (Fig. 18-13). Underlying soft tissue displacement may cause a slight movement of the bases and must be taken into account when evaluating the contact. If the record is unacceptable, the procedure must be repeated.

After the wax has been chilled, the trial dentures are placed on their casts and the locked articulator is closed in CR; the opposing teeth should fit into the indentations in every way (anteriorly, posteriorly, laterally, and vertically) (Fig. 18-14). When the original CR interocclusal record and the check are both correct, it is surprising how well these teeth will fit into the indentations.

If the opposing teeth do not fit exactly into the indentations in the new record, it means that the original mounting was incorrect or that the patient did not bite cleanly into the interocclusal wax. To evaluate this, it is necessary that the chilled trial dentures and wax record be returned to the mouth and their accuracy reevaluated as previously described. If the record still appears to be correct in the patient's mouth, then the original CR registration and/or

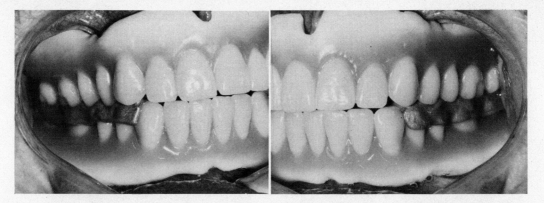

Fig. 18-13 Checking the accuracy of the interocclusal wax record clinically.

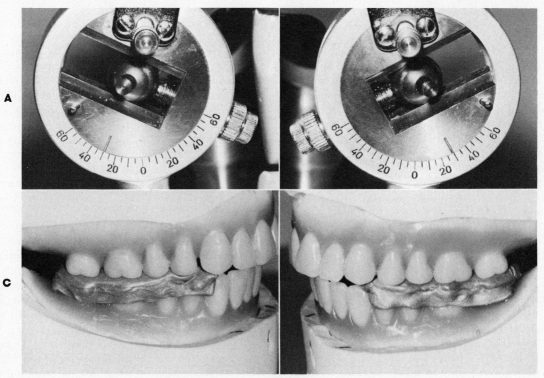

Fig. 18-14 With the condylar mechanisms locked in a centric position, **A** and **B,** the upper teeth should fit accurately into the wax index, **C** and **D.** When this occurs, it means that the original recording was correct.

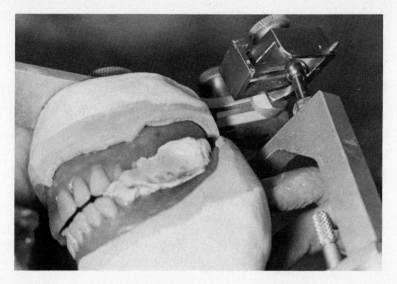

Fig. 18-15   A plaster interocclusal CR record is used to test the accuracy of preliminary mounting on the articulator. The location of the condylar sphere in contact with the posterior, lateral, and superior elements of the condylar housing indicates that the preliminary record and test record are clinically identical. Thus the casts on the articulator are assumed to be in CR.

mounting were incorrect. In these cases the mandibular cast must be separated from the mounting ring and the cast remounted by means of the last interocclusal wax record. The new mounting is again checked to prove or disprove its correctness.

If the initial registration (preliminary CR record) was made in plaster or a bite registra-

tion paste, the same recording medium should be used to verify the accuracy of the mounting on the articulator. Likewise, if wax was used, wax should be the verifying medium. However, it is easier to distort wax when the record is removed from the mouth and tested on the articulator (Fig. 18-15).

CHAPTER 19

Creating facial and functional harmony with anterior teeth

The anatomic structures that collectively form the face normally develop concurrently and are interdependent during function throughout life. Disruptive events in this homeostatic complex can range from relatively minor changes such as a deflective occlusal contact to major alterations in bodily form such as removal of the natural teeth, which drastically affects the form and function of the remaining living parts.

In this context of homeostasis, creating facial and functional harmony with anterior teeth becomes a biologic challenge of utmost significance. Not only must the teeth be of proper form, size, and color to harmonize with the face; they must also become a functioning component in a living environment that depends on their proper position for its normal physiologic activity. This proper position allows patients to preserve their facial identity as it existed when natural teeth were present. The ability of patients to maintain their normal facial expression will likely be the most important psychologic factor in acceptance of the dentures.

ANATOMY OF NATURAL APPEARANCE AND FACIAL EXPRESSION

The dentist who is treating a patient with complete dentures has as much to do with the beauty of the face as has any other medical specialist. The appearance of the entire lower half of the face depends on the dentures. It is usu-

ally not difficult on casual meeting to detect the person who is wearing poorly constructed dentures (Fig. 19-1). The characteristic thin drooping upper lip that appears lengthened and has a reduced vermilion border is typical of malpositioned anterior teeth and probably a reduced vertical dimension of occlusion. Tense wrinkled lips often reveal the patient's efforts to hold the denture in place. The drooping corners of the mouth tell the story of the misshapen and misplaced dental arch form of the anterior teeth, the thin denture borders, and often the reduced occlusal vertical dimension. The appearance of premature aging may be caused not by age itself but by the lack of support for the lips and cheeks due to the loss or improper replacement of teeth. The apparent extra fullness of the lower lip may be the result of too broad a mandibular dental arch or the elimination or reduction of the mentolabial sulcus. This may indicate that the lower anterior teeth have been placed too far lingually or that the labial flange of the lower denture base is overextended or too thick.

Normal facial landmarks

One must study normal facial landmarks before attempting to achieve the goal of a natural and pleasing facial expression with complete dentures. The facial landmarks of the lower third of the face have a direct relationship to the presence of the natural teeth (Fig. 19-2). The contours of the lips depend on their intrin-

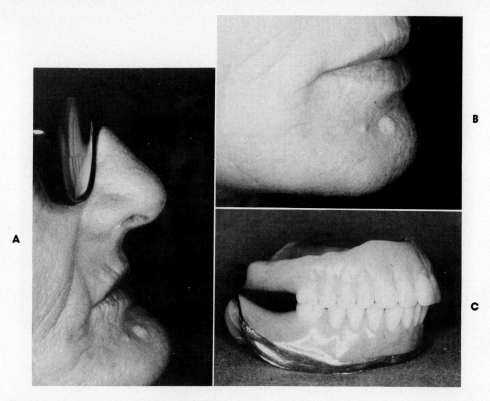

Fig. 19-1   A, The lower part of this face lacks proper contour because of inadequate support for the orbicularis oris and muscles related to it. **B,** Facial contours have been properly restored. The improvement in appearance is directly related to the position of the artificial teeth and the form of the supporting base material of the complete dentures, **C.**

sic structure and the support for them provided by the teeth and the soft tissues or denture bases behind them. When the natural teeth are lost, these landmarks and surrounding facial tissues become distorted. To reestablish normal appearance and function, artificial teeth must be replaced in the same position as the natural teeth that were lost.

The lips vary in length, thickness, shape, and mobility in different patients. Such variance accounts for the degree of visibility of the upper and lower anterior teeth during speech and other facial expressions. When the mandible is in the resting position, the lips usually contact each other and turn slightly outward, exposing the vermilion border. The vertical

groove in the middle of the upper lip is called the philtrum, and the horizontal depression midway between the lower vermilion border and the bottom of the chin is called the mentolabial sulcus, or groove (Fig. 19-2). Incorrect positioning of the anterior teeth or supporting base material of complete dentures will alter the normal appearance of the vermilion border, the philtrum, and the mentolabial sulcus in edentulous patients.

The nasolabial sulcus, or groove, is a depression in the skin on each side of the face, which runs angularly outward from the ala of the nose to approximately just outside the corners of the mouth (anguli oris) (Fig. 19-2). The zygomaticus originates on the zygomatic bone and an-

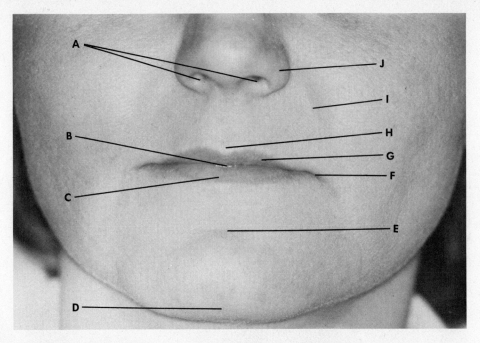

Fig. 19-2 Facial landmarks. *A*, Nares; *B*, rima oris; *C*, lower lip; *D*, mentum; *E*, mentolabial sulcus; *F*, angulus oris; *G*, upper lip; *H*, philtrum; *I*, nasolabial sulcus; *J*, ala nasi.

gles downward and forward to insert at the corner of the mouth into the orbicularis oris. The action of the two zygomatici in elevating the corners of the mouth for smiling produces the nasolabial sulcus (Fig. 19-3). Many older patients want to have the nasolabial sulcus obliterated because it becomes a wrinkle as the skin loses resilience. Removal of the nasolabial fold has been attempted by thickening the denture base under the fold, but the extra bulk in this location causes a very unnatural appearance. The sulcus is normal and should not be eliminated. The proper treatment is to bring the entire upper dental arch forward to its original position when the natural teeth were present and to maintain the original arch form of the natural teeth and their supporting structures. Thus the prominence of the nasolabial sulcus will be restored to its original contour.

In many patients the corners of the lip line (rima oris) will be as high as the center portion but the lip line will not necessarily be straight all the way across.

The upper lip rests on the labial surfaces of the upper anterior teeth, and the lower lip on the labial surfaces of the lower anterior teeth and incisal edges of the upper teeth. For this reason the edge of the lower lip should extend outward and upward from the mentolabial sulcus. A reproduction of the horizontal overlap of the natural anterior teeth in the denture is essential to maintaining proper contour of the lips (Fig. 19-4).

A study of the inclination of the osseous structure supporting the lower anterior teeth indicates that, in most patients, the clinical crowns of the lower teeth are labial to the bone that supports them. Likewise, a study of the

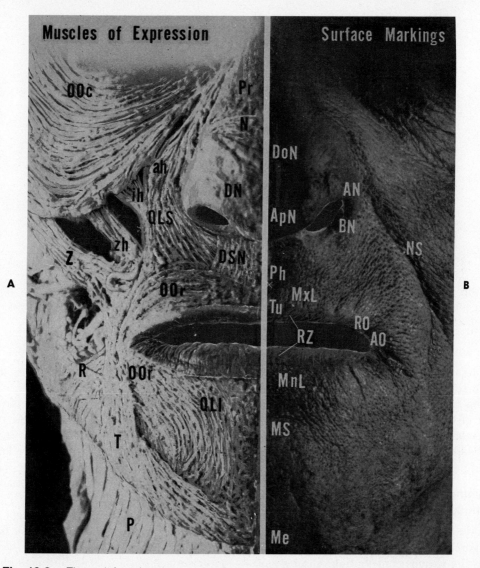

Fig. 19-3   The polyfunctional pyramid. **A,** Underlying superficial musculature. *OOc,* Orbicularis oculi; *Pr,* procerus; *N,* nasalis; *QLS,* quadratus labii superioris; *ah,* angular head; *ih,* infraorbital head; *zh,* zygomatic head; *DN,* dilator naris; *DSN,* depressor septi nasi; *Z,* zygomaticus; *R,* risorius; *OOr,* orbicularis oris; *T,* triangularis; *QLI,* quadratus labii inferioris; *P,* platysma. **B,** Surface anatomy. *DoN,* Dorsum nasi; *AN,* ala nasi; *ApN,* apex nasi; *BN,* basis nasi; *NS,* nasolabial sulcus; *Ph,* philtrum; *MxL,* maxillary lip; *Tu,* tubercle; *RO,* rima oris; *AO,* angulus oris; *RZ,* red zone or vermilion border; *MnL,* mandibular lip; *MS,* mentolabial sulcus; *Me,* mentum.   (From Martone AL, Edwards LF: J Prosthet Dent **11:**1009-1018, 1961.)

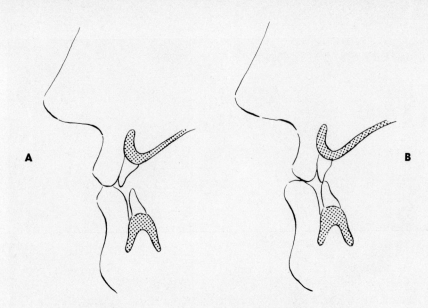

Fig. 19-4   A, Reproduction of a patient's former horizontal overlap with the correct facial contour. **B,** Horizontal overlap changed so the maxillary anterior teeth contact the mandibular teeth, with resultant damage to the upper lip.

inclination of osseous structure and the inclination of maxillary anterior teeth reveals that the upper lip functions on an incline (Fig. 19-5). Neglect of these factors in the replacement of natural teeth often will cause the lip to be ill-formed and in time lead to the formation of vertical lines in the lip.

Maintaining facial support and neuromuscular balance

The orbicularis oris and its attaching muscles are important in denture construction inasmuch as the various contributing muscles have bony origins and their insertions are into the modioli and orbicularis at the corners of the mouth (Fig. 19-6, *A*). Thus the functioning length of all these muscles depends on the function of the orbicularis oris. The muscles that merge into the orbicularis oris are the zygomaticus, the quadratus labii superioris, the caninus (levator anguli oris), the mentalis, the quadratus labii inferioris, the triangularis (depressor anguli oris), the buccinator, and the risorius.

The orbicularis oris is the muscle of the lips. It is sphincterlike, attaching to the maxillae along a median line under the nose by means of a band of fibrous connective tissue known as the maxillary labial frenum and to the mandible on a median line by means of the mandibular labial frenum.

The buccinator is a broad band of muscle forming the entire wall of the cheek from the corner of the mouth and passing along the outer surface of the maxilla and mandible until it reaches the ramus, where it passes to the lingual surface to join the superior constrictor of the pharynx at the pterygomandibular raphe (Fig. 19-6, *B*).

The two buccinators and the orbicularis form a functional unit that depends on the position of the dental arches and the labial contours of the mucosa or the denture base for effective action. With the loss of teeth, the function of the

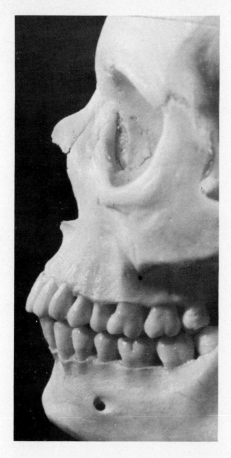

Fig. 19-5   The incisal edges and labial surfaces of the lower anterior teeth are labial to the bone supporting them. The inclination of the labial plate of bone and the labial surfaces of the upper anterior teeth causes the upper lip to function on an incline. It is easy to observe the lack of support of the lip that will result when artificial anterior teeth are positioned over the crest of the residual ridge. Resorption of the alveolar process in the mandibular anterior region after removal of the anterior teeth will move the residual bony ridge lingually at first and then labially as resorption continues.

orbicularis, buccinator, and attaching muscles is impaired. Since these muscles of expression are no longer supported at their physiologic length, contraction of the unsupported fibers does not produce normal facial expression, because the lips and face no longer move naturally or maybe even at all. Contraction simply takes up the droop in the fibers. However, when these muscles are correctly supported by complete dentures, impulses coming to them from the central nervous system cause a shortening of the fibers that allows the face to move in a normal manner. Thus the memory patterns of facial expression developed within the neuromuscular system when the patient had natural teeth are continued or reinforced so the pa-

tient's original appearance is maintained (Fig. 19-7).

Three factors affect the face in repositioning the orbicularis oris with complete dentures: (1) the thickness of the labial flanges of both dentures, (2) the anteroposterior position of the anterior teeth, and (3) the amount of separation between the mandible and the maxillae (Fig. 19-8). If the jaws are closed too far and the dental arch is located too far posteriorly, the upward and backward positioning of the orbicularis oris complex will move the insertions of these muscles closer to their origins. This will cause the muscles to sag when at rest and to be less effective when contracting. Such positions automatically drop the corners of the mouth,

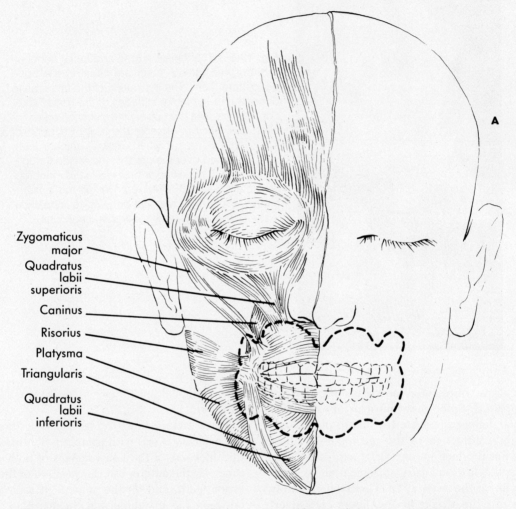

Zygomaticus major
Quadratus labii superioris
Caninus
Risorius
Platysma
Triangularis
Quadratus labii inferioris

Fig. 19-6   Muscles that maintain facial support. When artificial teeth and the denture base material restore the lips to their correct contour, the facial muscles will be at their physiologic length and contraction will create the normal facial expression of the patient. **A,** The facial muscles.

B

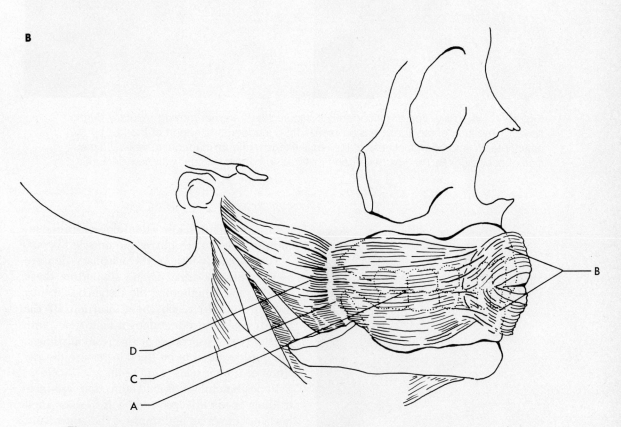

Fig. 19-6 cont'd   B, Functional unit of the buccinator. This muscle, *A,* and the orbicularis oris, *B,* depend on the position of the upper denture for their proper action. *C* is the pterygomandibular raphe and, *D,* the superior constrictor of the pharynx.

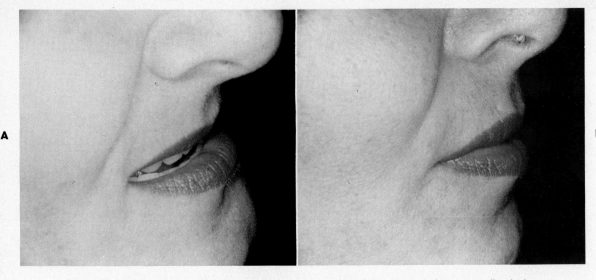

Fig. 19-7   A, These lips are incorrectly contoured and are not moving naturally during speech. The lack of facial expression results from inadequate support of the lips by the anterior teeth, improper thickness of the labial flanges, and an inadequate vertical dimension of occlusion. **B,** The lips have been restored to correct contour with new dentures.

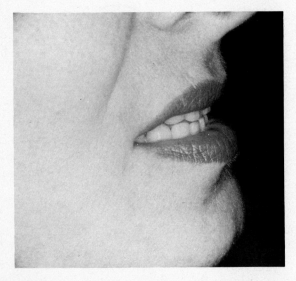

Fig. 19-8 Notice the activity of the lips during speech when they are properly supported by new dentures. Compare this with the lack of activity in the same patient (Fig. 19-7, *A*).

with a resultant senile edentulous expression, and may lead to atrophy of the muscle fibers.

The correct width of the maxillary denture borders plays a great part in supporting these muscles and lengthening the distance that they must extend to reach their insertion. If the mouth has been edentulous a long time, with considerable resorption of the residual ridges, the borders need to be thick to restore the position of the muscles (Fig. 19-9).

Repositioning anterior teeth that are protruding or slightly protruding to reduce their horizontal overlap and improve the appearance of the patient is a serious mistake. The muscles, teeth, and all associated structures grew simultaneously; and therefore the physiologic length of the muscles was determined early. In fact, the muscles of the face, cheeks, tongue, and lips helped align the natural teeth in the dental arches. To move teeth back in dentures is to invite a loss of facial expression that may

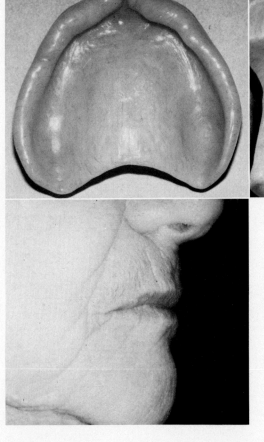

Fig. 19-9   **A** and **B,** The labial flange is thick at the borders. This thickness harmonizes with the available space in the patient's mouth because of resorption of the upper residual ridge. **C,** The bulk is needed for correct support of the upper lip.

be more damaging to the appearance of the patient than the slightly protruding teeth. Individual pronounced irregularities may be improved, as long as the position of the dental arch in its support of the orbicularis oris and attaching muscles is not perceptibly altered.

Thus normal facial expression and proper tone of the skin of the face depend on the position and function of the facial muscles. These muscles can function physiologically only when the dentist has positioned and shaped the dental arches correctly and has given the mandible a favorable vertical position. In addition, the dentures themselves must have a pleasing and natural appearance in the patient's mouth, a

condition that is dependent on arranging the artificial teeth in a plan that simulates nature. This, then, is the challenge of creating facial and functional harmony with anterior teeth.

BASIC GUIDES TO DEVELOPING FACIAL AND FUNCTIONAL HARMONY

After an acceptable vertical dimension of occlusion has been determined and the horizontal relation of the casts on the articulator has been verified for CR, the appearance of the patient is studied and modifications are made in the arrangement of the teeth to obtain a harmonious effect with the patient's face. The guides that are considered in developing facial and func-

Plate 19-1   The teeth used for both these patients are Vitapan hard acrylic resin (Vita Zahnfabrik, Bad Säckingen, FRG).

A and **B,** With preextraction records as a guide, this patient's upper canines are shade A3.5 but her other anterior and posterior teeth are A2. Frequently the upper natural canines will be darker than the other teeth.

C and **D,** Her high school graduation picture, showing her natural teeth, was used as a guide in selecting and arranging the anterior teeth for replacement dentures at age 64.

E and **F,** She requested a light shade, which was used, with a pleasing result.

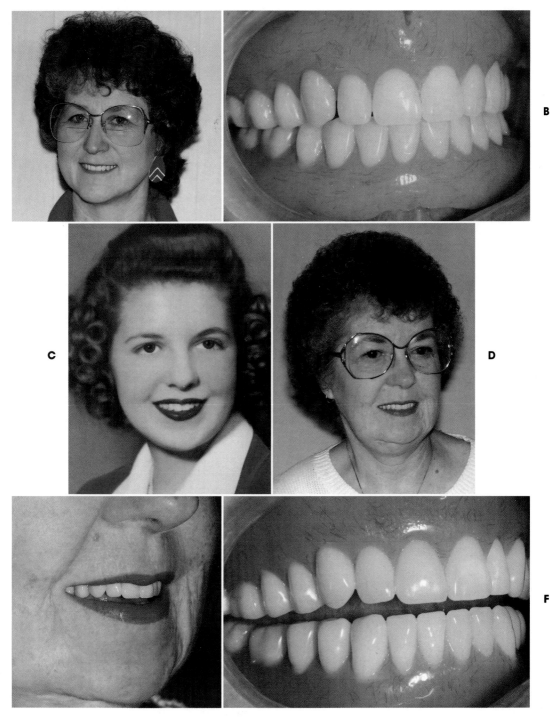

Plate 19-1 For legend see opposite page.

tional harmony include (1) the preliminary selection of artificial teeth, (2) the horizontal orientation of anterior teeth, (3) the vertical orientation of anterior teeth, (4) phonetics in the orientation of anterior teeth, (5) the inclination of anterior teeth, (6) harmony in the general composition of anterior teeth, (7) refinement of individual tooth positions, (8) the concept of harmony with sex, personality, and age of the patient, and (9) the correlation of esthetics and incisal guidance. Although these factors will be discussed individually, for simplicity they are interrelated in the actual clinical situation.

Preliminary selection of the artificial teeth

The preliminary selection of teeth must be critically evaluated for size, form, and color as they have been arranged in the trial denture. The six upper anterior teeth, when properly supporting the upper lip, should be of sufficient overall width to extend in the dental arch to approximately the position of the corners of the mouth and still allow for individual irregularities of rotation, overlapping, and spacing. The canines should extend distally so they can be the turning point in the dental arch. The form of the teeth should be harmonious with the face but not necessarily identical with the outline form of the face. The color of the teeth should blend with the face so the teeth do not become the main focal point of the face. The

anterior teeth are the principal ones to be considered in esthetics, although the posterior teeth, involving height of plane and width of arch, play their part also. Any records used in the initial selection of teeth should be consulted at this time to ensure that the desired result has been achieved (Plate 19-1). The dentist must make changes in the selection of teeth if such changes will improve the appearance of the dentures.

Horizontal orientation of the anterior teeth

The position and expression of the lips and the lower part of the face are the best guides for determining the proper anteroposterior orientation of anterior teeth. The other guides or measurements are secondary and must be ultimately related to the appearance of the patient.

The greatest harm done in esthetics is setting the maxillary anterior teeth back to or under the ridge, regardless of the amount of resorption that has taken place. A study of the anterior alveolar process will disclose that its direction is upward and backward from the labial surface of the maxillary incisors (Fig. 19-5). Therefore the crest of the upper ridge is considerably more posterior in a resorbed ridge than it was when the teeth were recently removed (Fig. 19-10).

Insufficient support of the lips resulting from anterior teeth that are located too far posteri-

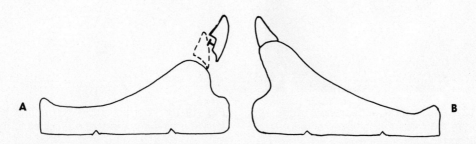

Fig. 19-10   **A,** Correct positioning of an artificial central incisor to restore the physiologic length of muscles for proper functioning. *Dotted outline* shows the tooth incorrectly positioned to follow the residual ridge. **B,** Position of the original natural central incisor.

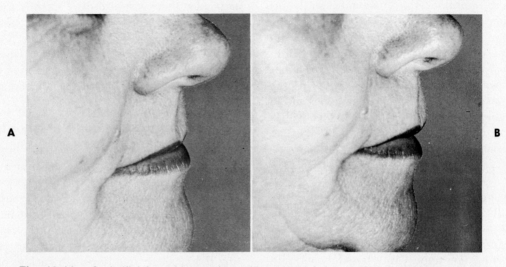

Fig. 19-11 **A,** Artificial anterior teeth positioned too far posteriorly. Notice the lack of tone in the skin of the upper lip. **B,** Artificial anterior teeth positioned correctly in an anteroposterior direction. Notice the improved skin tone.

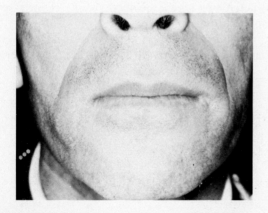

Fig. 19-12 A stretched appearance of the lips and philtrum indicates that artificial anterior teeth are positioned too far anteriorly.

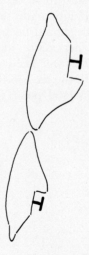

Fig. 19-13 Correct inclination of the teeth and incisal edges in a moderate prognathic relation.

orly is characterized by a drooping or turning down of the corners of the mouth, a reduction in the visible part of the vermilion border, a drooping and deepening of the nasolabial grooves, small vertical lines or wrinkles above the vermilion border, a deepening of the sulci, and a reduction in the prominence of the philtrum (Fig. 19-7, *A*).

A striking difference occurs when the anterior teeth are in proper position (Fig. 19-11). The vermilion borders become visible, the corners of the mouth assume a normal contour, many of the small vertical lines above the vermilion of the upper lip are reduced or eliminated, and the tone of the skin surrounding the dentures takes on a character similar to that of the skin in other parts of the face not affected by the position of the teeth. Although the nasolabial groove will still be present, the drooping appearance can often be considerably reduced. Nasolabial grooves should not be eliminated, and the dentist must be careful about what is told the patient in this regard. However, patients should be informed as to the other improvements that can be made by the dentures that will produce a more youthful appearance.

Excessive lip support resulting from anterior teeth located too far anteriorly is characterized by a stretched tight appearance of the lips, a tendency for the lips to dislodge the dentures during function, elimination of the normal contours of the lips, and distortion of the philtrum and sulci (Fig. 19-12). A photograph of the patient with natural teeth can be most helpful in the placing of artificial teeth. The teeth can be so arranged that the appearance and contours of the lips and lower part of the face resemble those seen in the picture (Plate 19-1, *C*).

The relation of the maxillary and mandibular anterior ridges to each other has an influence on the anteroposterior position of both the maxillary and the mandibular anterior teeth. A common error is to attempt to establish a standard vertical and horizontal overlap without regard to the ridge relation. This should not be done because the anteroposterior position of the teeth must correspond to the positions of the ridges. If the mandibular ridge is forward of the maxillary ridge, as in prognathism, the upper anterior teeth should be placed lingual to the mandibular teeth. The anterior teeth can then be set end to end, with the incisal edges at an angle that produces a seating action on the maxillary denture (Fig. 19-13).

A study of the position of natural teeth on diagnostic casts will provide information that can be transferred to the arrangement of artificial anterior teeth. As mentioned previously, the upper lip functions on an incline produced by the labial plate of the alveolar process and the crowns of the upper anterior teeth. The position of the natural anterior teeth makes their labial surfaces at least as far forward as the la-

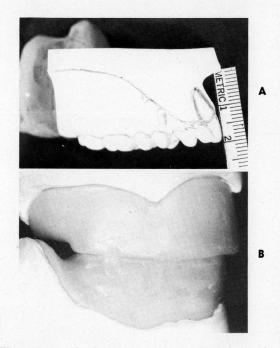

Fig. 19-14   **A,** Relation of the labial surface of the natural central incisor to the reflection in a sectioned cast. **B,** The inclination of the labial surfaces of wax occlusion rims should simulate the inclination observed in the natural situation. When the occlusion rims slope lingually toward the occlusal surface in the anterior region, they will rarely if ever provide proper support for the lips.

bial most part of the reflection (Fig. 19-14, *A*). This information can be transferred to the position of the artificial anterior teeth on the trial denture base. Such a guide will also be helpful in contouring the occlusion rims (Fig. 19-14, *B*) and in developing the preliminary arrangement of anterior teeth.

Observing the position of the anterior teeth when the trial denture base is out of the mouth can be helpful. The labial surfaces of many natural upper central incisors are approximately 8 to 10 mm in front of the middle of the incisive papilla. Measurements with a Boley gauge from the middle of the incisive fossa on the trial denture base to the labial surfaces of the artificial central incisors will show the relationship of these teeth to the incisive papilla (Fig. 19-15, *A*).

When the trial denture bases are viewed from the tissue-contacting surface, the labial portions of the anterior teeth should be apparent and a visualization of their imaginary roots

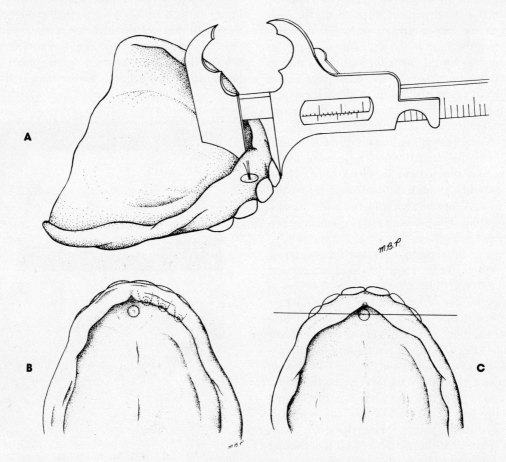

Fig. 19-15 Indications of correct anteroposterior positioning of artificial anterior teeth. **A,** By measurement from the middle of the incisive fossa on the trial denture base to the labial surfaces of the central incisors. **B,** By visualization of the imaginary roots of artificial anterior teeth. The imaginary roots will be further in front of the residual ridge when a great amount of resorption has occurred. **C,** By determining the relationship of a transverse line extending between the middle of the upper canines and the incisive fossa.

can be helpful. If the imaginary roots appear to be on the labial of the residual ridge (with allowance made for bone loss from that part of the ridge), the anterior teeth will be very near to their correct labiolingual positions. If the imaginary roots appear to extend into the crest of the residual ridge, the artificial teeth are positioned too far posteriorly on the trial denture base (Fig. 19-15, B). The location of the incisive fossa in relation to the crest of the ridge gives an indication of the amount of resorption of the upper residual ridge: the greater the resorption, the farther in front of the crest the imaginary roots should appear.

An imaginary transverse line between the upper canines as viewed from the tissue-contacting surface of the upper trial denture base should cross close to the middle of the incisive fossa when anterior teeth of the proper size are located correctly in the anteroposterior position (Fig. 19-15, C). If the line falls anterior to the incisive fossa, the overall width of the anterior teeth may be too small or the teeth may be positioned too far forward. If the line falls posterior to the papilla, the overall width of the anterior teeth may be too large or the teeth positioned too far back.

Vertical orientation of the anterior teeth

The amount of the upper anterior teeth seen during speech and facial expression depends on the length and movement of the upper lip in relation to the vertical length of the dental arch. If the upper lip is relatively long, the natural teeth may not be visible when the lip is relaxed or even during speech (Fig. 19-16, A);

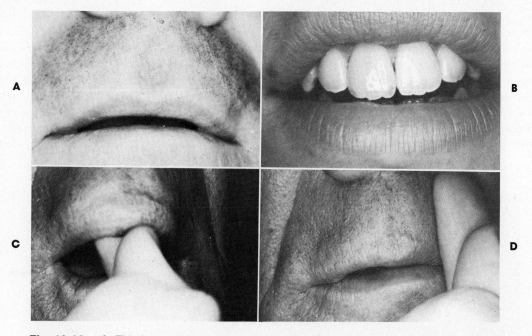

Fig. 19-16   A, This long upper lip obscures the natural upper anterior teeth even during speech. **B,** A relatively short upper lip exposes almost all the crowns of the upper central and lateral incisors. **C,** The upper lip is allowed to drape over the index finger, which has been placed on the incisive papilla. The thumb is in contact with the vermilion border. **D,** The amount of index finger that has been covered by the upper lip is an indication of the length of the upper lip relative to the upper residual ridge.

however, in this situation some teeth may be exposed when the person smiles. In other patients, with a relatively short upper lip, the full crowns may be visible below the upper lip (Fig. 19-16, *B*); in some of these patients, a large amount of the mucous membrane (or denture base) in addition to the teeth may be exposed when they smile.

Furthermore, the movement of the lips during function varies considerably among patients. Thus, when artificial teeth are placed in the same position as the natural teeth, the amount of upper teeth visible will vary for each patient. During a normal smile the incisal and middle thirds of the maxillary anterior teeth are visible in almost all patients and the cervical third in approximately half the patients. The incisal third of the mandibular anterior teeth will be visible in most patients. Mandibular anterior teeth are seen to a greater extent than maxillary anterior teeth in about half the patients during speaking. In addition, mandibular anterior teeth become more visible in persons 40 years of age and older and are seen to a greater extent in men than in women.

A simple test can be used to estimate the length of the upper lip in relation to the residual ridges. The index finger is placed on the incisive papilla with the relaxed upper lip extending down over the finger (Fig. 19-16, *C*). The amount of the finger covered by the upper lip gives an indication of the length of the lip relative to the residual ridge and the extent to which it will cover the upper anterior teeth (Fig. 19-16, *D*). An estimation of the amount of residual ridge resorption must be included in the calculation. Knowing the length of time the natural teeth have been out will help make this estimate.

However, the lower lip is a better guide for the vertical orientation of anterior teeth than the upper lip is. In most patients the incisal edges of the natural lower canines and the cusp tips of the lower first premolars are even with the lower lip at the corners of the mouth when the mouth is slightly open (Fig. 19-17, *A*). If artificial lower anterior teeth are located above or below this level, their vertical positioning will probably be incorrect (Fig. 19-17, *B*). In addition to any changes in position of the lower teeth, the position of the upper teeth and the vertical dimension of occlusion must be considered, because these are all closely interrelated. When the lower teeth are above the lip at the corners of the mouth, any one or a combination of the following may exist: (1) the plane of occlusion may be too high; (2) the vertical overlap of the anterior teeth may be too much; (3) the

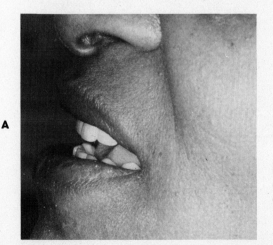

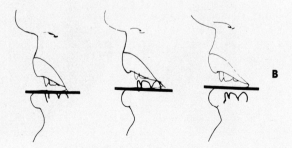

Fig. 19-17   A, Incisal edge of the natural lower canine at the level of the lower lip. **B,** Relationship of artificial lower teeth to the lower lip: *left,* correct height; *middle,* too high; *right,* too low.

vertical space between the jaws may be excessive. When the lower teeth are below the lip at the corners of the mouth, the opposite situations may exist. The use of other observations and guides will help in deciding what corrections should be made.

Observing the size of the trial denture bases can give clues to the vertical orientation of the anterior teeth. In most patients the lower and upper natural teeth occupy approximately the same amount of interarch space. If the dimensions of the lower trial denture, from the border of the base to the incisal edges of the teeth, appear to be significantly different from the same measurements on the upper trial denture, then the plane of occlusion may need to be raised or lowered to make the trial dentures more similar in height (Fig. 19-18). These measurements are made from the incisal edges to the denture borders. The vertical space between the jaws (vertical dimension of occlusion) must also be considered because of its close in-

terrelationship with the plane of occlusion. If there has been more shrinkage from one jaw than from the other, the amounts of base material between the incisal ends of the teeth and the basal surface of the denture may be quite different, even though the overall dimensions are similar.

A study of the location of artificial anterior teeth and their imaginary roots in relation to the residual ridges on the trial denture bases can help determine the position of the teeth. The artificial anterior teeth should be located vertically in the same positions as were previously occupied by the natural teeth. When it appears as though there is not sufficient interarch space to accommodate the upper and lower anterior teeth without significantly reducing their size by grinding, it is well to remember that at one time there was space for the natural teeth, with an adequate interocclusal distance in the patient's mouth. Insufficient space between the residual ridges is an

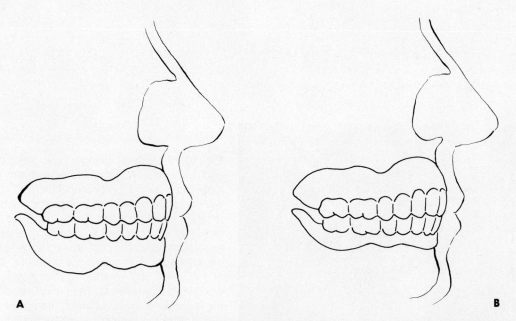

A **B**

Fig. 19-18 **A,** Upper and lower dentures of approximately the same height. **B,** Upper denture considerably larger than the lower. Often this discrepancy in size indicates an incorrect vertical positioning of the artificial teeth.

indication that either the artificial teeth are longer than the natural teeth or the vertical dimension of the face is too short.

Phonetics in the orientation of anterior teeth

Phonetics, the production of speech sounds, can be used as a guide to the positions of teeth. To do this, however, it is necessary to know how the various speech sounds are made. Anterior tooth position is critical to the production of some sounds and not at all to the production of others.

As the teeth are being arranged for esthetics, it is not the speech sound itself that is critical but the interrelationships of the tongue, teeth, denture base, and lips. The sounds made by patients at the time of tryin can never be as accurate as when hard denture base resin has been substituted for the trial bases and the patient has become accustomed to the dentures.

All speech sounds are made by controlled air. The source of the air is the lungs, and the amount and flow of the air are variable. The controls are the various articulations or "valves" made in the pharynx and the oral and nasal cavities. The structures involved in each valve constitute the basis for one classification of speech sounds. The valves for modifying the flow of air to produce speech sounds include (1)

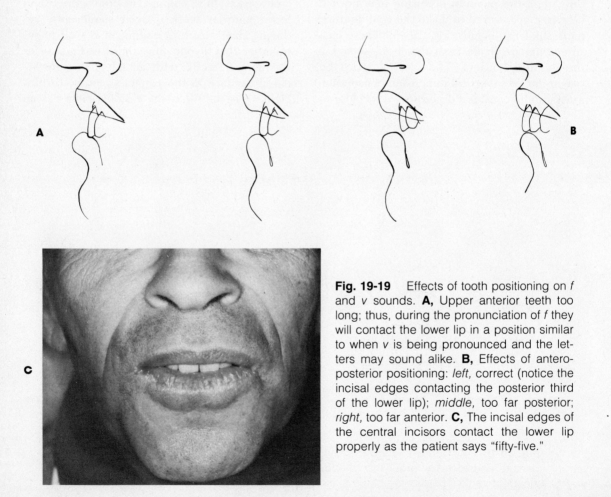

Fig. 19-19   Effects of tooth positioning on *f* and *v* sounds. **A,** Upper anterior teeth too long; thus, during the pronunciation of *f* they will contact the lower lip in a position similar to when *v* is being pronounced and the letters may sound alike. **B,** Effects of anteroposterior positioning: *left,* correct (notice the incisal edges contacting the posterior third of the lower lip); *middle,* too far posterior; *right,* too far anterior. **C,** The incisal edges of the central incisors contact the lower lip properly as the patient says "fifty-five."

the labial, (2) the labiodental, (3) the dental and alveolar (anterior), (4) the palatal, and (5) the velar (posterior). The first four of these groups of sounds can be affected by the position of the teeth.

A voice sound is one that is initiated in the vocal cords (such as vowels *a, e, i, o,* and *u* and the voiced consonants *b, d, g, j, v, m, n, l,* and *r*). The voice sounds may or may not be a part of the sounds produced by the action of the valves. This makes possible the production of at least two speech sounds at each of the valves. Some voice sounds, too, may be made without involving the use of air valves. These are modified when the resonance of the oral and nasal cavities is changed. Changes in resonance can change the sounds produced by some of the air valves.

Labial sounds. The labial sounds *b, p,* and *m* are made at the lips. In *b* and *p* air pressure is built up behind the lips and released with or without a voice sound. Insufficient support of the lips by the teeth and denture base can cause these sounds to be defective. Therefore the anteroposterior position of the anterior teeth and the thickness of the labial flanges of dentures can affect *b* and *p* sounds.

Labiodental sounds. The labiodental sounds *f* and *v* are made between the upper incisors and the labiolingual center to the posterior third of the lower lip. If the upper anterior teeth are too short (set too high up), the *v* sound will be more like an *f*. If they are too long (set too far down), the *f* will sound more like a *v* (Fig. 19-19, *A*).

However, the most important information to be sought while the patient makes these sounds is the relationship of the incisal edges to the lower lip. The dentist should stand alongside the patient and look down at the lower lip and the upper anterior teeth. If the upper teeth touch the labial side of the lower lip while these sounds are made, the upper teeth are too far forward or the lower anterior teeth are too far back in the mouth (Fig. 19-19, *B*). In this situation the relationship of the inside of the lower lip to the labial surfaces of the teeth should be observed while the patient is speaking. If the lower lip drops away from the lower teeth during speech, the lower anterior teeth are most likely too far back in the mouth (Fig. 19-20, *A*). If, on the other hand, imprints of the labial surfaces of the lower anterior teeth are made in the mucous membrane of the lower lip or if the lower lip tends to raise the lower denture, the lower teeth are probably too far forward and this means that the upper teeth are also too far forward (Fig. 19-20, *B*).

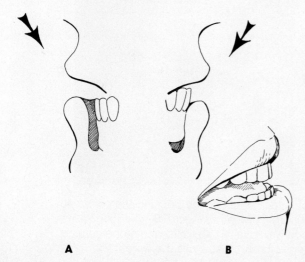

Fig. 19-20   Incorrect positioning of lower anterior teeth. **A,** Too far posterior; a space develops between the lip and the teeth during pronunciation of words containing labiodental sounds. *Arrow* indicates that the observation of this relationship is made by looking down at the lower lip and anterior teeth. **B,** Too far anterior; the lower lip crowds into the lower anterior teeth and may tend to raise the lower denture off the residual ridge during pronunciation of labiodental sounds. *Arrow* again indicates the observation made by looking down.

A   **B**

If the upper anterior teeth are set too far back in the mouth, they will contact the lingual side of the lower lip when *f* and *v* sounds are made. This may occur also if the lower anterior teeth are too far forward in relation to the lower residual ridge. Observing from the side and slightly above the patient will provide the necessary information for determining which changes should be made (see Fig. 19-19, *B*).

Dental and alveolar sounds. Dental sounds (such as *th* in *this*) are made with the tip of the tongue extending slightly between the upper and lower anterior teeth. This sound is actually made closer to the alveolus (the ridge) than to the tip of the teeth. Careful observation of the amount of tongue that can be seen with the words *this, that, these,* and *those* will provide information as to the labiolingual position of the anterior teeth (Fig. 19-21). If about ⅛ inch (3 mm) of the tip of the tongue is not visible, the anterior teeth are probably too far forward (except in patients who had a Class II malocclusion) or there may be an excessive vertical overlap that does not allow sufficient space for the tongue to protrude between the anterior teeth. If more than ¼ inch (6 mm) of the tongue extends out between the teeth when such *th* sounds are made, the teeth are probably too far lingual.

Other alveolar sounds (such as *t, d, n, s,* and *z*) are made with the valve formed by contact of the tip of the tongue with the anteriormost part of the palate (the alveolus) or the lingual side of the anterior teeth. If the teeth are too far lingual, the *t* in *tend* will sound more like a *d*. If they are too far anterior, the *d* will sound more like a *t*. The palate of a denture base that is too thick in the area of the rugae could have the same effect.

The sibilants (*s, z, sh, zh, ch,* and *j* [with *ch* and *j* being affricatives]) are alveolar sounds, because the tongue and alveolus form the controlling valve. The important observation when these sounds are produced is the relationship of the anterior teeth to each other. The upper and lower incisors should approach end to end but not touch. A phrase such as "I went to church to see the judge" will cause the patient to use these critical sounds, and the relative position of the incisal edges will provide a check on the total length of the upper and lower teeth (including their vertical overlap)

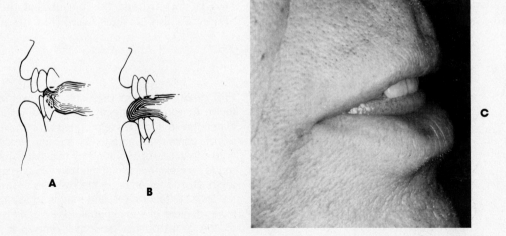

Fig. 19-21 Effects of vertical positioning of anterior teeth on the pronunciation of *th*. **A,** The tongue is prevented from extending properly between the teeth. **B,** The tongue extending between the teeth when they are properly positioned. **C,** Notice the proper tongue position when this patient, wearing complete dentures, pronounces the word *thick*.

(Figs. 19-22 and 19-23, *B*). More important, a failure of the incisal edges to approach exactly end to end indicates a possible error in the amount of horizontal overlap of the anterior teeth (Fig. 19-23). This test will reveal the error but will not indicate whether it is the upper teeth or the lower teeth that are incorrect labiolingually.

The *s* sounds can be considered dental and alveolar speech sounds because they are produced equally well with two different tongue positions, but there can be some variation even behind the alveolus. Most people make the *s* sound with the tip of the tongue against the alveolus in the area of the rugae, with but a small space for air to escape between the tongue and alveolus. The size and shape of this small space will determine the quality of the sound. If the opening is too small, a whistle will result. If the space is too broad and thin, the *s* sound will be developed as an *sh*, somewhat like a lisp. The frequent cause of undesired whistles with dentures is a posterior dental arch form that is too narrow.

A cramped tongue space, especially in the premolar region, forces the dorsal surface of the tongue to form too small an opening for the escape of air. The procedure for correction is to thicken the center of the palate so the tongue does not have to extend up as far into the narrow palatal vault. This allows the escapeway for air to be broad and thin. A lisp with dentures can be corrected when the procedure is reversed and a narrow concentrated airway is provided for the *s* sound.

About one third of patients make the *s* sound with the tip of their tongue contacting the lingual side of the anterior part of the lower denture and arching itself up against the palate to form the desired shape and size of airway. The principles involved in such a palatal valve are identical to those involved in the other tongue positions. However, the lower denture can cause trouble. If the lower anterior teeth are too far back, the tongue will be forced to arch itself up to a higher position and the airway will be too small. If the lingual flange of the lower denture is too thick in the anterior region, the result will be a faulty *s* sound. It can be corrected when the artificial teeth are placed in the same position as the natural teeth occupied and the lingual flange of the lower dentures is so shaped that it does not encroach on the space needed by the tongue.

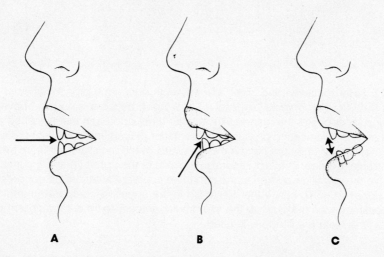

A **B** **C**

Fig. 19-22 Vertical length of anterior teeth during the pronunciation of sibilants: **A,** correct; **B,** excessive vertical overlap; **C,** inadequate vertical overlap.

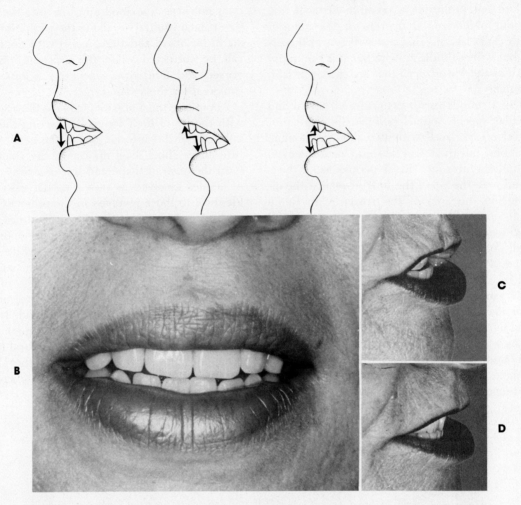

Fig. 19-23   Horizontal overlap of the anterior teeth during the pronunciation of sibilants. **A** shows *(left)* correct, *(middle)* excessive, and *(right)* deficient amounts of overlapping. In **B** the incisal edges of the mandibular anterior teeth approach the incisal edges of the maxillary anteriors, indicating proper anteroposterior placement for sibilant pronunciation. In **C** the mandibular anteriors have moved forward of the maxillary anteriors, with insufficient horizontal overlap. The lack of tone in the skin of the upper lip and the small vertical lines above the vermilion border suggest that the maxillary anteriors do not properly support the upper lip. In **D**, notice the difference in the upper lip compared to that in **C** and the relationship of the maxillary to the mandibular anterior teeth during sibilant pronunciation when the teeth are properly located.

Palatal and velar sounds. The truly palatal sounds (such as those in *year, she, vision,* and *onion*) present less of a problem for dentures. The velar sounds *(k, g,* and *ng)* have no effect on dentures.

Patient adaptations in phonetics. It is obvious that denture bases and the positions of teeth can affect the production of speech sounds, but fortunately people learn to adapt their speaking habits to correct errors that may be caused by faulty tooth placement in dentures. For this reason speech sounds are not a safe guide to tooth positions. The safe guide is to observe carefully the relationships of the lips and tongue to the teeth and the denture bases when certain sounds are made.

With these observations the patient should be encouraged to speak normally and not attempt to overcome any speech difficulty. When patients are aware of the dentist's real objective, they find it difficult to move the mouth normally. Dentists should watch the lips and tongue, paying minimal attention to the sounds of speech, to get the most information about tooth position from phonetics.

Fortunately, the relation of teeth and denture base surfaces to the production of sounds and the retention of dentures can be variable and yet not cause serious speech interferences. This variability is tolerated because patient adaptability in phonetics is unusual. If this were not true, it is doubtful whether any patients wearing complete dentures would ever be able to articulate and enunciate properly. On the other hand, the more nearly duplicated conditions are as regards the structures of the oral cavity, the better the speech of the denture patient will be. Functional contouring of the polished surface of the palate of the maxillary denture with mouth-temperature wax is an example of simulating previous conditions that can improve the speech of the patient.

Inclination of the anterior teeth

In some patients the upper anterior teeth are inclined labially relative to the frontal plane when the head is erect (Frankfort plane parallel to the floor). In others they are inclined more lingually (Fig. 19-24, *A*). Diagnostic casts, photographs, and what the patient remembers about the "slant of the upper front teeth" can help solve the problem concerning the inclination of the natural teeth.

A study of teeth in human skulls indicates that the roots of the anterior teeth are parallel to and very close to the labial surface of the bone. Usually there is an obtuse angle between the bone and the labial surfaces of the teeth. In some skulls the labial surfaces of the teeth are parallel to the bone but also slope labialward. When the labial surfaces are curved from cervical to incisal, the cervical third may appear to be continuous with the inclination of the labial plate of bone (Fig. 19-24, *B*). Diagnostic casts support this premise. When the natural teeth are removed with no unnecessary surgery, the original inclination of the labial plate of bone is preserved and will remain until considerable resorption has occurred, thus providing a guide to the inclination of the anterior teeth (Fig. 19-24, *C*). The inclination of the labial surface of the residual ridges as seen on edentulous casts can supply this information.

The profile form of the patient's face is often representative of the natural anterior tooth inclination within the oral cavity. The lips supply the pressures from the outside that help determine the anteroposterior position and inclination of the anterior teeth. Thus it is logical to assume that the inclination of the anterior teeth parallels the profile line of the face (Fig. 19-25). Suggestions for individual tooth position to provide harmony between the inclination of the teeth and the profile line of the face are described later in this chapter (p. 413).

Harmony in the general composition of anterior teeth

A number of factors are interrelated in the general composition of the anterior teeth for a normal and pleasing appearance. Although these factors vary among patients, there is suf-

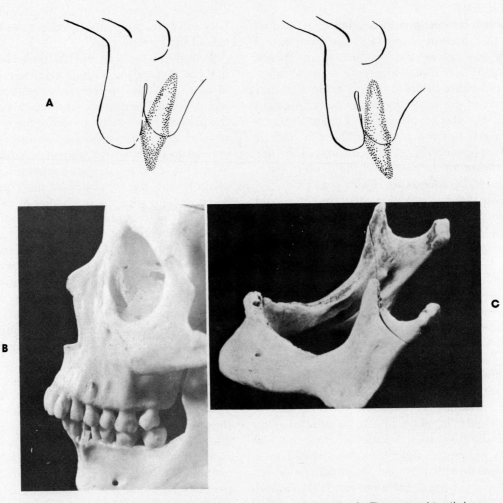

Fig. 19-24   Labial and lingual inclination of the anterior teeth. **A,** The natural teeth have varying degrees of inclination. **B,** Notice the inclination and position of the anterior teeth in relation to the inclination of the labial plate of bone. **C,** The inclination of this lower residual ridge provides the information that the lower anterior teeth, which it once supported, had a labial inclination.

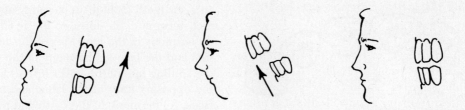

Fig. 19-25   The inclination of anterior teeth often parallels the profile line of the lower third of the face.

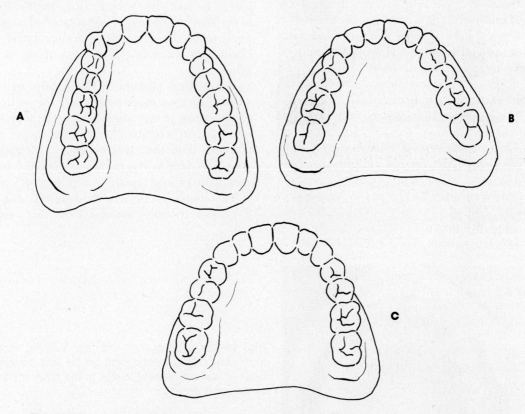

Fig. 19-26   Varying shapes of the natural dental arch: **A,** square; **B,** tapering; **C,** ovoid.

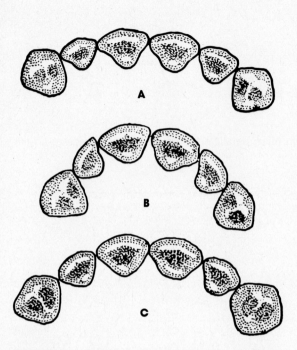

Fig. 19-27 Anterior arch forms: **A,** square; **B,** tapering; **C,** ovoid.

ficient constancy to warrant individual attention. The topics to be discussed in providing harmony within the general composition of the anterior teeth include (a) harmony of the dental arch form and the form of the residual ridge, (b) harmony of the long axes of the central incisors and the face, (c) harmony of the teeth with the smiling line of the lower lip, (d) harmony of the opposing lines of the labial and buccal surfaces, (e) harmony of the teeth and profile line, and (f) harmony of incisal wear and age.

Harmony of the dental arch form and form of the residual ridge. The anterior arches may be classified in a general way as square, tapering, and ovoid, to follow the form of the dental arch when the teeth are present (Fig. 19-26). However, they cannot be closely classified as such because of the frequent intermingling of the characteristics of one form with those of another.

The central incisors in the square arch assume a position more nearly on a line with the canines than in any other setup. The four incisors have little rotation because the square arch is wider than the tapering arch. This gives a broader effect to the teeth and should harmonize with a broad square face (Fig. 19-27, A).

The central incisors in the tapering arch are a greater distance forward from the canines

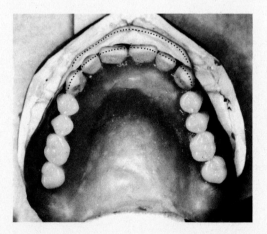

Fig. 19-28 *Dotted lines* indicate that the arch form of artificial anterior teeth on the trial denture base is basically similar to that of the anterior part of the residual ridge.

than in any other arch. There is usually considerable rotating and lapping of the teeth in the tapering arch because of less space. Therefore crowding results. The rotated positions reduce the amount of tooth surface showing, and the teeth do not appear as wide as in other setups. This narrowed effect is usually in harmony with a narrower tapering face (Fig. 19-27, *B*). In fact, the very narrowness of the tapered arch contributes to the narrowness and taper of the face. Natural teeth move in function, and this frictional movement wears the contact areas. Artificial teeth need to be ground on these corresponding contact areas to allow the necessary rotational positions and give the desired effect of a tapering setup.

The central incisors in the ovoid arch are forward of the canines in a position between that of the square and that of the tapering arch. The teeth in this form of arch are seldom rotated, and they therefore show a greater amount of labial surface than in the tapering setup and, as a result, have a broader effect that should harmonize with an ovoid face (Fig. 19-27, *C*).

The form of the palatal vault gives an indication as to the original form of the dental arch before removal of the natural teeth and resorption of the residual ridge. A broad and shallow edentulous palatal vault indicates that the dental arch form originally may have been square; a high V-shaped edentulous vault probably indicates a tapering dental arch; a rounded vault of average height may indicate an ovoid dental arch. Most patients exhibit some combination of these classifications.

The arch form of the artificial anterior teeth should be similar in shape to the arch form of the residual ridge, if one assumes there was no unnecessary surgery when the anterior teeth were removed (Fig. 19-28). This simple anatomic fact is often neglected, but it should be observed carefully. When the anterior teeth are arranged in an arch form that corresponds to the form of the residual ridge, often natural-appearing irregularities that may have been present in the patient's mouth will be reproduced.

Changing the shape and position of the artificial dental arch away from the form of the natural arch causes a highly unsatisfactory loss of face form and expression. A square arch form where the natural arch was more tapering will cause a stretching of the lips, with elimination of the natural philtrum. A tapering arch form where the natural dental arch was square will not adequately support the corners of the mouth for proper facial expressions.

The shape and position of the dental arch de-

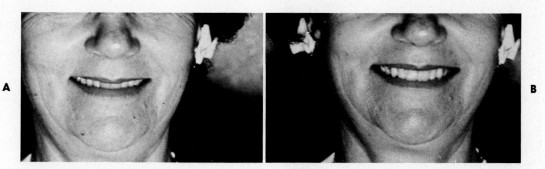

Fig. 19-29 **A,** Buccal corridor inadequate because of improper placement of the upper teeth. **B,** Anterior teeth in proper position to support the upper lip. Notice the adequate buccal corridor.

termine the size of the buccal corridor. The buccal corridor is the space between the buccal surfaces of the upper teeth and the corners of the mouth visible when the patient smiles. It varies considerably among patients, and its size is not critical. However, the presence of the buccal corridor helps eliminate an appearance of too many teeth in the front of the mouth. When the arch form of the posterior teeth is

too wide or the lips do not move to their full extent during smiling because of improper support, the size of the buccal corridor will be reduced or perhaps eliminated (Fig. 19-29).

Patients may request a change in the position or form of their dental arch, but the dentist should not compromise on this point because the unfavorable consequences can be laid to no one else.

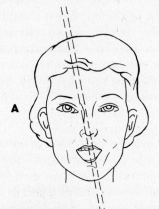
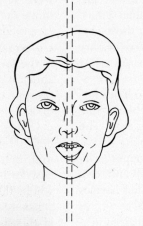
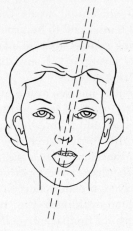

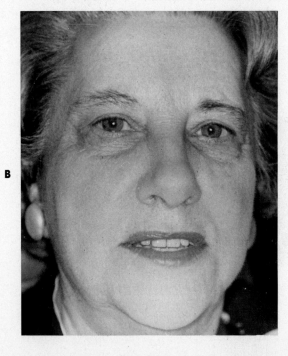

Fig. 19-30 The long axes of the central incisors should be parallel to the long axis of the face. **A,** The *middle drawing* shows that such parallelism provides a necessary harmony of lines. Notice the disharmony on the *left* and *right*. **B,** The long axes of artificial central incisors have been correctly aligned.

Harmony of the long axes of the central incisors and face. One of the early observations that should be made in developing the arrangement of anterior teeth for the individual patient is the relationship of the long axes of the central incisors to the long axis of the face. When the long axes of these teeth are not in harmony with the long axis of the face, the arrangement will not blend with the face because the incisal plane of the anterior teeth will not be parallel to the interpupillary line (Fig. 19-30, A). This will cause an unpleasant disharmony of lines. It is a simple task to reset the central incisors to make their long axes harmonize with the long axis of the face (Fig. 19-30, B). If the central incisors must be divergent at their incisal edges, the midline of the dental arch should be at the center of the face. Then the lateral incisors and canines will almost automatically fall into their proper alignment and the incisal plane will be in balance with the interpupillary line.

The long axes of the central incisors should be parallel to the long axis of the face, and the midline of the dental arch (the contact area between the central incisors) should be located near the middle of the face. This is determined by dropping an imaginary perpendicular from the midpoint on the interpupillary line. The midline position of the natural central incisors can be estimated also by observing the position of the incisive papilla on the cast and the corresponding fossa in the upper trial denture base, since the incisive papilla was located lingually and between the natural upper central incisors before their extraction.

The midline of the mandibular dental arch is between the central incisors and is usually aligned with the midline of the maxillary central incisors. When the lower anterior teeth are correctly located anatomically in the lower dental arch, an imaginary line drawn anteroposteriorly through the middle of the lower denture should pass between the lower central incisors (Fig. 19-31). The maxillary and mandibular midlines fail to coincide in most adults with natural teeth, however, so the prosthodontist must attempt to set the artificial teeth to coincide with this imaginary midline.

The application of these principles regarding the placement of central incisors and their inclinations may be modified to meet individual needs as indicated by preextraction records.

Harmony of the teeth with the smiling line of the lower lip. When a person smiles, the lower lip forms a pleasant curvature known as the smiling line. This can be used as a guide in arranging the upper anterior teeth.

When the line formed by the incisal edges of the upper anterior teeth follows the curved line of the lower lip during smiling, the two lines will be harmonious and will create a pleasing appearance. When the incisal edges of the upper anterior teeth form a curved line that is not in harmony with, or is opposite in contour to, the line formed by the lower lip during a smile, the contrast of the lines is disharmonious and will be displeasing in appearance (Fig. 19-32, A).

The vertical position of the upper canines is primarily responsible for the shape of the smiling line. When the canines are so arranged that their incisal edges are slightly shorter than the

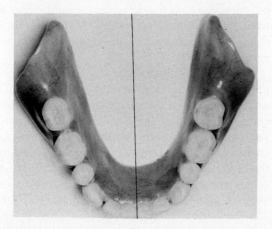

Fig. 19-31 Lower anterior teeth correctly positioned, as shown by the *imaginary line* passing through the middle of this lower denture between the lower central incisors.

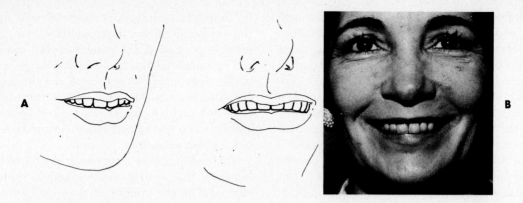

Fig. 19-32 Harmony of the line formed by the incisal edges of the upper anterior teeth with that formed by the curvature of the lower lip. **A,** Lines in harmony *(left)* and not in harmony *(right)*. Results are a pleasing and a displeasing appearance. **B,** Notice the harmony in this face.

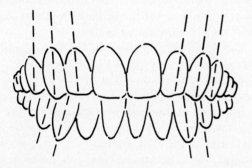

Fig. 19-33 Balanced opposing lines. Dissimilarities in the inclination, rotation, and position of the teeth on each side of the midline provide what is called asymmetric symmetry, which is essential for natural-appearing teeth.

incisal edges of the lateral incisors, the smiling line will tend to parallel the lower lip as the patient smiles (Fig. 19-32, *B*). A reverse smiling line is one of the most frequent causes of artificial-appearing dentures.

Harmony of the opposing lines of labial and buccal surfaces. Setting teeth with their long axes parallel to each other is what causes people to dread complete dentures, because the appearance is artificial. Many patients are sub-

consciously irritated by this artificial appearance of dentures and tend to find other faults with them that would otherwise be overlooked.

A well-balanced painting or drawing must have lines at opposing angles as well as some parallel lines. The same principle applies to having a pleasing picture of the teeth. For example, if the teeth on both sides of the arch were inclined to be parallel to each other, they would make a most unsatisfactory-appearing denture. There should be asymmetric symmetry in the arrangement of the teeth (Fig. 19-33).

The labial and buccal lines must have opposing equivalent angles, or nearly so, for a harmonious effect. If the maxillary right lateral incisor is set at an angle of 5 degrees to the perpendicular, the lateral incisor on the left side should be set 5 degrees to the perpendicular in the opposite direction. The scheme of opposing angles can be carried to the maxillary canines and the mandibular opposing canines (Fig. 19-33). Deviation in angulation may also be arranged in different teeth on the two sides. Extra inclination of a lateral incisor on one side may be balanced by inclination of the opposite canine; asymmetric symmetry is the objective.

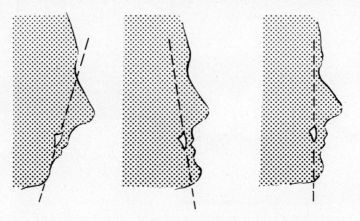

Fig. 19-34   The labial face of the central incisor parallels the profile line of the face. Notice how the incisal third of the tooth breaks lingually from the profile line.

There should be harmony between the labial and buccal lines of the teeth and the lines of the face. Square and ovoid faces should have teeth with lines that are more nearly perpendicular whereas tapering faces should have teeth with lines that are more divergent from the perpendicular.

An optical illusion may be created for patients who have a nasal deflection. Four of the maxillary teeth can be set at an opposite angle to the deviation, making it less apparent.

Harmony of the teeth and profile line of the face. As a general rule the labial surfaces of the maxillary central incisors are parallel to the profile line of the face. In prognathic patients with protruding mandibular incisors, the incisal edges of the maxillary teeth are out farther than the cervical ends of the teeth. In the opposite condition (in which the mandibular incisors are retruded to some extent), the incisal edges of the maxillary teeth are inclined lingually more than the cervical ends of the teeth (Fig. 19-34).

When the labial of the maxillary central incisors is parallel to the profile line of the face, the lateral incisors should be set at an opposite angle to prevent parallelism from being predominant. For example, in a patient with retrognathic jaw relations whose maxillary central incisors are out at the cervical ends, the lateral incisors could then be depressed at their cervical ends to oppose the line made by the labial surfaces of the central incisors. For the prognathic patient the incisal edges of the maxillary central incisors often are set labially. The maxillary lateral incisors could then be placed slightly out at the cervical ends to oppose the labial face line of the central incisors.

Most faces are a blend of two or three types of profiles. Arrangement of teeth for a harmonious appearance must be modified accordingly. The predominating facial form can be helpful as a guide for positioning the teeth.

Harmony of incisal wear and age. The incisal edges and proximal surfaces of anterior teeth wear concomitantly with age. This is another characteristic of natural teeth that must be incorporated in artificial teeth if they are to appear in harmony with the age of the patient. The incisal edges of denture teeth should *always* be ground to simulate the wear surfaces that would have developed by the time the patient reached his current age. Thus a young patient would likely exhibit less incisal wear (Fig.

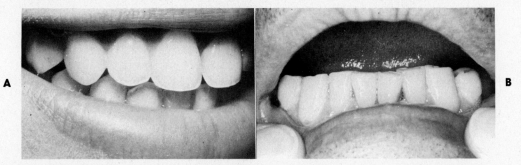

Fig. 19-35 The amount of wear on the incisal edges of anterior teeth should concur with the patient's age. **A,** Lack of wear is compatible with youth. **B,** Extreme wear indicates a much older person.

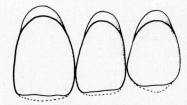

Fig. 19-36 A simple sketch by the dentist of the outline form of artificial teeth will be helpful in planning the incisal wear to be incorporated for a particular patient. *Dotted line* shows the original appearance of the incisal edges of artificial teeth; *solid line,* the incisal wear anticipated.

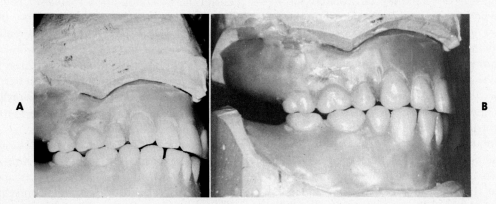

Fig. 19-37 **A,** Incisal wear on artificial anterior teeth. **B,** The pattern of wear in **A** has been developed to improve the appearance of the denture and assist in balancing the occlusion. Wear on the upper canine is placed to correspond with wear on the lower canine in a balanced occlusion.

19-35, *A*) and an older one more wear (Fig. 19-35, *B*).

A sketch of the anticipated pattern of wear to be placed on the incisal edges of anterior teeth can be beneficial. The outline form of the artificial teeth is sketched on a piece of paper, and the anticipated changes that are to be created to simulate wear on the incisal edges are depicted on the drawing (Fig. 19-36). In general, more lingually placed upper teeth or parts of teeth will wear increasingly whereas more labially placed upper teeth will wear somewhat less. The greatest amount of wear on the lower anterior teeth or parts of teeth will occur in the more anteriorly placed lower teeth. The simulation of wear on anterior teeth should be logically in harmony with the way it occurs when the upper and lower teeth pass over each other.

Developing incisal wear on artificial teeth during balancing and correcting of the occlusion is a logical approach to this phase of esthetics. Thus wear is placed on the teeth where it would have occurred during function and also where it assists in the mechanics of balancing the occlusion (Fig. 19-37).

The effect that the form of the tooth creates can be dramatically altered by reshaping the tooth to simulate wear. The same mold of anterior teeth can be altered to help create a young, soft, feminine appearance for one patient or an older, vigorous, masculine appearance for another (Fig. 19-38, *A*).

Most patients who need dentures are at an age

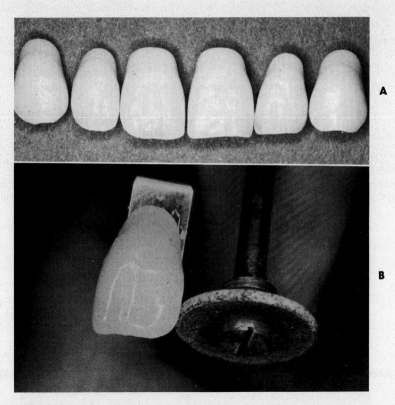

Fig. 19-38   A, One mold of teeth has been modified so the three teeth on the left depict youth and femininity while the three on the right are suitable for an older masculine individual. **B,** The contact areas and incisal edges of artificial teeth must be modified to provide a natural appearance.

when the contact areas of their natural teeth have been worn, whether or not the teeth overlap each other. Therefore the artificial teeth should be so altered that they do not have the appearance of ball contact points with large interproximal spaces. If the teeth selected have contact points that resemble those of a young person's teeth, they should be ground to provide a more natural appearance (Fig. 19-38, *B*).

Refinement of individual tooth positions

One of the essential factors in satisfying patients with complete dentures is that the dentures be pleasing and natural in appearance. Dentures are not pleasing unless the teeth are arranged in a plan that nature developed (Lombardi, 1973). If patients have some anterior teeth remaining, diagnostic casts should be made as preextraction records to be used in selecting and arranging the individual teeth. If dentists use preextraction records in construction of many dentures, they soon will learn nature's scheme in arranging teeth for patients who have lost all teeth before a record was made. With patients for whom no preextraction records are available, dentists can select another cast of natural teeth and follow this arrangement as a guide.

The selection and placing of artificial teeth will not appear natural unless the teeth are set with typical inclinations and rotations that the

eye has been accustomed to seeing. These inclinations and rotations can cause the same teeth to appear as oversized or normal. For example, if the canine is rotated so the eye sees only its mesial half, the tooth will look only half as large as it would if its entire labial surface were visible to the eye. Lateral and central incisors, especially in a tapering setup, do not show the entire labial surface when seen from directly in front. This reduction in the amount of surface showing harmonizes with a tapering face.

A beginning point for studying the labiolingual inclination of the maxillary anterior teeth in relation to the perpendicular is shown in Fig. 19-39. The labial surface of the maxillary central incisor is parallel to the profile line of the face, which is almost perpendicular. The labial surface of the lateral incisor is angled in at the cervical end more than that of the adjacent tooth. The labial surface of the canine is angled out at the cervical end more than that of any other maxillary anterior tooth. The degree to which the cervical end of the canine extends outward usually harmonizes with the lateral lines of the face. The labial surface of the mandibular central incisor is in at the cervical end more than the labial of the lateral incisor or canine is. The mandibular lateral incisor is out at its cervical end more than the central incisor, so as to be almost perpendicular. The mandibular canine is out at its cervical end to the same

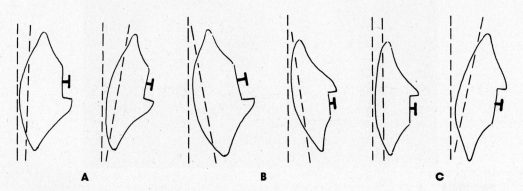

A   B   C

Fig. 19-39   Normal labiolingual inclinations of anterior teeth relative to the perpendicular. **A,** Central incisor; **B,** lateral incisor; **C,** canine.

degree as the maxillary canine, except at an opposite angle. The labiolingual inclinations of maxillary anterior teeth are intended to serve only as *guidelines* from which variations must be made if the individual patient's teeth are to appear natural.

A beginning point for studying the anterior teeth from the labial aspect in their mesiodistal inclination is shown in Fig. 19-40. The maxillary and mandibular central incisors are almost perpendicular whereas the laterals are inclined distally at their cervical ends more than any other anterior tooth. The canines are inclined toward the distal at their cervical ends more than the central and less than the lateral incisors are.

A beginning point for studying the rotational positions of the anterior teeth from an incisal aspect is shown in Fig. 19-41. The maxillary central incisor is slightly rotated from parallelism with the line of arch contour. The lateral incisor is rotated so its distal surface is turned lingually a considerable angle from the line of arch contour. The canine is rotated so the distal half of its labial surface points in the direction of the posterior arch. The mandibular incisors have a rotational position that generally parallels the arch contour.

A beginning point for studying the superoinferior position of the six anterior teeth in relation to the incisal plane is shown in Fig. 19-42. The maxillary lateral incisor and canine are slightly above the level of the incisal plane.

All these positions of anterior teeth from the various aspects serve only as beginning points and must be varied into harmonious irregularities that are not foreign to any that nature has established. For example, a maxillary canine is seldom in at the cervical end and will appear completely artificial if this irregularity is attempted. The patient cannot point out the exact cause of the unnaturalness but will be aware that something is wrong. Although these are the beginning positions for studying teeth in ideal alignment, dentures with teeth set precisely in these positions will also look artificial.

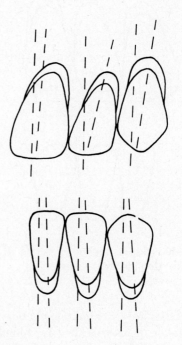

Fig. 19-40 Mesiodistal inclination of anterior teeth relative to the perpendicular.

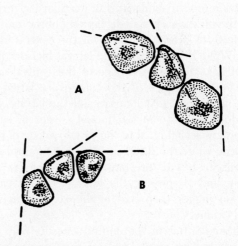

Fig. 19-41 Incisal views of anterior teeth showing their angle of rotation. **A,** Maxillary and, **B,** mandibular.

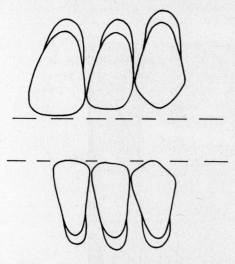

Fig. 19-42 Superoinferior positions of anterior teeth relative to the incisal plane.

Irregularities are essential to esthetics.

A number of irregularities are found so frequently that they appear natural when reproduced. To reduce the artificiality of dentures, it is well for the dentist to make the teeth somewhat irregular. When this is done, a study of the common irregularities of maxillary anterior teeth will show (1) a slight lapping of the mesial surfaces of lateral incisors over the central incisors, (2) a depressing of the lateral incisors lingually so the distal surface of the central and the mesial surface of the canine are labial to the mesial and distal surfaces of the lateral, (3) a rotating of the mesial incisal corner of each lateral incisor lingual to the distal surface of the central while the distal surface of the lateral remains flush with the mesial surface of the canine, and (4) placing the incisal edge of each lateral higher than that of the central incisor and canine.

Irregularities of the central incisors may be developed by overlapping of the labial incisal angle of one central incisor on the adjacent central incisor, by placing one central incisor slightly lingual to the other central incisor without rotation, and by placing one central slightly labial to and longer than the other.

The maxillary canine may be placed labially in the dental arch, giving this tooth considerable prominence. However, the canine must maintain a rotational position that does not expose the distal half of its labial surface to the eye when viewed from immediately in front. The canine must never be depressed at its cervical end. Rather, its labial surface should be more or less parallel to the side of the face when viewed from the front.

The mandibular anterior teeth can be made slightly irregular, with much effectiveness, if the irregularities are harmonious with nature's frequent irregularities. A setup that decreases the artificial appearance is one in which both central incisors are forward and rotated mesially, one or both lateral incisors are lingual to the arch curve and slightly longer than the adjacent teeth, and the mesial surfaces of the canines overlap the distal surfaces of the lateral incisors (Fig. 19-43).

To overlap teeth in rotational positions and at the same time avoid excessive labiolingual irregularities, the lingual side of the proximal surface of the overlapping tooth must be ground. The overlapping contacts in natural teeth have been worn by the movement of the teeth on their contact points in function. Therefore, to simulate worn natural overlapping, the dentist must grind the more labially placed of two overlapped teeth on its lingual contact area.

Harmony of spaces and individual tooth position. The use of spaces between teeth can be effective for emphasizing individual tooth positions and creating a natural-appearing arrangement of teeth. A space is not usually desirable between the upper central incisors unless one existed between the natural teeth. Even then, if the space was large, a smaller space in the denture can create a similar effect and be more pleasing (Fig. 19-44, *A*). Spaces between central and lateral incisors, between lateral inci-

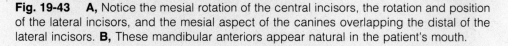

Fig. 19-43   A, Notice the mesial rotation of the central incisors, the rotation and position of the lateral incisors, and the mesial aspect of the canines overlapping the distal of the lateral incisors. **B,** These mandibular anteriors appear natural in the patient's mouth.

sors and canines, and between canines and pre-molars are effective irregularities that are visible, particularly when seen from the side (Fig. 19-44, *B* and *C*). The location of spaces should be chosen carefully to maintain proper balance in the overall composition. Spaces must be designed so they can be self-cleansing.

Concept of harmony with sex, personality, and age of the patient

Frush and Fisher have stated that "creating the illusion of natural teeth in artificial dentures . . . is based on the elementary factors suggested by the sex, personality, and age of the patient." Femininity is characterized by curved surfaces, roundness and softness in the form of the dentition, and a prominent smiling-line alignment of the anterior teeth. Masculinity is characterized by boldness, vigor, and squareness in the dentition and a straightness of the incisal line of teeth. The personality spectrum is divided into delicate, medium, and vigorous, with connotations of personality variations in the masculine or feminine classifications. It is related to the molds, colors, position of teeth, and form of the supporting matrix for the teeth. Age is depicted in dentures by worn incisal edges, erosion, spaces between teeth,

and variations in the form of the matrix around the cervical end of a tooth (Frush and Fisher, 1956ab, 1957, 1958).

Individual tooth form and position also are related to these concepts. The size and position of the central incisors dominate the arrangement of the six upper anterior teeth. Rotation of the distal surfaces anteriorly and placement of one central incisor bodily ahead of the other make the appearance of these teeth more vigorous (Fig. 19-45, *A*). Smaller lateral incisors with rounded incisal angles appear more feminine than larger ones (Fig. 19-45, *B*). Rotation of the lateral incisors will harden or soften the composition. Canines are positioned to complete the smiling line, rotated so their mesial surface faces anteriorly, abraded according to physiologic age, set with the cervical end out, and aligned with the long axis in a vertical direction when viewed from the side (Fig. 19-45, *C*).

The concept of the influence of sex, personality, and age provides additional information for developing harmony between the composition of tooth arrangement and the patient. Dentists must take full advantage of all concepts to create dentures that restore the natural appearance of their patients (Fig. 19-46).

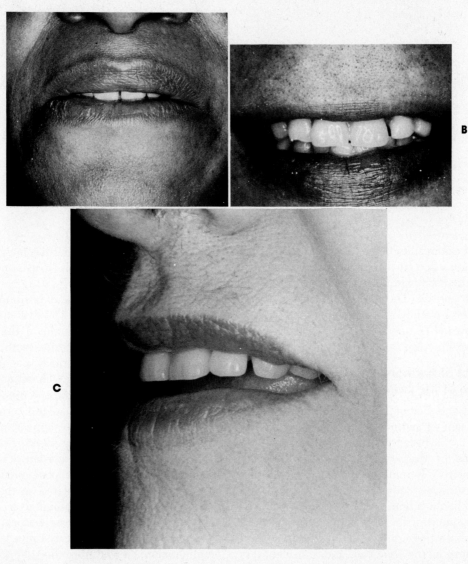

Fig. 19-44 **A,** Space between the upper central incisors can be effective in maintaining the identity of a patient if it was present between the natural central incisors. **B,** Space between the central and lateral incisors helps create a natural appearance in the arrangement of artificial anterior teeth. **C,** Space between the lateral incisor and canine provides a good esthetic effect when seen from the side. However, it is not visible when seen from the front. (Compare with Fig. 19-30, *B.*)

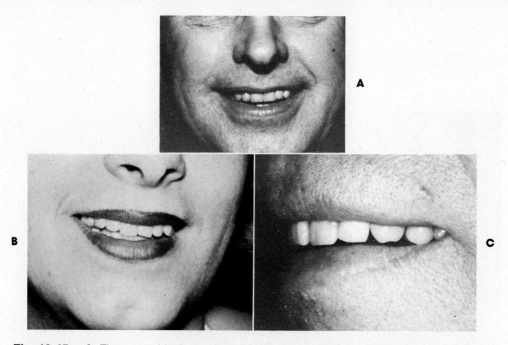

Fig. 19-45   A, The central incisors dominate this arrangement of artificial anterior teeth. **B,** The rounded incisal edges and relative sizes of the upper lateral incisors provide a composition that is feminine in appearance. **C,** Notice the location of the upper left canine relative to the smiling line. Wear on this tooth is compatible with the patient's age. Notice also the anteriorly facing mesial surface and the vertical long axis of this tooth.

Correlating esthetics and incisal guidance

The best plan of occlusion to enhance stability of complete dentures is one with a shallow incisal guidance inclination. The reduction in vertical overlap of the anterior teeth may detract from the appearance of dentures because it is likely to place the maxillary anterior teeth too high or the mandibular anterior teeth too low in the oral orifice. The simplest way to overcome this difficulty and still maintain a pleasing esthetic appearance would be to increase the horizontal overlap (Fig. 19-47). However, if this is done, the lip support or the occlusal vertical dimension will be changed. These procedures may not be feasible if the esthetics and mechanics are to be protected.

The dentist can reduce the vertical overlap of anterior teeth by increasing the interridge distance. However, this must not be done to the extent that it would encroach on the interocclusal distance. A compromise involves slightly shortening the upper and lower canines while maintaining the full length of the incisors. In this situation, occlusal balance in the protrusive position may not be possible, although it can be achieved in the lateral occlusions. Protrusive balance is less important than lateral balance because incision is performed consciously. The patient can control the amount and direction of force applied when biting into food. On the other hand, chewing is done at a subconscious level. Patients do not

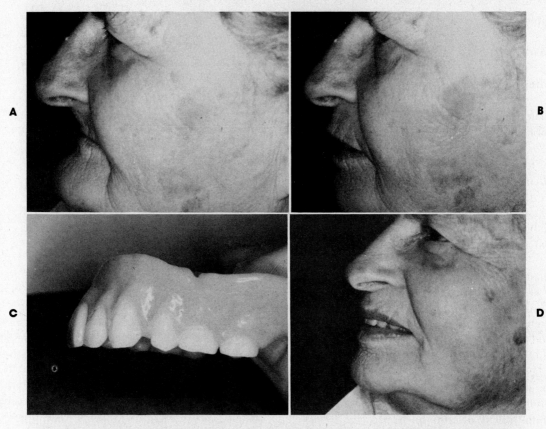

Fig. 19-46 **A,** Total lack of support of a patient's face. Notice the prominent chin. **B,** The lips have been restored to a natural position, accompanied by an improved appearance of the chin and restoration of the mentolabial sulcus. **C,** The upper anterior teeth are arranged on an incline relative to the upper lip. Notice their distance in front of the residual alveolar ridge. **D,** The lips move naturally because the muscles that control facial expression have been restored to their proper physiologic length. The teeth also appear natural because of their correct size, form, color, and arrangement.

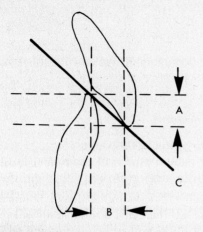

Fig. 19-47 Vertical, *A*, and horizontal, *B*, overlaps. *C*, Incisal guidance angle.

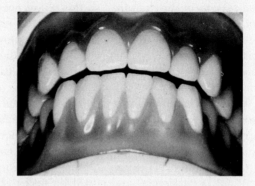

Fig. 19-48 Opposing anterior teeth should not contact when the posterior teeth are in CO.

think of the amount and direction of the force they apply. Consequently they cannot protect themselves from forces that would dislodge their dentures. The angle of incisal guidance for lateral occlusion must be adjusted so the posterior teeth contact at the same time that the upper and lower canines are end to end.

Even when the vertical overlap of the anterior teeth must be severe for proper esthetics, the opposing anterior teeth should not be in contact when the posterior teeth are in centric occlusion (Fig. 19-48). Such contact will eventually cause excess pressures from occlusion of the anterior teeth when the residual ridges resorb and the vertical dimension of occlusion is decreased. Excessive force usually cannot be tolerated by the anterior part of the residual ridges and will likely cause increased resorption of bone and development of hyperplastic tissue in this region.

PATIENT ACCEPTANCE OF THE ARRANGEMENT OF ANTERIOR TEETH

Patients must be given the opportunity to observe and approve the final arrangement of the anterior teeth at the tryin appointment.

The dentures should not be completed until approval is obtained. Even when patients indicate that they "do not care how their teeth look," they must be given full opportunity to inspect and approve the arrangement. These patients often become extremely concerned with their appearance when they begin to wear the dentures.

Patients should not be permitted to observe the trial dentures in the mouth until the dentist is satisfied with the composition as it is created. The premolars should be in the proper arch form, and the wax denture bases should be carved to approximate the final form. Initial reactions of patients can be long-lasting, and an unsatisfactory reaction to a partially completed arrangement of anterior teeth may cause continued problems even though the final appearance of the dentures is perfectly satisfactory.

Since the dentures will be seen most often by other people during normal conversation, patients should first observe themselves in this situation. The patient is positioned 3 to 4 feet (1 to 1.3 m) in front of a large mirror with the trial dentures in the mouth and given the opportunity to observe the dentures during normal conversation and facial expression. The reaction at this time can be critical to the eventual success of the dentures, so this phase must not be done hurriedly or haphazardly. The patient should be encouraged to bring the most critical family member or friend with him/her to assist in evaluating the appearance of the trial dentures.

The dentist should listen carefully to all comments made by the patient and never dismiss any of them as silly or of no consequence. Some changes that the patient may suggest can be incorporated. However, other suggestions may not be advisable, and it will be necessary to explain that they are not anatomically feasible but would prevent the muscles in the cheeks and lips from properly moving the face. Many patients will be pleased with the appearance of the dentures and request few, if any, changes when the position of the artificial teeth approximates that of the natural teeth.

When the dentist and staff and the patient and any critical friends are satisfied with the appearance, it is helpful to have the patient sign a statement that will be placed in the patient's chart as follows:

I have been given the opportunity of looking at the final arrangement of the artificial teeth (while positioned in wax). Any necessary changes have been made and I am happy with the general appearance of the dentures.

This protects the dentist against the occasional patient who will claim that he/she was not given the opportunity to view the teeth while arranged in wax or that the requested changes were not done.

BIBLIOGRAPHY

Frush JP, Fisher RD: How dentogenic restorations interpret the sex factor, J Prosthet Dent 6:160-172, 1956a.

Frush JP, Fisher RD: How dentogenics interprets the personality factor, J Prosthet Dent 6:441-449, 1956b.

Frush JP, Fisher RD: Age factor in dentogenics, J Prosthet Dent 7:5-13, 1957.

Frush JP, Fisher RD: The dynesthetic interpretation of the dentogenic concept, J Prosthet Dent 8:558-581, 1958.

Lombardi RE: The principles of visual perception and their clinical application to denture esthetics, J Prosthet Dent 29:358-382, 1973.

CHAPTER 20

Completion of the tryin: eccentric jaw relation records, articulator and cast adjustment, establishing the posterior palatal seal

When the final occlusion is developed and corrected on the articulator, it is essential that the movements of the articulator simulate mandibular positions or movements of the patient within the range of normal functional contacts of teeth. Thus the condylar elements of the articulator must be so adjusted that they approximate the condylar-guiding factors within the temporomandibular joints. These adjustments of the condylar elements of the articulator are made by means of interocclusal eccentric records.

PROTRUSIVE AND LATERAL RELATIONS

There seems to be confusion in the minds of many dentists as to what a protrusive registration is intended to attain. The idea that the angle and lines of the bony fossa completely govern the path of the condyle is erroneous. A study of the anatomy and function of the joint reveals the fact that the condylar path is governed partly in its shape and function by the meniscus. The meniscus is attached in part to the lateral pterygoid and moves forward during opening and lateral mandibular movements. The path is controlled further by the shape of the fossa, the attachments of the ligaments, the biting load during movement (muscular influence), and the amount of protrusion. Variation in registrations can be caused by several factors. The registration may vary according to the biting pressure exerted after the mandible has

been protruded. The condyle, not being locked on a path, is subject to change in its path with a variation of pressure. Undoubtedly, there is some leeway for adaptability to conform with the changing conditions of the teeth. Many parts of the body are phenomenal in their ability to adapt to unusual conditions, and the TMJ is one of them. Not many complete dentures could be worn if this were not true. However, registration of a normal comfortable movement of the condyle in its path, with subsequent harmonious centric and eccentric occlusion to conform with this, greatly augments lasting function of dentures. There thus does not seem to be much excuse for failure to register this path, since it is not difficult or time consuming in proportion to the results obtained.

CONTROLLING FACTORS OF MOVEMENT

Edentulous patients bring only one controlling factor to the movement of the mandible, a fact that seems to be misunderstood generally. The misconception derives from the fact that many dentists think the condyle paths control the movement of the mandible entirely. In the laws of articulation the incisal guidance provided by the anterior teeth is an important part of the control. This guidance is always decided by the dentist, whether consciously or not. With semiadjustable articulators like the Dentatus, Hanau, and Whip Mix, incisal guidance is controlled by the inclination of the incisal guidance mechanism, which is determined by the horizontal and vertical overlap of the anterior teeth. The incisal guidance is more influential in controlling movements of the mandible than the condylar paths are, because the condylar paths are farther away from the cusp inclines, which both the incisal angle and the condyle angle influence.

ECCENTRIC RELATION RECORDS

The path of the condyle in protrusive and lateral movements is not on a straight line. The shape of the mandibular fossa is an ogee curve as viewed in the sagittal plane. This double curve will cause the apparent path of the condyle to be different with varying amounts of mandibular protrusion. The ideal amount of protrusion for making the record is the exact equivalent of the amount of protrusion necessary to bring the anterior teeth end to end. However, the mechanical limitations of most articulators require a protrusive movement of at least 6 mm so the condylar guidance mechanisms can be adjusted.

Methods of registering the condyle path may be classified as intraoral and extraoral. Extraoral methods are generally exemplified by the Gysi and McCollum techniques. The intraoral methods may be listed as (1) plaster and Carborundum grind-in, (2) chew-in by teeth opposing wax, (3) chew-in modified by a central bearing point, (4) Needles styluses cutting a compound rim, (5) Needles technique modified by a Messerman tracer, (6) protrusive registration in softened compound, (7) protrusive registration in plaster, and (8) protrusive registration in softened wax.

Lateral and protrusive condylar inclinations may be registered when straight protrusive movements are made. Many dentists consider these short-range lateral movements sufficiently indicative for practical purposes. However, for a complete registration, lateral records are necessary to indicate the limit of the range of movement, as shown by the Gothic arch (needle point) tracings.

Wax interocclusal records may be made on the occlusion rims before the teeth are set up or on the posterior teeth at the tryin appointment. Records made on occlusion rims must be considered tentative because the vertical and horizontal overlaps of the anterior teeth have not as yet been determined and the exact amount of protrusion and the level at which the anterior teeth are to contact are still unknown. These preliminary records permit tentative adjustment of the condylar guidances on the articulator.

Plaster interocclusal records are made after the anterior teeth have been arranged for esthetics and after both CR and the vertical dimension have been verified. If the horizontal overlap is sufficient to obtain enough protrusive movement of the lower jaw that the articulator can be adjusted, this record will be adequate. It will also be an accurate record of the relation of the jaws during incision. If the horizontal overlap of the incisors is too small to permit sufficient mandibular movement for adjustment of the condylar guidance, the patient must be instructed to protrude the jaw farther when the record is made. The minimum amount of protrusion for condylar guidance adjustment is 6 mm. This limitation is necessary because of mechanical deficiencies of most articulating instruments.

Lateral interocclusal records can be made to set the condylar inclination and the mandibular lateral translation on the articulator. However, with complete dentures it is more difficult to secure accurate and reproducible lateral records than protrusive records, in part because of the displaceability of the ridge mucosa. In addition, most semiadjustable articulators are not able to accept many lateral eccentric records. It is therefore generally accepted that making lateral interocclusal records for complete denture patients is not practical and probably not warranted.

Eccentric interocclusal records may be made with the guidance of extraoral tracings. While the tracing device is still attached to the occlusion rims, the amount of protrusive movement is determined by observation of the distance between the apex of the tracing and the needle point. The amount and direction of the lateral movement can be determined by observing the distance of the needle point from the apex of the tracing while the needle is on one of the arcs of the tracing. When the needle point is 6 mm from the apex, the mandible in the first molar region will be approximately 3 mm lateral to its position in CR. The molar tooth will have moved laterally 3 mm, because it is approximately midway between the tracing and the working-side condyle.

Protrusive interocclusal records for the Whip Mix articulator

After tryin the trial dentures are placed on the articulator. The lateral condylar guidances are set at 0 degrees so the articulator will be moved in a straight protrusive direction. The horizontal condylar guidances are set at 25 degrees to give an indication of the space that will exist between the posterior teeth when the mandible is protruded.

The lower member of the articulator is moved forward approximately 6 mm with the teeth out of contact and then closed until the incisal edges of the lower anterior teeth reach the vertical level of the incisal edges of the upper anterior teeth. The 6 mm of forward movement that is necessary to permit proper adjustment of the horizontal condylar path of the articulator may bring the lower anterior teeth several millimeters in front of the upper anterior teeth.

The horizontal relation of the lower to the upper anterior teeth and the relationship of the midlines of the upper and lower anterior teeth are observed carefully, since they will be the guides to the dentist that the patient has closed in approximately the proper position when the protrusive record is made in the mouth (Fig. 20-1, A). Interfering opposing posterior teeth that contact before the lower anterior teeth reach the desired verti-

cal relation should be removed from the wax occlusion rim.

When the dentist has become familiar with the relation of the lower to the upper anterior teeth in the protrusive position, the trial dentures are removed from the articulator and placed in the patient's mouth. The trial dentures are held in position by the dentist in the same way as for making the interocclusal CR record.

The patient is instructed to move his jaw straight forward and then to bite lightly on his front teeth. The dentist determines the amount and nature of the forward protrusion by the previous observation of the relationship of the anterior teeth on the articulator. The patient practices closing in the protrusive position under the guidance of the dentist until both become familiar with the procedure (Fig. 20-1, B).

A small amount of recording material that does not distort easily when set (impression plaster) is placed on the occlusal surfaces of the lower posterior teeth (Fig. 20-1, C). Then, as in the practice sessions, the patient protrudes his mandible and closes into the recording material. He is instructed to stop the closure before the opposing teeth make contact and to hold the jaw lightly and steadily in the desired position until the recording material sets (Fig. 20-1, D). The relationship of the lower to the upper anterior teeth in the patient's mouth should closely approximate the relationship observed on the articulator and during the rehearsal sessions.

The trial dentures and interocclusal record are removed from the mouth. The lateral condylar guidances on the upper member of the articulator are set at 20 degrees so they will not interfere if the mandible has not moved forward in straight protrusion, and the horizontal condylar guidances are set at 0 degrees. Then the trial dentures and interocclusal protrusive record are returned to the articulator (Fig. 20-2, A). The horizontal condylar housings are rotated individually

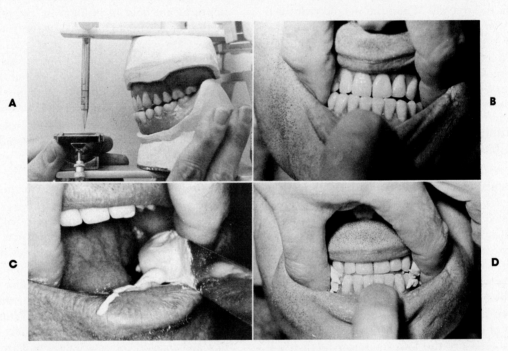

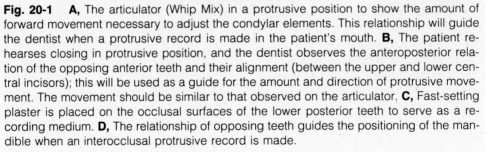

Fig. 20-1 A, The articulator (Whip Mix) in a protrusive position to show the amount of forward movement necessary to adjust the condylar elements. This relationship will guide the dentist when a protrusive record is made in the patient's mouth. **B,** The patient rehearses closing in protrusive position, and the dentist observes the anteroposterior relation of the opposing anterior teeth and their alignment (between the upper and lower central incisors); this will be used as a guide for the amount and direction of protrusive movement. The movement should be similar to that observed on the articulator. **C,** Fast-setting plaster is placed on the occlusal surfaces of the lower posterior teeth to serve as a recording medium. **D,** The relationship of opposing teeth guides the positioning of the mandible when an interocclusal protrusive record is made.

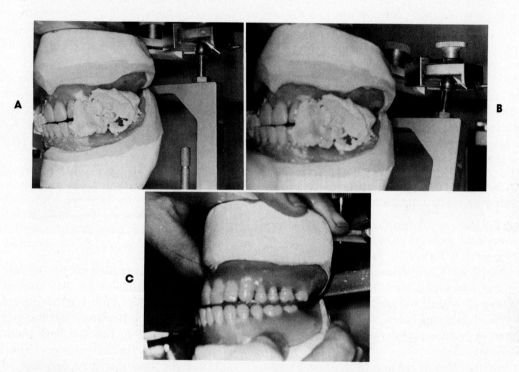

Fig. 20-2   Trial denture bases positioned by an interocclusal protrusive record are returned to the Whip Mix articulator. **A,** The horizontal condylar guidance mechanism is not in contact with the condylar sphere *(arrow).* **B,** The condylar mechanism is rotated into contact with the condylar sphere *(arrow),* thus establishing horizontal condylar guidance on the articulator. **C,** An interocclusal protrusive record has been made in wax, with the articulator adjusted as in **B.**

until the guidance plates contact the condylar spheres (Fig. 20-2, *B* and *C*), and the angulation of the protrusive movement for both sides is recorded.

The advantages of the protrusive registration made in plaster, or a recording material of similar consistency, are that the resistance to the biting force is minimal and uniform and there is nothing that guides the patient's mandible except the memory patterns of mandibular protrusion and the instructions by the dentist. Also the recording material will not be distorted during adjustment of the articulator. The disadvantage of plaster is related to the difficulty many patients experience in holding their mandibles in a steady protrusive position long enough for the material to set.

Protrusive interocclusal record for the Dentatus or Hanau articulator

Three thicknesses of Aluwax are placed over the occlusal surfaces of the mandibular posterior teeth (Chapter 18) rather than the two described for CR verification. The edges of the wax are sealed on both the buccal and the lingual with a warmed spatula (Fig. 20-3). The chilled upper trial denture should be placed in position on the upper cast mounted in the articulator.

Next just the Aluwax portion of the lower trial denture is immersed in a water bath of 130° F (54° C) for 30 seconds (Fig. 20-4). The lower trial denture is placed on the lower cast, and the articulator is set ¼ inch (6 mm) in protrusion with the condyle paths registering 25 degrees. At this position the upper member of the articulator is pressed into the warm wax to approximately a third its depth. The mandibular trial denture is removed from the cast, and the wax record is chilled thoroughly.

Both the trial dentures are now placed in the patient's mouth, and the patient is taught how to protrude into these indentations. The patient is rehearsed in this protrusive action to prepare for making such a protrusive movement later when the wax is softened.

The mandibular trial denture is now removed from the mouth and the wax record is resoftened in hot water, care being taken not to destroy the indentations.

The trial denture is reinserted into the mouth, and the patient is told to feel carefully and move into these markings in the manner rehearsed previously (Fig. 20-5). (Instructions have already been given not to exert occlusal pressure into these indentations until told to do so.)

The position of the teeth relative to the indentations is carefully observed, and when the teeth coincide with these markings the patient is instructed to bite but not to bite through the wax.

As an alternative the patient can be instructed to relax his jaw muscles while the dentist elevates the mandible with the index finger placed beneath the inferior portion of the chin (Fig. 20-6). With either approach, to avoid any tooth interference, the anterior teeth should remain slightly out of contact.

The wax record is chilled in the mouth, removed, and examined for any contact between the teeth. The trial dentures are replaced on the articulator, and the articulator is protruded so the maxillary teeth will fit partially into the indentations. The locknuts for the condylar guidance slot adjustments are loosened. While pressure is exerted on the upper articulator member with one hand and the condylar guidance slot is worked back and forth with the other hand, a condylar path inclination is found that permits the teeth to stay in contact with the wax throughout (Fig. 20-7). This adjustment is repeated for the opposite side. It will readily be seen that too steep a path prevents contact in the posterior part of the arch and too horizontal a path prevents contact in the anterior part of the arch. As stated earlier, the correct degree of condylar path incline can be attained by having the teeth contact wax throughout the arch; the condylar guidance slot is locked in the position thus obtained.

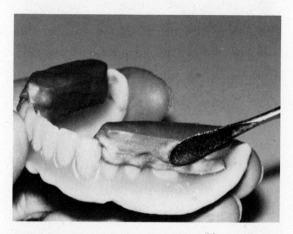

Fig. 20-3 Three layers of Aluwax sealed with a warm spatula.

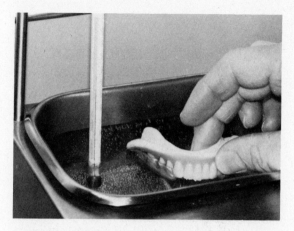

Fig. 20-4 Only the Aluwax portion is immersed, in 130° F (54° C) water for 30 seconds.

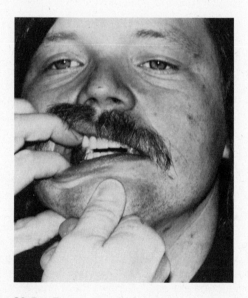

Fig. 20-5 The mandible is guided into the index previously made on the articulator.

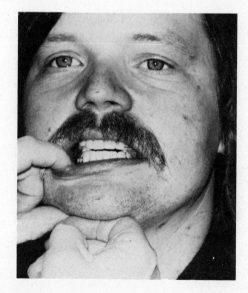

Fig. 20-6 The patient is to bite carefully into the wax but to stop before making contact with the anterior teeth.

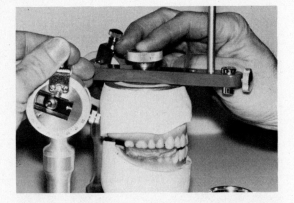

Fig. 20-7 Pressure on the Dentatus articulator with one hand and back and forth movement of the condylar guidance slot with the other permit a condylar path inclination to be found that gives uniform contact of the wax index and opposing teeth.

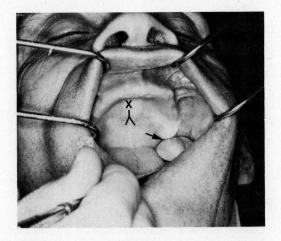

Fig. 20-8 The pterygomaxillary (hamular) notch *(arrow)* in the mouth is often deceiving. To be certain of its location, the dentist can palpate it with a mouth mirror. *X* denotes the foveae palatinae.

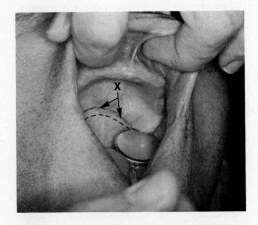

Fig. 20-9 The vibrating line has been traced on the palatal tissues with indelible pencil. The *X with arrows* marks where it passes through the hamular notch on both sides slightly anterior to the foveae palatinae. The denture can end posterior to this line *(dotted arc)* because of the gradual slope of the palate.

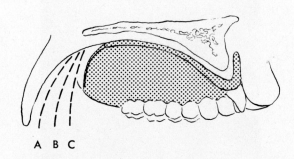

A B C

Fig. 20-10 The vibrating line and width of the posterior palatal seal depend on the soft palate form *(A, B,* or *C).* Form *C* allows only a narrow posterior palatal seal; *A* allows the widest seal.

A protrusive record is first made on the articulator so the correct amount of protrusive distance (which is also centered) will guide the patient's mandible to the desired protrusive position. Unless the patient has a guide and is rehearsed, it will be extremely difficult to keep the mandible from closing too far or not far enough in protrusive occlusion, to the right or left in lateral occlusion, or in a combination of protrusion and lateral occlusion. Such a record will give an unsatisfactory setting to the articulator. The record is made with a protrusive distance of ¼ inch (6 mm), because it is believed that with a shorter distance the condyle will not move down its path sufficiently to be recorded on the instrument. A protrusive movement of more than ¼ inch is usually beyond the range of the patient and registration of a greater distance is not necessary.

An alternative procedure involves the use of impression plaster for making the protrusive interocclusal record as described for the Whip Mix articulator.

ESTABLISHING THE POSTERIOR PALATAL SEAL

The posterior palatal seal is completed before the final arrangement of the posterior teeth, because this final arrangement is a laboratory procedure and is done in the absence of the patient.

The posterior border of the denture is determined in the mouth, and its location is transferred onto the cast. A T burnisher or mouth mirror is pressed along the posterior angle of the tuberosity until it drops into the pterygomaxillary (hamular) notch (Fig. 20-8). The locations of the right and left pterygomaxillary notches are marked with an indelible pencil. On the median line of the anterior part of the soft palate are two indentations formed by the coalescence of ducts known as the foveae palatinae. The shape of these depressions varies from round or oval to oblong. The dentist can make them more readily discernible by having

the patient hold his nose and attempt to blow through it (Valsalva maneuver). This will accentuate the foveae palatinae and vibrating line.

The vibrating line of the soft palate, normally used as a guide to the ideal posterior border of the denture, is usually located slightly anterior to the foveae palatinae. However, it may be on or slightly posterior to the foveae palatinae. The slight deviation from these markings is estimated by having the patient say "ah" and thus vibrate his soft palate. The dentist observes closely and marks the vibrating line with an indelible pencil (Figs. 20-9 and 20-10). The two pterygomaxillary notch markings are joined to the median line mark. The trial denture base is now inserted so the indelible pencil line will be transferred from the soft palate to the trial denture base, and the excess baseplate is reduced to this line (Fig. 20-11). The trial denture base is placed on the cast, and a knife or pencil is used to mark a line following the posterior limits of the baseplate (Fig. 20-12). This line should extend laterally 3 mm beyond the crest of the hamular notch.

The anterior line that indicates the location of the posterior palatal seal is drawn on the cast in front of the line indicating the end of the denture (Fig. 20-13). The width of the posterior palatal seal itself is limited to a bead on the denture that is 1 to 1.5 mm high and 1.5 mm broad at its base (Fig. 20-14). A greater width creates an area of tissue placement that will have a tendency to push the denture downward gradually and to defeat the purpose of the posterior palatal seal. In other words, the posterior palatal seal should not be made too wide. Placement of tissue should be such that when the dentures move in function, as they always do, the placed tissue will move with the dentures and not break the seal.

A V-shaped groove 1 to 1.5 mm deep is carved into the cast at the location of the bead. A large sharp scraper is used to carve it, passing through the hamular notches and across the palate of the cast (Figs. 20-15 and 20-16). The groove will form a bead on the denture that

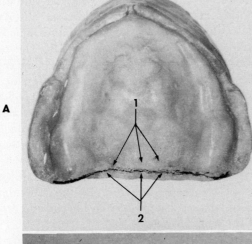

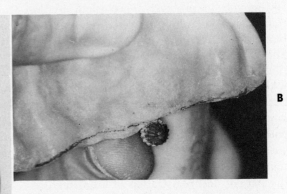

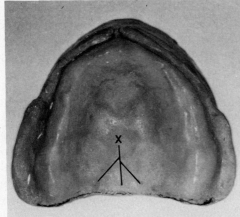

Fig. 20-11 **A,** The indelible pencil line across the palate in Fig. 20-9 has been transferred to the denture base and can be seen rather indistinctly, *1,* anterior to the solid line marking the end of the denture, *2.* **B,** The trial denture base is shortened posteriorly with a vulcanite bur as far as this line. **C,** The trial denture base showing the anticipated length of the completed denture. *X* denotes the location of the vibrating line that was transferred from the patient's mouth.

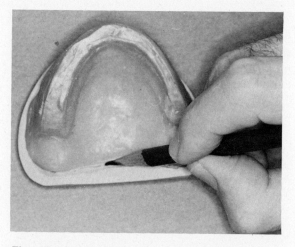

Fig. 20-12 Posterior extent of the trial denture base traced on the cast.

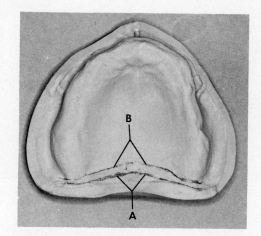

Fig. 20-13 The posterior line, *A,* indicates the end of the denture posteriorly across the palate. The anterior line, *B,* marks the location of the posterior palatal seal that will be carved into the cast and transferred as a bead onto the denture.

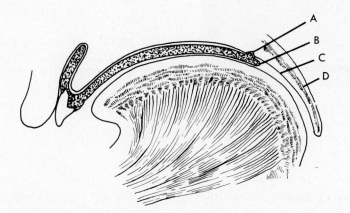

Fig. 20-14 Denture in place in the mouth. A bead on the posterior extent, *A,* is 1 mm high, 1 mm broad at the base, and 2 mm anterior to *B,* the end of the denture. *C,* Movable soft palate; *D,* muscles of the soft palate.

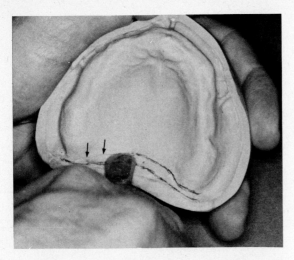

Fig. 20-15 A groove is carved into the cast *(arrows)* with a large sharp scraper to form the posterior palatal seal.

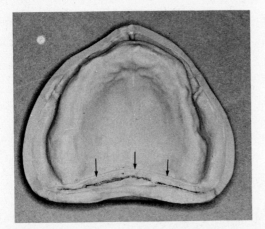

Fig. 20-16 The groove in the cast *(arrows)* forms a bead on the finished denture (Fig. 20-14).

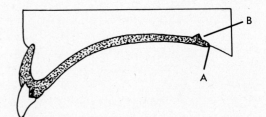

Fig. 20-17 The denture ends on the cast at *A.* The bead, *B,* located 2 mm in front of the vibrating line, is extended laterally through the center of the hamular notches.

provides the posterior palatal seal (Fig. 20-17). The bead will be 1 to 1.5 mm high, 1.5 mm wide at its base, and sharp at its apex. The depth of the groove in the cast will be determined by the thickness of the soft tissue against which it is placed and will establish the height of the bead.

The narrow and sharp bead will sink easily into the soft tissue to provide a seal against air being forced under the denture. If the bead has been made too high, the sharpness will make this apparent within 24 hours of the insertion of the dentures, and it can be easily relieved. The narrowness of the bead makes the seal with minimal downward pressure on the denture.

CHAPTER 21

Arranging posterior teeth for functional harmony

The arrangement of artificial posterior teeth for functional harmony depends on a thorough understanding of occlusion. Occlusion is any contact between the incising or masticating surfaces of the upper and lower teeth. There are many kinds of occlusion that are significant in complete denture prosthodontics. The specifications for each kind of occlusion are related to other conditions at the time the occlusal contact is made. For example, centric occlusion is the relation of opposing occlusal surfaces that provides the maximum planned contact or intercuspation, or both, and it should exist when the mandible is in centric relation to the maxillae. All other occlusions are eccentric occlusions. Protrusive occlusion refers to the occlusion existing when the mandible is moved forward from centric occlusion. Lateral occlusion refers to the occlusion existing when the mandible is moved laterally. Balanced occlusion refers to occlusion with simultaneous contacts of the occlusal surfaces of all or some of the teeth on both sides of the arch, regardless of the mandibular position.

The side toward which the mandible is moved is called the working side for purpose of identification. For the same purpose, the side opposite the working side is called the nonworking or balancing side.

The setting of teeth includes orientation of the plane, shaping and positioning of the arch, inclinations and rotations for esthetics, and the mechanics for obtaining proper tooth inclination for a balanced occlusion. Occlusion is too often construed as the only important objective in the setting of teeth. Such is not the case because, for example, the posterior dental arch could be too wide and still be in perfect balance. Nevertheless, despite perfect balance, the wide arch would cause failure of the dentures because of excessive leverage. The occlusal plane could be balanced and yet be too high or too low, with a ruinous result. Occlusion has to do with cuspal and incisal inclinations and their relation to other inclinations and jaw movements.

IMPORTANCE OF OCCLUSION

Occlusion is probably the most important subject in all disciplines of dentistry. Consideration of occlusal stresses, both vertical and lateral, and their components in the making of single tooth restorations is of prime importance in the preservation of a tooth, the teeth, and the restoration. Care should be used when finishing restorations not to take a tooth out of harmony or to leave it underfilled or overfilled. On the other hand, the entire occlusion should be tested for possible disharmony, which could be improved with a knowledge of what would constitute proper harmony in centric and eccentric positions in that dental arch.

MAINTENANCE OF THE ARCHES

In fixed restorations that replace one or several teeth, it becomes extremely important to establish optimally distributed stresses to preserve the supporting structures around the abutment teeth, which now have an extra load to bear. The future of that entire arch depends on the harmonious relation of all the teeth in centric and eccentric positions. There are times when the recuperative powers of the supporting tissues are so good that the supporting structures may tolerate an inharmonious occlusion. However, as age increases and resistance to disease decreases, when the supporting structures are overloaded, they usually break down because of improper distribution of stresses. Repeated fracture of facings is generally a result not of failure in mechanical attachment or strength but of excessive loading caused by disharmony of cuspal inclines.

MAINTENANCE OF OCCLUSAL HARMONY

A contributing factor in the breakdown of supporting structures is unbalanced centric and eccentric occlusions.

In most parts of the body nature heals, compensates, or both, any disease and injury. However, nature does not heal dental caries, nor is it capable of taking care of the ravages of malocclusion. Therefore in repairing and restoring dental function, it is as important to understand occlusion in all its phases as it is to restore any tooth destruction caused by dental caries.

Orthodontically, any movement of a tooth or teeth, however slight, will cause a change in the relationship of the inclines of the moved teeth to the remainder of the arch. Therefore as soon as the teeth are not held by an appliance, inharmonious inclinations begin shifting them out of their acquired positions. For this reason, harmony of inclines throughout the dental arch is of paramount importance.

Differences in artificial occlusion and natural occlusion

It must be understood, however, that occlusion that is acceptable for natural teeth may not be acceptable for complete dentures. For example, with complete dentures, protrusive and lateral contact is preferred; with natural occlusion, this exact type of relationship is seldom needed.

The dentist must test and correct the occlusion of the entire mouth for harmony of centric and eccentric relationship before and after the construction of a partial denture. The remaining teeth are loaded to their maximum, and therefore distribution of vertical and lateral stresses must be executed carefully if the restoration and remaining teeth are to function efficiently and cause no destruction of supporting structures.

Reduced inclines in dentures

The difficulties and handicaps of reduced anchorage in complete dentures demand the utmost in occlusal harmony. The dentist has the power to establish all factors of occlusion except the condylar path. Therefore the opportunity exists for establishing a reduced amount of displacing cusp inclinations while still maintaining a harmony between the factors that does not disturb the stability of the complete dentures.

Rationale for arranging posterior teeth in a balanced occlusion

During mastication the teeth make contact to a variable extent on both the chewing side and the nonchewing side. A combination of tissue resiliency and denture movement during function accounts for the high frequency of the nonchewing, or balancing, side contacts. Denture movements occur regardless of the type of posterior occlusal forms used. Sheppard (1964) suggested the expression "enter bolus, enter balance" to account for this observation. Balanced occlusion can even be of questionable significance during mastication if interferences are built into the occlusion because of inaccurate jaw relation records. Studies in dentulous patients indicate that interferences on the nonchewing side have a damaging potential. Interceptive occlusal contacts on the nonchewing side are known to interfere with the delicate integrated neuromuscular coordination used in chewing. Not only are these interferences confusing and distressing to the patient, they also significantly impair the patient's masticatory efficiency.

Longitudinal studies conducted in the early 1960s and in 1971 have shown that after 2-year and 1-year periods of wearing complete dentures, defective occlusion was observed in several of the patients' dentures. When these observations are seen in the context of Tallgren's review (1972), the changes in occlusion or articulation are understandable. Changes in occlusal balance occur, regardless of the type of posterior tooth form used.

Although proof is lacking to support the validity of bilateral balance, a balanced occlusion is essential during tooth contact when no food is in the mouth. The horizontal movements of the mandible generated on an articulator do not simulate functional jaw movements; they in fact simulate parafunctional jaw movements (Fig. 21-1, *A* to *C*), and artificial teeth are balanced to provide maximum denture stabilization during these anticipated mandibular activities. Such a balanced occlusion can usually be readily obtained with anatomic teeth. This objective can also be achieved with nonanatomic teeth by the use of a compensating curve or ramp type of arrangement and probably with the flat plane type of tooth arrangement as well (Fig. 21-1, *D* to *G*). Several clinicians dismiss the flat plane type of arrangement as ensuring contact in CR only. The premise must be postulated, however, that during jaw movements the combination of exerted muscle forces and resiliency of the supporting mucosal tissues will actually allow for a bilateral contact or balanced occlusion to develop in many patients over a limited range of mandibular movement. The exact range of freedom of parafunctional tooth contacts has not been determined. It is tempting to presume that this area is within the range of bilateral nonanatomic tooth contacts as arranged and so readily achieved on a flat plane.

There is a dearth of evidence to support any specific method or philosophy of articulation as being optimal. On the other hand, numerous clinical observations have been made that successful denture wearing is probably more dependent on a good patient-dentist relationship, coupled with a careful clinical technique, than on any particular technique per se.

There exists a distinct cosmetic limitation to the use of cuspless teeth. The concept of a flat occlusal plane that allows for maximum horizontal mandibular movements is predicated on the use of a neutral or 0-degree incisal guidance. Most edentulous patients can be adequately treated by use of an incisal guidance with no vertical overlap of the anterior teeth. In most patients sufficient horizontal overlap of the incisors can be used to permit some jaw movement in a protrusive direction without seriously compromising the patient's esthetic appearance. However, when proper appearance of the patient requires a vertical overlap of the anterior teeth, cusped posterior teeth must be used (such as in a modified Angle Class II, Division 2, type of anterior tooth arrangement). If an extra expenditure of time and effort should be required for using anatomic teeth in these situations, it would, of course, be justified.

The actual morphologic shortcoming of a cuspless posterior tooth can frequently be compensated by slight reshaping of the mesial and distal corners of the premolars with a sandpaper disk to develop the appearance of a cusp. A more pleasing esthetic result can then be obtained (Fig. 21-2, *A* and *B*).

An alternative to the nonanatomic design is the Synoform posterior tooth (Vita Zahnfabrik), which has a very shallow cusp inclination (Fig. 21-2, *C* and *D*). This might be considered by some patients more esthetically pleasing than the purely nonanatomic design.

TEMPOROMANDIBULAR JOINT DISTURBANCES

The TMJs influence the inclinations of teeth, and likewise the inclinations of teeth influence the TMJs. If the teeth and the joints are in harmony as to their inclinations in centric occlusion and during eccentric movements, the

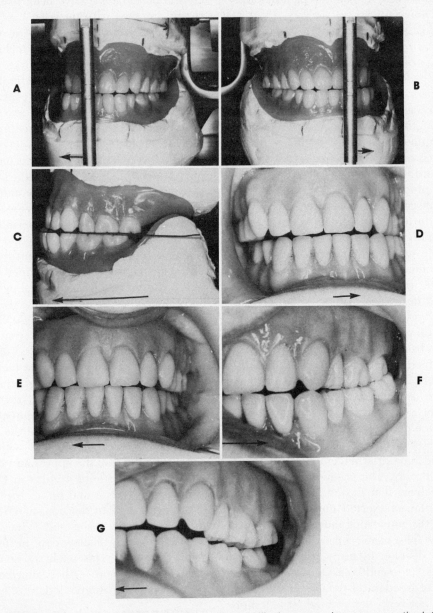

Fig. 21-1 **A** to **C,** Right, left, and protrusive mandibular excursions on an articulator to simulate bruxing or parafunctional movements of the mandible. **D** and **E,** Intraoral views of left and right excursions with posterior teeth set on a flat plane. **F** and **G,** Left intraoral working and balancing contacts with posterior teeth set so the second molars serve as a ramp to maintain balancing contacts. These simulated movements are done in the mouth for parafunctional, rather than functional, purposes.

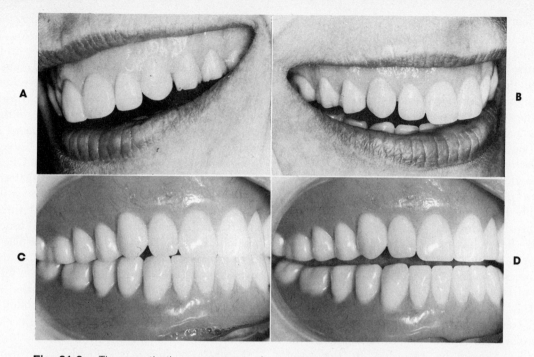

Fig. 21-2   The unesthetic appearance of a nonanatomic premolar, **A,** is remedied by recontouring its mesial and distal marginal ridges, **B.** Using a very shallow-cusped posterior tooth, **C** and **D,** will also improve the esthetic effect.

joints can be expected to remain healthy. However, when the inclinations are not in harmony because of loss and shifting of teeth, excessive wear of cusps, or incorrectly constructed inlays, crowns, fixed partial dentures, or removable partial and/or complete dentures, a pathologic condition may result. When these two factors are not in harmony, the TMJs may be the stronger of the two (in which case the teeth and supporting structures will be destroyed) or the reverse may be true (and the TMJs will bear the brunt of the malocclusion). This diseased condition of the joints may be manifested by clicking sounds, neuralgia, obscure headaches, joint pain and discomfort during mastication, a burning sensation of the tongue, and sometimes trismus of varying degrees. The presence of these symptoms must not be construed as the result of occlusal disharmony; yet such disharmony must always be investigated as a potential etiologic factor. The dental literature provides numerous examples of the correlation between occlusal disharmonies and TMJ dysfunction.

FACTORS OF CENTRIC OCCLUSION

Generally speaking, *occlude* in medical science means "to close." Therefore the term *occlusion* in dentistry refers to the position of the teeth in contact. Centric occlusion means strictly the teeth in contact when the mandible is in centric relation to the head. However, centric occlusion is usually defined as the position of the maxillary and mandibular dental arches wherein the teeth make maximum contact. (It must be remembered that CO is the normal termination of masticatory closure.) This definition, then, includes the position of the mandible when the teeth have been worn out of CO. Thus centric occlusion and centric relation with tooth contact may not coincide. Centric occlusion and centric relation in a child when the teeth are in contact under normal conditions will be identical. As wear progresses and destruction takes place, the mandible gradually assumes a different position from centric relation. This is an extremely important factor in the registration of occlusal relations in complete denture construction of maxillary dentures, mandibular dentures, or both. It may readily be demonstrated by means of motion pictures showing the position of the mandible under heavy biting stress. In other words, although a patient chewing lightly may use habitual eccentric occlusion and that may be protrusive or lateral or both, when a resistant bolus of food is encountered the mandible tends to work completely back to the retrusive position. Therefore the relation of the mandible to the maxillae should be recorded in the most retruded position for maximum stability and efficiency.

UNDERSTANDING CENTRIC RELATION

Centric relation is defined as the most posterior position of the mandible relative to the maxillae at the established vertical dimension. This definition takes into consideration the three-dimensional nature of CR and the fact that the horizontal position of the *body* of the mandible varies with changes in its vertical position, even though the condyles remain maximally retruded. It is more accurate than other definitions that are related to a technique used for locating or recording CR. In this definition centric relation is specified as the "most retruded position of the mandible from which lateral movements can be made at a given degree of jaw separation." It is based on the use of a Gothic arch (needle-point) tracing technique for making the registration. It cannot be appropriately applied to certain methods of recording CR, however. Interocclusal record techniques and hinge axis techniques do not permit any lateral movement when the CR record is made.

Vertical force applied while the CR record is being made may be uneven and will cause more displacement on one side than the other; the CR established from this uneven record will be incorrect, even though the bones of the jaws are in centric relation when the record is made. Also, the record may be incorrect, even though the mandible is in the position of CR, if the soft tissues of one part of the basal seat are thicker and therefore softer and more easily displaced than those of other parts. In these situations the teeth of the dentures will touch first on the side where the greater displacement occurs, even though the bones of the mandible and the cranium are precisely in CR. The centric jaw relation must be recorded in such a way that the teeth will meet simultaneously at their first contact in centric occlusion.

Eccentric occlusion is defined as protrusive and right and left lateral contacts of the inclined planes of the teeth when the jaw is not moving.

Articulation can be defined as the relationships of the teeth during movements into and away from eccentric position while the teeth are in contact. It is occlusion in motion.

CRITICAL COMPONENTS IN THE ARRANGEMENT OF POSTERIOR TEETH

The maxillary and mandibular natural teeth have a normal cuspal relation to each other that maintains their positional and functional interrelationship. In centric occlusion this causes certain cusps to rest in the opposing fossae. These cusps perform a definite function (Fig. 21-3). Nature maintains a harmony of inclines in eccentric positions. For instance, in left lateral movement wherein the left side becomes the working side and the right side the balancing side, the mandibular buccal cusps slide out between the opposing maxillary buccal cusps to maintain contact. The maxillary lingual cusps on the left (working) side move between the

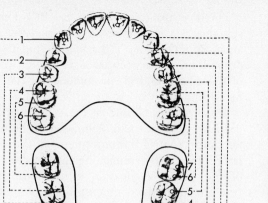

Fig. 21-3   Lines connecting the cusp, or point, on one denture to the fossa on which it rests in CR on the opposing denture. Three *arrows* indicate the directions in which this point or cusp travels during a working-side movement, a balancing-side movement, and a protrusive movement.

opposing mandibular lingual cusps to maintain contact. The mandibular left anterior teeth slide out on the inclines of the maxillary left incisors to maintain contact. The lingual cusps of the maxillary teeth on the right (balancing) side slide on the inclines of the lingual surfaces of the mandibular buccal cusps to maintain contact on this side. In such a left lateral movement, the lingual inclines of the maxillary buccal cusps and the buccal inclines of the mandibular lingual cusps on the left side and the lingual inclines of the left maxillary anterior teeth are in harmony with the lingual inclines of the mandibular buccal cusps on the right side. The inclination of the condylar path on the right side is also in harmony with these inclines during such movement. Other eccentric movements, if all conditions are normal, have comparable harmonies of cusp inclines in the various comparable positions.

Generally speaking, the same laws of occlu-

sion apply in natural teeth as in complete dentures. However, the vertical overlap, and therefore the incisal guide angle, is already established in natural teeth whereas in complete dentures the vertical overlap is partly in the hands of the dentist. It can be made at the sharp angle of 60 or more degrees or at the flatter angle of 5 or even 0 degrees, at the dentist's discretion, and still have harmonious occlusal balance. Nevertheless, not all inclines are desirable, even though they balance. The laws of occlusion can be made to apply, regardless of the factors in natural or complete dentures. Occlusal balance and harmony apply to and can be attained in all combinations of controlling factors, however.

Two controlling end factors that must be considered in complete denture occlusion are the condylar inclination and the incisal guide angle. In the edentulous patient only one factor, the *condylar inclination,* is determined by the patient. The dentist has no control over the condylar inclination that the patient possesses and cannot change or modify it to fit a theory. Any lack of harmony between tooth inclines and condylar inclines can result in disturbances to the temporomandibular articulation and to lasting stability of the dentures. The other controlling end factor, the *incisal guide angle,* is established by the dentist in the choice of setting but within the limits of esthetics. It is understood that the more closely the incisal guide angle approaches 0 degrees the more stable the dentures will be because of the reduction of lateral inclines. However, there are limitations in this reduction that the dentist must consider—those of esthetics, ridge fullness, and ridge relation—any of which can change the incisal guide angle.

LAWS OF PROTRUSIVE OCCLUSION

The five principal factors in the laws of occlusion for protrusive movement, as stated by Hanau, are inclination of the condylar guidance, prominence of the compensating curve, inclination of the plane of orientation, inclination of the incisal guidance, and height of the cusps.

The order of the factors has been revised, principally for clarity and convenience. A few words have been changed (such as *height* to *inclination*) because the inclination of the cusp is more important in arranging teeth. The phrase *plane of orientation* has been changed to *orientation of the occlusal plane* because this describes more adequately the action that takes place. The word *orient* means "to find the proper bearings or relations of." Thus *orientation of the plane* is a factor that must be determined whereas *plane of orientation* implied that this factor already had been determined.

The five principal factors are therefore restated as (1) inclination of the condylar guidance, (2) inclination of the incisal guidance, (3) orientation of the occlusal plane, (4) inclination of the cusps, and (5) prominence of the compensating curve.

The first and second of these (inclination of condylar guidance and inclination of the incisal guidance) control the movements of the articulator whereas the remaining three (orientation of the plane, inclination of the cusps, and prominence of the compensating curve) may be changed by the dentist to attain harmony among all five factors (Fig. 21-4).

Fig. 21-5 presents the first factor of occlu-

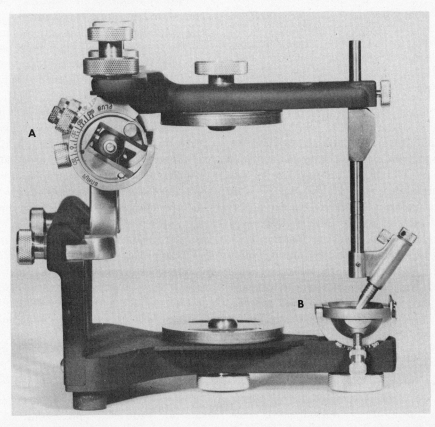

Fig. 21-4 The condylar inclination, *A,* and the incisal guide incline, *B,* are the controlling end factors that are determined before the three other factors are established by the dentist.

sion, condylar inclination, which is the only factor given by the patient. This factor is obtained by means of protrusive registration. In Fig. 21-6 the condylar factor has been transferred to the condylar guidance setting on the articulator.

Fig. 21-7 shows the second factor of occlusion, incisal guide angle, as set by the dentist to determine the controlling path of the articulator. This factor is influenced by the amount of vertical and horizontal overlap that the dentist selects, which is really a cosmetic decision. The greater the horizontal overlap, the more it will reduce the angle of inclination as long as the vertical overlap remains the same; and, of course, the less the vertical overlap, the less the angle of inclination will be.

The mandible is guided into entirely different positions by changing the incisal inclination. The posterior teeth are closer to the action of the incisal inclination than to the action of the condylar inclination (Fig. 21-8). Therefore greater influence is exerted on the teeth by the incisal inclination than by the condylar guidance.

In Fig. 21-9 are shown mandibles with different vertical overlaps. The mandible in Fig. 21-9, *A*, has a very shallow vertical overlap, with a resultant lowered cusp inclination; in Fig. 21-9, *B*, the mandible has a steep vertical overlap and a consequent steep cusp inclination. Thus it can be seen how the cuspal inclination is automatically determined from a rotational center established by lines drawn at right angles to these two end factors, the incisal and condylar guidance surfaces.

Remember: All actions in protrusive movement of the articulator are on arcs from a center that has been established by the intersection of lines drawn at right angles to the guiding surfaces. They thus are controlled by the condylar guidance surface and the incisal guidance surface. Whereas a steep vertical overlap places the rotational center below and posterior to the mandible, a shallow vertical overlap places it above the mandible (Fig. 21-9). These

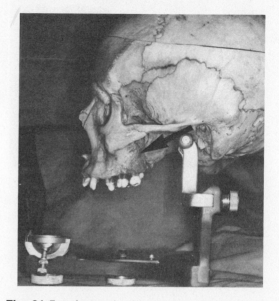

Fig. 21-5 *Arrow* simulates the condylar path inclination, which is the only control over jaw movement that an edentulous patient has.

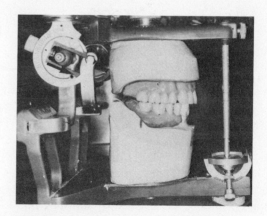

Fig. 21-6 An articulator mounting with the condylar path inclination in Fig. 21-5 transferred to the articulator.

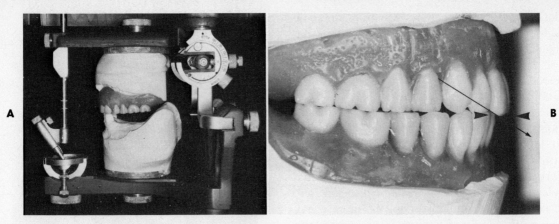

Fig. 21-7 The incisal guide angle, which is controlled by the dentist, is established on the articulator. **A,** A flat incisal guide table and, **B,** one of approximately 15 degrees (at the incisor level, *arrowheads*). This angle was based on the dentist's choice of incisor tooth overlap as dictated by cosmetics.

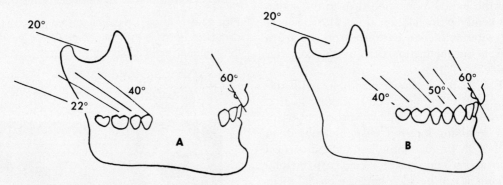

Fig. 21-8 **A,** Resultant cusp angulation if, hypothetically, the teeth were moved closer to the condyle influence. **B,** Same condylar and incisal inclinations, with the resultant cusp angulation when the teeth are moved forward closer to the incisal guide influence.

are theoretical factors that help give a better understanding of articulator and jaw movements. However, in reality they need not be worked out in the construction of a denture because the articulator automatically establishes them.

Nevertheless, it must be reemphasized, the condylar surface and the incisal surface estab-

lish and determine movement. The other three factors (orientation of the plane, inclination of the cusps, and prominence of the compensating curve) may be changed so they will move on concentric curves, as represented in Fig. 21-9, lines *2* to *4*. Notice that the tooth inclines can be changed by inclining the occlusal plane up or down at the back, tipping the long axes

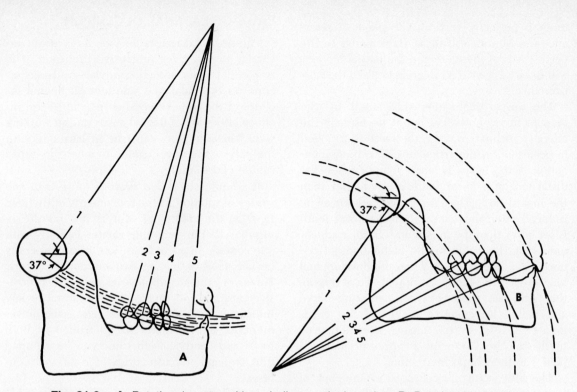

Fig. 21-9   **A,** Rotational center with a shallow vertical overlap. **B,** Rotational center below the mandible with a steep vertical overlap. An occlusion developed as in **B** will tend to push the upper denture forward more than an occlusion developed with the rotational center above the level of the occlusal plane.

of the teeth, or grinding the cuspal inclinations. Notice further that teeth can be set on varying levels and still be in harmony of movement with the articulator. However, locating an occlusal plane high or low to favor the weaker of the two ridges can cause both esthetic and mechanical trouble. If the soft tissues surrounding the dentures are to function as they did for natural teeth, the occlusal plane must be oriented exactly as it was when the natural teeth were present.

Thus the orientation of the occlusal plane becomes the third fixed factor of occlusion. By positioning the anterior teeth correctly for esthetic appearance and locating the posterior end of the occlusal plane approximately two

thirds the way up the retromolar pad, the dentist fixes the orientation of the occlusal plane. Any necessary alterations for balancing the occlusion must therefore be made on other factors affecting the occlusion (that is, the cuspal inclination or the prominence of the compensating curve).

The inclination of the cusps of the teeth, the fourth factor of occlusion, refers to the angle between the total occlusal surface of the tooth and the inclination of the cusp in relation to that surface. For example, the designation "33-degree tooth" indicates that the mesial slopes of the cusps make a 33-degree angle with a plane touching the tips of all the cusps of the tooth. In other words, if the long axis of the tooth is perfectly vertical, the plane of reference (horizontal) will be at right angles to the vertical axis of the tooth and the mesial inclines will likewise have a 33-degree angle to the horizontal.

The cuspal inclination designated by the manufacturer, however, is not necessarily the effective inclination when the tooth is arranged in occlusion on the articulator. The basic inclination of the cusps is made steeper when the distal end of a lower tooth is set higher than the mesial end. The cuspal inclination can be reduced when the distal end of the lower tooth is set lower than the mesial end. Similar adjustments can be made in the inclinations of the buccal and lingual cusps when the buccolingual long axes of the teeth are tipped. Thus tipping the teeth can produce a compensating curve and make the effective height of the cusps greater or less. By this means, even 0-degree teeth can be arranged to present inclined planes to their opposing teeth.

The fifth factor of occlusion, prominence of the compensating curve, is valuable insofar as it allows the dentist to alter cusp height without changing the form of the manufactured tooth. Thus the cusps can be made longer or shorter (steeper or flatter) simply by inclining the long axis of a tooth to conform to the end guidelines.

If the tooth itself does not have cusps, the compensating curve can be used to produce the equivalent of cusps. The mesial inclines of lower teeth can be thought of as actual segments of a compensating curve cut into pieces, with the pieces arranged in a more or less straight line. If each of these pieces is arranged to line up with all the others, the result will be a compensating curve with a single continuous surface. Such a surface can be used with 0-degree teeth.

It must be understood that although the factors of occlusion are described separately for clarity they are adjusted simultaneously in the setting of the teeth to obtain harmony and balance with the movement of the articulator.

LAWS OF LATERAL OCCLUSION

The principal factors for lateral occlusion are similar to those for protrusive occlusion. The two end factors are (1) condylar guidance incline on the balancing side and (2) lingual inclines of the upper buccal cusps and buccal inclines of the lower lingual cusps on the working side. These inclines must be in harmony with the path of the lower canine to meet the upper canine end to end.

It is understood that there is more than one center of rotation in the movements of the jaw. In fact, the rotational centers are infinite in number. If the mandible rotates laterally with one condyle in a fixed position, it can generally be classified as having two rotational centers. However, the mandible can start in a protrusive position and then shift to a lateral or any intermediate position. Nevertheless, the movements of the mandible are controlled by both tooth and condyle factors and can be grouped into two general categories of rotational centers.

In any given eccentric position it is possible to draw lines at right angles to the cusps on which the mandible has stopped and establish the rotational center for that position. For instance, the mandible in Fig. 21-10 has moved to the left, and the mandibular teeth have stopped at a certain point on the opposing cusp incline on the left side. A line drawn upward at right angles to the buccal incline of the mandibular lingual cusp on the working side and another at right angles to the lingual surface of the mandibular buccal cusp on the balancing side will meet at *B*. All inclines involved in this left lateral position must be on the curves of arcs drawn from this rotational center. The rotational center shifts according to the direction in which the mandible (or mandibular member of the articulator) moves from centric position. This rotational center is established by lines drawn at right angles to the working-side inclines, the balancing-side inclines, and the balancing-side condyle. These parallel arcs of concentric circles at varying distances (*B1, B2, B3*)

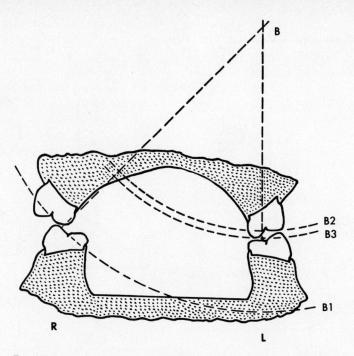

Fig. 21-10   Establishing the center of rotation in a lateral movement by lines drawn at right angles to the cusp inclines. *B1*, *B2*, and *B3* are concentric around *B*.

from the center are all in harmony during movement.

The rotational center may also slide laterally while the mandible is in lateral occlusion. This lateral movement or shift of the mandible is the result of the movement of the condyles along the lateral inclines of the mandibular fossae. It is known as the Bennett shift. According to the findings of Gysi, 15 degrees is the average Bennett shift. (It is well to remember that a rotational center can shift laterally and still form an arc from the shifting rotational center.) In Fig. 21-11 the effect of incisal and condylar inclination on posterior tooth cusp inclination on both the working and the balancing sides can be seen. Notice the difference in working-side and balancing-side inclines. In the example cited this difference is attributable to the fact that the condyle on the working side neither rises nor falls but merely rotates (except for the Bennett shift). Therefore the working-

side inclines are not as steep as the balancing-side inclines. Notice further how the angle of inclination on the working side is less in the posterior area and greater toward the incisal area, how the degree of inclination changes with the distance away from the condyle and toward the incisal area, and how the inclination changes with the distance away from the condyle and toward the incisal area. If the inclination of the incisal guidance were zero, all the working-side inclines would be 0. Since in this instance the incisal guidance is 30 degrees, we start with a smaller degree of angulation in the posterior region and gradually increase toward 30 degrees as the incisal area is approached.

The balancing-side inclines are steeper than the working-side inclines because there are two factors of angulation: the incisal (30 degrees) and the condylar (10 degrees). The dentist controls the setting of the incisal inclination, and

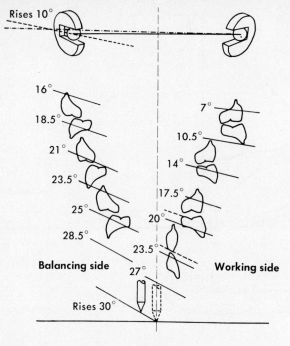

Fig. 21-11 Influence of incisal guidance and condylar inclines on the working and balancing sides. The condylar guidance is 10 degrees; the incisal guidance, 30 degrees.

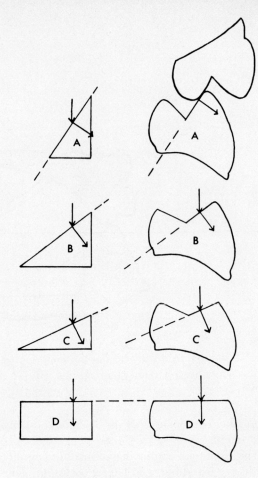

Fig. 21-12 Resultant forces of inclines.

the patient registers the condylar inclination; then the articulator automatically controls the inclinations of the teeth in all positions after the dentist has moved the teeth so they are in contact in all movements (that is, in harmony and occlusal balance).

In the discussion of occlusion it was pointed out that the edentulous patient provides the condylar inclination but can do nothing regarding incisal inclination. It was noted further that the condylar inclination is not the only influential factor; in fact, it is not even as great a factor as the amount of vertical overlap or incisal guidance (the dentist's decision) is. With an edentulous patient there is no way of knowing what the incisal guidance factor in the natural dentition was or what it should be in the completed dentures. Therefore, of necessity, the

dentist must select the amount of vertical overlap or incisal inclination. A study of the geometric influences of inclines shows that reducing cusp inclination is a great stabilizer of dentures. The obvious question pertains to the advisability of having flat occlusal surfaces throughout. This theoretically cannot be done and still have bilateral balance, since the condyles do not presumably move horizontally. Therefore, again in theory, there must be some inclination of the occluding surfaces to harmonize with the downward movement of the mandible. Since the stability of dentures varies with cuspal inclination, an inclination that is as flat as possible is selected for complete dentures.

A brief study of the effect of vertical forces on varying degrees of inclination will emphasize the desirability of the greatest possible cusp reduction for stabilization. Fig. 21-12 shows this graphically. In *A*, notice that the tooth and cuspal incline cause the buccal surface to shift; in *B*, less shifting influence occurs; in *C*, still less; and in *D*, no shifting influence is seen. These diagrams show readily that inclines disturb the stability of dentures and should be reduced to a minimum. Occlusion is one of the retentive and stabilizing forces that impressions cannot overcome, no matter how great an amount of initial retention they may possess.

A related factor that may seem contradictory to the foregoing must be mentioned here: Reduction of cuspal inclines does not necessarily eliminate lateral forces on teeth and dentures. Mastication by cusped teeth is accomplished with essentially vertical closing forces. The cusps cut, tear, and shear, as well as crush, food. Teeth with 0-degree cusps cannot shear food *unless* some horizontal movement is included in the chewing cycle. This horizontal movement, induced by the muscles of mastication, transmits horizontal forces to the supporting structures and may cause more denture movement than the cuspal inclines.

In Fig. 21-13 are shown the directional movements of the mandible as described by the cusps over their opposing surfaces. Circle *a* is the opposing maxillary cusp moving over the surfaces of a mandibular first molar. The anteroposterior arrow, *P*, shows the direction of contact between the cusp and the inclined plane in a straight protrusive movement. Arrow *B* indicates a lateral movement that is diagonal in the balancing direction. Arrow *W* shows the movement of the cusp in the working direction. It must not be taken for granted that the mandible makes only these three grooved movements, however. Movements that are composites of *B* and *P* or *P* and *W* are

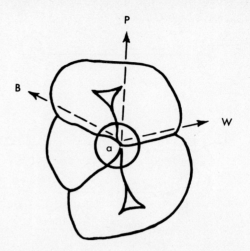

Fig. 21-13 Directional movement of the maxillary cusp on a posterior mandibular tooth. *a*, The maxillary cusp; *B*, direction of balancing movement; *W*, direction of working-side movement; *P*, direction of protrusive movement.

also made, which means that the mandible can move and occupy any part of the space between *B* and *W*.

Well-formed, unworn, and healthy natural teeth in normal occlusion guide the mandible through these general directional movements. With the dental arch intact and with good supporting structures, the periodontium of such teeth will stand the shock of guiding the mandible. On the other hand, the support for denture bases is such a small fraction of the support for natural teeth (Chapter 1) that denture bases need only a small fraction of the lateral and protrusive cusp inclines of natural teeth. Such a realization almost implies an ideal of 0-degree guidance for the incisal and condylar factors of occlusion. Hence the final argument between the two occlusal morphology schools (anatomic versus nonanatomic) hinges on the dentist's perception of the importance of a patient-determined versus a dentist-determined condylar guidance.

If the plan of occlusion is to have the least

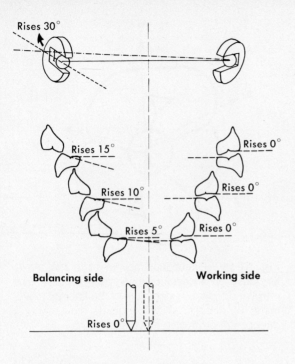

Fig. 21-14 Cuspal inclinations with a steep condylar guidance (30 degrees) and with horizontal (0-degree) incisal guidance.

possible cuspal inclines, teeth should be selected and arranged according to this plan. Posterior teeth should have no more than a 5-degree angle in the premolars and should then become progressively steeper in the second molar region, depending, of course, on the condylar guidance. However, if the vertical overlap of the anterior teeth develops an incisal guidance steeper than 5 degrees, teeth with steeper cuspal inclinations must be used.

This plan of occlusion for complete dentures calls for the reduction of all inclines or cusps that interfere with the movement between incisal guidance and condylar guidance. Denture bases can ill afford cusps that travel in established grooves. This means that the incisal pin is not limited to the outside path of a Gothic arch but can travel anywhere within this outside path. It should travel on any combination

of protrusive and lateral movements without striking the slightest rise or unevenness. Occlusion should be smooth running.

In Fig. 21-14 is shown a scheme for selecting, setting, and grinding to fit a plan of horizontal incisal guidance and whatever condylar guidance the patient may have (30 degrees in the illustration). As can be seen, the working-side inclines on all the teeth are horizontal. These inclines are determined by the horizontal movement of the working-side condyle, which merely rotates and does not rise or fall, and by the incisal guidance, which moves sideways but does not rise or fall. The balancing-side inclines start at 0 degrees, or nearly so, in the premolar region and increase progressively as they approach the 30-degree balancing condyle inclination.

OCCLUSAL SCHEMES USED IN COMPLETE DENTURES FOR THE EDENTULOUS PATIENT

The form of posterior teeth should be selected in the context of the dentist's broad objectives to fulfill the requirements of (1) esthetics, (2) harmonious function, and (3) maintenance of hard and soft tissues of the edentulous arches. Every dentist aims at fulfilling these objectives, regardless of the posterior tooth form selected. Posterior tooth forms have aroused a great deal of controversy among clinicians and researchers. Generally, most of the participants in the debate on the ideal posterior tooth form believe that the argument is settled and their opponents are wrong. Direct evidence is lacking to support any one concept.

There are several schools of thought on the choice of occlusal forms of posterior teeth for prosthetic restoration (Fig. 21-15), though only the two major ones are described here. These are the anatomic and nonanatomic techniques of posterior tooth morphology.

Anatomic teeth

The proponents of anatomic teeth insist that nature designed the tooth in a form best suited

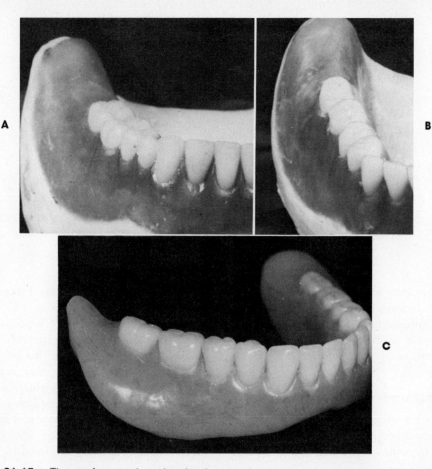

Fig. 21-15   Three of several occlusal schemes that represent varying concepts of arranging posterior teeth. **A,** Anatomic occlusion using 33-degree posterior teeth set with a compensating curve. **B,** Occlusion using posterior teeth set with a buccolingual reverse curve on the premolars and first molars and with the second molars shaped and positioned to provide balancing contacts. **C,** Very shallow-cusped posterior teeth arranged in a flat occlusal plane with the second molars positioned to provide balancing contacts. (Refer to Fig. 21-2, *C* and *D*.)

for the function of mastication. Cusped teeth have cutting blades so arranged that part of the nearly vertical closing force can shear food. Their contours can crush and triturate food when the proper forces are applied. Adequate sluiceways or escapes for food are present, which avoids the need for excessive pressures. The chewing efficiency of anatomic teeth for

some foods is greater than that of the modified tooth forms. The cuspal inclinations facilitate the development of bilateral balance (contact) in the various eccentric occlusions. Cusps provide thickness of the occlusal pattern in eccentric occlusions, which is an aid in the development of balanced occlusion (Fig. 21-16).

Cusped teeth provide a resistance to denture

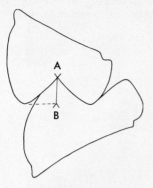

Fig. 21-16 *A-B* represents the thickness of the occlusal pattern in eccentric occlusions.

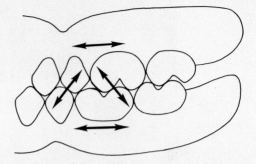

Fig. 21-17 Any possible tendency toward rotation produced by balancing tooth inclines is neutralized by the opposing inclines of cusps on the working side.

rotation in relation to each other and to their bases that is lacking in flat-cusped teeth (Fig. 21-17). The interdigitating cusps on the working side provide neutralizing incline plane contacts that tend to prevent rotation of the denture bases.

Nonanatomic teeth

Dentists who support the second school of thought, the concept of nonanatomic teeth, base their hypotheses on the following evidence:

Tooth contacts during mastication occur on the chewing and, even more frequently, the nonchewing sides. These contacts may occur irrespective of the form or arrangement of artificial teeth used. Tooth contacts also occur during swallowing and sleep. Most tend to be fleeting in nature, with the possible exception of the prolonged contacts occurring during parafunctional activity. A good deal of evidence supports the conclusion that patients do most of their chewing in centric occlusion, indicating that this is the position aimed for during jaw closure. Tooth contacts do not always occur in the same horizontal position, however. Patient posture and denture base dislodgment, or movement, influence the location of contacts. A cuspless occlusal scheme eliminates the pos-

sibility of deflective occlusal contacts when there is no food in the mouth.

The use of the patient's CR position does not imply that the patient is expected to masticate and swallow exclusively in this position. Many jaw closures also occur not only in proximity to but also anterior to CR, which supports the concept that an area of freedom of tooth contact in the occlusion anterior and lateral to CR should be provided in any occlusal scheme. Such freedom is easily achieved by using cuspless teeth.

The use of cuspless teeth involves less laboratory time and effort and can thus reduce the cost of treatment or save working hours for the dentist. The economic burden to the patient and the expense of the dentist's time are vitally connected with the phase of denture construction. This argument may be significant in the context of today's socioeconomic realities.

Advantages cited for nonanatomic teeth include (1) versatility of use, hence their employment in Class II and Class III jaw relationships; (2) permitting closure of the jaws over a broad contact area; (3) creating minimal horizontal pressures; (4) allowing for easier servicing of the complete dentures; and (5) allowing construction of dentures with a simple technique and articulator.

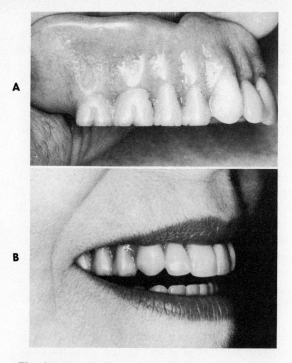

Fig. 21-18   **A,** Extraoral and, **B,** intraoral views of a nonanatomic posterior tooth arrangement illustrating the poor cosmetic effect achieved. See Fig. 21-2 for a solution to this problem.

Those who prefer the nonanatomic occlusal forms claim that damage to the basal seat of the dentures is caused by the intercuspation of cusped teeth as the vertical dimension of occlusion is lost through shrinkage of the ridges. This loss of denture foundation permits the jaws to close beyond the level at which occlusal contact was made when the dentures were first inserted. Such action causes the body of the mandible (and the lower teeth) to move forward. Because of the forward movement of the mandibular body, the mesial inclines of the cusps of the lower teeth make their first contact against the distal inclines of the cusps of the upper teeth. Thus the teeth can no longer contact in centric occlusion although the mandible is in CR. Such a malrelation forces the

upper denture forward and the lower denture backward.

On the other hand, nonanatomic teeth suffer from a number of disadvantages: (1) their anatomic form is esthetically inferior to that of cusped teeth (Fig. 21-18); (2) some patients complain of an inability to penetrate food effectively, which renders the dentures mechanically inefficient; and (3) they probably require the application of force in a nearly horizontal direction of jaw movement to shear food, and this results in lateral forces against the residual ridges.

Other tooth forms

Several other schools of thought on posterior tooth form and arrangement are also in evidence, each receiving varying support from different teaching centers and practitioners. In the absence of conclusive research on this matter, it appears reasonable to suggest that any tooth form, properly used, can fulfill the dentist's and patient's objectives of a functional and esthetically pleasing result. Such a result should also be accompanied by a commitment to the objective of minimal supporting-tissue changes in a longitudinal context. The latter objective is often described, though rarely encountered.

TECHNIQUES FOR ARRANGING CUSPED TEETH IN A BALANCED OCCLUSION
Setting each mandibular posterior tooth before the corresponding maxillary tooth is set

The anterior teeth are set first to their correct positions as indicated by esthetics. If the ridge relations are normal and the vertical and horizontal overlaps are approximately 1.5 mm each, the mandibular first premolar is set first. If the horizontal overlap is more than 1.5 mm, the maxillary first and second premolars are set first, and the mandibular first premolar is set after all the posterior teeth have been set. In either situation, the primary consideration is that the first premolar follow the form of the residual ridge. Its buccal surface should be parallel to the buccal surface of the canine, and it should be set slightly farther buccally than the canine but *never* farther buccally than the buccal flange.

When the ideal situation is assumed, the mandibular first and second premolars are set to conform to the shape of the residual ridge. Then the maxillary first premolar is set into CO with the two lower premolars. If a space develops between the maxillary canine and premolar, the maxillary second premolar is set in alignment in the upper arch. Then the two mandibular premolars are removed, and the mandibular second premolar is set in CO with the maxillary premolars. The mandibular first premolar is fitted between the canine and premolar after the necessary amount is ground from its mesial surface. The first three premolars set are the key to the relative anteroposterior intercuspation of all the remaining posterior teeth.

Once the premolars are set and properly related to each other, positioning of all the remaining posterior teeth is quite simple.

Each mandibular tooth is set before the corresponding maxillary tooth. It is positioned buccolingually so a perpendicular erected to the buccal side of the crest of the residual ridge will bisect its buccal cusp. The vertical height of its occlusal surface is adjusted so it will be on a line from the mandibular canine to near the top of the retromolar pad. After it is set, the maxillary tooth is placed to occlude with it. If the wax in the position where the tooth is to be set is pooled with a hot spatula and the cervical end of the tooth is heated, the tooth can be set slightly too long. Then the articulator is closed so the opposing teeth push the tooth up to the desired level. The index finger holds the cervical end of the tooth in place while the articulator is closed. This will develop the desired lingual cusp contact. The same procedure is used for setting all the remaining teeth.

A similar procedure can be used to set the teeth into a balanced occlusion. The tooth is set into the wax so it will be too long; then the articulator is closed in the lateral position, opened, and closed in the centric position, opened, and closed in the lateral position

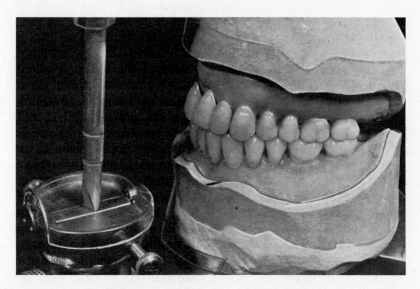

Fig. 21-19   Teeth in centric occlusion.

again. This will cause the tooth to rotate on its long axis or tip, and the inclines of its cusps will guide it into the proper position. The finger must keep the cervical end of the tooth from skidding laterally, and the articulator must be opened and closed into the desired position. The teeth must *not* slide on each other as the articulator is moved from one position to the other.

When the teeth are being set into a balanced occlusion, the amount of lateral movement to be used is that necessary to bring the maxillary and mandibular canines into an end-to-end relation to each other.

No attempt is made to balance the occlusion until the tryin is complete, esthetics are satisfactory, the CR record is correct, and the condylar guidance has been set. In CO the cusps are resting in their opposing fossae, with which they are designed to balance (Figs. 21-19 and 21-20).

Final balancing of the teeth is attained when three factors are changed: the compensating curve, the orientation of the plane, and the inclination of the cusps after the two end factors

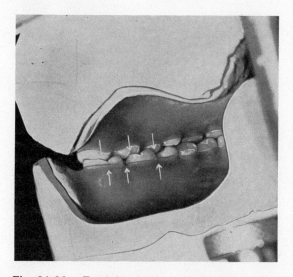

Fig. 21-20   Teeth in centric occlusion, lingual aspect. *Arrows* show the cusp-fossa alignment.

(incisal guidance and condylar guidance) have been established.

Balancing of the teeth must not be allowed to change the contacting of the pin on the incisal guide table. To do so would permit a change in one of the controlling factors.

When the articulator moves into lateral position, it should show the cusps of the maxillary teeth traveling across the intercusp spaces and grooves of the mandibular teeth as points *A* of the maxillary teeth (Fig. 21-21) travel across points *B* of the mandibular teeth on the buccal inclines of the working side.

On the lingual inclines of the working side, points *A* travel across points *B* on the mandibular teeth, as shown in Fig. 21-22. On the balancing side the lingual cusps of the maxillary teeth should be in contact with the buccal cusps of the mandibular teeth (Fig. 21-23).

Setting the maxillary teeth first

The maxillary posterior teeth are set up, starting with the first premolar and continuing to the second molar, without placing the teeth in close proximal contact. This slight opening of the contact points allows the mandibular teeth to better assume their correct (and important) mesiodistal relation to the maxillary teeth. To set the maxillary teeth in their correct buccolingual position, a straightedge is placed over the crest of the mandibular ridge (indicated by markings on the artificial borders of the mandibular cast in Fig. 21-24). A line is scratched in the wax, with a straightedge as a guide (Fig. 21-25). The lingual cusps of the maxillary teeth are placed over this line (Fig. 21-26). The mandibular teeth then assume their buccolingual and mesiodistal position by intercuspating with the maxillary posterior teeth. Since intercuspation is very exacting, it is best done by placing the mandibular first molar in position first. To place the first molar and still preserve the location of the crest of the ridge on the remainder of the occlusion rim, a block of wax approximately the size of the tooth is removed (Fig. 21-27). By placing the mandibular first molar in

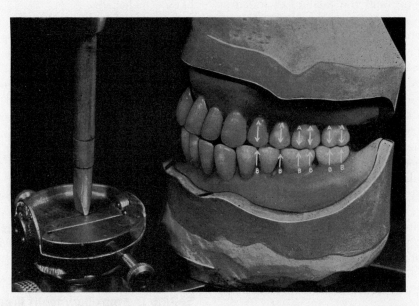

Fig. 21-21   Teeth in left lateral position on the working side. Points *A* pass across points *B*.

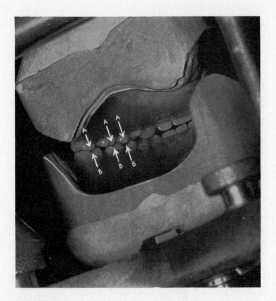

Fig. 21-22   Teeth in working position, lingual aspect. Points *A* pass across points *B*.

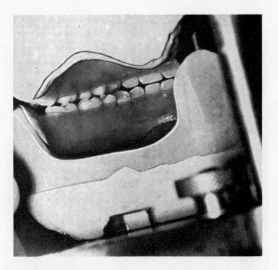

Fig. 21-23   Teeth in balancing position.

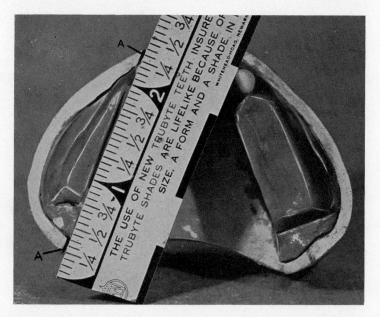

Fig. 21-24   A line to indicate the crest of the mandibular ridge between *A* and *A*.

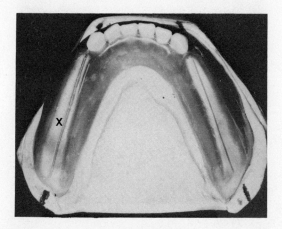

Fig. 21-25   The line, *X*, between points on the border of the cast is used as a guide for positioning mandibular teeth on a curve conforming to the shape of the residual ridge.

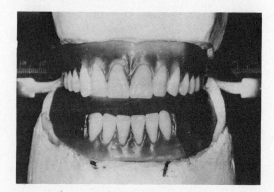

Fig. 21-26   The lingual cusps are placed directly over lines on the mandibular occlusion rim (*X* in Fig. 21-25).

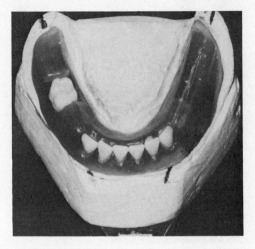

Fig. 21-27   First molar in place.

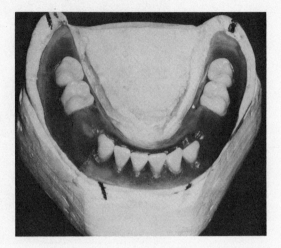

Fig. 21-28   Second molars in place.

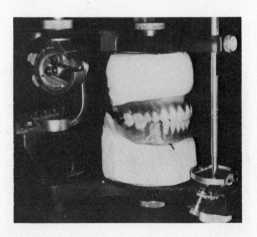

Fig. 21-29   Second molar in place.

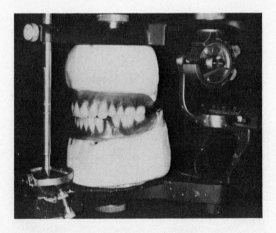

Fig. 21-30   Mandibular second premolar in place.

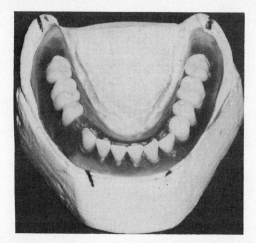

Fig. 21-31 The mandibular first premolar was too wide for the space available.

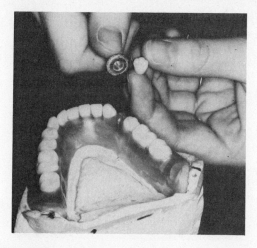

Fig. 21-32 Grinding the mandibular first premolar to fit the remaining space.

position without adjoining teeth, it is possible to determine its correct anteroposterior position more easily. If the dentist were to start with the mandibular first premolar, the inconstant vertical overlap might crowd the tooth into difficult intercuspation with the maxillary teeth and this would be carried into placement of all the mandibular posterior teeth. Therefore placement of the mandibular first premolar is left to the last, to take up all the variation in vertical and horizontal overlap of the anterior teeth. The first premolar is then ground to fit the remaining space.

The teeth are not arranged for balance at this time; they are set only in their correct centric positions to the opposing teeth. Inclinations for balance are completed after the posterior teeth are all in position.

The second molar is now placed, and has only one possible interference in assuming its correct anteroposterior position (Figs. 21-28 and 21-29).

The mandibular second premolar is next placed, after another block of wax has been cut away in this area (Fig. 21-30).

The mandibular first premolar is the last

tooth to be placed, and it frequently needs to be ground because vertical overlap of the patient is usually greater than the amount of vertical overlap with which the teeth were originally set in creating the master molds by the manufacturer (Fig. 21-31). (Manufacturers could not make as many molds as there are varying ridge relations.) For this reason, teeth must be ground and shaped to fit the space available (Fig. 21-32).

Another reason why the mandibular first premolar is chosen as the last tooth in the arrangement is that it has only the buccal cusp in occlusion and does not affect esthetics as greatly by being reduced in size as the maxillary first premolar would, which shows more plainly as the lips move.

One common error that causes anatomic teeth to be set inefficiently as to leverage and esthetics is attempting to use a given mold of teeth without altering a single tooth. This usually crowds the mandibular anterior teeth too far forward, gives a wide effect in the premolar regions, and upsets the correct intercuspation and occlusion. The sequence recommended in this discussion allows latitude by placing the

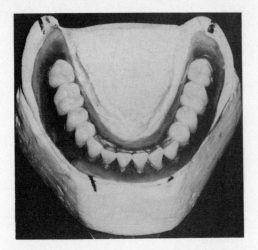

Fig. 21-33 All the mandibular teeth in place.

teeth in two sections: anterior and posterior. Then, in arranging the posterior teeth, the mandibular first premolar is the only one that needs to be ground and adjusted to take up the ridge-relation variance. This is believed to require a minimum amount of effort for the achievement of acceptable leverage and esthetics (Fig. 21-33).

TECHNIQUES FOR ARRANGING CUSPLESS TEETH IN OCCLUSION

Cuspless occlusal schemes may be designed with either a compensating curve or a flat plane.

Compensating curve

The arrangement of posterior teeth in a compensating curve of occlusion is quite similar to that described for anatomic teeth. The established contours of the occlusion rims and the markings on the casts are used as guides. The teeth are arranged to contact maximally on a compensating curve and to harmonize with the controlling end factors (the right and left condylar inclinations and the incisal guidance).

With cuspless teeth it is necessary to use a 0-degree incisal guidance to develop balancing contacts in the protrusive position (Fig. 21-34). Practical experience has shown that it is not always possible to arrange nonanatomic teeth in balanced occlusion with a compensating curve alone. The difficulty lies in the absence of cusp height in nonanatomic teeth. In these situations protrusive lateral balance can be attained on the articulator by use of a second molar ramp (Fig. 21-35, *A* and *B*). Even then, complete balance in all excursions is not feasible, and the dentist has to settle for a three-point balance effect (Fig. 21-35, *C*). If a vertical overlap of the anterior teeth is needed for esthetic reasons, a sufficient horizontal overlap must be introduced to prevent disclusion of posterior teeth in a protrusive contact movement (Fig. 21-36).

It must be emphasized that using nonanatomic teeth with a compensating curve, with or without a balancing ramp, entails laboratory procedures that are not as time consuming as those employed in the use of posterior teeth with cusps.

Flat plane

The technique for arranging cuspless teeth in a flat plane of occlusion is predicated on several premises that are distinct departures from what has been described in this chapter.

Complete denture patients should avoid incising with their anterior teeth. If they recognize this limitation, no balancing contact will be necessary for protrusive occlusions. To assist patients in this effort, the anterior teeth are set with an incisal guidance as close to 0 degrees as possible. Most patients can tolerate such incisal guidance without a serious esthetic compromise. Occasionally, however, the patient's or dentist's desire to achieve an optimal cosmetic result will necessitate a vertical overlap of the anterior teeth. This can generally be accommodated by the use of a sufficient horizontal overlap to allow a range of uniform posterior tooth

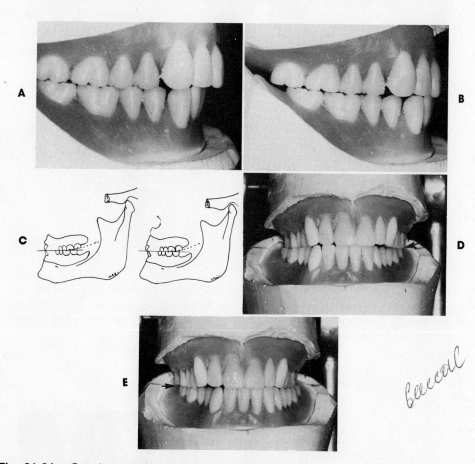

buccal

Fig. 21-34   Cuspless teeth are arranged on the articulator to contact maximally on a compensating curve in, **A,** CR and, **B,** a straight protrusive excursion. Both the incisal guide table on the articulator and the incisal guidance of the artificial teeth equal 0 degrees. No vertical overlap of the anterior teeth is present, **C.** Right and left mandibular lateral protrusive excursions are simulated on the articulator in **D** and **E.** Notice the balancing-side contacts in both *(arrows).*

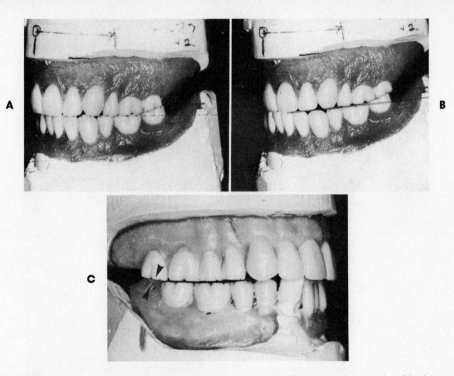

Fig. 21-35 Occasionally a three-point balanced occlusion must be used, with the second molars set on a ramp, **A** and **B.** If it is not technically feasible to use an artificial tooth, the wax can be carved to provide a balancing-side contact *(arrowheads),* **C.**

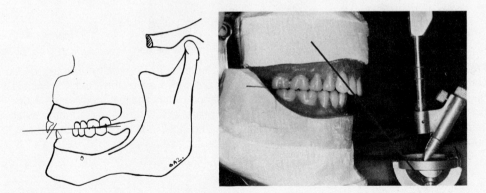

Fig. 21-36 Sufficient horizontal overlap is present in these anterior teeth to balance the required vertical overlap introduced for cosmetic reasons.

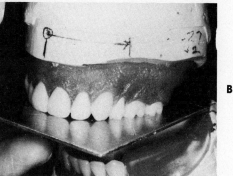

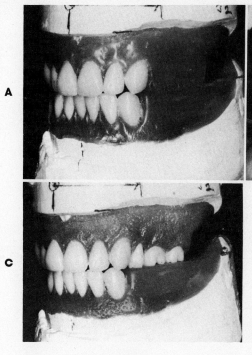

Fig. 21-37 **A,** Anterior teeth positioned with a zero-degree incisal guidance. **B** and **C,** The maxillary setup is completed so the incisal edges of the anterior teeth and the occlusal surfaces of all posterior teeth are flat against a flat plane.

contact anterior to the CR position (Fig. 21-36).

The condylar inclinations on the articulator are set at 0 degrees while the cuspless teeth are arranged (Fig. 21-37, A). In this manner, incising is avoided and cusp projections above the occlusal plane are absent in the posterior segments. The Hanau or Whip Mix articulator is thereby reduced to a simple hinge articulator. With the mandibular occlusion rim on its cast on the articulator, the maxillary posterior teeth are set in the maxillary wax rim. The teeth are positioned to occlude with the flat surface of the mandibular occlusion rim and to approximate the position of the maxillary occlusion rim contour that was previously determined. The markings established by the dentist on the maxillary cast are also used as guides in the arrangement of the teeth. The completed maxillary setup will usually show the in-

cisal edges of the anterior teeth and the occlusal surfaces of all posterior teeth to be flat against a flat plane (Fig. 21-37, B and C). Occasionally the maxillary anterior teeth can be placed slightly lower in relation to the posterior occlusal plane to improve cosmetics. In this situation, however, the horizontal overlap must be adequate to allow a gliding range of posterior teeth without "tripping" the dentures.

Next, the mandibular teeth are arranged so they will maximally contact the upper teeth (Fig. 21-38). Each tooth, in turn, is placed in a soft wax socket made in the occlusion rim, which has been heated with a spatula, and the articulator is closed while the tooth is oriented buccolingually to conform to the contoured lower occlusion rim, to the markings on the cast, and to the maxillary teeth. The anteroposterior relation of the upper and lower teeth to

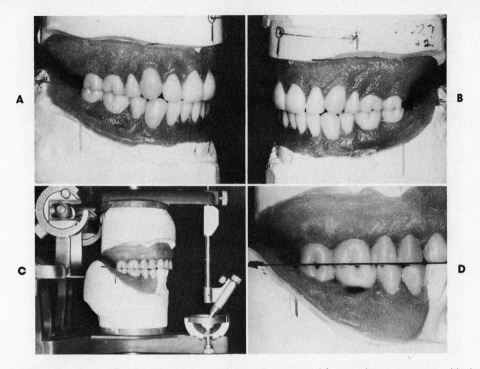

Fig. 21-38   A and **B,** Mandibular posterior teeth arranged for maximum contact with the maxillary teeth. **C,** In this case the condylar guidance and the incisal guide table on the articulator are set at 0 degrees. **D,** The completed posterior tooth arrangement conforms to a flat plane.

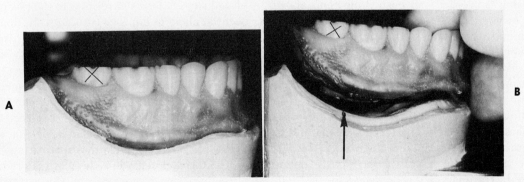

Fig. 21-39   A, The last artificial mandibular tooth should never be set on the slope of the ridge. **B,** The cast is marked where the mandibular ridge begins to curve upward.

each other is not critical because of the absence of cusps that would require intercuspation. Any combination of premolars or molars can be used to fill the available space. The posterior limit of the extent of these teeth is the point at which the mandibular ridge begins to curve upward (Fig. 21-39). Sometimes the large size of a patient's mouth or the patient's preoccupation with the number of teeth present on the denture will necessitate placing second or even third molars on this slope. In such situations, these teeth must not make contact with their antagonist or antagonists. In the horizontal plane the maxillary teeth usually overlap the mandibular ones. Flat-cusped teeth are readily arranged to accommodate a unilateral or a bilateral crossbite situation.

BIBLIOGRAPHY

Bergman B, Carlsson GE, Ericson S: Effect of differences in habitual use of complete dentures on underlying tissues, Scand J Dent Res 79:449-460, 1971.

Bergman B, Carlsson GE, Hedegård B: A longitudinal two-year study of a number of full denture cases, Acta Odontol Scand 22:3-26, 1964.

Feldmann EE: Tooth contacts in denture occlusion—centric occlusion only, Dent Clin North Am 15:875-887, 1971.

Ramfjord SP: Dysfunctional temporomandibular joint and muscle pain, J Prosthet Dent 11:353-374, 1961.

Schuyler CH: Fundamental principles in the correction of occlusal disharmony, natural and artificial, J Am Dent Assoc 22:1193-1202, 1935.

Sheppard IM: Incisive and related movements of the mandible, J Prosthet Dent 14:898-906, 1964.

Tallgren A: The continuing reduction of the residual alveolar ridges in complete denture wearers: a mixed-longitudinal study covering 25 years, J Prosthet Dent 27:120-132, 1972.

Zarb GA, Lewis DW, Scrivener EW: A clinical study of the effects of complete dentures on the oral tissues, IADR Abstr 413, p 152, 1970.

CHAPTER 22

Appearance and functional harmony of denture bases

Three principal factors are concerned in the functional harmony of denture bases. They are the basal or impression surface, the leverage position and occlusal surface of the teeth, and the shape or form of the polished surfaces of the dentures (Fig. 8-1).

An increase in size of the basal surface increases the amount of adhesion, the amount of border seal, and the amount of biting resistance. These are discussed in Chapters 7 and 9.

The most important of all factors are the occlusal surfaces. These are discussed in Chapter 21 and therefore will not be considered here except as they pertain to the other two factors.

The third factor, which is usually overlooked, is the shape of the polished surfaces. This should be given careful consideration. The two end factors in determining inclination of the polished surface are the width of the border and the buccolingual position of the teeth. The middle factor is the fullness given the wax to obtain convexity or concavity.

Figs. 8-1 and 8-2 show the inclined plane action of the muscles of the cheek and tongue in gripping a bolus of food. This action may be described by the illustration of a patient chewing a small pickled onion, with the tongue and cheek holding the onion in place over the occlusal surfaces of the teeth while closing pressure is exerted on it. This force exerted in the direction of the occlusal plane by the tongue and cheek can act as either a placing or a displacing agent, depending on the shape of the polished surface.

A further study of Figs. 8-1 and 8-2 shows the power of inclined plane forces on the shape given the polished surfaces as a mechanical aid or detriment in retention. For instance, when the lingual and buccal borders of a mandibular denture are being shaped, they can be made concave so the tongue and cheek will grip and tend to seat the denture. In the opposite case (in which the lingual and buccal surfaces are made convex by waxing and a narrow impression base is used) the inclined plane forces resulting from pressures of the tongue and cheeks will tend to unseat the denture. The buccolingual position of the teeth is important, because the farther toward the cheek the teeth are the greater the unseating inclined plane action becomes. A buccal position of the teeth would necessitate shaping the surface of the denture base in such a manner that the muscle action of the cheeks would tend to unseat the mandibular denture.

The buccal surface of mandibular dentures in the first premolar region should be shaped carefully so as not to interfere with the action of the modiolus, connecting the facial muscles with the orbicularis oris. This connecting point of muscles can displace the mandibular denture if the polished surface inclines toward the cheek or if the arch in the premolar region is too wide. These factors seem to be little understood.

WAXING

As has been stated, the form of the polished surfaces of a denture influences its retentive

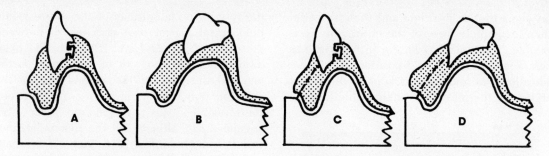

Fig. 22-1 **A** and **B,** The amount of wax to be added. **C** and **D,** The correct reduction.

quality. In addition, it influences the esthetic values of the denture. The wax surfaces around the teeth are known as the "art portion" of the polished surface and should, for esthetic reasons, imitate the form of the tissues around the natural teeth. Any fancy or artificial festooning is distinctly out of place. A slight projection of the root to follow the individual tooth can be made, however. The upper part of the polished surface, known as the "anatomic portion," should be formed in such a way as to lose none of the original border width of the impression. A small surplus can be allowed, to compensate for the loss of base material during finishing.

The form of the denture bases between the teeth and the border should be shaped in such a manner as to aid retention by the mechanical directional forces of the muscles and tissues (Figs. 8-1 and 8-2). Generally speaking, fullness on the buccal and labial surfaces of mandibular and maxillary dentures is desirable; and the opposite is true on the palatal surface of the maxillary denture, to provide all possible space for the tongue. The speech of the patient will be handicapped unless a contour comparable to that of the palate before the natural teeth were lost is developed. The thickness of the palatal part of the base will vary with the loss of bone from the residual alveolar ridge. The lingual flange of the mandibular denture should have the least possible amount of bulk, except at the border (which must be quite thick). This thick-

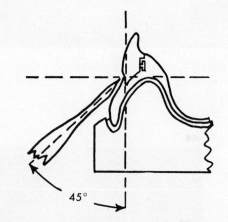

Fig. 22-2 The angle at which the knife should be held for cutting the gingival line.

ness is under the narrower portion of the tongue, and it greatly enhances the seal by contacting the mucolingual fold.

An excess of baseplate wax is added on the buccal and labial surfaces of the mandibular and maxillary trial dentures. The bulk of this is cut back to the outer border of the cast (Fig. 22-1), and then the small end of a knife is held at a 45-degree angle to the tooth surface to form the wax gingival margin (Fig. 22-2). The common tendency is to cut this line too straight from interproximal to interproximal, not leaving enough wax in the interproximal spaces (Fig. 22-3). It is well to have a surplus of wax along the gingival line and then to retrim when a complete view of the entire waxing is possible. Triangular markings can be placed as a guide to the length and position of the root indications, as long as it is kept in mind that the root of the maxillary canine is the longest,

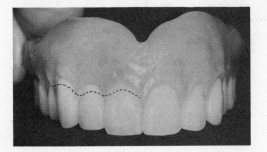

Fig. 22-3 Gingival line cut with the proper contour. The *dotted line* shows incorrect cutting.

the root of the lateral incisor the shortest, and the central incisor root of a length between these two (Figs. 22-4 and 22-5). On the mandibular denture the root of the canine is the longest, the root of the central incisor the shortest, and the lateral incisor root between these two. The wax is scraped out of these triangular areas, after which the root indications will become manifest (Fig. 22-6). The sharp and rough indications are now rounded with a large scraper and the spatula (Figs. 22-7 and 22-8). They should not be overemphasized.

The lingual surface of the mandibular denture may be made slightly concave without extending the concavity under the lingual surface of the teeth. A projection of the tooth beyond the polished surface acts as an undercut into which the patient's tongue will slip, thereby causing the denture to be unseated (Fig. 22-9).

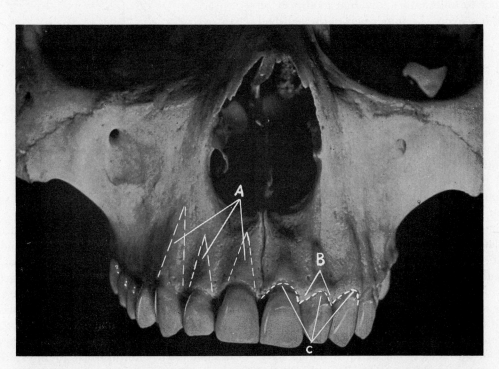

Fig. 22-4 *A,* Root indications on the skull; *B,* continued gingival prominences; *C,* contour of the gingival line.

The palatal surface of the maxillary denture should be waxed to a uniform thickness of 2.5 mm. Thus, when the processed resin is smoothed and polished, the palate will be as thin as possible and yet sufficiently thick to provide adequate strength. Lingual festooning restores part of the lingual surface of the tooth that is not supplied in artificial teeth. Wax is added and carved on the lingual side of the artificial teeth to imitate the normal lingual contours of each tooth (Figs. 22-10 and 22-11).

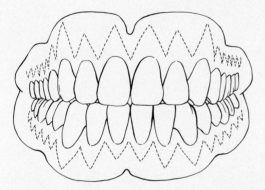

Fig. 22-5 Location and lengths of root indications to be made in wax.

MATERIALS USED FOR DENTURE BASES*
Acrylic resin

The material most often used in making denture bases is polymethyl methacrylate (PMMA) and is commonly called acrylic resin, or just acrylic. PMMA is modified by the addition of cross-linking monomers that increase craze-resistance and rigidity. Pigment is added for color. PMMA is a solid polymer composed of long straight chains of molecular units of methyl methacrylate. Methyl methacrylate is a liquid monomer. Denture base resins are supplied as a liquid monomer and powder polymer. The liquid wets the powder and forms a binder when it hardens.

Two methods of polymerizing or hardening the resin are employed, heat cure and chemical cure. The heat cure is accomplished when heat attacks the initiator (benzoyl peroxide) in the powder, which acts on the methyl methacrylate to form a polymer. The chemical cure differs only insofar as an activator in the liquid attacks

*We wish to acknowledge the assistance of Dr. Carl W. Fairhurst, Regents Professor and Coordinator of Dental Physical Sciences, Medical College of Georgia School of Dentistry, Augusta.

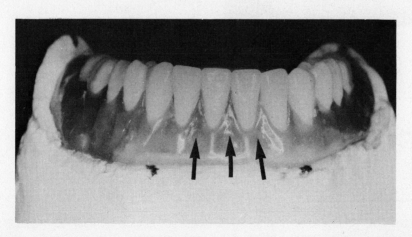

Fig. 22-6 Preliminary removal of wax from between the root indication lines (*arrows*).

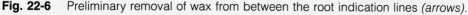

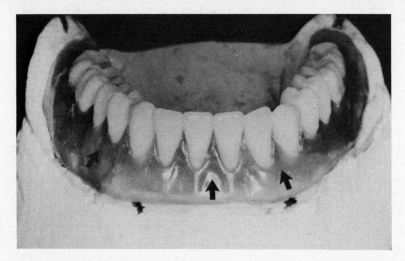

Fig. 22-7   Depressions between the root indication lines *(arrows)* that will be smoothed with the wax spatula.

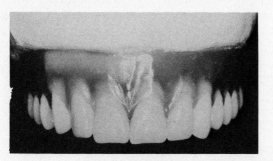

Fig. 22-8   The entire waxup, with root indications given a final smoothing.

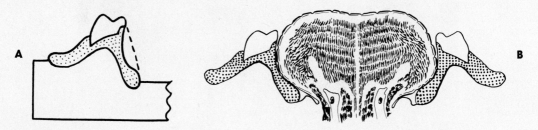

Fig. 22-9   **A,** Proper form of the lingual polished surface contour. **B,** Position of the tongue relative to the lingual surface of the denture base.

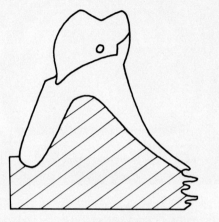

Fig. 22-10 The normal lingual contour of artificial posterior teeth is established during the waxing procedure.

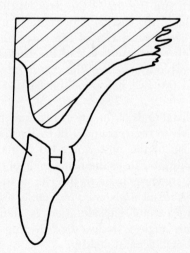

Fig. 22-11 The lingual contour of the upper central incisor is reestablished in the waxing procedure. This particular contour will aid phonetics and provide a natural feel to the patient's tongue.

the initiator when the liquid and powder are in contact.

The strength of the available denture resins varies considerably. If the denture base will have minimal thickness, with a greater risk of fracture, Lucitone 199,* a grafted type of PMMA, is recommended.

Metal

Metal denture bases may be made from a number of different materials such as gold, aluminum-manganese, platinum, Stellite (cobalt-chromium) alloys, and stainless steel (Fig. 22-12).

The *advantages* of metal denture bases are principally as follows:

1. Better thermal conductivity as compared to resins
2. Increased tissue tolerance because of a less-irritating surface and less stimulation from heat and cold
3. Reduced bulk across the palate, an important factor to the patient since more tongue space is created
4. Increased accuracy of fit of the denture base on the mucosa of the basal seat
5. Increased weight, causing increased stability of lower dentures

Some *disadvantages* of metal bases are the following:

1. Greater initial and greater restorative costs
2. Difficulty and expense of rebasing and regrinding the occlusion
3. Less margin of error permissible in the posterior palatal seal
4. Increased weight for a maxillary denture

FORMATION AND PREPARATION OF THE MOLD

After the trial dentures have been waxed, they are prepared for flasking. A Hanau ejec-

---

*Caulk/Dentsply, Milford DE, 19963.

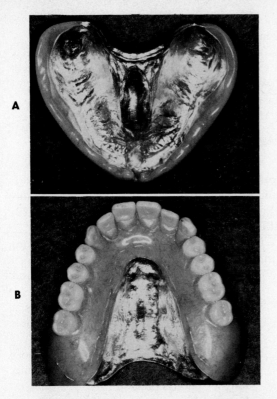

Fig. 22-12   Metal bases for complete dentures. **A,** Gold or Stellite (cobalt/chromium) covers the palate and residual ridges, with the borders formed in acrylic resin. **B,** Notice the distribution of metal and acrylic resin and also that the lingual surfaces of the teeth have been restored with acrylic. The posterior palatal seal area need not be made of metal. A "mesh" area here will provide excellent retention for an acrylic posterior palatal seal.

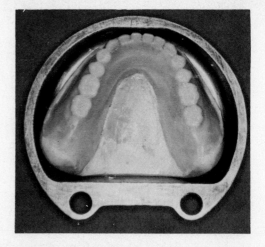

Fig. 22-13   The lower wax denture pattern and its cast in the bottom half of the lower flask. (From Javid NS, Boucher CO: J Prosthet Dent **29**:581-585, 1973.)

tor-type flask is used to facilitate removal of the trial denture after processing without danger of breaking the denture.

The trial denture is tested in the flask to establish its height in relation to the height of the bottom half of the flask (Fig. 22-13). The top half of the flask is placed in position to ensure that the teeth are not too high in relation to the top of the flask. Approximately ⅛ to ¼ inch (3 to 6 mm) of space should be available between the teeth and the top of the flask. If the teeth are too high, the cast must be reduced in thickness. The artificial rim of the cast should be flush with the bottom half of the flask to prevent possible breakage of the cast in later separation of the two halves of the flask (Fig. 22-14).

The distal ends of the lower cast may be high in relation to the remainder of the cast and extend close to the posterior edge of the flask. This condition causes the distal ends of the cast to be at an acute angle to the rim of the flask. Thus the distal ends are vulnerable to breakage, and careful consideration is demanded when this angle is reduced so the top half of the flask will separate easily.

A mix of artificial stone is placed in the bottom half of the flask, and the cast, which has been painted with separating medium (Fig. 22-15), is placed down into the stone until its rim is nearly level with the top edge of the flask. The stone is leveled between the edge of the cast and the rim of the flask.

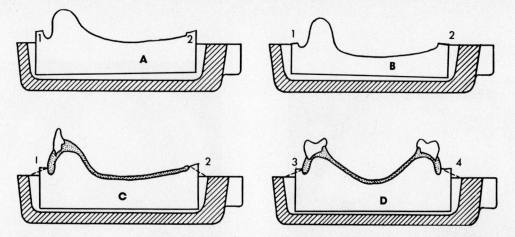

Fig. 22-14 First half of flasking of the maxillary trial denture. **A,** Cast too high in areas *1* and *2*. **B,** Areas *1* and *2* at a favorable level. **C,** Areas *1* and *2* should be beveled. **D,** Areas *3* and *4* to be beveled.

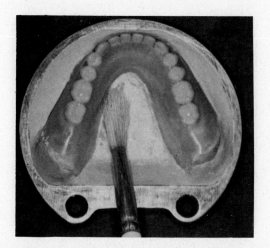

Fig. 22-15 Separating medium applied with a camel's hair brush on the exposed stone of the land. (From Javid NS, Boucher CO: J Prosthet Dent **29:**581-585, 1973.)

After separating medium has been applied to the exposed stone in the flask, a core of artificial stone 2 to 4 mm thick is developed around the labial and buccal surfaces of both wax dentures, on the lingual of the lower wax denture and the palatal of the upper. The top of the cores should be 2 to 3 mm below the occlusal plane of the teeth (Figs. 22-16 to 22-18). **V**-shaped grooves are placed in the cores so they will separate with the top half of the flask.

Separating medium is applied on the exposed surfaces of the core, and the top half of the flask is set in position. The two flask halves must meet exactly. Then a mix of artificial stone is poured up to the level of the incisal edges of the anterior teeth and the tips of the cusps of the posterior teeth (Fig. 22-19). The exposed stone is painted with separating medium, the flask is completely filled with artificial stone, and the lid of the flask is set in position.

The flask is placed in boiling water and allowed to remain 4 to 6 minutes according to its size. Then it is removed from the water and

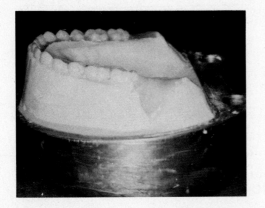

Fig. 22-16 Buccal and lingual cores around the lower denture with *V*-shaped grooves. (From Javid NS, Boucher CO: J Prosthet Dent **29:**581-585, 1973.)

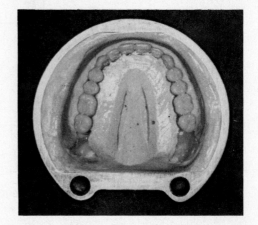

Fig. 22-17 Buccal and lingual cores around the upper denture with *V*-shaped grooves. (From Javid NS, Boucher CO: J Prosthet Dent **29:**581-585, 1973.)

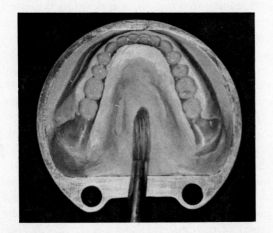

Fig. 22-18 Labial, buccal, and lingual cores coated with a separating medium. (From Javid NS, Boucher CO: J Prosthet Dent **29:**581-585, 1973.)

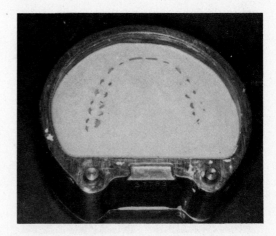

Fig. 22-19 After the upper half of the flask has been put in place, a heavy mixture of dental stone is poured to the level of the tips of the cusps. (From Javid NS, Boucher CO: J Prosthet Dent **29:**581-585, 1973.)

A

B

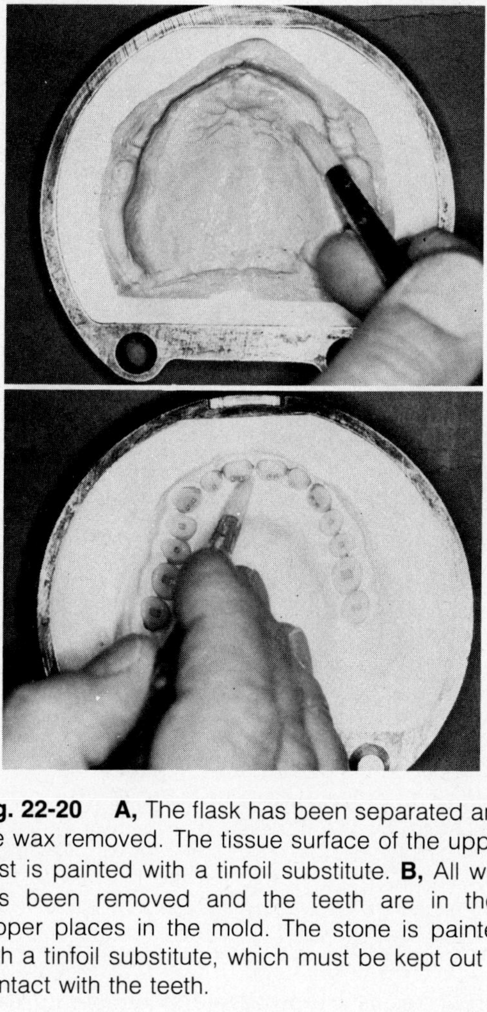

Fig. 22-20   A, The flask has been separated and the wax removed. The tissue surface of the upper cast is painted with a tinfoil substitute. **B,** All wax has been removed and the teeth are in their proper places in the mold. The stone is painted with a tinfoil substitute, which must be kept out of contact with the teeth.

opened from the side opposite the greatest undercut. After it is opened, the surplus wax is washed out with a stream of boiling water. When the water has been drained from the flask, the mold is washed again with boiling water containing a powdered detergent and then with clean boiling water. Liquid detergents have a greater tendency to leave a residue, which is undesirable, especially with acrylic resin teeth, and solvents such as chloroform are not used because of their effect on the acrylic.

After the stone is dry, but while still hot, the inside of the mold and the cast are painted with a tinfoil substitute; a camel's hair brush is often used for this (Fig. 22-20). The tinfoil substitute must not come in contact with the teeth or pool in the mold around the teeth. It is allowed to dry, and a second coat is painted on the inside of the mold. The flask is allowed to cool to room temperature.

When acrylic resin teeth are used, the exposed surfaces must be kept very clean. A wax residue on the teeth seems to be the principal contaminant and the main cause for adhesive failure.

PACKING THE MOLD

An acrylic resin dough is made by mixing the powder (polymer) and liquid (monomer) in accordance with the manufacturer's directions. Monomer is a sensitizer that can cause an allergic contact eczematous reaction on the skin or mucous membrane. Consequently it is advisable to wear rubber gloves and work under proper ventilation. When the monomer is completely polymerized, it no longer elicits an allergic reaction. When the mixture has reached a doughy consistency, it is placed between two plastic sheets and formed into a roll about 1 inch (2.5 cm) in diameter. The roll is flattened to be about ¼ inch (6 mm) thick, and pieces are cut to approximate the length of the flanges and the size of the palate (Fig. 22-21, *A*). The pieces are positioned around the buccal, labial, and palatal surfaces of the upper mold (Fig. 22-21, *B* and *C*) and around the buccal, labial, and lingual surfaces of the lower mold (Fig. 22-22, *C*). The flask is closed in a press with a sheet of separating plastic between the two halves until they are almost in approximation (Fig. 22-21, *D*). Then the flask is opened, the excess flash resin is cut away precisely at the denture border, and additional resin is added at any places that are deficient (Fig. 22-22). This trial packing procedure is repeated until the mold is filled and no flash is formed. Then the flask is closed completely without the separating

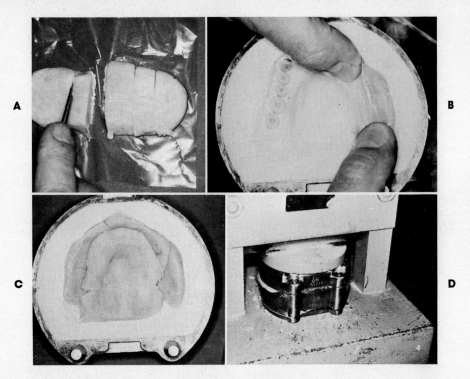

Fig. 22-21 **A,** Acrylic resin dough is formed into a cylindrical mass and cut into pieces the approximate size of the mold. **B,** A section of the dough is placed in the mold for the upper denture. It is carried to place with cellophane to prevent contamination. **C,** The dough has been distributed throughout the upper mold. **D,** The flask is closed slowly in an automatic press.

sheet. The slightest discrepancy in closure of the two halves of the flask will cause an error in the occlusion.

The flask is transferred to a spring clamp. The clamp is closed tightly but not fully compressed. This will allow the resin to expand upon processing and then finally contract while still under pressure. After a wait of 30 to 60 minutes to allow the liquid to penetrate the powder thoroughly, the flask and clamp are placed in a curing unit. The denture is processed for 9 hours in water held at a constant temperature of 165° F (73.5° C). Conventional acrylic resins are processed at temperatures of 135° to 180° F. No significant distortion takes place when the acrylic is processed at or below the manufacturer's recommended temperature. However, the amount of monomer remaining in the cured resin clearly affects the degree of cytotoxicity of the denture base material.

The flask must cool to room temperature before deflasking begins. It is crucial that sufficient time be allowed for cooling inside the flask. If this precaution is not taken, increased distortion of the acrylic will occur.

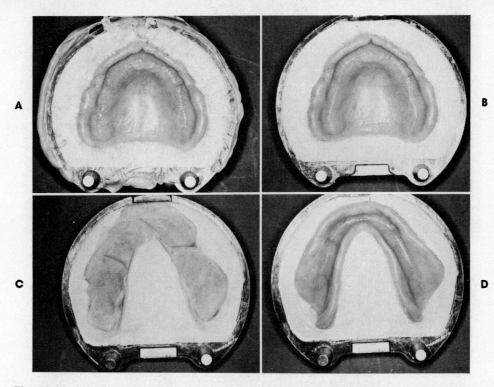

Fig. 22-22   A, Excess acrylic resin in the mold has been forced between the two halves of the flask during the initial trial packing. **B,** Excess in the upper mold removed through a series of trial packing. **C,** The dough is distributed throughout the lower mold. **D,** Excess removed through a series of trial packings.

PRESERVING THE ORIENTATION RELATIONS

Deflasking is completed, and the processed dentures are left on the casts. The casts and dentures are returned to the mountings on the articulator, and the processing changes are observed. The processing changes are usually not corrected at this time, since new interocclusal records will be made from the patient.

The upper cast is attached to the upper mounting, and a record of its relationship to the articulator is made in plaster of Paris on the remounting jig. Fast-setting plaster is spread on the jig, and the teeth of the upper denture are pressed into the plaster while the cast is in its keyed position on the articulator. The plaster on the jig is allowed to set (Fig. 22-23).

SHAPING AND POLISHING THE CURED RESIN BASES

The dentures are removed from the artificial stone casts. The feather edges of the denture base material are removed with files, scrapers, and burs. Care must be taken with rotating instruments because enough heat can be generated during grinding to cause distortion of the

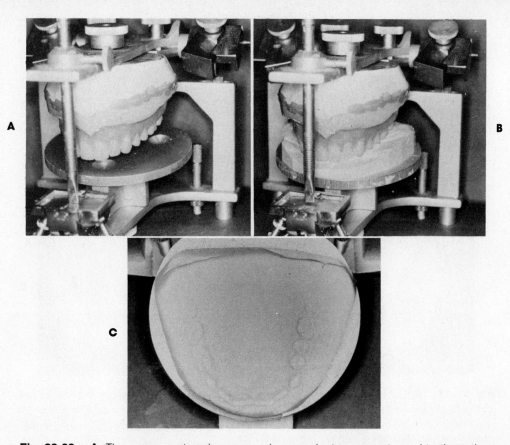

Fig. 22-23 **A,** The upper cast and processed upper denture are returned to the articulator mounting an attached with sticky wax. The remounting jig is positioned on the lower member of the articulator. **B,** The upper denture is closed into the plaster on the remounting jig so the occlusal surfaces of the teeth will make an imprint in plaster. **C,** Plaster record of the teeth on the upper denture. This will permit the denture, after deflasking, to be repositioned in proper relation to the upper member of the articulator.

denture base. The feather edges around the gingival line of the teeth are cut down by means of burs and chisels to conform with the desired contour. Special care also must be taken when acrylic resin teeth have been used. Any difficulty during polishing of the dentures is caused by the fact that they are not properly prepared for polishing. With burs, stones, chisels, and sharp scrapers, the surface is shaped

until it is a smooth and clean. No plaster and no deep scratches should remain after the preparation for polishing. It is impossible to retain the desired contour of the dentures if abrasives such as pumice are used for finishing.

A rag wheel and felt cone with pumice are good for smoothing the palatal portion of the upper denture. A single-row brush wheel and a rag wheel about ¼ inch (6 mm) in width are

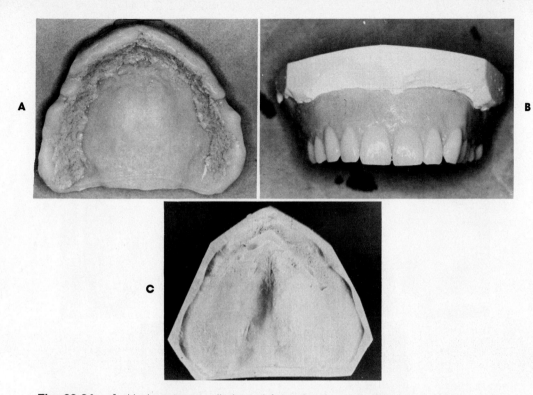

Fig. 22-24   A, Undercuts are eliminated from the tissue surface of the denture when they are filled with wet tissue paper. **B,** Upper remounting cast poured in the upper denture. **C,** Upper denture removed from the upper remounting cast. It must be possible for the denture to be easily returned to and fit accurately on the cast.

used with pumice to smooth the labial and buccal surfaces of the denture without destroying the contour. A final high polish is given all the surfaces with a rag wheel and polishing material (tripoli, tin oxide and water).

CONSTRUCTION OF REMOUNTING CASTS

Remounting casts serve as an accurate, convenient, and time-saving method of reorienting the completed dentures on the articulator for occlusal corrections. All undercuts on the tissue surface of the dentures are filled with wet

tissue paper, Mortite (a caulking compound), or wet pumice (Fig. 22-24, *A*).

Remounting casts of fast-setting plaster or artificial stone are poured into the denture. After the plaster has set, the excess is trimmed down to the border (Fig. 22-24, *B*) and the dentures are removed from the casts. The block-out material is then scraped from the undercut areas, and the dentures are cleaned. The casts are examined to ensure that the grooves formed by the border of the dentures are not deeper than 1 mm. Excessive depth of the grooves jeopardizes exact placement of the dentures each

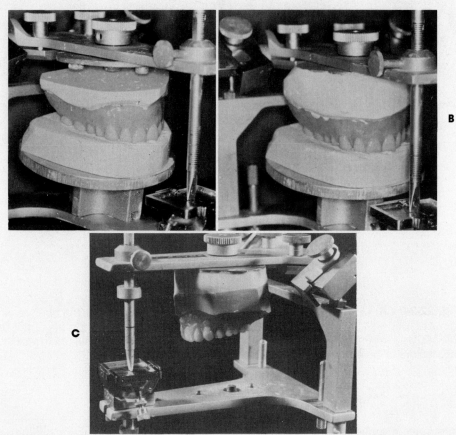

Fig. 22-25   A, The upper denture and remounting cast have been repositioned in the plaster imprints of the teeth on the remounting jig. **B,** The remounting cast attached to the mounting ring on the upper member of the articulator by fast-setting plaster. **C,** Remounting jig and plaster index removed from the lower member of the articulator. The upper completed denture and remounting cast are located in the same relation on the articulator as established originally by the face-bow record.

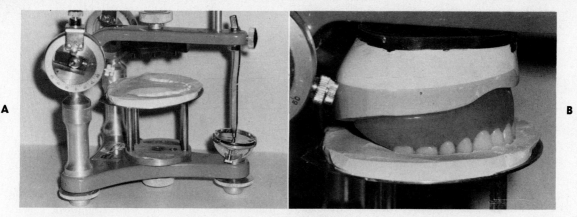

Fig. 22-26   A, Occlusal index previously made on the Dentatus articulator before the waxed-up maxillary denture was removed from the original mounting. **B,** Remounting cast attached to the mounting ring on the upper member of the articulator with fast-setting plaster.

time they are removed and placed back on the cast (Fig. 22-24, *C*).

With the remounting jig and index positioned on the mandibular member of the articulator, the maxillary denture and remounting cast are placed in the plaster indentations. The maxillary remount cast is attached to the maxillary member of the articulator by means of fast-setting plaster (Fig. 22-25).

Alternative procedure

To save time and expedite the laboratory phase, the plaster index can be made when the waxup is completed just prior to removal of the casts from the articulator. After processing of the acrylic, the dentures are removed from the master casts and are then finished and pol-

ished. When the remounting casts have been made, the occlusal index is placed on the articulator (Fig. 22-26, *A*). The maxillary denture can then be attached to the upper member of the articulator with fast-setting plaster (Fig. 22-26, *B*). An inexpensive type of mounting plate can be used so the mountings will be permanent if desired. This is an acceptable alternative to using the more expensive metal mounting plates.

BIBLIOGRAPHY

Johnstone EP, Nicholls JI, Smith DE: Flexure fatigue of 10 commonly used denture base resins, J Prosthet Dent 46:478-483, 1981.

Spratley MH: An investigation of the adhesion of acrylic resin teeth to dentures, J Prosthet Dent **58**:389-392, 1987.

CHAPTER 23

Completing the rehabilitation of the patient

The moment new dentures are placed in a patient's mouth, all the procedures involved in denture construction are subject to review and reevaluation. The choice of procedures, the technical effectiveness of the procedures used, and the skill needed in carrying out the procedures are exposed to three evaluations. These are by the dentists who rendered the service, the patients who are to use the dentures, and the friends and associates of the patients who will be viewing the result.

DENTISTS' EVALUATIONS

Evaluations made by dentists should be the most critical, for these are the only professionals who can know the possibilities and limitations in the treatment of the patient. In this moment of truth, dentists must know and recognize and admit (at least to themselves) any deficiencies in the prosthodontic service provided. If they are not completely honest with themselves at this point, are not informed about the type of observations that should be made, and are not extremely critical of the results of the treatment, they are not rendering a truly professional service. Worse than this, the quality of the denture service they provide to other patients will deteriorate. If, as a part of the treatment of edentulous patients, dentists make complete dentures that they consider to be perfect, their next dentures are likely to be not as good. In other words, if dentists cannot find anything at all that they would try to change in treating the same patient again with complete dentures, they are not being as criti-

cal of their own efforts as they should be. The maintenance of quality of prosthodontic service depends on a constant vigilance and self-discipline. The forgetting curve takes its toll in technical skills and procedures just as it does in didactic knowledge. A critical evaluation by the dentist of every prosthodontic service rendered will tend toward a constant improvement of the service. This is an essential part of the care of denture patients after new dentures have been provided.

PATIENTS' EVALUATIONS

Patients' evaluations of their new dentures are made in two phases. The first is the reaction to the completed dentures the first time they are placed in the mouth. This can range from hopeful confidence to fear and apprehension. The patient's frame of mind will depend largely on the dentist, but it may be affected by previous experiences in denture wearing and by comments of other people. If adequate diagnoses were made before any treatment was started, all misconceptions and inaccurate information will have been brought to light. At this time wise dentists will have allayed their patients' fears and corrected any misinformation, and instructions regarding the use of dentures will have been started. These dentists will have demonstrated to their patients that they are treating them properly and that they have used the utmost care in the technical procedures involved in building the dentures. Thoroughness in each step from diagnosis to insertion is apparent to patients—and this builds confidence. Patients sense carelessly or hastily performed techniques, just as they recognize care used in making impressions and jaw relation records and in arranging the teeth for esthetics. A failure to spend adequate time at the tryin appointment leads to trouble on insertion of the dentures. If confidence cannot be earned and established *before* the day the dentures are placed in the mouth, the treatment after this time will be more complicated.

FRIENDS' EVALUATIONS

When patients leave the dental office with their new teeth, it is with mixed emotions. They want their friends to notice their improved appearance; they hope their friends and relatives will compliment them and confirm their judgment in the choice of dentist they have made; and, of course, they still wonder how they will progress with eating and speaking. They need help. If people comment about the new teeth, some patients may wonder if the teeth look natural; and if they do not comment, the patients may wonder if their friends are just being kind. In reality, when people comment about teeth, it usually is because the dentist has failed to achieve a natural-appearing result.

The evaluations by friends of patients are most likely to be inaccurate. Friends cannot know how the dentures feel; they cannot judge the efficiency of the dentures in eating and speaking; they cannot know the difficulties encountered by the dentist because of the poor foundation on which the dentures may have been built. They cannot understand the possible lack of coordination of the patient or the ineptness of some patients in attempting to follow instructions or to use the dentures. The patients themselves may recognize these difficulties as partly their responsibility, but the comments of friends may cause them to blame the dentist for problems that may have been beyond the dentist's control. Such well-meaning friends can add to a patient's difficulties because they have not been exposed to the information supplied to the patient by the dentist during the course of construction of the dentures. The only apparent way to guard against patients' being misinformed by their friends is to take the lead and make certain that patients have been correctly informed. This process can be a continuing one and should start at the time the diagnosis is made. Enlisting the aid of a patient's most critical friend or relative in critiquing the appearance at the tryin is also very helpful.

TREATMENT AT THE TIME OF DENTURE INSERTION

The insertion of new dentures in a patient's mouth involves more than seating the dentures and telling the patient to call if there is any trouble. It is at this time that the dentist's evaluation is started. Also there are certain technical procedures that must be carried out. The dentures, having been processed and polished, are not completed. Inaccuracies in the materials and methods used to get the dentures to this stage must be recognized and eliminated *before* the patient wears the dentures.

The inaccuracies may be the result of (1) technical errors or errors in judgment made by the dentist, (2) technical errors developed in the laboratory, or (3) inherent deficiencies of the materials used in the construction of the dentures. Regardless of the source of the inaccuracies, they should be corrected *before* the patient is permitted to use the dentures.

Prior to the placing of dentures in the patient's mouth, the denture *flanges* should be examined to ensure that they are not too thick and the denture *borders* should be examined for roundness with no obvious overextension. If carefully border-molded impressions have been made, the flanges and borders should require no alteration—provided, of course, the laboratory operations have respected those borders. If a penciled outline on the cast has been used to indicate the extent of the flanges, more changes in border form will be necessary than if an accurately border-molded impression has been used. If the laboratory technician has disregarded the borders recorded by the impression on the cast or has disregarded the instructions relating to the flanges and borders, some alteration may be necessary at the time of insertion.

The dentist's objective, however, should be to make the impressions and casts so perfectly that there is no doubt in the mind of the technician as to the form and extent of borders and flanges when the dentures are polished.

The patient should have been instructed to keep any previous dentures out of the mouth for 12 to 24 hours immediately before the insertion appointment. This is essential if the new dentures are to be seated on healthy and undistorted tissues. If the tissues have been distorted by old dentures, the new ones cannot seat perfectly even if they fit perfectly. Improper seating of dentures at this time can cause the appearance of errors in occlusion or fit that would not exist if the tissues were undistorted. Unnecessary adjustments of any type to correct such apparent errors, if made at this time, can cause irreparable damage to the dentures. This caution is predicated on the requirement that the patient be without *any* teeth for 24 hours (sometimes longer) to get the tissues healthy before the final impressions are made and that no teeth be used by the patient until the jaw relation records are verified at the tryin.*

The occlusion of all complete dentures should be perfected before the patient is allowed to wear the dentures. This is true regardless of the technique or instruments used in making the impressions, making the jaw relation records, arranging the teeth in a balanced occlusion, and processing the dentures. Construction of dentures for a patient involves

---

*As mentioned in Chapter 18, many patients will find leaving the dentures out of their mouth for 12 to 24 hours an unreasonable request. An acceptable alternative is to have the existing dentures relined with a soft temporary material to minimize tissue distortion problems.

many separate but related procedures. An error in any one can contribute to an error in the occlusion of the completed dentures.

ELIMINATION OF BASAL SURFACE ERRORS

All surfaces of the completed dentures must be critically examined for small projections caused by imperceptible discrepancies in the cast or in the investing materials. A magnifying glass used in addition to digital inspection of the denture bases can be effective in locating such irregularities. All denture borders, and especially the frenal notches, must also be examined carefully for sharp edges. Sharp borders in the frenal notches must be carefully rounded before the initial placement of the dentures.

Pressure indicator paste can be helpful when bilateral undercuts on the residual ridge interfere with the initial placement of dentures or when pressure spots were present in the final impression. The paste is brushed on the tissue surface of the denture base in a thin layer so the brush marks are visible and run the same direction. In this manner tissue interferences during placement of the dentures or excessive pressure on the residual ridge can be more easily interpreted than without the paste (Fig. 23-1). Then the painted surface is sprayed with a silicone liquid.

The denture is carefully placed on the residual ridge and pressure is applied by the dentist on the teeth to reveal any pressure spots in the denture base that would displace soft tissue (Fig. 23-2). A repeat recording should be made for verification of pressure spots, and the denture base carefully relieved (Fig. 23-3). When tissue interferences are present, the denture coated with pressure indicator paste is seated on the residual ridge until resistance is met. The marks in the paste indicate where the denture base should be relieved to accommodate the interference (Fig. 23-4). Pressure indicator paste should be used for every new denture,

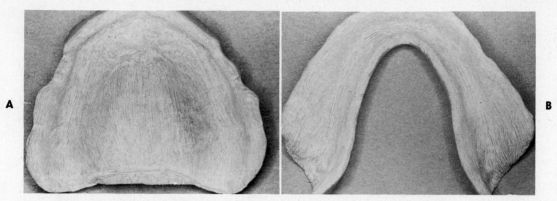

Fig. 23-1   A, Pressure indicator paste distributed in a thin even layer across the tissue surface of the upper denture. **B,** Paste distributed in the lower denture. Notice the brush marks running in the same direction. This method of distribution aids in determining interferences that might prevent proper placement of the denture and impede the detection of any harmful pressure spots.

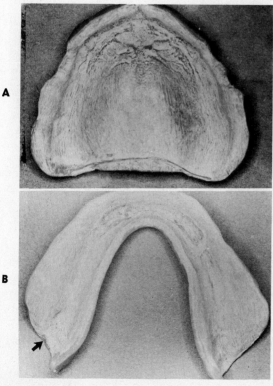

Fig. 23-2   A, Marks showing through the pressure indicator paste reveal the location of pressure spots exerted by the denture on the residual ridge. The spot in the region of the left hamular notch was also present on the final impression. The posterior palatal seal bead is visible through the pressure indicator paste and shows that the desired seal is being provided. **B,** Pressure areas visible through the alveolar groove anteriorly and the retromolar fossa *(arrow)*. These should be relieved, since they are not in a primary stress-bearing area for the lower denture. The exposed borders of the lingual flange are not necessarily significant at the time of initial placement of the lower denture but may become more so if they are related to unnecessary movement of the denture or soreness in the alveololingual sulcus at a later date.

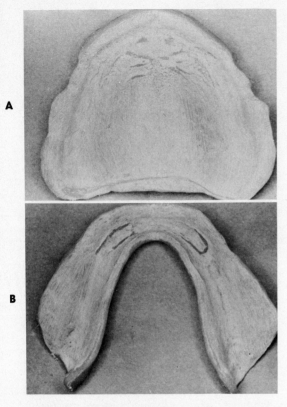

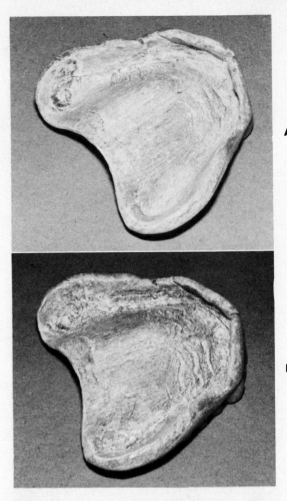

Fig. 23-3 The pressure spots in Fig. 23-2 have been carefully relieved with a no. 8 round bur. A minimum of denture base material was removed.

Fig. 23-4 **A,** Interference in the left posterior buccal flange area is noted prior to seating the maxillary denture in its correct position. **B,** After careful adjustment a new recording of the indicator paste indicates proper seating of the denture.

and any necessary adjustments should be made before proceeding with the occlusal adjustment.

ERRORS IN OCCLUSION

The errors in occlusion that may be observed can result from a number of factors. These include a change in the state of the TMJs, inaccurate maxillomandibular relation records by the dentist, errors in the transfer of maxillomandibular relation records to the articulator, failure to seat the occlusion rims correctly on the casts, ill-fitting temporary bases, failure to use the face-bow (with subsequent need to change the vertical dimension on the articulator), incorrect arrangement of the posterior teeth, failure to close the flasks completely, use of too much pressure in closing the flasks, or warpage of the dentures by overheating them during polishing. All these are errors in technique on the part of the dentist or laboratory technician.

Each procedure has the possibility of an error that might not be noted until the dentures

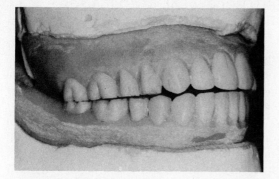

Fig. 23-5 Processed dentures are replaced on the articulator while still on their casts. The changes that occurred in processing of the acrylic have caused errors in the occlusion.

are placed in the patient's mouth. Even then, errors in occlusion might not be apparent unless other procedures are used to test for them. These errors in occlusion must be eliminated before the dentures are worn, or the soft tissues interposed between the bone and the dentures will be distorted in the attempt to eliminate the errors.

Occlusion errors may be the result of unavoidable changes in the denture base material itself (Fig. 23-5). Acrylic resins shrink when they change from a moldable to a solid form. They have a high coefficient of thermal expansion, and in cooling after polymerization they shrink and this causes warpage. The greatest amount of warpage occurs when the dentures are removed from the casts. Further warpage may occur if too much heat is generated in polishing the dentures. Subsequently the resin absorbs water in use, and this expands the resin. All these processing changes are inevitable, though some can be minimized by careful and special techniques.

True, these changes are relatively small and the soft tissue covering of the maxillae and mandible will give enough, or be displaced enough, to allow dentures to be seated and tolerated by most patients. Nevertheless, any discrepancies can alter the relationships of the

teeth to each other and must be eliminated before the dentures are worn by the patient.

Maxillomandibular relations are bone-to-bone relations and as such represent the status between two solid objects, the maxillae and the mandible. These bones are covered by mucosa and submucosal tissues, which are resilient and displaceable. Because of this displaceability, some dentists have considered that the dentures will settle into the tissues and small errors in occlusion will correct themselves. If this is true, it is done at the expense of the health of soft tissues and eventually at the expense of bone, because bone is a more plastic tissue than mucosa. Bone, in time, will change to relieve soft tissues of excess pressure. Thus failure to correct occlusion before the patient wears the dentures can cause destruction of the residual alveolar ridges.

Part of the error in occlusion can be eliminated by replacing the casts with the processed dentures still on them (in their original mountings on the articulator) and modifying the occlusal surfaces of the teeth by selective grinding (Fig. 23-5). This will eliminate most of the errors that are due to processing changes. However, it will not eliminate errors produced by the impressions or jaw relation records nor will it eliminate errors that develop when the dentures are removed from the casts or are polished. Therefore new interocclusal records of centric and eccentric relations should be made at the time new dentures are first inserted in the patient's mouth.

Further errors in occlusion may develop after dentures have been worn. The resins of which the denture bases are made absorb water. When this occurs, the bases expand and warp slightly, altering the relationships of the inclined planes of the cusps of anatomic (cusped) teeth. When the residual ridges supporting the dentures are favorable, this altered relationship may not be noticeable to the patient. However, if one or both of the residual ridges are badly resorbed, the patient may experience soreness under the dentures as a result of malocclusion. In this situation the dentures should be remounted on the articulator with new interocclusal records of centric and eccentric relations and the occlusion should be corrected by further selective grinding.

Checking for occlusion errors

The technique for checking to determine whether there are errors in occlusion is not difficult, but it does require willingness to see an error. Dentists must approach this observation with a negative attitude. They must *assume* that an error exists and *try* to find it. If they simply tell the patient to bite and then look at the teeth, the error in occlusion will not be detected. With these instructions, the patient will close the teeth together, and they will touch and slide into centric occlusion without this touch and slide being noticed by either the dentist or the patient. The dentures may shift on the ridges or the mandible may move into an eccentric position without detection.

The mandible is guided into CR by a thumb placed directly on the anteroposterior part of the chin, with directions to the patient to open and then close until the first feather touch is felt on the back teeth. At the first contact the patient opens and repeats this closure, stopping the instant he feels tooth touch, and then "closes tight." The procedure will reveal errors in CR by the touch and slide of teeth on each other (Fig. 18-1). The *amount* of occlusal error and the *location* of the deflective contact are not important in this test; they can be determined after the dentures have been remounted on the articulator. They are usually minute, and their accurate localization requires remounting. If articulating paper is used in the mouth to locate interceptive or deflective occlusal contacts, shifting of the denture bases or eccentric closures by the patient, as well as the presence of saliva, will prevent the articulating paper marks from recording errors. Occlusion errors are easily detected and corrected on the articulator.

INTEROCCLUSAL RECORDS FOR REMOUNTING DENTURES

The dentures must be remounted on the articulator for the selective grinding necessary in perfecting the occlusion, and interocclusal records of CR and protrusions are necessary for this procedure.

The errors in occlusion should be eliminated on the articulator rather than in the mouth. If these corrections are attempted in the mouth, it is difficult to see the errors because the soft tissues will be distorted and obscure the errors and the articulating paper will not mark efficiently. Because the soft tissues under the dentures are resilient, the denture bases shift in relation to the underlying bone when there is an error in occlusion and the teeth are rubbed together. The articulating paper marks are likely to be incorrect and, more important, the control of jaw position depends entirely on the ability of the patient to place and move the jaw correctly. Much of the selective grinding done according to articulating paper marks made in the mouth actually increases the amount of error in the occlusion. When new interocclusal records are made and the completed dentures are remounted on the articulator, the errors in occlusion are easily visible, easily located, and easily corrected by selective grinding. Properly made interocclusal records will not cause the denture bases to slip or rotate in relation to their bony foundations. Furthermore, on the articulator the dentures will be firm on their remount casts. The points of contact and errors of occlusion can be observed visually, with magnification if desired, and articulating paper marks are quite easily made on the dry teeth.

There is another advantage to making these corrections away from the patient. The interocclusal records, of course, are made in the patient's mouth; and from the patient's standpoint this is just another step in the construction of the dentures. On the other hand, if the grinding of occlusion is attempted in the presence of the patient, the operation *appears* to the patient to be one of correcting an error made by the dentist. Thus there is a psychologic advantage in doing the grinding in the laboratory.

INTEROCCLUSAL RECORD OF CENTRIC RELATION

Two pieces of Aluwax are placed over the mandibular posterior teeth. A thickness is chosen to eliminate the danger of making contact with the opposing teeth when biting pressure is exerted. The teeth must be completely dry, and the wax is pressed firmly on them to eliminate voids. The two thicknesses of wax are sealed with a warm spatula (Fig. 23-6). The upper denture is placed in the patient's mouth, and just the Aluwax portion is immersed in a water bath of 130° F (54° C) for 30 seconds (Fig. 23-7). Both the temperature and the time are critical in achieving a uniformly softened wax. Aluwax retains heat longer than baseplate wax, thereby providing time for the next step.

The mandibular denture is seated with the index fingers bilaterally positioned on the buccal flanges. The mandible is guided into CR by placing a thumb on the anteroinferior portion of the chin in such a way that some guidance is directed toward the condyles. The thumb must be on the point of the chin, not under it. The patient is guided in a hinge movement, closing lightly into the wax. As contact with the wax approaches, the fingers are raised from the buccal flanges and the patient is instructed to close into the wax until a good index is made (Fig. 23-8). Care must be taken to prevent the patient from penetrating the wax and making tooth contact; a minimum amount of occlusal pressure should be exerted.

The lower denture is carefully removed from the mouth and placed in ice water to chill the wax thoroughly (Fig. 23-9). Next the dentures are removed from the ice water and dried. The imprint of the opposing teeth must be crisp and about 1 mm deep, with no penetration by a maxillary tooth to strike a mandibular tooth

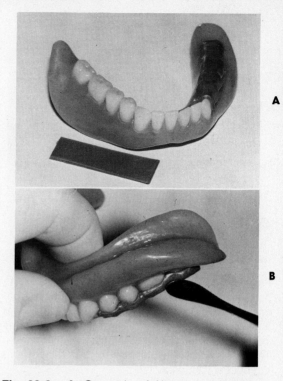

Fig. 23-6 **A,** One strip of Aluwax has been applied to the thoroughly dried teeth. A second strip will be added to it. **B,** The two thicknesses of wax are sealed with a warm spatula.

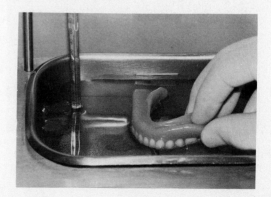

Fig. 23-7 The Aluwax is immersed in 130° F (54° C) water for 30 seconds.

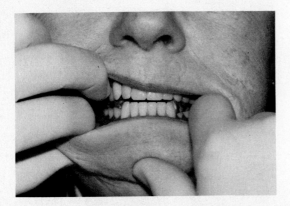

Fig. 23-8   The mandible is guided into CR with the thumb on the anteroinferior part of the chin and the index fingers seating the lower denture in a downward and forward direction. The patient is instructed to close lightly into the softened wax. The index fingers should be slightly raised from the buccal flanges at this point.

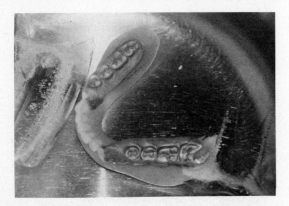

Fig. 23-9   The Aluwax attached to the mandibular denture is chilled in ice water.

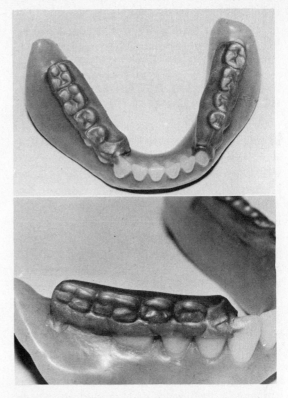

Fig. 23-10   The occlusal record is approximately 1 mm deep and free of any penetration by the underlying teeth.

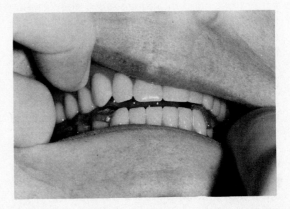

Fig. 23-11   Checking the accuracy of the chilled interocclusal wax record. There should be no tilting or torquing of the dentures from initial contact to complete closure.

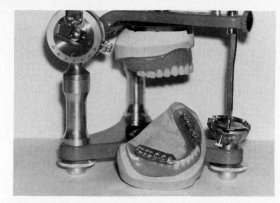

Fig. 23-12 The mandibular denture with the wax interocclusal record attached is positioned on the mandibular mounting cast. The maxillary denture has been previously positioned on the upper member of the articulator with the occlusal index (Fig. 22-26).

(Fig. 23-10). If this occurs, it will likely cause a shifting of the bases or a change in the maxillomandibular relation horizontally and vertically.

The Aluwax is thoroughly chilled before the dentures are returned to the patient's mouth and the patient is guided into CR as previously described. The record is acceptable if there is no tilting or torquing of the dentures from initial contact to complete closure (Fig. 23-11). Underlying soft tissue displacement may cause a slight movement of the bases and must be taken into account when evaluating the contact. If the record is unacceptable, the procedure must be repeated.

REMOUNTING THE MANDIBULAR DENTURE

The maxillary denture will have been mounted on the articulator by means of the remount occlusal index (Fig. 22-26), which will have preserved the face-bow orientation of the dentures. As a result the condylar setting recorded at the tryin should be valid.

After chilling and thoroughly drying the dentures and the wax, the mandibular denture is

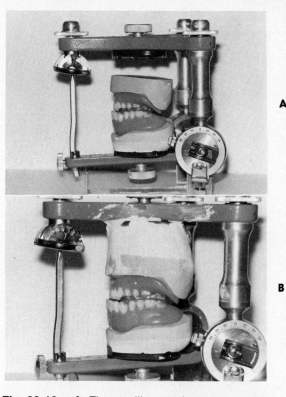

A

B

Fig. 23-13 A, The maxillary teeth are secured to the wax index with a drop of sticky wax in the canine and second molar areas. **B,** Fast-setting plaster has been used to secure the mandibular remount cast to the articulator.

positioned on the remount cast (Fig. 23-12). Next, the maxillary denture teeth are carefully positioned in the wax index and secured with a drop of sticky wax in the canine and second molar regions bilaterally (Fig. 23-13, *A*). (Sticky wax can be used to secure both dentures to their remount casts if necessary.) The incisal pin should be adjusted to allow for the thickness of the interocclusal wax record by raising the upper member of the articulator an appropriate amount. It is important that the condylar controls be locked into centric position. A creamy mix of fast-setting plaster is used to secure the mandibular denture to the lower member of the articulator (Fig. 23-13, *B*).

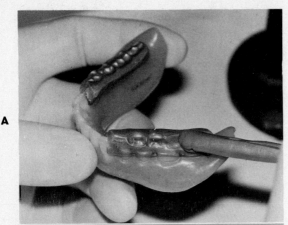

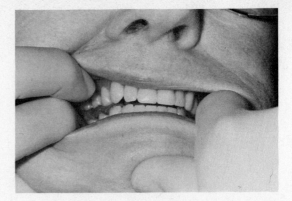

Fig. 23-15   A new CR record is made.

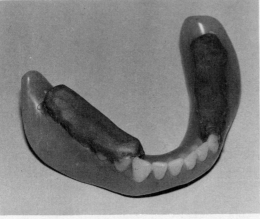

Fig. 23-14   A, The occlusal indentations filled with molten Aluwax. **B,** Surface of the Aluwax smoothed with a warm spatula.

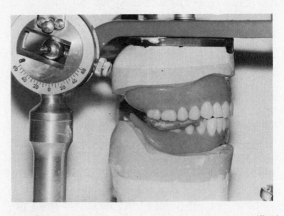

Fig. 23-16   The original cast mounting is verified when the maxillary teeth fit precisely into the wax index on the articulator with locked centric controls.

VERIFYING CENTRIC RELATION

CR should be verified for accuracy before proceeding, to prevent inappropriate tooth adjustment with a faulty recording. If the original wax record has become loose, new Aluwax should be placed as previously described. However, if the original record remains securely attached to the mandibular denture, a small amount of molten wax can be dripped into the occlusal index (Fig. 23-14, *A*). When all the indentations have been filled, the wax is smoothed with a warm spatula (Fig. 23-14, *B*). The wax is softened in the water bath and a new CR record is made as previously described (Fig. 23-15). After chilling and drying of the wax record, the dentures are returned to the articulator. With the articulator locked in CR the maxillary teeth should fit precisely into the new wax record (Fig. 23-16). If *all* the teeth drop simultaneously into the wax record, the mounting is correct.

If the opposing teeth do not fit exactly into

the indentations in the new record, it means that either the original mounting was incorrect or the patient gave an incorrect relation when making the record. To evaluate this, the dentist returns the dentures with the chilled wax record to the mouth and evaluates the accuracy as previously described. If the record still appears correct in the patient's mouth, the original CR registration and/or mounting were incorrect. In this situation the mandibular cast should be separated from the mounting ring and the cast remounted according to the last interocclusal wax record. The new mounting is again checked in the same manner to validate its correctness.

PROTRUSIVE INTEROCCLUSAL RECORD

The original face-bow orientation of the dentures can be preserved by means of the remount occlusal index, and the condylar setting recorded at the tryin appointment should still be valid. If there is any question as to the accuracy of the original condylar setting, a new protrusive record is made (as described in Chapter 20, Figs. 20-3 to 20-7).

ALTERNATIVE USE OF PLASTER INTEROCCLUSAL RECORDS

When plaster has been used to secure interocclusal records at the clinical tryin appointment for both CR and protrusions, the same recording medium should be used.

With the maxillary denture seated on its remount cast, the interocclusal record of CR places the mandibular denture in the desired relation to the upper denture (Fig. 23-17, A). The undercuts in the mandibular denture are blocked out with disposable tissue or caulking compound. Then plaster or stone is built up on the lower member of the articulator to such a height that when the articulator is closed the plaster will engage the borders of the mandibular denture (Fig. 23-17, B to D).

Articulator adjustment

After the mounting plaster has set, the protrusive interocclusal records are substituted for

the centric interocclusal records and the condylar guidances on the instrument are readjusted (Fig. 23-18). The horizontal condylar guidances are loosened, and the mechanism is rotated until both dentures are perfectly seated in the mounting plaster and the protrusive interocclusal records. The horizontal condylar inclination on each side is recorded on the mounting plaster. These numbers are then used with the formula for setting the lateral condylar guidance. The horizontal condylar guidance, divided by 8, plus 12 equals the lateral condylar guidance:

$$\frac{H}{8} + 12 = L$$

The thumb nut above the condylar guidance mechanism is loosened, and the mechanism is rotated around the vertical axis until the numbers correspond to the resultant of the formula. Then the thumb nut is tightened.

Eliminating occlusal errors in anatomic teeth

Final correction of any occlusal disharmony that may exist in dentures from any cause is made at this time by means of selective grinding. Selective grinding permits the desired factors of tooth form and occlusion to be retained.

Articulating paper of minimum thickness is used for marking the actual contacts of the teeth. Thicker paper gives deceptive results. The paper is interposed between the teeth, and markings are obtained by tapping the teeth together (Fig. 23-19). This can be done on both sides at the same time if two pieces of thin articulating paper are fastened together in front with a paper clip. After the first action on the articulating paper, only a few high spots appear. These are removed after a test to determine whether the mandibular or the maxillary teeth should be reduced at the contact points (Fig. 23-20).

Grinding is done with mounted Chayes stones no. 16, 11, and 5. The marking process and the grinding are repeated until practically all the teeth contact in CO. During this centric

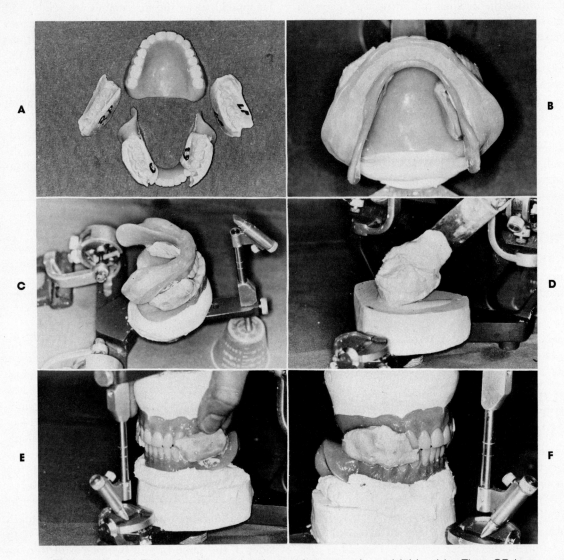

Fig. 23-17 A, Protrusive interocclusal records are made and laid aside. Then CR interocclusal records are made. **B,** Undercuts blocked out on the mandibular denture with caulking compound, and the denture seated on the CR record with the maxillary denture. **C,** The assembled dentures in mounting plaster on the upper member of the articulator. **D,** Impression plaster is placed on the original mounting plaster. **E,** The mandibular denture is held in place in the interocclusal record and lowered into the soft plaster on the articulator. **F,** It is attached to the articulator in CR. If a remount cast had been made, it would have placed in the same manner.

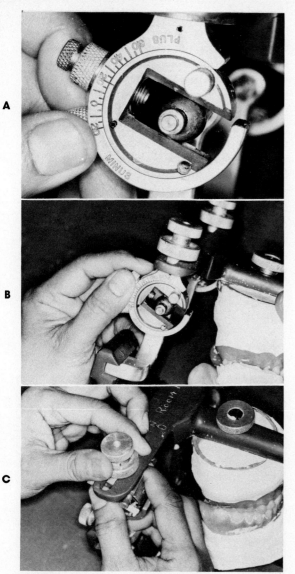

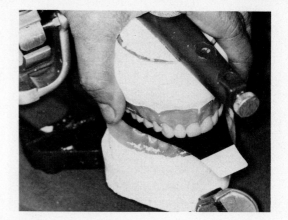

Fig. 23-19 Completed dentures mounted on the articulator preparatory to preliminary occlusal corrections. Articulating paper in place marks the occlusal contacts in CR.

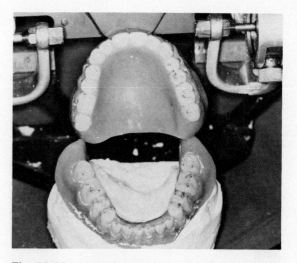

Fig. 23-18 **A,** Protrusive interocclusal records in place, and the horizontal condylar guidance loosened and rotated to a neutral position. **B,** The horizontal condylar guidance is adjusted so both dentures stay seated on their plaster mountings and in the protrusive interocclusal records. **C,** The lateral condylar guidance is adjusted by rotation.

Fig. 23-20 Articulating paper marks made in CR show interceptive or deflective occlusal contacts in CO. Grinding should be done only in fossae and not on the cusps.

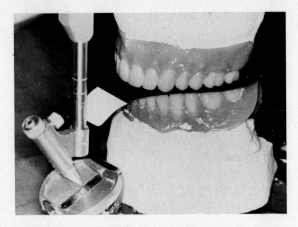

Fig. 23-21 Articulating paper is used to locate deflective occlusal contacts in left lateral occlusion. Notice the position of the incisal guide pin, which has resulted from movement of the articulator into a left working position.

grinding procedure, the incisal guide pin is relieved of contact on the incisal guidance table to allow for the slight reduction in vertical dimension that must necessarily take place.

After the centric deflective occlusal contacts have been removed, the pin is placed in contact with the incisal guide table and is kept in contact throughout the remainder of the grinding procedure. Thin articulating paper is placed over the teeth on both sides, the articulator is moved into one of the lateral positions, and the contacts are marked on both sides for the same lateral movement (Fig. 23-21). The markings will show contacts of the maxillary and mandibular buccal and lingual cusps and the maxillary and mandibular incisors on the working side (Fig. 23-22). Marks will also appear on the lingual cusps of the maxillary teeth and the buccal cusps of the mandibular teeth. If the pin rises away from the incisal guide ta-

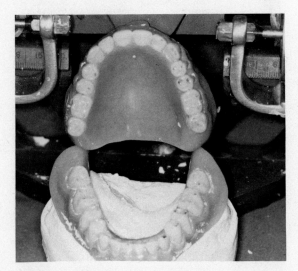

Fig. 23-22 Marks on the buccal cusps of the upper left posterior teeth and the lingual cusps of the lower left posterior teeth indicate contacts in left lateral occlusion. These surfaces are ground to develop uniform contacts. The lingual cusps of upper teeth and the buccal cusps of lower teeth are not ground, even though they show marks from the articulating paper.

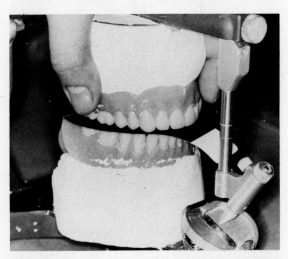

Fig. 23-23 The articulator is moved between right lateral occlusion and CO, with articulating paper between the teeth to locate deflective occlusal contacts in the lateral excursion. Notice the position of the pin on the incisal guidance table.

ble during this lateral movement, the buccal cusps of the maxillary teeth and the lingual cusps of the mandibular teeth on the working side are reduced with a mounted stone. The balancing-side marks are reduced on the lingual of the mandibular buccal cusps to eliminate balancing-side deflective occlusal contacts. The registration of these markings is continued with the same lateral movement, including the intermediate movements, and grinding of these high spots is continued until the pin stays in contact in all lateral and intermediate movements. This marking and grinding procedure is repeated for the right lateral movement (Figs. 23-23 and 23-24).

Grinding to correct lateral occlusions is limited to altering the lingual inclines of the maxillary buccal cusps and the buccal inclines of the mandibular lingual cusps on the working side and the lingual inclines of the mandibular

buccal cusps on the balancing side. After CO has been perfected, the lingual cusps of the maxillary teeth and the buccal cusps of the mandibular teeth must not be shortened.

If the grinding has been done in right and left lateral and intermediate movements, grinding in protrusion will also have been accomplished. Testing with articulating paper should show contact throughout the arches of the maxillary and mandibular dentures (Fig. 23-25). Inasmuch as denture teeth are fastened together as a unit, it is permissible to relieve the centric contact of the four incisors. This relief may be made at the time of setting the teeth, which will permit the use of a vertical overlap without increasing the incisal guide angle.

Carborundum paste for correcting occlusion. Carborundum paste should not be used to eliminate errors in the occlusion of cusped teeth. If it is used in centric and eccentric oc-

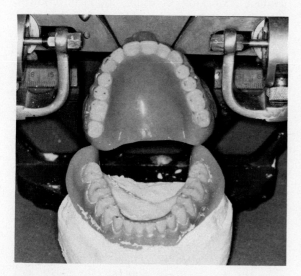

Fig. 23-24 Articulating paper markings in right lateral excursion. Marks on the buccal cusps of upper right posterior teeth and the lingual cusps of lower right posterior teeth indicate the contacts in right lateral occlusion. These surfaces are ground to develop uniform contacts. The lingual cusps of the upper teeth and the buccal cusps of the lower teeth are not ground, even though they show marks from the articulating paper.

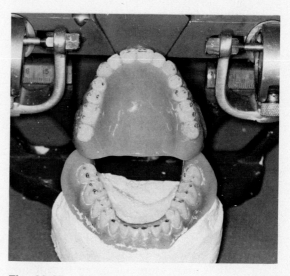

Fig. 23-25 Markings made by movements in all directions indicate uniform contacts.

clusions, the vertical dimension will be reduced and the contact areas of tooth surfaces will be increased unnecessarily. The stresses of mastication will then be distributed improperly, and the loss of sharpness of the cusps will cause a decrease in the size and number of food exits. If Carborundum paste is used at all, smoothing of minute irregularities must be limited to one or two gliding movements of the articulator (Fig. 23-26).

Types of occlusal error in centric occlusion and their correction. Three types of occlusal error can exist in CO, and each can be corrected by specific grinding for that error.

1. Any pair of opposing teeth can be too long and hold the other teeth out of contact. For correction of this error, the fossae of the teeth are deepened by grinding so the teeth will, in effect, telescope into each other (Fig. 23-27, *A*). The cusps are not shortened.

2. The upper and lower teeth can be too nearly end to end. For correction of this error, grinding is done on the inclines of the cusps in such a way as to move the upper cusp inclines buccally and the lower cusp inclines lingually. In the process the central fossae are made broader, the lingual cusp of the upper tooth is made more narrow when it is ground from the lingual side, and the buccal cusp of the lower tooth is made more narrow when it is ground from the buccal side (Fig. 23-27, *B*). The cusps are not shortened.

3. The upper teeth can be too far buccal in relation to the lower teeth. For correction of this error, the lingual cusp of the upper tooth is made more narrow by broadening the central fossa, and the buccal cusp of the lower tooth is moved buccally by broadening the central fossa (Fig. 23-27, *C*). In effect, the upper lingual cusp is moved lingually and the lower buccal cusp is moved buccally so the teeth telescope into each other. The cusps are not shortened.

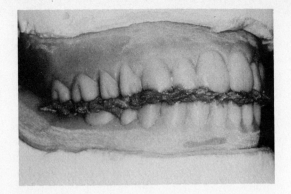

Fig. 23-26 Final smoothing can be done by abrasive paste in one or two gliding movements of the articulator.

Types of working-side occlusal errors and their correction. Six types of errors can exist in the occlusal contacts on the working side. Each of these will cause other teeth to be held out of contact in working occlusion, and each requires selective grinding of specific cusp inclines for its elimination.

1. Both the upper buccal cusp and the lower lingual cusp are too long. For correction of this error, the length of the cusps is reduced by grinding to change the incline extending from the central fossa to the cusp tip. The central fossa is not made deeper, but the upper buccal cusps and the lower lingual cusps are made shorter so the other teeth will touch in that position (Fig. 23-28, *A*).

2. The buccal cusps make contact but the lingual cusps do not. For correction of this error, the buccal cusps of the upper teeth are ground from the central fossa to the cusp tip to shorten the cusp and change the lingual incline of the cusp so it will be less steep (Fig. 23-28, *B*).

3. The lingual cusps make contact but the buccal cusps do not. For correction of this error, the lower lingual cusps are shortened by changing the buccal incline of the lower lingual cusp so it is not as steep. The upper lingual cusp is not

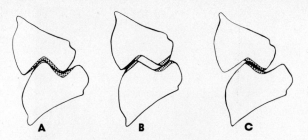

Fig. 23-27 Correction of errors in CO. Grind the shaded areas: **A,** teeth too long; **B,** teeth too nearly end to end; **C,** too much horizontal overlap.

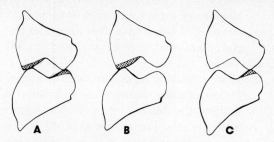

Fig. 23-28 Correction of errors on the working side. Shorten interfering cusps as indicated by the shaded areas: **A,** buccal and lingual cusps too long; **B,** buccal cusps too long; **C,** lingual cusps too long.

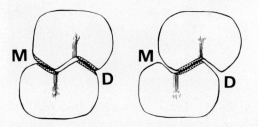

Fig. 23-29 Correction of errors in the mesiodistal relationship. Grind where areas are shaded: *M,* mesial surface; *D,* distal surface.

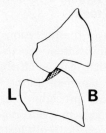

Fig. 23-30 Eliminating deflective occlusal contact on the balancing side. Grind the lingual incline of the lower buccal cusp: *L,* lingual surface; *B,* buccal surface.

shortened, and the central fossa is not made deeper (Fig. 23-28, *C*).

4. The upper buccal or lingual cusps are mesial to their intercuspating positions. This error may occur along with any of the three just listed. For its correction, grinding is done so the mesial inclines of the upper buccal cusps are moved distally when the cusps are narrowed and the distal inclines of the lower cusps are moved forward. The same cuspal inclination is maintained in this procedure (Fig. 23-29, *left*).

5. The upper buccal or lingual cusps are distal to their intercusping positions. This error may also occur along with buccolingual errors. For its correction, grinding is done from the distal of the upper cusps and from the mesial of the lower cusps (Fig. 23-29, *right*).

6. The teeth on the working side may not contact. The cause of this error is excessive contact on the balancing side.

Types of balancing-side errors and their correction. There are two types of balancing-side errors:

1. The balancing-side contact is so heavy that the working-side teeth are held out of contact. For correction of this error, paths are ground through the buccal cusps of the lower teeth to reduce the incline of the part of the cusp that is preventing the teeth on the working side from contacting (Fig. 23-30). As much as

possible of each interfering cusp is preserved. No grinding is done from the lingual cusps that may be involved in this contact.

2. There is no contact on the balancing side. To correct this error, it is necessary to shorten the buccal cusps of the upper teeth and the lingual cusps of the lower teeth on the *working* side. In this process the lingual inclines of the buccal cusps of the upper teeth and the buccal inclines of the lingual cusps of the lower teeth are made less steep. No grinding is done in the central fossae (Fig. 23-28, *A*).

Eliminating occlusal errors in nonanatomic teeth

Examination of the occlusion at the time of denture insertion often reveals one or more discrepancies that may be attributable to teeth coming out of alignment during the final stages of the laboratory procedure. An interocclusal CR record is made in a bite registration material with the opposing teeth just out of contact. The dentures are mounted on the articulator, and the following procedures are undertaken:

1. After being detected by articulating paper between the teeth, gross premature (interceptive occlusal) contacts in CR are removed by grinding (Fig. 23-31). The same procedures are used to locate and remove all occlusal interferences in lateral and protrusive occlusions. The grinding is done on the occlusal surfaces of teeth that appear to have been tipped or elongated in processing. In eccentric occlusion no grinding is done on the distobuccal portion of the lower second molar. All balancing-side grinding is done on the lingual portion of the occlusal surface of the upper second molar.

2. Abrasive paste is placed on the teeth on the articulator. These teeth are milled when the upper member of the articulator moves in and out of protrusive and right and left lateral excursions. When

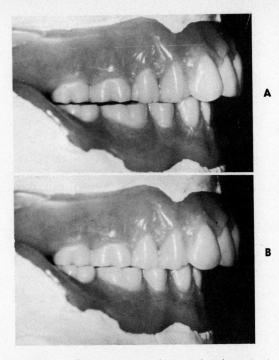

Fig. 23-31 Gross interceptive occlusal contact in the premolar region, **A,** is removed so maximal intercuspation occurs in CR, which is then transferred to the articulator, **B.**

the teeth slide smoothly through all excursions, the dentures are removed from the articulator and washed. Seldom is any correction necessary to attain a bilaterally balanced occlusion.

3. Spot grinding is done to correct any small discrepancies in CR that remain after the grinding with abrasive paste. The dentist adjusts them after identifying the discrepancy with articulating paper—using a light tapping motion with the articulator—and grinding the marks to ensure even occlusal contact in centric occlusion.

Final evaluation of the contacts

When the occlusal adjustment has been completed, the contacts of the teeth are carefully evaluated in CR and the various excursive movements (Figs. 23-32 and 23-33, *A* to *E*). Af-

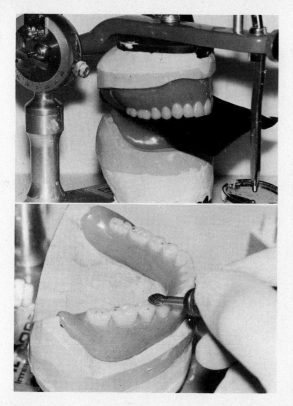

Fig. 23-32 Marking and adjusting occlusal premature contacts for the patient in Figs. 23-6 to 23-16.

ter careful polishing and cleaning of the dentures, they should be placed in the patient's mouth for evaluation of the contacts (Fig. 23-33, *F*). If all steps have been completed correctly, the contacts will be the same clinically as was achieved on the articulator.

ADVANTAGES OF BALANCED OCCLUSION IN COMPLETE DENTURES

What is the advantage of balanced occlusion in dentures when a bolus of food on one side so separates the teeth that they cannot possibly be in balancing contact on the opposite side? This question has aroused in the minds of many dentists the suspicion that balancing occlusion is a fetish of college professors and a few spe-

cialists. Many dentures are not balanced, since a large proportion of the profession is not thoroughly convinced of the value of balanced occlusion in relation to the effort involved in securing it. If a bolus of food were between the teeth on one side most of each of the 24 hours, there would not be much object in having an exactly balanced occlusion. However, teeth make contact many thousands of times a day in both eccentric and centric positions, with no food in the mouth during nonfunctional mandibular movements. Even while chewing, the teeth cut through to contact every few fractions of a second. A balanced occlusion ensures even pressure in all parts of the arch, which maintains the stability of the dentures when the mandible is in centric and eccentric (parafunctional) positions.

SPECIAL INSTRUCTIONS TO THE PATIENT

Educating patients to the limitations of dentures as mechanical substitutes for living tissues must be a continuing process from the initial patient contact until adjustments are completed. However, certain difficulties that will be encountered with new dentures and the information related to the care of dentures should be reinforced at the time of initial placement of the dentures. Forewarning makes the patient more tolerant of problems and less likely to relate them incorrectly to the fit of the dentures. Explanations provided after problems develop are often interpreted as excuses by the dentist for dentures that function less than satisfactorily.

Individuality of patients

Patients must be reminded that their physical, mental, and oral conditions are individual in nature. Thus they cannot compare their progress with new dentures to other persons' experiences. What is annoying and painful to some may be of secondary importance to others. Chewing and speech patterns with new dentures that are considered successful by

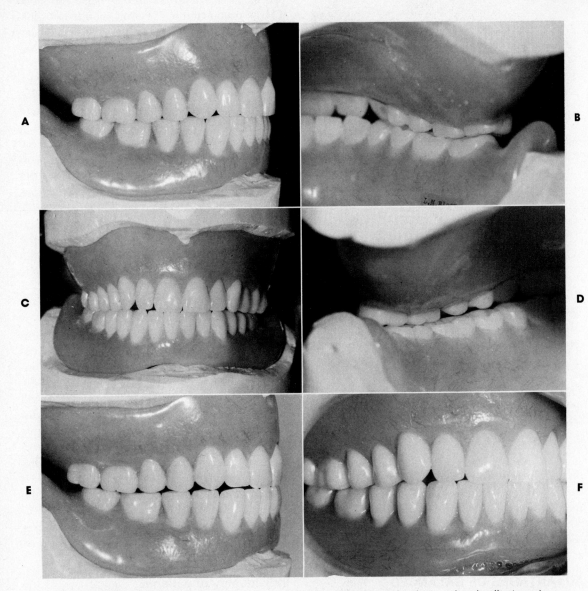

Fig. 23-33 Occlusal contacts on the articulator following selective occlusal adjustment. **A** and **B,** Centric occlusion, buccal and lingual views. **C** and **D,** Right lateral occlusion, labial and lingual views. Notice in the lingual how balance has been achieved in the molar region. **E,** Protrusive position. Here multiple balancing contacts exist because of the shape of the compensating curve. **F,** In this clinical view, notice the uniformity of contacts as established on the articulator **(A).** Color photographs of this patient are presented in Plate 19-1, *D* to *F*.

some persons may be interpreted as totally unsuccessful by others. In addition, adaptability to new dentures is modified by age. Persons who make the adjustment to new dentures during middle age will probably experience considerably more difficulty with dentures 15 years later, even though the new dentures may be technically superior to the original ones.

Patients tend to forget the severity of problems with the passage of time. Many persons indicate that their dentures have always been comfortable, even though they may have had a difficult adjustment period. Such remarks can be discouraging to patients with new dentures unless they have been advised of this possibility.

Appearance with new dentures

Patients must understand that their appearance with new dentures will become more natural with time. Initially the dentures will feel strange and bulky in the mouth and will cause a feeling of fullness of the lips and cheeks. The lips will not adapt immediately to the fullness of the denture borders and may initially present a distorted appearance. Muscle tension may cause an awkward appearance, which will improve after the patient becomes relaxed and more confident.

Patients should be instructed to refrain from exhibiting their dentures to curious friends until they are more confident and competent at exhibiting them at their best. When patients are not careful in following these instructions, they may likely become unfairly critical of the dentures and develop an attitude that will be difficult for the dentist to overcome. During the edentulous or partially edentulous period, gradual reduction of the interarch distance and collapsing of the lips will have occurred. These changes have usually been so gradual that the family and friends were not aware that they existed. Therefore a repositioning of the orbicularis oris and a restoration of the former facial dimension and contour by the new dentures may seem like too great a change in the pa-

tient's appearance. This can be overcome only with the passage of time, and patients are advised to persevere during the period.

Mastication with new dentures

Learning to chew satisfactorily with new dentures usually requires at least 6 to 8 weeks. Patients will become discouraged unless they are aware that this learning period is to be expected. New memory patterns often must be established for both the facial muscles and the muscles of mastication. Once the habit patterns become automatic, the chewing process can take place without conscious effort. The muscles of the tongue, cheeks, and lips must be trained to maintain the dentures in position on the residual ridges during mastication. Patients can be told that "these muscles must learn what they should and should not do."

Mastication is additionally impaired because of the excess flow of saliva for the first few days after placement of new dentures. However, in a relatively short time the salivary glands accommodate to the presence of the dentures and the production of saliva returns to normal.

Patients should begin chewing relatively soft food cut into small pieces. If the chewing can be done on both sides of the mouth at the same time, the tendency of the dentures to tip will be reduced. Patients should be told that during this early period, mastication is best attempted on simple types of food such as crackers, soft toast, or chopped meat and that no attempt should be made to masticate more resistant foods. Also, during the learning period, patients are advised to avoid observation by friends or members of the family, since the patients will be awkward in the beginning phases of chewing and susceptible to embarrassment and discouragement. Kindly but misplaced joking remarks and comments by members of the family may readily lead a patient to denture consciousness that will be reflected in the attitude toward the dentist and the dentures.

When biting with dentures, patients should be instructed to place the food between their teeth toward the corners of the mouth, rather than between the anterior teeth. Then the food should be pushed inward and upward to break it apart rather than downward and outward as would be done if natural teeth were present. Inward and upward forces tend to seat the dentures on the residual ridges rather than displace them.

Occasionally, edentulous patients have gone without dentures for long periods and have learned to crush food between the residual ridges or perhaps between the tongue and the hard palate. These persons usually experience increased difficulty in learning to masticate with new dentures, and the time for adjustment will likely be extended.

Patients should be told that the position of the tongue plays an important role in the stability of a lower denture, particularly during mastication. Patients whose tongues normally rest in a retracted position relative to the lower anterior teeth should attempt to position the tongue farther forward so it rests on the lingual surfaces of the lower anterior teeth. This will help develop stability for the lower denture.

Speaking with new dentures

Fortunately, the problem of speaking with new dentures is not as difficult as might be expected. The adaptability of the tongue to compensate for changes is so great that most patients master speech with new dentures within a few weeks. If correct speech required exact replacement of tissues and teeth in relation to tongue movement, no patient would ever learn to talk with dentures. The necessity of additional bulk over the palate would cause a lasting speech impediment. Even a 0.5 mm change at the linguogingival border of the anterior teeth would cause a speech defect, especially in the production of s sounds, if it were not for the extreme adaptability of the tongue to these changes. Therefore, tooth positions that restore appearance and masticatory function usually do not produce phonetic changes that are too great to be readily compensated.

However, a study of tongue positions is valuable and gives an appreciation of the value of positioning the dentures in the relation formerly occupied by the natural teeth.

Speaking normally with dentures requires practice. Patients should be advised to read aloud and repeat words or phrases that are difficult to pronounce. Patients usually are much more conscious of small irregularities in their speech sounds than those to whom they are speaking.

Oral hygiene with dentures

Patients must be convinced of the importance of maintaining good oral hygiene for the health of the oral cavity. Plaque, stain, and calculus accrue on dentures and oral mucosa of edentulous patients in a similar fashion as in the mouths of dentulous patients. Dental plaque is an etiologic factor in denture stomatitis, inflammatory papillary hyperplasia, chronic candidiasis, and offensive odors, and it must be removed.

Patients should be instructed to rinse their dentures and their mouths after meals whenever possible. Once a day it is essential that the dentures be removed and placed in a soaking type of cleanser for a minimum of 30 minutes. This time interval is required for effective killing of microorganisms on the dentures as well as removal of all stain. Kleenite* has been shown a very effective cleanser for both its cleaning ability and its ability to kill microorganisms. Leaving the dentures in the cleanser overnight is even better. When the dentures are removed from the soaking cleanser, they should be brushed gently with a soft brush and rinsed thoroughly. They should be brushed over a basin partially filled with water or covered with a wet washcloth to prevent breakage in case they are dropped. Patients should be discouraged from using toothpastes, since most contain an abrasive material that will wear away the surface of acrylic resin. An inexpen-

---

*Richardson-Vicks Inc, Wilton CT, 06897.

sive alternative soaking cleanser is one that can be made up using 1 teaspoon of Clorox and 2 teaspoons of Calgon in 8 ounces of water. The time intervals are the same as for Kleenite.

The mucosal surfaces of the residual ridges and the dorsal surface of the tongue should also be brushed daily with a soft brush. This will increase the circulation and remove plaque and debris that can cause irritation of the mucous membrane or offensive odors.

Preserving the residual ridges

The residual ridges were not intended to bear the stresses of mastication created by complete dentures. Therefore patients, especially when their general health is somewhat impaired, may expect some irritation and discomfort of the oral tissues. No two patients' mouths will react alike, since some tissues tolerate stress better than others. Thus it is impossible to predict exactly what to expect. Patients must be aware of these varying and unpredictable conditions.

If some irritation of the tissues is experienced, patients are advised to remove their dentures and rest the mouth for a time. More harm than good is done by telling patients that they must keep their dentures in the mouth constantly during this initial adjustment period, since they may become highly nervous and fatigued and be unnecessarily discouraged as to their final successful wearing of the dentures. However, patients are requested to wear the dentures for several hours before an adjustment appointment so any sore spots will be visible and accurate corrections of the dentures can be made. Patients must be cautioned concerning the critical nature of adjustments to the dentures. They must be convinced that the *dentist* is the only person qualified to undertake this most important aspect of denture service. Obviously, patients should never attempt to adjust the dentures themselves.

Patients should be told that dentures must be left out of the mouth at night to provide needed rest from the stresses they create on the residual ridges. Failure to allow the tissues of the basal seat to rest may be a contributing factor in the development of serious oral lesions such as inflammatory papillary hyperplasia or may increase the opportunity for the growth of fungus infections such as candidiasis. When dentures are left out of the mouth, they should be placed in a container filled with water to prevent drying and possible dimensional changes of the denture base material.

Residual ridges can be ruined by the use of denture adhesives and home-reliners, and patients should be cautioned about this. If these materials are used, patients soon feel insecure without them. Adhesives, and especially home-reliners, invariably modify the position of the denture on the residual ridge and can result in a change of both vertical and centric relations; the residual ridges can be irreparably damaged in a short time.

The special instructions must include directions for continued periodic oral examinations for edentulous patients. The tissues supporting dentures change with time, and the rate of change depends on both local and general factors. Good dentures eventually become ill-fitting and can damage the mouth without the patient's being aware that anything is wrong. Pathosis, which may or may not be associated with the dentures, can develop in the edentulous oral cavity. All edentulous patients should be examined by a dentist at least once a year and should be placed on a recall list for that purpose.

Educational material for patients

Since the education of patients is so critical to the success of new dentures, many dentists provide written instructions or other formal educational material that has been developed. In studying the material, patients become aware that dentures are not permanent, that the mouth changes, and most important that the care they provide themselves may be a deciding factor in the success they experience with dentures.

Denture patients need guidance after they have their new teeth. Much of this can be given verbally while the dentures are being constructed. However, this is not enough. People remember less of what they hear than of what they see. For this reason, it is wise to provide denture patients with printed information about their new teeth, about the care and cleaning of the teeth, about using them, and (not least important) about the periodic inspections that will be necessary later.

A number of books or pamphlets dealing with the care and use of dentures are available. One or more of these should be given each patient to read during the construction of the dentures. The information contained in them will help patients learn to use their new teeth and to recognize that periodic professional dental supervision is needed after the dentures have been fitted. These supplements to treatment are more important than some of us may recognize. After all, everyone knows how to make toast in an electric toaster, yet when you buy one you get a set of directions for its use. If patients are to have adequate care after they get their new teeth, they should have some readily available source of information about them.

BIBLIOGRAPHY

Moore TC, Smith DE, Kenny GE: Sanitization of dentures by several denture hygiene methods, J Prosthet Dent **52:**158-163, 1984.

CHAPTER 24

Maintaining the comfort and health of the oral cavity in a rehabilitated edentulous patient

Treatment with complete dentures is not truly successful unless the patient wears them. Therefore complete denture service cannot be adequate unless patients are cared for after the dentures are placed in the mouth.

In many instances the most crucial time in the success or failure of dentures is the adjustment period. The dentist is responsible for the care of the patient throughout this period, and it occasionally requires a number of appointments. It is important that the dentist and the patient have a clear understanding as to the financial implications of the adjustment period. This relates to the philosophy of the dentist in patient management.

The complete cooperation of the patient during the adjustment period is essential. In educating patients, the dentist must explain to them the problems that they are likely to face during the adjustment phase and the procedures that both the patient and the dentist must follow to alleviate these problems.

TWENTY-FOUR HOUR ORAL EXAMINATION AND TREATMENT

An appointment for a 1- to 3-day adjustment should be made routinely. Patients who do not receive this attention have more trouble than those who are cared for the first several days following the insertion of the new dentures. This is the critical period in the denture-wearing experience of the patient. When the patient returns for the first adjustment, the dentist can ask, "How are you getting along with the sore mouth?" This invites patients to describe their experiences and soreness, if any. The dentist must listen carefully to the patient and on the basis of these comments can learn approximately where to look for trouble. The statements may also furnish valuable information about psychologic problems that may be developing.

Examination procedures

The occlusion should be observed before the dentures are removed from the mouth. To do this, the mandible is guided into CR by placing a thumb directly on the anteroinferior portion of the chin and directing the patient to "open and close your lower jaw until you feel the first feather touch of your back teeth." At the first contact, the patient is directed to open and repeat this closure, "only this time stop the instant you feel a tooth touch and then close tight" (Fig. 18-1). If the teeth *touch and slide,* there is an error in CO. When such an error is detected, the dentures are placed on their remount casts on the articulator, and the occlusion is rechecked there. If the same error is found on the articulator, it is eliminated by selective grinding. If there is an error in the mouth and none is found on the articulator, new interocclusal records of the centric and protrusive relations must be made. The mandibular remount cast is removed from the articulator, and the lower denture is remounted before the occlusion is corrected.

After the occlusion has been tested, a thorough visual and digital examination of the oral cavity is performed so the location of sore spots can be determined. The examination begins with the mucosa of the upper buccal vestibule and proceeds around through the labial and the buccal vestibules on the other side of the mouth, with careful observation of the frena. The hamular notches and the hard and soft palates are examined for signs of abrasion. The area of the coronoid process is palpated, and the patient is asked if any tenderness is felt in this region.

The lower dental arch and associated dental structures are systematically examined both visually and digitally. The tissues lining the vestibular spaces and the alveololingual sulci, particularly the mylohyoid ridges and the retromylohyoid spaces, are observed carefully. The sides of the tongue and the mucosal lining of the cheeks must also be inspected.

Adjustments related to the occlusion

A number of problems can result from errors in the occlusion. Soreness may develop on the crest of the residual ridge from pressures created by heavy contacts of opposing teeth in the same region. Soreness may also be seen on the slopes of the residual ridge as a result of shifting of the denture bases from deflective occlusal contacts (Fig. 24-1). Before unnecessarily shortening or excessively relieving the denture base, the dentist must observe the occlusion carefully in the mouth and on the articulator, giving particular attention to the possibility of heavy balancing contacts that could cause rotation of the denture bases. The correction is made on the articulator by developing a pathway on the lower tooth for the offending upper cusp. Such occlusion errors are almost impossible to locate in the mouth because of movement of the denture bases on the supporting soft tissues.

Small lesions on the buccal mucosa of the cheek in line with the occlusal plane indicate that the patient is biting the cheek during mastication. The lesion will be located on the mucosa adjacent to the offending teeth. This problem can usually be corrected by reducing the buccal surface of the appropriate lower tooth to create additional horizontal overlap, thus providing an escapeway for the buccal mucosa.

A patient may complain, "My dentures are

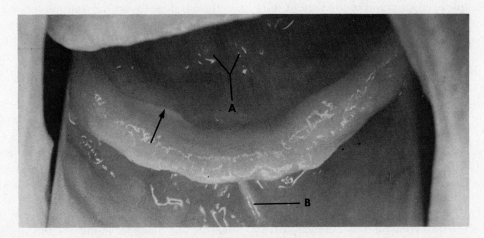

Fig. 24-1   A lesion *(arrow)* on the lingual slope of the lower residual ridge is likely due to errors in the occlusion that caused the denture base to shift and thus impinge on the mucosa. *A,* Sublingual caruncles; *B,* lower labial frenum.

tight when I first put them in my mouth, but they seem to loosen after several hours." This symptom usually is an indication of errors in the occlusion that can be corrected after new interocclusal records are made, the dentures are remounted, and the occlusion is adjusted on the articulator. The dentures become loose because the deflective occlusal contacts cause a continual shifting of the tissues in the basal seat. Although this problem may develop by the time of the 1- to 3-day adjustment, it is more likely to be seen a little later on.

Adjustments related to the denture bases

A number of problems with new dentures are related to the denture bases themselves. Lesions of the mucosa in the reflections are most often caused by denture borders that are too sharp or denture flanges that are overextended. Sometimes the labial notch of the denture will be sharp or of insufficient size, and the frenum becomes irritated. Usually the notch needs to be deepened slightly and also rounded and made smooth (Fig. 24-2). Widen-

ing of the notch may not be necessary and could lessen denture retention. The notch is deepened with a fissure bur. Then the denture base material is made round and smooth by a sharp scraper and a Burlew disk, followed by pumice on the tip of a felt cone or a brush wheel.

Soreness created by extra length of the anterior part of the lingual flange should not be confused with soreness on the slopes of the ridge resulting from occlusion. An indelible pencil mark is placed either on the sore spot in the mouth or on the denture base and is transferred for accurate location of the site for reduction of the denture border (Fig. 24-3). The denture border is carefully shortened with a

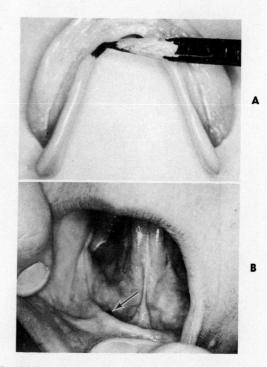

Fig. 24-3   **A,** An indelible mark is placed on the border of the lingual flange at the site judged to correspond to the spot where the patient complained of soreness. **B,** The mark is transferred to the mucosa in the floor of the mouth and will be used to locate where the border should be relieved.

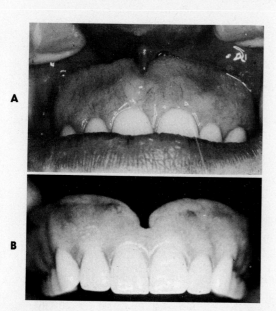

Fig. 24-2   **A,** The labial notch must accommodate the action of the labial frenum. **B,** It must be sufficiently deep, with borders that are rounded and smooth.

sharp acrylic bur and polished with pumice and a rag wheel.

Lesions in the region of the hamular notch must be considered carefully. If the irritated tissue is posterior to the notch, the denture base is too long and must be shortened. However, if the soreness is in the notch itself, the posterior palatal seal is likely creating too much pressure, and the inside of the tissue surface of the denture base will need to be relieved (very cautiously). A mistake in judgment at this point can reduce or eliminate the seal of the upper denture, so the notch must be carefully palpated before this diagnostic determination is made (Fig. 24-4).

Soreness may develop along the crest of the lower ridge when spiny projections of bone remain in this region (Fig. 24-5, A). Precautions

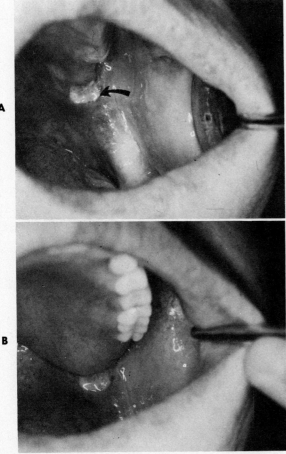

Fig. 24-4 **A,** The sore spot *(arrow)* is posterior to the hamular notch, indicating that the denture base is too long in this region. **B,** After adjustment of the denture, notice that the spot is posterior to the border.

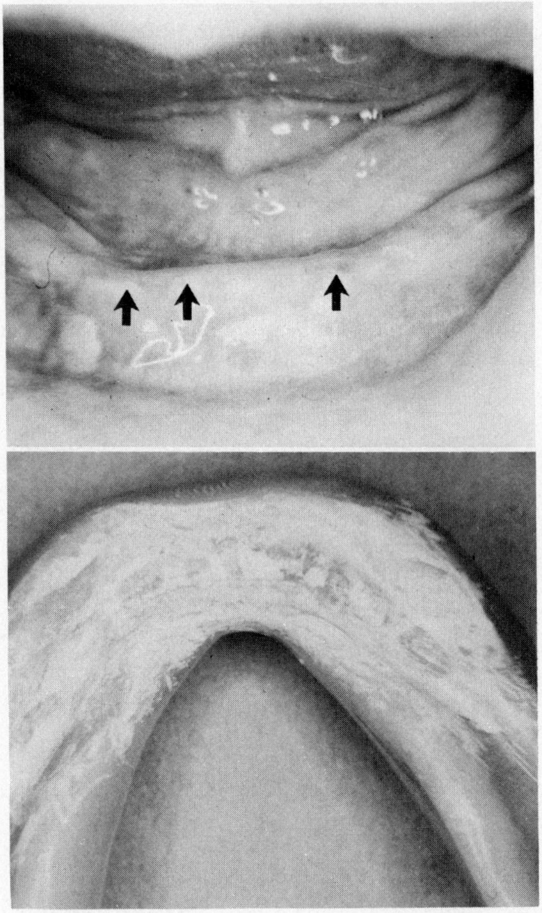

Fig. 24-5 **A,** Spiny projections of bone *(arrows)* underlie the mucosa covering the crest of this lower residual ridge. **B,** Pressure spots in the indicator paste show where relief will be needed. The denture base will be adjusted with a no. 8 round bur.

taken in the impression procedure may not always be adequate. The denture base is coated with pressure indicator paste, the denture is placed in the mouth, and pressure is directed on the teeth in a vertical direction (Fig. 24-5, *B*). The denture base is relieved with a round bur in the locations indicated.

Lesions of the mucosa lining the retromylohyoid fossa can be caused by excessive length or pressure of the denture flange (Fig. 24-6, *A*). Often patients will complain of soreness when they swallow or state that they feel as if they have a sore throat. The denture base should be shortened, or the tissue surface relieved, to reduce pressure depending on the location of the lesion (Fig. 24-6, *B*). Complaints of soreness during swallowing are also frequently related to irritation in the region of the mylohyoid ridges.

Since additional stress is placed on the buccal shelf of the lower jaw during impression-making procedures, a differential diagnosis of

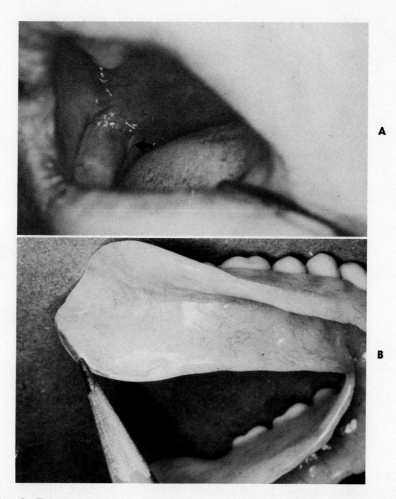

Fig. 24-6   A, This lesion on the mucosa lining the retromylohyoid fossa *(arrow)* was caused by excessive length and pressure from the denture base. **B,** A pencil mark indicates the site for correction of the lesion.

soreness in this area may be necessary. If the irritation is related to the length of the buccal flange (Fig. 24-7, *A*), which can be determined when the denture border in the mouth is compared to the location of the lesion, the length of the flange should be shortened. However, if the sore spot is on the mucosa overlying the buccal shelf, then the denture base in this region is relieved. Pressure indicator paste can be helpful in determining the location of the

lesion (Fig. 24-7, *B*). The denture base is relieved slightly with a sharp acrylic bur, and in this instance the length of the flange is not reduced.

Excessive pressure from the lower buccal flange in the region of the mental foramen may cause a tingling or numbing sensation at the corner of the mouth or in the lower lip. This results from impingement on the mental nerve and occurs particularly when excess resorption

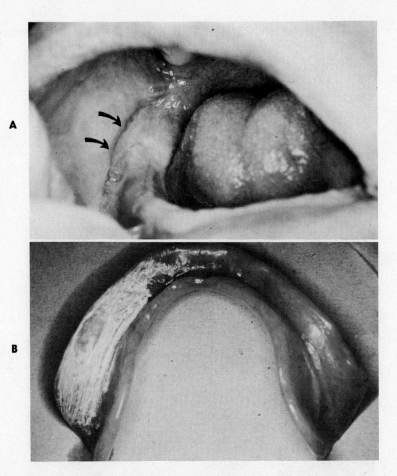

Fig. 24-7 **A,** This line of irritation *(arrows)* was caused by an overextended buccal flange of the lower denture. **B,** The pressure spot in indicator paste represents the part of this denture base that has been placing excessive pressure on the buccal shelf (not related to **A**).

has caused the mental foramen to be located near the crest of the lower residual ridge. A similar situation can occur in the upper jaw from pressure on the incisive papilla transmitted to the nasopalatine nerve. The patient may complain of burning or numbness in the anterior part of the upper jaw. Relief may be required in the upper denture base in this region.

Patients may return for the initial adjustment appointment complaining that their dentures cause them to gag. This problem may actually be related to the dentures themselves, or there may be a psychologic component. When the problem is denture related, usually the upper denture is the culprit, although on occasion the lower denture or both will be involved. Most often the gagging relates to the posterior border of the upper denture. The border may be improperly extended, or the posterior border seal may be inadequate (Fig. 24-8). Gagging occurs when the posterior border seal is disrupted as the tissue distal to the vibrating line moves upward and downward during function. When the vibrating line has been properly located, it is not necessary (and usually not desir-

able) to extend the posterior border of the upper denture more than 2 mm beyond this point. If the posterior palatal seal is inadequate, modeling compound can be added to reshape this part of the upper denture and help alleviate the situation. Then the modeling compound can be replaced with acrylic resin. The occlusion may also be a factor, since shifting of the denture bases affects the posterior palatal seal.

On occasion, patients will state that the upper denture comes loose when they open their mouth wide to bite into a sandwich or to yawn. Generally this complaint indicates that the distobuccal flange of the upper denture is too thick and interferes with normal movements of the coronoid process (Fig. 24-9). The borders of the upper buccal flanges should properly fill the buccal vestibule. However, the distal corners of the denture base below the borders must be thin to allow the freedom necessary for movement of the coronoid process.

Again, in discussions with patients, it may be revealed that the upper denture tends to loosen during smiling or other forms of facial expression. Excessive thickness or height of the flange of the upper denture in the region of the buccal notch or distal to the notch may cause this problem (Fig. 24-10). As the buccal frenum moves posteriorly during function, it encroaches on a border that is too thick and the denture becomes loosened. Reduction of the width of the border posterior to the upper buccal notch will often relieve this problem.

Modifications of the denture base must be carefully made. To grind away parts of the base unnecessarily can cause further difficulty. The overextended parts of the denture base must be carefully reduced with a sharp bur according to the amount of inflammation observed. Then the borders must be polished wherever they have been modified. An unpolished border may lead to further inflammation even though it is not overextended. If the border is polished by the dentist, any modification by the patient will be apparent.

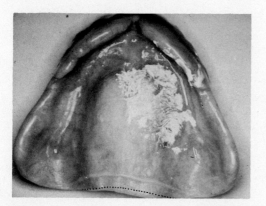

Fig. 24-8 Overextended posterior border of an upper denture. When the border was shortened to the approximate length indicated by the *dotted line,* the denture no longer caused the patient to gag.

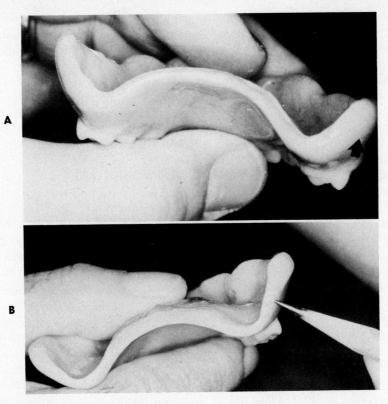

Fig. 24-9 **A,** The distobuccal flange of this upper denture is too thick below the border *(arrow).* **B,** This flange is of proper thickness.

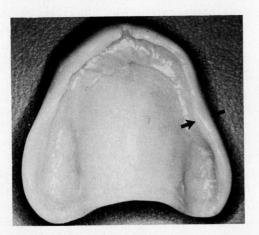

Fig. 24-10 Notice the excessive thickness of the right buccal border in the region of the buccal notch *(arrows).* The buccal frenum, moving posteriorly over this border during facial expression, can loosen or unseat an upper denture.

SUBSEQUENT ORAL EXAMINATIONS AND TREATMENTS

Dentures require inspection and sometimes further adjustment after they have been used by the patient. During the first several weeks the acrylic resin absorbs water, and this can change the size and shape of the dentures. Even though the alterations are small, they may be sufficient to change the occlusion. Minute changes in the occlusion can create discomfort by making the dentures shift or slide in function. Soreness reported by patients in this situation is most likely on the lingual side of the mandibular ridge in the region of the canine and first premolar, and is most likely due to deflective occlusal contact between the last molar teeth diagonally across the mouth, often between the balancing inclines of the lower second molars.

In most instances the occlusal error can be observed and corrected by placement of the dentures in their original remount casts on the articulator. If, however, the bases have so changed that they no longer fit the remount casts the way they did originally, it will be necessary to make new remount casts and new interocclusal records. The remount jig record will permit the upper denture to be remounted without making a new face-bow transfer record.

After the new records are made, the occlusion is corrected by selective grinding with the same procedure as was used at the time of their insertion. It is interesting that the occlusal changes will likely be small but the soreness they produce is very real and disturbing. Dentists should not succumb to the temptation to grind from the denture base without determining the real cause of the trouble.

Sometimes generalized irritation or soreness of the basal seat will develop (Fig. 24-11). Although this condition may be attributable to a number of factors (such as an excessive vertical dimension of occlusion, nutritional or hormonal problems, or unhygienic dentures), it more likely is due to the occlusion. As indicated previously, errors in occlusion should be suspected whenever a patient states that the dentures are "tight when I first put them in my mouth in the morning but seem to loosen later in the day." A collection of calculus on the teeth on one side of the denture also indicates the need for correcting the occlusion.

Certain symptoms at an adjustment appointment suggest an insufficient interocclusal distance. The patient may comment, "After I've worn the new dentures for several hours, my gums get sore and the muscles in the bottom part of my face seem tired." On removal of the dentures, the mucosa of the basal seat will often exhibit a generalized irritation. These symptoms indicate that when the patient's mandible is in the resting position there is not sufficient space between the opposing teeth to allow the supporting structures of the residual ridge and the involved muscles to rest normally. If this is true, several options exist: Sometimes creating a small amount of additional interocclusal distance will solve the problem, and the dentist can do this by returning the dentures to the articulator and grinding the artificial teeth to reduce the vertical dimension

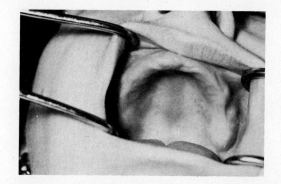

Fig. 24-11 Notice the generalized irritation and erythema of the basal seat of this upper residual ridge. The occlusion is often the primary contributing etiologic factor. The dentures must be remounted on the articulator with new interocclusal records, and the occlusion must then be readjusted.

of occlusion; esthetics and the amount of clearance between the anterior teeth are the limiting factors in this procedure, and another 1 to 1.5 mm of interocclusal distance can thus be created. Other times it may be necessary to reset the artificial teeth of one or both dentures; the decision as to which teeth should be moved is based on esthetics and the vertical dimension of occlusion. Finally, in some instances, the dentures will have to be remade.

Periodic recall for oral examination

When patients are dismissed at the end of adjustment appointments, they are instructed to call for an appointment if they have any problems. Some difficult patients should be scheduled for appointments periodically, perhaps at 3- to 4-month intervals. This will help their morale and may tend to eliminate their seeking adjustment appointments on a weekly basis or even more often.

Every denture patient should be placed on a recall program, just as any patient is. The dentist should not hesitate to inform a patient that occlusal corrections, relining, new dentures, or other fairly involved procedures may be necessary as changes in the mouth continue to occur. A 12-month interval is the suggested time between recall appointments for most complete denture patients.

BIBLIOGRAPHY
Phillips RW: Skinner's Science of dental materials, Philadelphia, 1982, WB Saunders Co, p 200.

Rehabilitation of the partially edentulous patient

CHAPTER 25

Tooth-supported complete dentures

The loss of teeth, especially mandibular teeth, frequently leads to a rapid reduction in the height of the alveolar process (Fig. 25-1, *C*). This morphologic change is considered a major oral disease entity, yet the effort to preserve the patient's oral health is limited by an incomplete understanding of the biomechanical and systemic factors influencing the reduction of residual ridges.

Dentists have long recognized the difference that the presence of teeth makes to alveolar ridge integrity (Fig. 25-1, *A* and *B*). It appears that the presence of a healthy periodontal ligament helps maintain alveolar ridge morphology.

Over the past several years reports have described the favorable results obtained by constructing complete dentures over retained teeth or roots, or both, that may or may not have been prepared. Much exists in the literature about the benefits that a patient obtains from such overdenture techniques—better preservation of ridge height and improved denture stability. Longitudinal support, however, has been lacking for the claim that retention of tooth roots and their periodontal ligaments ensures better levels of alveolar bone. Nevertheless, at least one pilot study has lent credence to the observation that overdentures do contribute to alveolar bone maintenance.

Retained roots are accepted by the tissues and develop a nonfunctional type of periodontal ligament attached to a cellular cementum. Evidence of this comes from clinical, radiographic, and histologic studies of retained root tips showing that submucosal retention of vital roots improves the contour of edentulous ridges; it also meets the expectations of patients and has even earned the endorsement of dentists. However, although it deserves continued investigation, the technique will not be described further in this chapter since it is still at a rather early stage of development.

INDICATIONS AND CONTRAINDICATIONS FOR OVERDENTURES

Overdentures, which may be of the partial or complete type, were initially prescribed for patients with congenital or acquired intraoral defects (Fig. 25-2). In recent years they have been used in patients with badly worn down teeth (Fig. 25-3), patients with only a few teeth remaining (Fig. 25-4, *A* to *D*), and patients with aberrant jaw size or position (Fig. 25-4, *E* to *K*).* The cosmetic and functional results obtained have been excellent, and the retention of a few of the patient's own teeth is frequently of immense psychologic value. The tooth-supported complete denture is a viable and simple alternative to complete denture therapy. Its application is virtually unlimited, and depends on the dentist's judgment, skill, and versatility and, above all, on the patient's motivation to maintain an impeccable oral environment. *Covering teeth and gingival tissues with overdentures is not conducive to maintaining a*

---

*One report (McDermott and Rosenberg, 1984) underscores the value of overdentures in patients who have undergone irradiation.

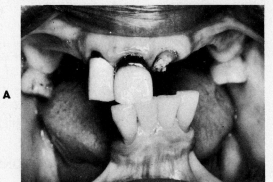

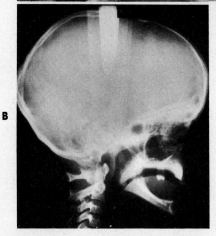

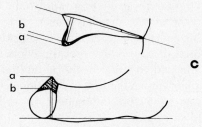

Fig. 25-1 **A,** Dramatic residual ridge reduction of the mandibular edentulous segments contrasts sharply with integrity of the alveolar ridge where the incisors are present. **B,** Virtual absence of the upper and lower alveolar ridges in the mandible of a 13-year-old boy whose dentition was congenitally absent. **C,** Measurements of alveolar resorption. The anterior height of the upper and lower alveolar ridges at two stages of observation (*a* and *b*). The difference (*a* − *b*) represents reduction of the ridges between observations. *Shaded area* denotes the resorption. (**C** modified from Tallgren A: J Prosthet Dent **27:**120-132, 1972.)

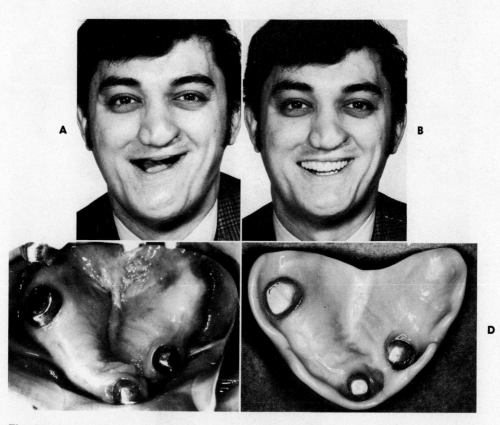

Fig. 25-2   A and **B,** A young man whose cleft lip and palate have been surgically repaired. **C,** Mirror reflection of the maxillae showing the remaining teeth restored with gold copings, which in turn were related to fitted copings embedded in the maxillary denture, **D.**

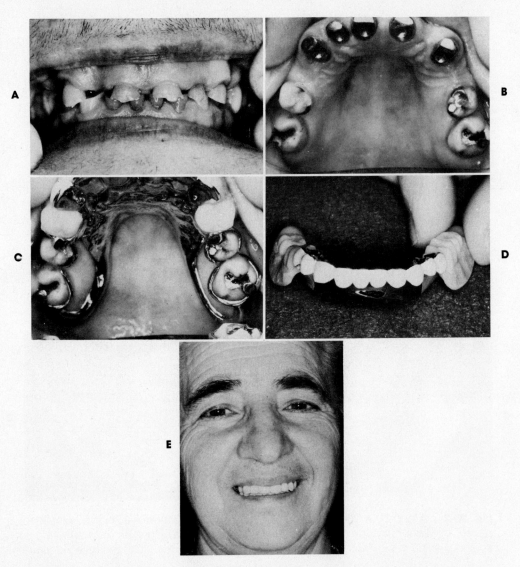

Fig. 25-3   A, Badly broken-down dentition of a 62-year-old woman. **B** and **C,** The maxillary anterior teeth have been restored with gold copings, and a maxillary cast removable partial denture has been built over the copings. **D,** The mandibular dentition was restored with a part-overlay cast removable partial denture. **E,** The restored vertical dimension greatly improves the appearance of the patient.

plaque-free environment, however. Therefore, not surprisingly, clinical experience with overdenture patients reveals a significant frequency of caries and gingival disease around the abutments. Caries can develop in a short time, with some patients more susceptible than others, although the problem appears to have been significantly reduced by the application of fluoride

solutions to prepared abutment teeth.

Contraindications are relatively few and are related essentially to an absence of patient motivation. Most patients who are candidates for their first complete dentures have at least one or two teeth that can be saved by periodontal treatment (to improve the crown/root ratio) and endodontic therapy.

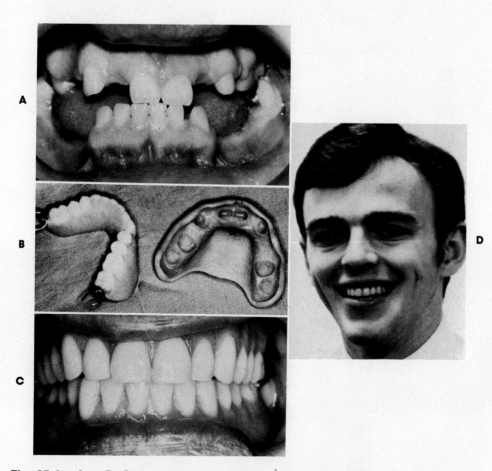

Fig. 25-4 **A** to **D,** Congenitally missing teeth have undermined both the appearance and the functional efficiency of this patient. Overdentures were used to create a normal appearance. **E, F, I,** and **J,** Pretreatment views of a patient whose complaint of mandibular dysfunction and poor cosmetics was attributable to a reduced vertical dimension of occlusion. **G, H,** and **K,** A maxillary overdenture resolved the problem. (**A** and **D** courtesy Dr. A.H. Fenton, University of Toronto.)

Continued.

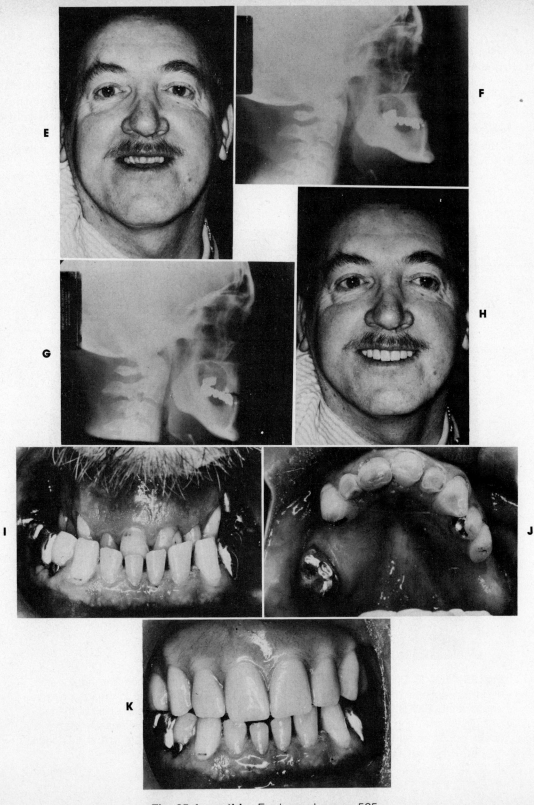

Fig. 25-4, cont'd   For legend see p. 525.

SELECTION OF ABUTMENT TEETH

The critical factor in the selection of abutment teeth appears to be the status of the periodontium and the alveolar bone surrounding the teeth (Fig. 25-5). It is easy to argue that as many teeth as possible should be retained, but consideration also should be given to the following factors:

1. *Cost.* A considerable expense may be incurred if several teeth are to be retained,

treated endodontically, and covered with gold copings. Furthermore, isolated teeth seem preferable to several adjacent teeth (for example, in the anterior part of the mandible), since it can be argued that the latter may lead to a greater risk of gingival damage from interproximal increased plaque accumulation.

2. *Preference for anterior teeth.* The anterior alveolar ridge seems more vulnerable

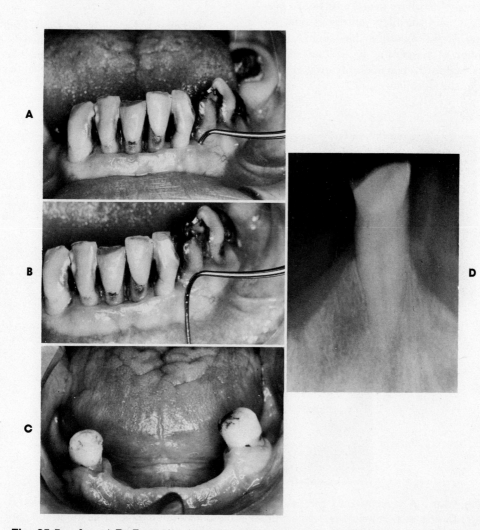

Fig. 25-5   **A** and **B,** Extensive bone loss has eliminated the possibility of using these teeth for abutment service. A healthy periodontium, seen clinically in **C** and radiographically in **D,** qualifies these teeth for use as abutments.

to reduction than the posterior alveolar ridges. Broken-down crowns on posterior teeth can also be restored with pin-amalgams or composites and used as removable partial denture abutments rather than overdentured ones without a cosmetic compromise.

3. *Endodontically treated teeth.* These seem to lend themselves to the technique with minimal alterations.

4. *Preference for mandibular overdentures.* However, maxillary overdentures are prescribed, and maxillary anterior roots retained, if the mandible has such a large number of remaining teeth that its occlusal support is considerably greater than that in the maxillae.

PREPARATION OF ABUTMENT TEETH

Various methods and devices have been proposed for preparing abutment teeth to receive an overdenture. It is our impression that the essential feature in this technique is not the type of attachment used but the following basic principles:

1. An abutment root or tooth must be chosen that is surrounded by healthy periodontal tissues (Fig. 25-6). The healthy tissues may already be present or may be achieved by appropriate periodontal therapy.

2. Maximum reduction of the coronal portion of the tooth should be accomplished. A better crown/root ratio is thereby established, and minimal interference will be encountered with the placement of artificial teeth. The routine

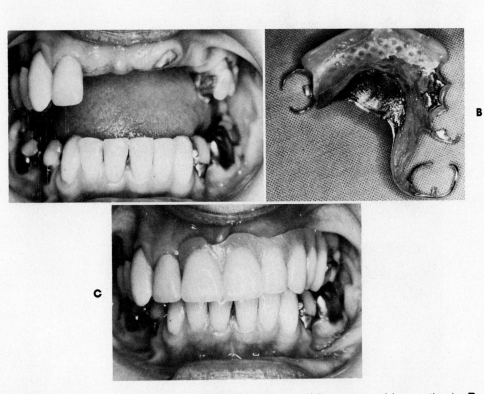

Fig. 25-6   **A,** Healthy roots can be retained and covered by a removable prosthesis, **B** and **C.** This design will help maintain bone in the canine area as long as the tissue surrounding the residual roots is maintained in a sanitative phase.

use of endodontically treated teeth helps achieve this. However, some patients have advanced pulpal recession, usually combined with extensive tooth wear, and this allows coronal reduction without the need for endodontic treatment (Fig. 25-7).

3. The need for a gold coping or a crown-and-sleeve-coping retainer (as described by Yalisove) depends on several factors. Fre-

quently a devitalized and broken-down tooth can be restored with an alloy or a composite and rounded off and polished with fine sandpaper disks (Fig. 25-8).

Occasionally a gold coping is necessary and can be prepared with or without a post or retentive pins depending on the amount of tooth structure remaining above the gingival attachment. The gold coping (Fig. 25-9) does involve

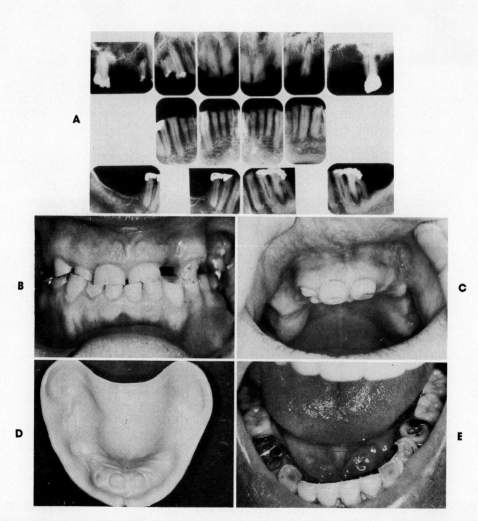

Fig. 25-7 Advanced pulpal recession, **A,** in a patient whose dentition showed considerable wear and neglect, **B.** Three maxillary anterior teeth were retained, **C,** and an overdenture was constructed, **D.** The badly worn anterior mandibular teeth were reduced, polished, and partially "restored" with a cast removable partial denture of the overlay type, **E.**

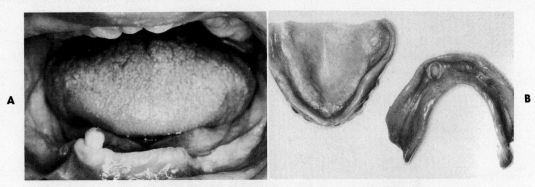

Fig. 25-8 **A,** A devitalized single tooth is covered with a composite restoration, and the crown/root ratio is improved by reducing the crown and rounding it off with sandpaper disks. **B,** A complete denture is then constructed over this abutment tooth. (Courtesy Dr. A.H. Fenton, University of Toronto.)

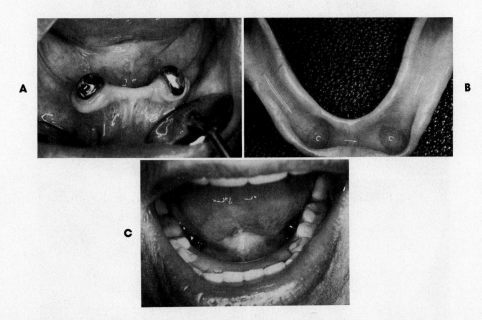

Fig. 25-9 **A,** Gold copings to protect and partially restore the mandibular canines. **B,** An overdenture has been hollowed out in these areas to conform to the abutment contours. **C,** The cosmetic merits of the complete denture are in no way compromised.

an additional expense, but some patients are uncomfortable with the sight of "unprotected" roots in their mouth. The patient's susceptibility to caries must also be considered, and if doubt exists it is better to use a gold coping on abutment teeth. Tooth preparation is similar to that for a complete gold crown, with a combination of shoulder and chamfered gingival margins as dictated by the amount of residual tooth structure. It must be emphasized that the main objective in using gold is the preservation of alveolar bone and not the introduction of a technique for more retentive dentures. Consequently a simple, short, convex abutment preparation (with or without a casting) appears to be the ideal root surface preparation.

4. The patient must be well motivated to maintain the hygienic phase of periodontal care. Regular follow-up visits are essential, and oral health maintenance measures are periodically reviewed and revised as necessary. Fluoride gel is prescribed for daily application to the inside of the overdenture to bring the fluoride into intimate contact with the natural tooth structure.

Extensive experience with fluoride gel in young caries-susceptible cleft palate patients supports this directive. However, 1% neutral pH sodium fluoride liquid or gel may cause irritation or a burning sensation in the tissues of some patients, and in these cases the frequency of application can be reduced from daily to two or three times per week.

5. The occasional need for removal of one or more abutment teeth must be expected. The cause is usually a periodontal abscess, and removal of the affected tooth with appropriate filling in of the contacting site in the overdenture can be done readily and inexpensively.

CLINICAL PROCEDURES

The procedures will vary depending on whether a tooth-supported complete denture is being constructed or a tooth-supported immediate-insertion complete denture is planned.

Tooth-supported complete denture

The important principles of complete denture construction must be respected before the

mechanical ingenuities of particular types of attachments are considered. These principles are identical to those already described in previous chapters, and they should be meticulously followed and carried out. A well-executed complete denture technique does not need to rely on mechanical contraptions, frequently of a stress-breaking variety, to achieve the objectives embarked upon in the treatment of complete denture patients.

One problem of tooth-supported complete denture service is the occasional tendency for patients to demonstrate an untoward gingival response around the abutment teeth (Fig. 25-10). The following may cause gingival irritation: (1) movement of the denture base (more apparent in mandibular dentures), with the development of a loading factor at the gingival margins; (2) poor oral hygiene with failure to remove plaque or to pay sufficient attention to tissue rest and periodic recall assessments; and (3) excess space in the prosthesis around the gingival margins of the abutment teeth, which leads to the development of a "dead space" (a potential source of inflammation).

Clinical experience has shown that a slight space around the gingival margin is essential, to avoid overloading this particularly vulnera-

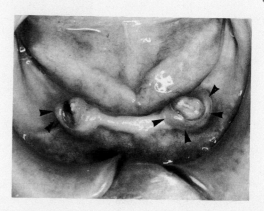

Fig. 25-10 Gingivitis (arrowheads) around the abutments of an overdenture caused by inadequate hygiene measures of the patient.

ble site, especially with mandibular dentures since they appear to become unstabilized more easily than maxillary dentures. On the other hand, a dead space may lead to a combined hypertrophic/hyperplastic response of the gingival margin similar to that elicited by a relief chamber in a complete maxillary denture. One way to avoid this is to hollow out an area in the resin overdenture and line it with a tissue conditioner at the time of denture placement. The resiliency of the liner, combined with its need for frequent replacement, can create an optimal schedule for recall appointments. However, there also may be subsequent deterioration of the material and, with it, the risk of gingival tissue damage. Our preference, therefore, is to use an autopolymerizing hard acrylic resin overdenture.

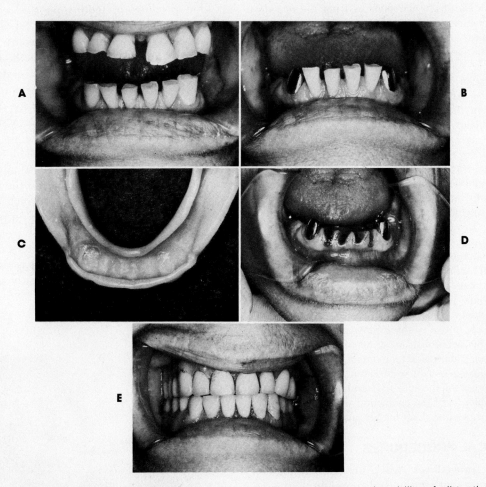

Fig. 25-11 **A,** This patient with advanced periodontal disease and mobility of all teeth except the mandibular canines is a candidate for immediate dentures. The decision was made to retain the canines as abutments for a mandibular overdenture. Thus the dentist was able to restore the canines, **B,** prepare the dentures, **C,** and the mouth surgically, **D,** and finally insert an immediate overdenture, **E.** (Courtesy Dr. Francis Zarb, University of Toronto.)

Tooth-supported immediate-insertion complete denture (Fig. 25-11)

The procedures for immediate tooth-supported complete dentures are identical to those described in Chapter 26, except that the coronal reduction of the selected abutment teeth is done at the time the remaining teeth are extracted. The teeth to be retained are prepared on the master cast to the approximate shape of the eventual coping and the remaining teeth are trimmed away in the usual manner. The processed immediate denture thus demonstrates depressions on its impression surface that will conform to the teeth that are being retained. The endodontic treatment is completed one or more appointments before the immediate denture insertion, or just before the combined surgical-prosthetic appointment. Some dentists prefer the latter because removal of the tooth crown facilitates the endodontics. Immediate denture insertion and follow-up are carried out in the usual manner. The need for refining the impression surface of the denture in the operated and coping sites by the addition of a treatment resin is essential because rapid tissue changes are to be anticipated. When healing has occurred, any necessary copings are prepared and the prosthesis is refitted.

LONGITUDINAL STUDIES

The worthy preoccupation of dentists with retaining patients' teeth has led to a dramatic surge of interest in the overdenture concept. Several reports have been published, and many anecdotal claims made, but there has been a lack of well-documented long-term clinical follow-up of these patients. Current research seems to endorse the claim that overdentures are a dramatically effective alternative to conventional complete denture therapy, and their use in routine practice is assured. However, the very nature of overdenture design

and its relationship to plaque must always be kept in mind if this excellent treatment modality is to fulfill its potential.

BIBLIOGRAPHY

Atwood DA: Reduction of residual ridges: a major oral disease entity, J Prosthet Dent **26**:266-279, 1971.

Brewer AA, Fenton AH: The overdenture, Dent Clin North Am **17**:723-746, 1973.

Carlsson GE, Persson G: Morphologic changes of the mandible after extraction and wearing of dentures: a longitudinal clinical and x-ray cephalometric study covering 5 years, Odontol Rev **18**:27-54, 1967.

Crum RJ, Rooney GE Jr: Alveolar bone loss in overdentures: a 5-year study, J Prosthet Dent **40**:610-613, 1978.

Dolder EJ: The bar joint mandibular denture, J Prosthet Dent **11**:689-707, 1961.

Fenton AH, Hahn N: Tissue response to overdenture therapy, J Prosthet Dent **40**:492-498, 1978.

Guyer SE: Selectively retained vital roots for partial support of overdentures, J Prosthet Dent **33**:258-263, 1975.

Herd JR: The retained tooth root, Aust Dent J **18**:125-131, 1973.

McDermott IG, Rosenberg SW: Overdentures for the irradiated patient, J Prosthet Dent **51**:314-317, 1984.

Preiskel HW: Prefabricated attachments for complete overlay dentures, Br Dent J **123**:161-167, 1967.

Preiskel HW: An impression technique for complete overlay dentures, Br Dent J **124**:9-13, 1968.

Tallgren A: The reduction in face height of edentulous and partially edentulous subjects during long-term denture wear; a longitudinal roentgenographic cephalometric study, Acta Odontol Scand **24**:195-239, 1966.

Tallgren A: The effect of denture wearing on facial morphology; a 7-year longitudinal study, Acta Odontol Scand **25**:563-592, 1969.

Toolson LB, Smith DE: A five-year longitudinal study of patients treated with overdentures, J Prosthet Dent **49**:749-756, 1983.

Toolson LB, Taylor TD: A 10-year report of a longitudinal recall of overdenture patients, J Prosthet Dent **62**:179-181, 1989.

Warren AB, Caputo AA: Load transfer to alveolar bone as influenced by abutment designs for tooth-supported dentures, J Prosthet Dent **33**:137-148, 1975.

Welker WA, Jividen GJ, Kramer DC: Preventive prosthodontics—mucosal coverage of roots, J Prosthet Dent **40**:619-621, 1978.

Yalisove IL: Crown and sleeve-coping retainers for removable partial prostheses, J Prosthet Dent **16**:1069-1085, 1966.

Zarb GA, Bergman B, Clayton JA, MacKay HF: Prosthodontic treatment for partially edentulous patients, St Louis, 1978, The CV Mosby Co.

CHAPTER 26

Immediate denture treatment

Immediate dentures are constructed before all the remaining teeth have been removed and are inserted immediately after the removal of these teeth. They may be either a single complete denture or maxillary and mandibular complete dentures. When both maxillary and mandibular immediate dentures are proposed, it is advisable to construct them simultaneously. This will ensure that cosmetic or occlusal irregularities in the otherwise dentulous arch will not interfere with tooth positioning in the immediate prosthesis.

INDICATIONS FOR IMMEDIATE DENTURES

The dentulous or partially edentulous patient whose remaining natural teeth must be extracted is the prime candidate for immediate denture service (Fig. 26-1). In the past decade there has been an impressive decrease in the number of patients requiring immediate complete dentures. Nevertheless, the clinical protocol for providing this service deserves emphasis. Patients in such a predicament should be spared the humiliation of being without teeth while waiting for their edentulous tissues to heal so they can be fitted with complete dentures. Furthermore, patients for whom total extractions are required will benefit from this treatment:

1. The combination of analgesic administration, gentle surgery, and the denture's splinting action appears to reduce the pain that accompanies the procedure. The discomfort and inconvenience associated with learning to manipulate the dentures can be endured at the same time that recovery from the surgery is progressing.
2. The patient is spared the inconvenience and distress of several months of inability to masticate food and the inevitable nutritional compromise.
3. Appearance is affected minimally, since cheek and lip support is maintained. The morphologic face height is also maintained, and the tongue does not spread out as a result of lost contact with the teeth.
4. It is easier for the dentist to place the teeth in their former identical positions. As a result more faithful reproduction of individual tooth variation, arch contours, and tooth positions is possible. The dentist can use the remaining teeth as guides for orienting the anterior teeth in their vertical and anteroposterior positions and for duplicating the anterior dental arch width. In this manner the positions of the anterior teeth can be accurately reestablished.
5. The availability of tissue conditioners and acrylic resin border-molding materials provides enormous scope for easy and correct modification of the immediate prosthesis. These materials can be applied both at the insertion stage and at subsequent appointment stages, with a net effect of ensuring immediate and continuous excellence of prosthesis fit and comfort for the patient. *It has even been*

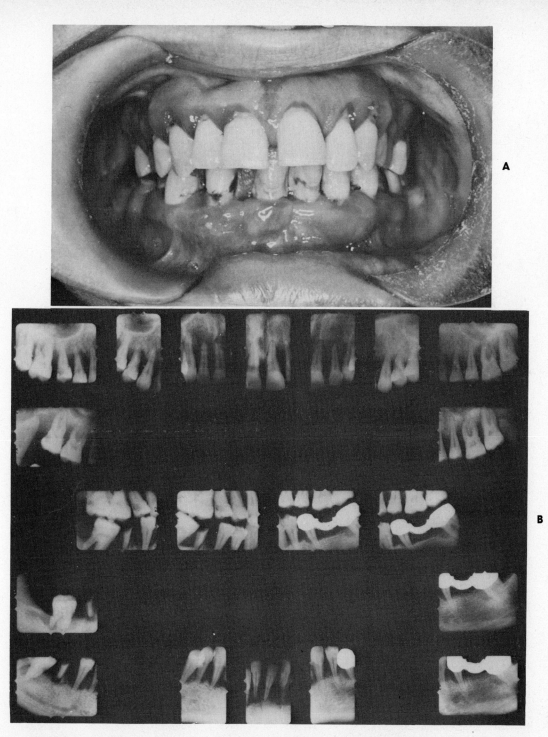

Fig. 26-1 **A** to **D,** An otherwise attractive natural tooth arrangement has been ruined by appalling neglect in this mouth. Immediate dentures had to be prescribed.

Continued.

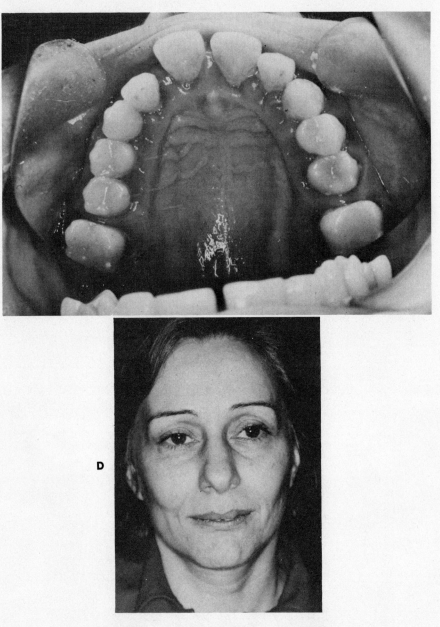

Fig. 26-1, cont'd   For legend see p. 535.

suggested that advances in these dental materials have virtually eliminated all contraindications to the immediate denture service.

After a full arch extraction, bone often seems to resorb more rapidly without the stimulation supplied by an immediate denture base for functional rebuilding. Dentists have used this argument to justify the immediate denture service as opposed to a waiting period without teeth after extraction and before the construction of complete dentures. However, longitudinal studies do *not* indicate that the choice between the two methods is critical when viewed in the context of bony resorption. The rate and magnitude of resorption are a complex and imperfectly understood consequence of tooth loss that appears to be influenced more by denture-wearing habits (and hence loading of the denture-bearing tissues) than by timing of the prosthetic service. Histologic examinations also have failed to demonstrate significant differences between the two methods. It appears, then, that the most compelling reason for immediate denture service is its clinically demonstrated predictability of effectiveness. Most patients seem to adapt readily to immediate dentures.

CONTRAINDICATIONS TO IMMEDIATE DENTURE SERVICE

There are a few minor disadvantages to immediate denture service, since more "maintenance work" is required than with conventional dentures. The maintenance effort is related to establishing the fit of the dentures and the stability of the occlusion in the context of ongoing changes in the recently operated supporting tissues. Interim relines with tissue conditioners are needed, their number (one to three in the first year) depending on the rapidity of alveolar bone resorption and on patient reports regarding comfort and function. It must be emphasized, however, that the relines are simple to carry out and not particularly time-consuming. The major changes in the denture-supporting tissues take place within 8 to 12 months, and at this time a reline with a hard acrylic resin is usually done. (See Chapter 28.) Quite obviously, the patient undergoing immediate denture treatment needs to be advised of these additional procedures, to ensure complete understanding of the responsibilities for regular appointment follow-up and the professional fees entailed.

DELAYED AND TRANSITIONAL DENTURES

Rarely, some dentists will elect to treat a patient who is in poor oral health with systemic disease (usually renal or cardiac) by delaying the insertion of immediate dentures. In this approach the prepared dentures are inserted 3 to 4 weeks (or even longer) after the extractions. The objective is to avoid the "make and break" contact of the denture with the surgically treated tissues, which may cause transient bacteremia during the early postoperative period. Some patients may occasionally be prescribed transitional dentures. These are interim immediate dentures that are usually fabricated by a modified and abbreviated form of the technique described in this chapter. The objective is to use these dentures for just a few months until stability of the denture-supporting tissues is achieved. Subsequently, new dentures must be fabricated. This approach does have its merits, which include all the advantages proposed earlier, plus the added benefits of (1) producing a definitive denture and (2) leaving the patient with a spare denture after the definitive one is completed. Various clinical and laboratory methods have been described to enable this approach to be only slightly more time-consuming and expensive than the conventional immediate denture approach.

TREATMENT PLANNING

Candidates for immediate denture treatment usually present with different numbers of teeth in various locations (anteriorly, posteriorly, or both) and with diverse occlusal relationships.

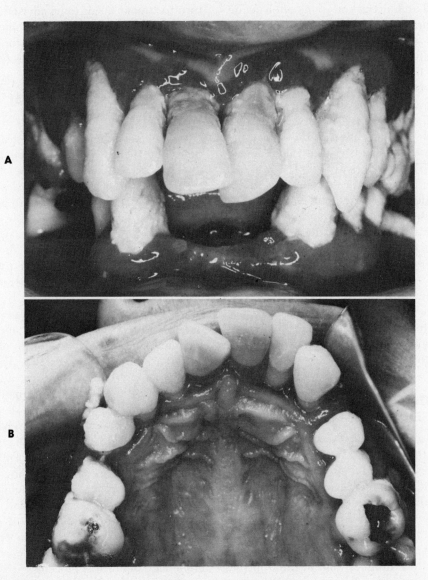

Fig. 26-2 **A** and **B,** Clinical and, **C** and **D,** radiographic views of advanced periodontal disease in two patients who are candidates for immediate denture service. In these situations a two-stage surgical approach is impractical and should be avoided.

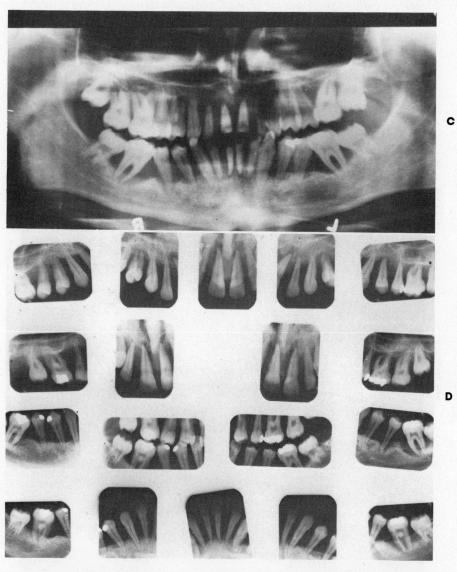

Fig. 26-2, cont'd For legend see opposite page.

It is possible to prescribe a two-stage surgical approach for a patient in good oral health with most of the original teeth still present (Fig. 26-2). The posterior teeth are extracted first, leaving bilateral centric stops on the provisionally retained natural teeth (usually the anteriors and/or the canines and premolars, Fig. 26-3). After a 6-week healing period the impressions are started. This protocol makes it easier to establish the height and width of the posterior borders for the finished dentures.

It is also possible to avoid the two-stage ap-

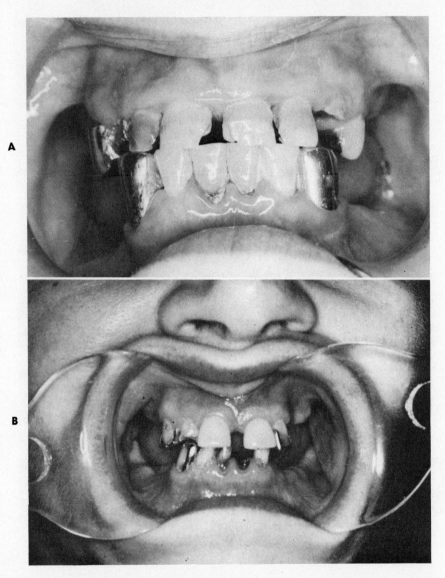

Fig. 26-3   The presence of centric stops in two patients prevents overreducing the interarch distance and facilitates the establishment of a vertical dimension of occlusion for immediate denture construction.

proach and make impressions with the posterior teeth still in the mouth, opting for a one-stage procedure. However, then the chances of making accurate impressions of the potential basal seat areas may be somewhat curtailed, although, it should be emphasized, the ready availability of provisional relining materials now enables dentists to bypass the two-stage procedure and accurately reline dentures at the time of their immediate insertion.

With either approach a general scaling/curettage of the oral tissues is necessary before the prosthetic appointments. Rendering the mouth plaque free will reduce edema and facilitate the surgical procedure and postoperative course. Quite often an occlusal adjustment of the remaining natural teeth will be called for, since the factors that necessitated tooth extraction (extensive caries, periodontal disease, extrusion, drifting) are often associated with occlusal discrepancies that affect the registration of maxillomandibular relations. The establishment of a CO coinciding with CR will ensure that the patient's incorrect maxillomandibular relationship is not carried over into the prosthetic occlusion.

The diagnostic casts, or the final working casts, will supply all the necessary information regarding the teeth (other than their shade and color). A record can be made of the anterior teeth to show the individual characteristics that the dentist may elect to include in the tooth setup (Fig. 26-4).

CLINICAL PROCEDURES

With some modifications, the procedures for making immediate dentures are virtually the same as those described for making complete dentures.

Preliminary impressions and diagnostic casts

Impressions are made in a stock perforated tray. The tray is adapted to the soft tissues forming the reflections by bending the flanges and adding utility wax on the borders (Fig. 26-5, *A*). The center of the palatal surface of the maxillary tray is also covered with wax, to effect a closer approximation of the tray to the palatal tissues (Fig. 26-5, *B*). The wax borders

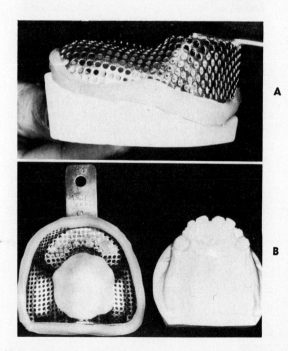

Fig. 26-5 **A,** Peripheral border utility wax is added to a stock tray. Wax is also added to the center of the palatal surface of the maxillary tray, **B.**

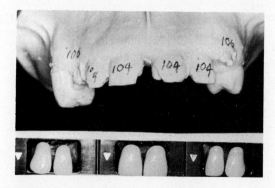

Fig. 26-4 Noting the tooth characteristics on the diagnostic cast is a useful aid for the dentist in selecting an appropriate replacement.

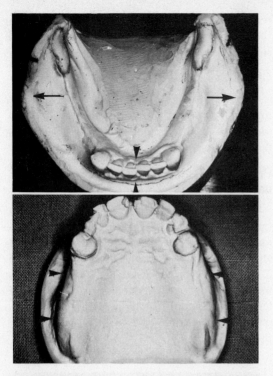

Fig. 26-6   Diagnostic casts made from impressions in stock trays. The extra width of the trays tends to distort the border tissues *(arrows).*

ensure proper extension of the impression and adequate support of the alginate (irreversible hydrocolloid) impression material. If the wax shows through the first impression surface because of tissue contact, it will not harm the impression since it is soft and exerts but minimal pressure. The diagnostic casts prepared in this manner are usually quite adequate for the construction of custom trays. They are rarely accurate enough to be used as final working casts, however, since stock trays do not fit properly and tend to distort the border tissues (Fig. 26-6).

Custom trays, final impressions, and casts

The fabrication of custom trays depends on the final impression technique to be used. We have employed two methods, with consistently good results:

The first (Fig. 26-7) is a method that utilizes custom autopolymerizing (cold-curing) resin trays made over a *cast* with a wax spacer. A tripod-stop effect is established on the incisal edges of the remaining teeth anteriorly and in the posterior palatal seal and buccal shelf areas posteriorly. The tray is tried in the mouth for extension and adaptation and is corrected where needed; its borders are molded as described in Chapter 8. The tray is ready for the final irreversible hydrocolloid impression when several retentive perforations have been made and an adhesive applied to the tissue surface. If a rubber or silicone impression material is to be used, space is provided in the tray over the ridge crest and over the center of the palate and the recommended adhesive is applied. Either of these impression materials gives excellent results.

The second (Fig. 26-8) is a combination method that utilizes cold-curing resin trays made to conform to the *edentulous segments* only. The trays have positive stops on the lingual surfaces of the remaining teeth and in the buccal shelf and posterior palatal seal areas. Roughened handles on the tongue side of the buccal areas provide retention for this section of the superimposed irreversible hydrocolloid in a stock tray. The procedure for border molding the buccal, lingual, posterolingual, and posterior palatal seal areas is as described earlier. The tray is relieved by placing several escape holes (see Fig. 7-26) and is lined with the preferred impression material (rubber, silicone, ZOE). The sectional impression is checked in the usual manner (Chapters 8 and 10), all excess material is removed, and the impression is replaced in the mouth. A perforated stock tray that will accommodate the anterior teeth and the overlying mucolabial fold is selected and filled with irreversible hydrocolloid. Alginate is placed in the labial vestibule before insertion of the loaded tray into the mouth. When the irreversible hydrocolloid has set, the two sectional

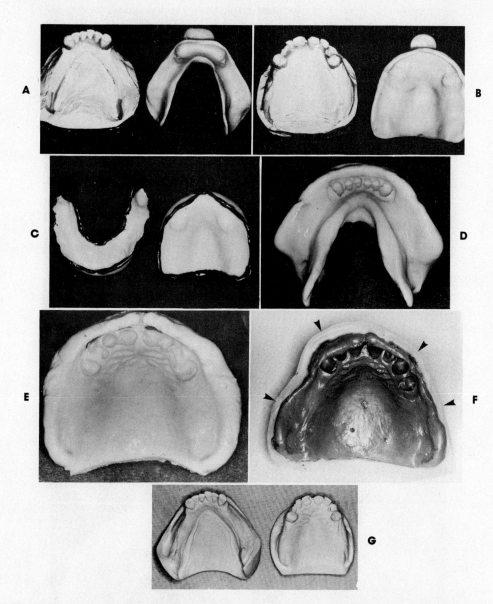

Fig. 26-7 **A** and **B,** Blocked-out undercuts and interproximal areas on casts made from impressions in custom autopolymerizing resin trays. Notice that the wax spacers have been removed. **C,** The trays have been border molded with low-fusing modeling compound. **D** and **E,** Irreversible hydrocolloid impressions. **F,** Thiokol rubber impression of the maxillae. The impression is prepared for boxing *(arrowheads)* before the stone is poured. **G,** The completed working casts.

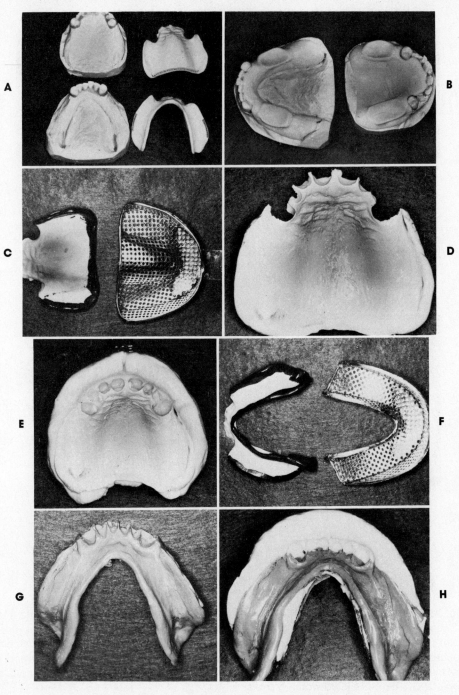

Fig. 26-8 For legend see opposite page.

Fig. 26-8 The combination-method impression technique uses custom trays, **A** and **B,** that conform to the edentulous segments of the jaws. The wax spacer has been removed from the tissue side of the custom trays, and the darker areas show where the resin contacted the mucosa. **C** to **H,** Border-molded resin trays and wash impressions made of ZOE paste in the maxillae and of Thiokol rubber in the mandible. (Any light-bodied impression material can be used.) The secondary impression in the stock tray is made of irreversible hydrocolloid.

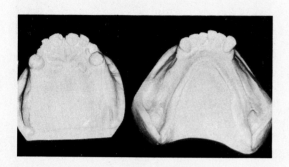

Fig. 26-9 Final working casts made by the combination-method impression technique.

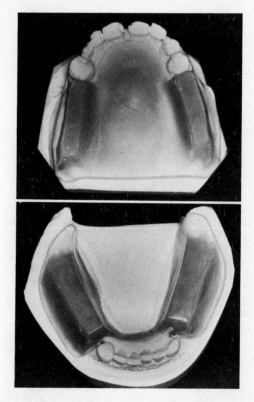

Fig. 26-10 Cold-curing tray resin used as a recording base along with the wax occlusion rims.

impressions are usually removed together. Failure to do this, however, is not disastrous; it merely necessitates reorienting the resin tray into the irreversible hydrocolloid. This technique can yield good final working casts (Fig. 26-9).

Jaw relation records

Jaw relation records are made from the occlusion rims. Again, both the laboratory and the clinical procedures are practically identical to those in complete denture construction. The objective of an accurate transfer of maxillomandibular relations is complicated slightly by the fact that it is not always possible to extend the anterior part of the trial denture base onto a stable area on the lingual surfaces of the anterior teeth. An extremely stable trial denture base is of paramount importance, however, and it is well worth the additional time to produce a trial base that fits the tissues very closely. Hard baseplate wax, reinforced wax, or cold-

curing tray resin may be used (Fig. 26-10). (The indications for jaw relation records and the materials used are discussed in Chapter 11.)

The natural mandibular teeth can be a helpful guide in establishing the height of the occlusal plane, and the occlusion rims are con-

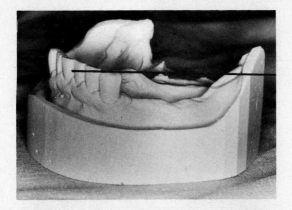

Fig. 26-11 The remaining mandibular teeth and retromolar pad are useful landmarks in establishing the height of the occlusal plane.

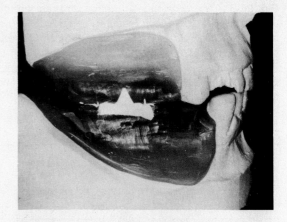

Fig. 26-13 After the occlusion rims have been trimmed so they meet evenly when the jaws are in CR, they are grooved and a fast-setting plaster record is made.

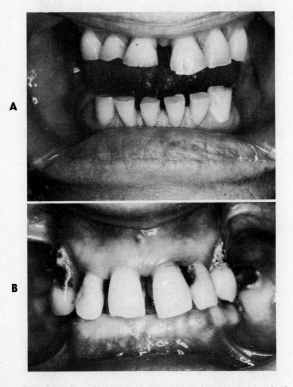

Fig. 26-12 **A,** Loss of the posterior teeth has led to a dramatic decrease in the vertical dimension of occlusion. **B,** The vertical dimension is reestablished in a manner similar to that used when treating a completely edentulous patient.

structed to that height (Fig. 26-11). Reference was made earlier to the importance of correcting any tooth-guided malposition of the mandible that patients might have acquired during the years when they were becoming edentulous. If dentures are constructed with centric occlusion in an acquired eccentric position, deflective occlusal contacts can loosen the dentures and presumably destroy underlying bone. *An occlusal adjustment of the remaining natural teeth is frequently necessary before final impressions are made, to ensure that CO and CR coincide.*

A study is made when the jaw relations are recorded to determine whether the occlusal vertical dimension is to be reproduced exactly (Fig. 26-12). An uneven loss of teeth, loosening of the remaining teeth, and tooth wear have often led to a reduced vertical dimension of occlusion. If the vertical dimension is to be increased, the amount of change should be determined at this time. The technique for registering CR is similar to that described in Chapter 18. The maxillary occlusion rim is so contoured that in CR it contacts the mandibular occlusion rim evenly and the optimal interocclusal dis-

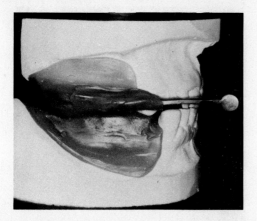

Fig. 26-14 The face-bow fork is sealed to the buccal surfaces of the maxillary occlusion rim. Notice that the projections in the concavity of the fork have been removed to facilitate insertion of the fork into the rim's buccal aspect.

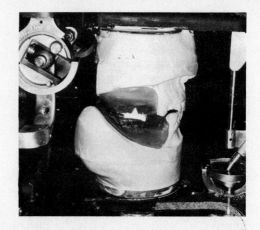

Fig. 26-15 The face-bow and CR record transfers have been completed, and the casts are mounted on the articulator.

tance is achieved. Notches 5 mm deep are cut into the rims, and a CR registration is made with fast-setting plaster (thick and creamy) (Fig. 26-13), beeswax, or ZOE paste. If a face-bow is to be used, the fork, specially prepared for removable partial and immediate dentures by grinding away its two anterior prongs, is attached to the occlusion rim (Fig. 26-14). The face-bow transfer is then made in the usual manner, and the articulator mounting is completed (Fig. 26-15).

Protrusive relation records and articulator adjustment. The making of protrusive relation records and adjusting the articulator are optional procedures and depend on dentist preference. Their use is also justified on the basis of whether cusped or cuspless teeth are to be used.

Cusped teeth. Whenever cusped teeth are employed, the articulators may be adjusted arbitrarily, or else protrusive records are made following one of two procedures:

In the first, approximately four layers of baseplate wax, cut in the shape of the arch, are placed over the maxillary anterior teeth and occlusion rims. The wax is softened, and the ar-

ticulator is set 6 mm in protrusion, with an approximate condylar reading of 10 to 20 degrees. Then the articulator is closed into the soft wax. In making a protrusive record, it is difficult to control the amount of distance the mandible goes forward when the record is made. For this reason the record is made first on the articulator and is then chilled and placed in the mouth to rehearse the patient in what is desired. After the patient has an understanding of protruding the mandible into the wax indentations, the wax is again warmed in water at 135° F (57° C). Water is used instead of a flame so the indentations will be preserved to guide the mandible. When the lower teeth are inserted lightly into the indentations, the patient is told to apply occlusal pressure. The wax is thick enough that the mandibular position can be recorded without penetration of the wax. The wax is chilled in the mouth, and the wax record and occlusion rims are placed in the casts on the articulator to test the adjustment. The locknuts for the condylar guidance adjustments are loosened so the slot adjustments will move readily to adapt to the inclination that the patient has recorded in the warm wax. If the path on the articulator is too steep, the record will not touch the occlusion rim in back. If the path is too flat, the occlusion rims and teeth will not contact in front. These adjustments are placed at an inclination that will allow the entire surfaces of the mandibular and maxillary rims to be in contact. When the dentist is satisfied, the condylar guidance slot adjustment locknuts are tightened and the protrusive wax record is removed. The mandibular wax occlusion rim is removed from the metal framework, and the metal framework is again placed on the cast and is luted in position. The baseplates and occlusion rims of both casts can now be disposed of since there are no further tryins in this immediate denture procedure.

In the second, and equally effective, method of making a protrusive maxillomandibular relation record for immediate dentures, impression plaster is used. This method has the advantages of requiring minimal pressure at the time the record is made. The patient protrudes and closes easily on the front teeth. However, closure must be stopped just before the teeth touch. When the plaster has set, the occlusion rims are removed from the mouth and this record is used to adjust the condylar guidances on the articulator.

Cuspless teeth. The use of cuspless or nonanatomic teeth is described in Chapter 21. The same principles governing their selection for conventional complete dentures may be applied to immediate denture service.

Positioning the posterior teeth

The articulated casts can now be used for setting the posterior teeth. The principles described earlier are adopted, and the teeth are set in tight centric occlusion (Fig. 26-16). The trial denture bases are tried in the patient's mouth, and CR is confirmed. If the previous maxillomandibular relation record was incorrect, CR and CO will not coincide. The mandibular posterior teeth are removed from the trial base, a new CR record is made, and the mandibular cast is remounted. The teeth are

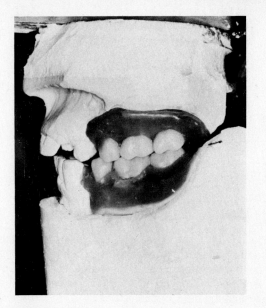

Fig. 26-16 The trial denture bases with the posterior teeth set in tight intercuspation can now be returned to the mouth for confirmation of the original CR record.

then reset to the new articulator mounting and retried in the mouth before the patient is dismissed.

Tooth selection

Tooth selection is easily carried out, since the patient's remaining natural teeth are an excellent starting point for form, size, and shade selection.

Positioning the anterior teeth

Positioning of the anterior teeth depends on whether the dentist wants to duplicate the patient's natural tooth arrangement. Whereas this is desirable for the majority of patients, some do present with rather unesthetic arrangements, which are usually the result of advanced periodontal disease and drifting of the teeth (Fig. 26-2, *A* and *B*). Quite clearly in these situations a positioning of the prosthetic teeth will be demanded that offers the maximum cos-

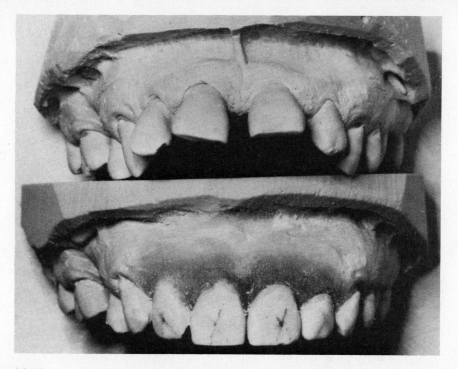

Fig. 26-17 It was proposed that these anterior teeth be immediately replaced so the patient would have an optimal cosmetic result. The stone teeth were waxed onto the diagnostic cast in their preferred position to serve as a guide for the final tooth placement. (Courtesy Dr. A.H. Fenton, University of Toronto.)

metic result (Fig. 26-17). The casts are rendered edentulous, and the desired tooth arrangement is created irrespective of where the natural teeth were. When the dentist decides to position the anterior teeth in their original locale, there are two methods that can be used:

In the first (Fig. 26-18), alternate teeth are cut away on the cast and the labial portion of each root is excavated to a depth of approximately 1 mm on the labial side and flush with the gingival margin on the lingual or palatal side. The slight depression carved in the labial region will accommodate the ridge laps of the artificial teeth. Quite obviously, in mouths with periodontal disease accompanied by gingival recession and bone loss, little or no labial stone has to be removed. Minimal trimming to the

cast will allow the construction of a denture that provides adequate matrix for a full and rounded ridge in the immediate area. The best results are obtained if very little or no bone is removed at the time the dentures are inserted. The selected teeth are placed in their specific positions and modified as required.

The right central incisor is usually placed first and is secured with wax. Then alternate teeth are removed and replaced until all have been set. By removing only one tooth at a time, the dentist can duplicate in its replacement any delicate irregularities that may exist. The muscles of facial expression depend on duplication of the dental arch; hence one tooth is placed at a time. The lateral incisors are then cut away on the cast and replaced, and the re-

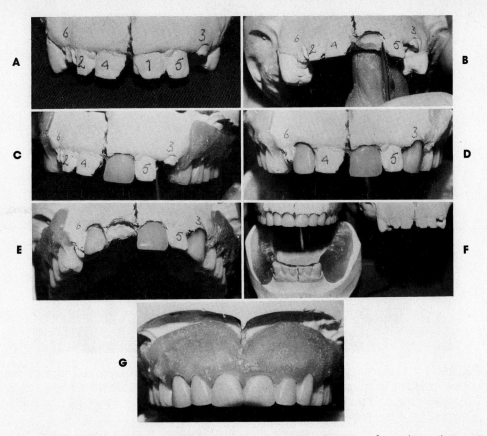

Fig. 26-18   The teeth to be extracted are numbered on the cast, **A,** and are then cut away, **B,** and replaced, **C** to **F.** In the replacement there is minimal excavation of bone from the cervical of each labial root, to allow for a ridge-lapping effect of the replacement teeth. The completed tooth setup, **G,** is a noticeable improvement over the original.

maining maxillary teeth (left central incisor and right and left canines) are set exactly as on the stone cast. A Boley gauge is used for measuring the distance between the labial surfaces of the canines on the stone cast so their replacements will have an identical distance between the labial surfaces.

By this method it is fairly easy to attain accurate duplication of the total appearance, the positions of individual teeth, and the position of the dental arch. However, final cast trimming must be completed at the wax boil-out stage and, for reasons of convenience, is frequently done by the dental technician. The risk of un-

necessary simulated bone trimming may then be created.

In the second method (Fig. 26-19) of tooth positioning the casts are trimmed to a line drawn corresponding to the depth of the gingival sulcus and the teeth are broken off the cast at their cervical aspects. The ridge is rounded in all areas (except interproximally) as for a non–bone trimming. This is done first on one half of the remaining segment and then on the other. The segments of artificial teeth can be set alternately, or the entire cast may be rendered edentulous and the diagnostic cast used as a guide for tooth placement (Fig. 26-20).

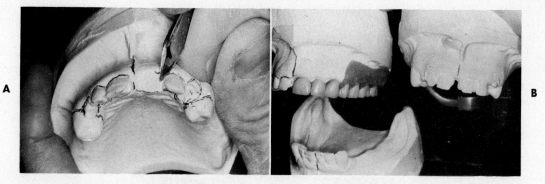

Fig. 26-19   A, The casts are trimmed to a line corresponding to the depth of the gingival sulcus. **B,** Half the trimming is done, and this segment is set, with the diagnostic cast used as a guide. Then the other side is completed in similar fashion.

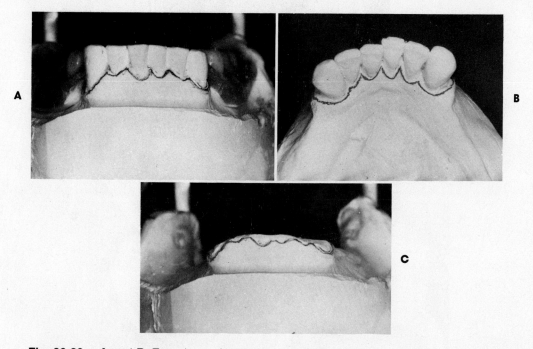

Fig. 26-20   A and **B,** Two views of an entire cast that is to be rendered edentulous according to a line representing the depth of the gingival sulcus. **C,** The teeth have been broken at the cervical aspects and the residual ridge has been rounded off.

By this method the dentist has the advantage of seeing that the cast preparation is correctly done rather than delegated to a technician.

The patient whose pictures have been used to illustrate the two methods of tooth positioning desired a more even arrangement of her artificial teeth than had existed in the natural dentition. This desire was respected (Fig. 26-21), and her incisal guidance (as determined by the vertical and horizontal overlap) accordingly modified. Her condylar guidance was obtained from the interocclusal record, and her artificial occlusion was adjusted to harmonize with the two end factors governing movements of the articulator (p. 444, Chapter 21). If cuspless (nonanatomic) teeth had been selected, a more neutral incisal guidance would have been developed with but minor alteration of the anterior cosmetic tooth arrangement.

When deep or sharp vertical overlaps of the natural teeth exist, reproducing these may be detrimental to complete denture stability. A

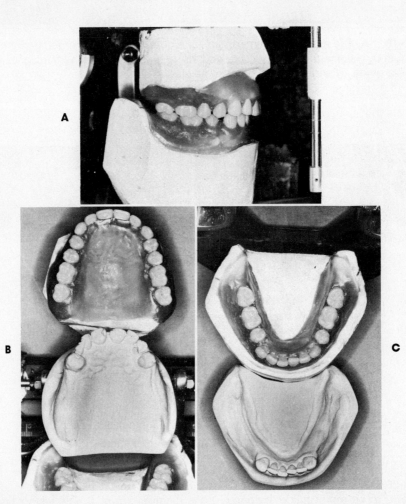

Fig. 26-21   A, Tooth setup completed. **B** and **C,** Both dental arches have been designed to conform to guides established by the residual dentition. The incisal guidance has been modified to suit the cosmetic needs of the patient as determined by the dentist.

deep vertical overlap results in a steep incisal guide angle, which in turn necessitates sharp inclines on all the anterior and posterior teeth. Thus steep inclines are a disturbing factor in the stability of dentures, particularly if the immediate maxillary denture is opposed by a natural (or restored) mandibular dentition (see Chapter 27), although good esthetics can be maintained by introducing some horizontal overlap and reducing some vertical overlap. In other words, the incisal guidance is kept to a minimum.

Waxing and flasking

The upper labial border of the denture is filled in with wax according to the fullness of the border on the cast. An adequate thickness of the denture border is necessary to protect the patient's tissues if edema follows the removal of teeth and insertion of the denture. The fullness of the border is reduced after completion of the denture, when all danger of swelling from the surgery is past. There can be no tryin of the trial denture other than to check the accuracy of the cast mounting before the anterior teeth are set. The rest of the waxing is done according to the principles described in Chapter 22.

Flasking is performed in the usual way. After the wax boil-out and cleansing, a careful study of the radiographs is done so the amount of bone that has been destroyed by disease can be determined. It is possible to avoid this step, however, by preparing the casts as described in the second method of tooth positioning. The ridge area is trimmed to the desired form, or the cast is trimmed. Occasionally it will be necessary to estimate further the amount of bone to be removed during the surgical process if (and when) an alveolectomy is indicated. The cast is trimmed to reduce and smooth the anterior alveolar prominence for favorable reception of the denture. Any slight projections left in the finished denture to conform to ridge irregularities can be removed from the inside of the finished denture before it is inserted in the

patient's mouth. A well-rounded and full ridge that is convex or balloon-shaped will assure the denture's going to place and allow the ridge in the mouth to retain this desired form.

Preparation of the surgical template

A transparent surgical template may be used as a guide for shaping the ridge at the time the teeth are removed and the denture is inserted. The template will reveal places on the ridge where additional bone must be removed and will minimize the amount of surgery needed.

After the cast has been trimmed, an impression of it is made in alginate (irreversible hydrocolloid). The cast and flask are thoroughly soaked in water, and the impression material is placed in the same tray in which the original impression was made. (If the original impression was made in an individual acrylic resin tray, this impression tray will fit the cast perfectly.) The loaded tray is forced into position on the cast in such a way that no air is trapped in the impression material. When the material has set, the impression is removed and plaster is poured into it to form a cast. A hole is drilled through the center of the duplicate cast, and a clear resin template can then be made by a vacuum-formed technique (Fig. 26-22).

The surgical template is a prescription for the surgical procedure and is an essential adjunct when any amount of bone trimming is necessary.

Processing, occlusal corrections, and final preparation of the immediate denture(s)

Relief, if needed, is placed over any hard areas (such as the median palatal raphe) by use of a sheet of 20- or 24-gauge tin or lead that has been thinned on the edges and burnished to place. The dentures are processed, and resultant changes in occlusion are corrected before removal of the dentures from their casts for finishing. Articulating paper locates any deflective occlusal contacts in centric occlusion, and these are ground away with small mounted stones.

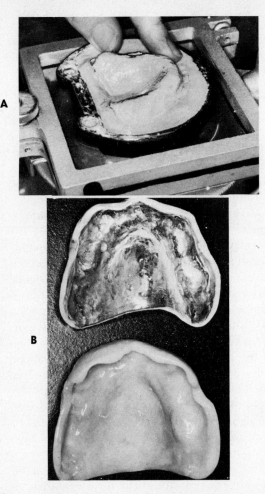

Fig. 26-22 **A,** A maxillary clear resin template is made by a vacuum-formed technique. **B,** The completed template compared to the finished maxillary denture.

Eccentric occlusions are not corrected at this time, since the final occlusal corrections will be made only after the tissues have healed completely.

Before any surgery is undertaken, the labial flange of the denture must be thinned to a minimum; however, the border must remain well-rounded. The prominences on the inner surface, representing the locations of fresh tooth sockets, are trimmed, and identical changes are made in the transparent surgical template. It is necessary that no early pressure be placed in the regions of immediate extractions. The anterior portion of the socket is particularly sensitive because the labial plate is so thin and sharp. The inner surface of the denture is reduced wherever socket prominences protrude. It must also be recessed in the area of the sharp labial plate. A stone capable of cutting both porcelain and resin (such as one of tungsten-carbide composition*) should be used. Since the shape of this inner surface can be only an approximation of the postsurgical contour, an excess of denture material must be removed to spare the patient undue tissue discomfort and also to allow the ridge to fill to a broader bearing surface.

The inclination of the maxillary incisors causes an undercut in the labial region that need not be removed. The denture can be inserted with an upward/backward path, thus allowing the undercut to remain and give a better bearing surface.

Unilateral or bilateral undercuts of the posterior alveolar ridge are frequent. It is always tempting to eliminate these surgically, but they can often be well managed by selecting an alternate path of insertion and withdrawal of the denture combined with judicious trimming of the width of the resin flange in the undercut area (Fig. 26-23).

Surgery and insertion of the dentures

The surgical extraction procedure is well described in oral surgery textbooks.

The transparent surgical template is placed in the mouth *after* all the teeth have been removed but *before* any surgical trimming of bone or soft tissue is done (Fig. 26-24). When the template is securely seated against the palate or on the mandibular residual ridge, spots at the surgical site that are blanched from the

---

*Brasseler USA Inc, Savannah GA, 31419; Midwest Dental Products Corporation, Des Plaines IL, 60018; Pfingst & Co Inc, South Plainfield NJ, 07080.

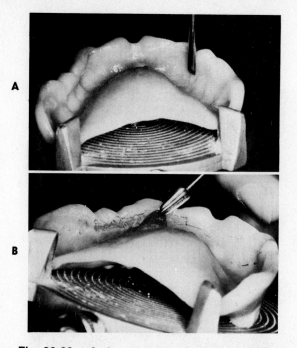

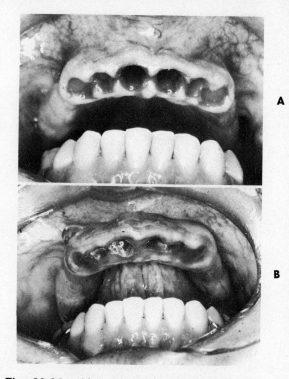

Fig. 26-23   A, A surveyor rod is used to demonstrate the entire undercut buccal segment of the denture and to explore variations in its path of insertion and withdrawal. Reduction of the resin undercut, **B,** is usually adequate to ensure patient comfort.

Fig. 26-24   After the teeth are extracted, **A,** a template is tried in place, **B,** before any surgical bone trimming is done.

pressure can be seen. The template is removed, and soft tissue or bone is trimmed as indicated to relieve the spots. In this procedure the surgical template must be seated perfectly, or it will not reveal the regions that must be trimmed. If the bone and soft tissues are not properly shaped to the contour of the template and denture, the denture will not seat in its correct position. Failure to trim enough tissue to enable the template to go to place or trimming excess tissue will cause the denture to be in an incorrect position. These errors will make the occlusion incorrect, causing unnecessary discomfort. The denture must seat in the mouth in exactly the position it was intended to occupy. The tissue flaps are approximated and sutured, and the denture (which has been

previously sterilized in a cold sterilizing solution) is placed in the mouth. The patient is asked to close for the first check of occlusion. If the denture has been seated correctly after surgery, there should be no gross deflective contacts. Occlusal changes resulting from processing will have been removed while the denture was on the articulator. The patient is instructed to keep the denture in position for 24 hours, at which time the dentist will remove it for the first time.

Tissue conditioners can be used to advantage at this stage. If the denture is loose (usually because of an ultraconservative trim of the stone cast or an unanticipated need for extra surgical trimming of the socket sites), a temporary liner will compensate for the fit discrepancy and en-

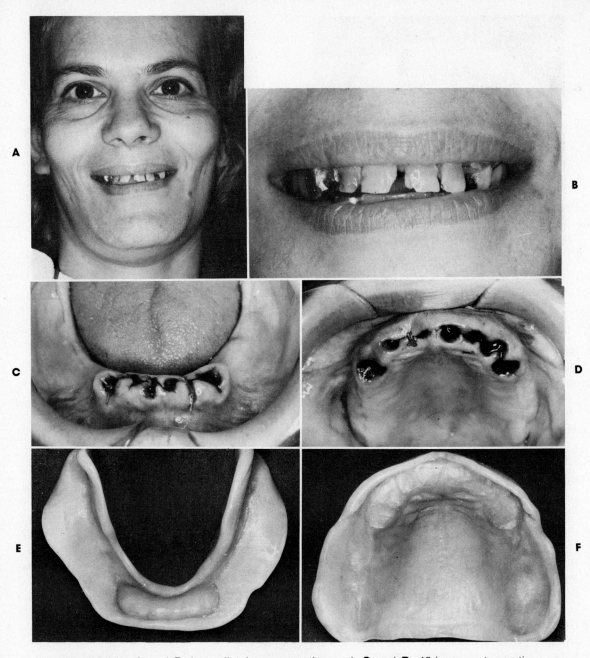

Fig. 26-25 **A** and **B,** Immediately preoperative and, **C** and **D,** 48-hour postoperative views. **E** and **F,** Tissue surfaces of the completed dentures.

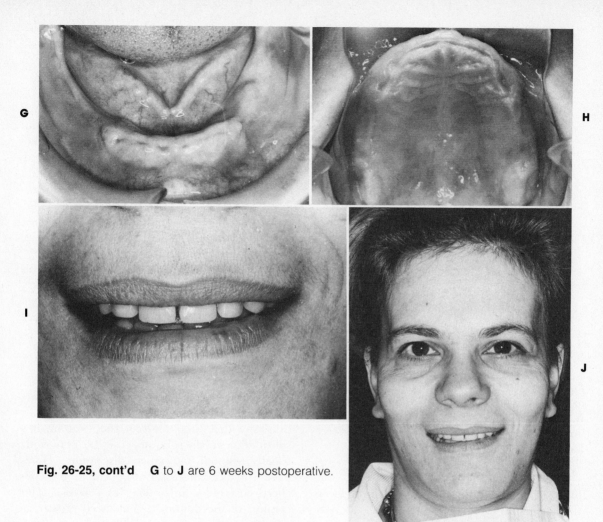

Fig. 26-25, cont'd   G to **J** are 6 weeks postoperative.

sure both comfort and stability. It must be emphasized, however, that any projections of tissue conditioner material into socket sites may interfere with normal socket healing and should be trimmed. *Nevertheless, the ease and versatility with which tissue conditioners have been employed in this treatment technique have virtually eliminated all contraindications to their use.*

Postoperative patient instructions
(Fig. 26-25)

Dentures must be left in the mouth during the first 24 hours. The patient is cautioned that leaving them out at first may result in swelling that will cause reseating to be either impossible or extremely painful. Any pain from the trauma of extraction will not be alleviated by removal of the dentures from the mouth. Within the

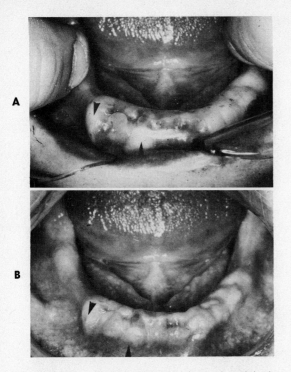

Fig. 26-26 Pressure areas *(arrowheads)* that must be relieved on the tissue side of the denture. **A,** The surgical template employed postoperatively to identify such areas. **B,** Intraoral view of the pressure areas.

first 24-hour period ice packs may be held on the face for 15 minutes each hour. This is only a precautionary suggestion; as a general rule, patients suffer no undue discomfort. If a patient cannot sleep because of nervousness or discomfort, a sedative should be prescribed.

An immediate denture acts as a splint over the surgical field and helps prevent a breakdown of the blood clot, which is often destroyed by fluids in the mouth; therefore, troublesome hemorrhaging is rather rare.

The patient is advised to do no chewing during the first 24 hours, and a liquid diet is prescribed. Because the occlusion has not been finally adjusted, mastication cannot be efficient. Stability of the denture will improve when the occlusion is perfected, and this cannot happen until the swelling subsides. Occlusal adjustment is usually done 48 hours to 1 or 2 weeks after the denture is inserted.

At the end of 24 hours the mouth is examined for border impingement and excessive pressure spots at the site of recent extractions. It is not difficult to detect a spot that has not been trimmed sufficiently after removal of the remaining teeth. It will be manifest as a typical strawberry-red macula. When one is encountered, a ring is marked around it with an indelible pencil and the mark is transferred to the inner surface of the denture as the denture is pressed to place. The area on the denture is then relieved with a stone or scraper.

Over the next 2 to 3 weeks the denture is again examined as required for possible excessive border extension. In the postsurgical period the template can be employed to confirm areas of pressure from the denture base (Fig. 26-26).

Perfecting the occlusion

Overt occlusal discrepancies can be eliminated at the end of the 48-hour period, because by that time most of the swelling has subsided and the denture can be removed, usually without too much discomfort. However, it may be necessary to postpone final occlusal correction for as long as 2 weeks. The comfort of the denture is enhanced greatly as soon as imperfections in the occlusion have been corrected.

This may be done intraorally, as with natural dentitions, or (preferably) in the laboratory. The interocclusal record of CR is made in the same manner as for complete denture patients. The impression plaster is placed on the lower premolars and molars, and the patient is instructed to pull the lower jaw back as far as it will go and to *close* on the back teeth. The word *bite* is avoided at this time because it implies protrusion. Closure is stopped before any teeth touch. When the plaster is set, the interocclusal records are marked for identification and are laid aside.

If a partial lower denture or the natural teeth oppose the immediate denture, an irreversible hydrocolloid impression of the entire arch is made in a stock metal tray with the partial denture in place. The denture is seated in the impression, and the undercuts are blocked out with wax (or Moldine). Then a stone cast is made. This cast is mounted on the articulator by means of the interocclusal record of CO, and the condylar guidances are adjusted according to a protrusive interocclusal record. The occlusion is corrected on the articulator described for complete dentures (Chapters 23 and 24).

SUBSEQUENT SERVICE FOR IMMEDIATE DENTURES

After the usual adjustments, the denture must be cared for in accordance with individual conditions, which vary greatly. The patient should come into the office at least every 3 months for an evaluation of changes that have taken place. If retention difficulties are encountered during this initial period, a tissue conditioner can be used on the tissue surface of the denture. (The use of tissue conditioners is described in Section V.) This material has the property of flowing for a sufficient time to allow equilization of tissue and occlusal pressures. When it hardens, the tissue conditioner can frequently endure the stresses of usage for many weeks (and even months if properly cared for). This procedure can be repeated if required and will enable the dentist to maintain the fitting status of the dentures during the time of rapid tissue changes. The danger of a changing occlusal relationship is largely controlled in this manner.

Research has shown that socket calcification is complete 8 to 12 months following tooth extraction and the bone volume of the alveolar ridge is reduced 20% to 30% during those 12 months. This suggests that a time lapse of almost a year is required before bone completely regains its physical properties. An interval of 8 to 12 months should therefore elapse before a hard acrylic resin refitting of the immediate dentures is performed.

A tendency for increased vertical resorption in the operated maxillary ridge under a complete immediate denture opposed by remaining natural teeth has also been demonstrated. Mastication takes place mainly in the premolar and molar regions when these teeth have been artificially replaced, and this explains why maxillary immediate denture construction combined with a simultaneous reconstruction of the lower jaw (if posterior mandibular teeth are missing) results in less mobility of the maxillary denture and more normal mastication as well as leads to a lower rate of resorption in the anterior region of the upper jaw.

Research also has revealed mandibular postural changes following varying denture-wearing periods. Such changes may be regarded as adaptations to an initially pronounced alteration in mandibular position. Furthermore, it has been shown that the preservation of a residual mandibular dentition opposing an immediate complete upper denture prevents significant changes in jaw and occlusal relationships and the resulting changes in muscle activity.

IMMEDIATE MAXILLARY DENTURES FOR THE PATIENT REQUIRING AN EXTENSIVE ALVEOLECTOMY

Good evidence exists favoring a philosophy of minimal or no bone surgery in immediate denture preparation. Despite this, a patient's jaw morphology may dictate moderate or even extensive bone trimming to achieve the desired cosmetic or functional results. The following three specific situations deserve comment:

1. Patients with an Angle Class II, Division 1, jaw appearance may desire a maxillary alveolectomy to improve their cosmetic appearance. The results obtained are frequently dramatic (Fig. 26-27). It must be pointed out, however, that the modification in lip support will become more evident as the patient gets older. The resultant effect is in-

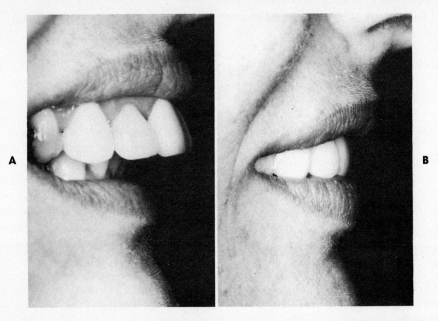

Fig. 26-27 A prominent premaxillary segment, **A,** has been dramatically modified by maxillary alveolectomy and prosthodontics, **B.**

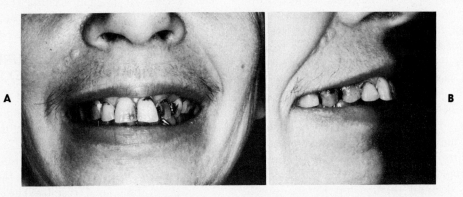

Fig. 26-28 **A** and **B** are pretreatment views of an Angle Class II, Division 1, malocclusion.

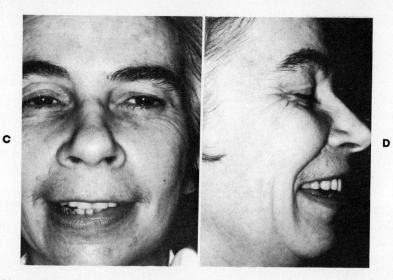

Fig. 26-28, cont'd   C and **D** were taken 7 years following maxillary alveolectomy and denture placement. Notice the inadequately supported labial border. The best position for artificial teeth is in the same location as the natural teeth (unless, of course, the natural teeth are out of their normal position because of periodontal disease or occlusal problems).

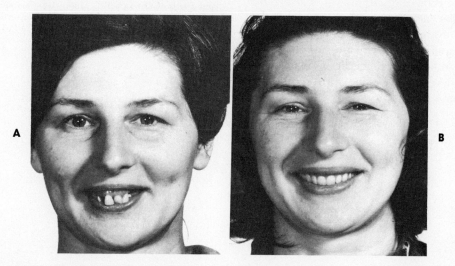

Fig. 26-29   A prominent labial alveolar ridge, **A,** has been reduced surgically, **B,** to allow the teeth to be positioned more superiorly but still in basically their same horizontal position. Notice the reduced prominence of the gingival tissues around the anterior maxillary teeth.

adequate support of the vermilion border (Fig. 26-28) and an apparent collapse of the corners of the mouth. This procedure must therefore be done with extreme caution because of the premature aging effect on the lower third of the face as a result of improper support of the lips. It has been our frequent experience that these patients require a more labial arrangement to their artificial teeth when the dentures are remade after several years.

2. Patients with a short active upper lip and a prominent labial alveolar ridge may require a modified alveolectomy to avoid a shortening or thickening of the upper lip after an immediate denture is inserted. (Fig. 26-29).

3. Patients with diametrically opposed alveolar undercuts may present the dentist with a temptation to correct one of the undercuts. However, if they are 1 mm or smaller, mucosal resiliency will usually compensate for them. If they are more pronounced, a survey of the edentulous region of the master cast will be necessary. Then a path of denture insertion and withdrawal is selected to cover the largest possible area of labial or buccal residual ridge. Usually a combination of mucosal resiliency, cast surveying, and careful relief of the acrylic resin engaging the undercut will suffice to overcome this problem.

BIBLIOGRAPHY

Appelbaum MC: The practical dynamics of the interim denture concept: a comparison with the conventional immediate denture technique, J Am Dent Assoc **106**:826-830, 1983.

Carlsson GE, Bergman B, Hedegård B: Changes in contour of the maxillary alveolar process under immediate dentures; a longitudinal clinical and x-ray cephalometric study covering 5 years, Acta Odontol Scand **25**:1-31, 1967.

Carlsson GE, Persson G: Morphologic changes of the mandible after extraction and wearing of dentures; a longitudinal clinical and x-ray cephalometric study covering 5 years, Odontol Rev **18**:27-54, 1967.

Drummond JR, Duthie N, Yemm R: An immediate denture technique for replacing the last natural teeth, Br Dent J **155**:297-299, 1983.

Holt RA, Stratton RJ, Donoghue T: Prevention of cross-contamination during immediate denture delivery, Quintessence Int **11**:787-789, 1985.

Langer A: The interim immediate denture, Quintessence Int **4**:411-419, 1983.

Lassila V: Adaptation in maxillary immediate denture treatment, Proc Finn Dent Soc **81**:210-214, 1985.

Smith DE: Interim dentures and treatment dentures, Dent Clin North Am **28**:253-271, 1984.

Tallgren A, Tryde G, Mizutani H: Changes in jaw relations and activity of the masticatory muscles in patients with immediate complete upper dentures, J Oral Rehabil **13**:311-324, 1986.

Wictorin L: An evaluation of bone surgery in patients with immediate dentures, J Prosthet Dent **21**:6-13, 1969.

Young L Jr, Gatewood RR, Moore DJ, Sakumura JS: Surgical templates for immediate denture insertion, J Prosthet Dent **54**:64-67, 1985.

CHAPTER 27

Single complete dentures opposing natural teeth

MAXILLARY SINGLE DENTURES

When designing complete maxillary and mandibular dentures, the dentist has complete control over the articulation of teeth. This is rarely the case when a single complete denture is opposed by a residual natural dentition (such as a maxillary denture opposite the natural mandibular teeth, or vice versa). In such situations the objective of a balanced occlusion and denture stability cannot always be met without significant correction or alteration of the opposing natural tooth inclines and the occlusal plane. Patients needing new or replacement maxillary single dentures frequently have these problems; but with careful attention paid to the extra demands on the dentist's skills in occlusal design, good results can generally be obtained.

Reenumerating the objectives of a prosthetically restored occlusion, we arrive at the following: (1) an acceptable interocclusal distance; (2) a stable jaw relationship with bilateral tooth contacts in retruded closure; (3) stable tooth quadrant relationships, providing axially directed forces; (4) multidirectional freedom of tooth contacts throughout a small range of mandibular movements.

In the fabrication of complete dentures, these objectives are relatively easy to accomplish since they translate into an arrangement of bilateral segments of prosthetic teeth that will allow for bilateral horizontal contact during a small range of mandibular movements. This strategy can thereby significantly reduce the risk of dislodgment of dentures that carry the prosthetic segments. All these factors are un-der the control of the dentist and technically relatively easy to accomplish. However, the design of a prosthetic occlusion for a single denture opposing a natural or restored mandibular dentition poses more of a technical challenge, since the dentist's control over the occlusal design and arrangement is reduced and may even sometimes be compromised.

The most common cause of difficulty with the occlusion of a maxillary denture and opposing natural teeth is the inclination of some parts of the occlusal plane of the natural teeth. If the entire occlusal plane is not reasonably level, horizontal forces that reduce the stability of the denture will be directed against it. For example, in an arch in which the mandibular first molars have been lost, the second and third molars will have tipped forward so their occlusal surfaces face upward and forward instead of just upward (Fig. 27-1). If the opponents of these teeth have been lost, the second and third molars may have become elongated as well. The common error is to set the maxillary artificial teeth to meet the occlusal surfaces of the tipped teeth in the same way as they would if the natural teeth were in their correct alignment. This causes a forward thrust to be exerted on these molars whenever food is between them. Such forward thrust is the resolution of vertical functional and parafunctional forces, and it affects the denture whenever the mandible is moved to the opposite side.

The forward thrust developed by the inclined occlusal surfaces causes the maxillary denture to tend to rotate. Obviously, rotation

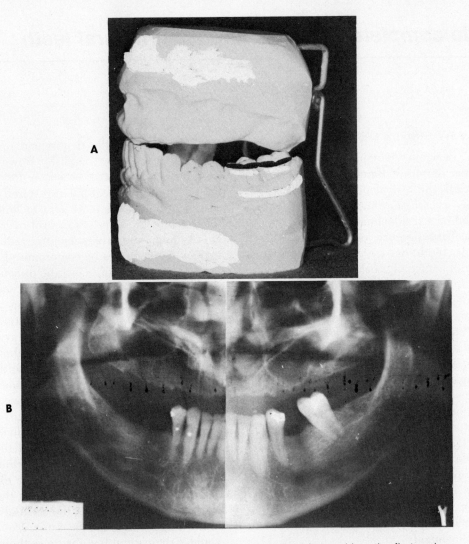

Fig. 27-1   A, The second and third molars have tipped forward into the first molar position. It is therefore necessary to modify the occlusal morphology of these molars by extensive tooth grinding or the placement of cast restorations. If either is not possible, one or both teeth may have to be considered for extraction. **B,** A similar situation demonstrated in a panoramic radiograph. Here the molar is extruded and must be reduced occlusally to avoid interference with the maxillary occlusal scheme.

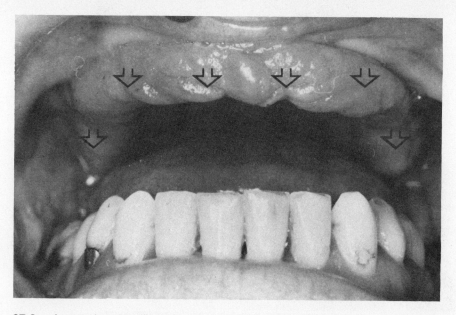

Fig. 27-2 A complete maxillary denture worn for 12 years opposing a natural mandibular dentition. The entire maxillary ridge has resorbed and been replaced by hyperplastic tissue *(arrows)*.

of a denture will break the intimate contact of the denture base with its basal seat and retention will be lost. The resultant compromise in denture stability may then produce increased resorption of the residual ridge. The occlusal plane of the natural teeth must be made reasonably level, or the artificial teeth must be set to contact only the highest parts of the natural teeth.

An excellent and well-fitting denture base is easily loosened when the mandible is moved into eccentric positions if there are steep inclines or deflective contacts in these positions. Therefore the teeth must be prepared so cross-arch balancing contacts are not lost.

For economic reasons it may be necessary to build a maxillary denture without replacement of some missing mandibular teeth. The question then arises, how far is it permissible to go and still have a favorable prognosis? It is essential that some posterior teeth and some anterior teeth be present on both sides of the arch, but

building a maxillary denture against only six or even eight teeth in the anterior part of the mandibular arch may invite failure. Close contact is necessary among all the anterior teeth in such a setup, and this necessitates steep inclines, which are likely to displace the denture. True, some patients wear maxillary dentures against this combination of teeth in the mandibular arch despite the tipping action that is constantly taking place. However, our clinical experience indicates that when occlusal forces are localized to a small portion of the maxillary ridge bone reduction is more likely and frequently is accompanied by the development of replacement hyperplastic tissue (Fig. 27-2).

When a fixed or a removable partial denture is planned for the mandibular arch, it is important that the occlusal scheme be an integrated one (that is, *one developed when both arches are treated together*, Fig. 27-3). If the mandibular arch is not to be restored prosthetically, careful planning on articulated casts will ensure

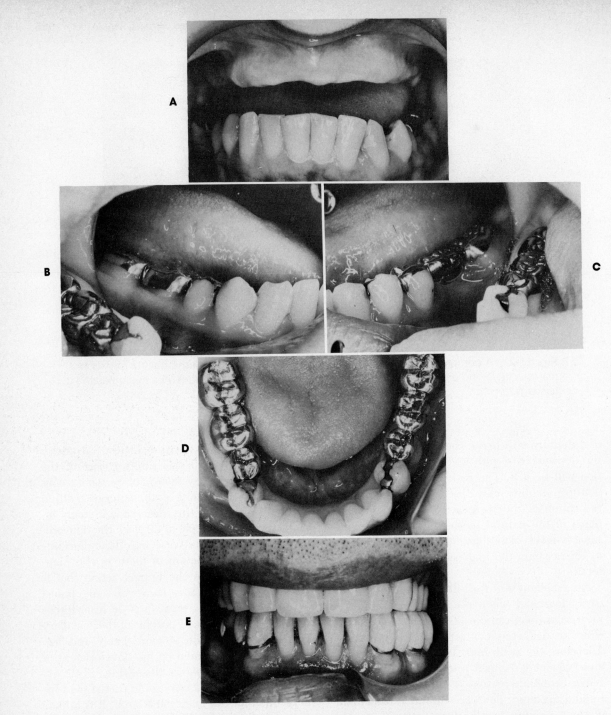

Fig. 27-3 The mandibular natural teeth in **A** to **D** have been restored; therefore these fixed partial prostheses were designed and fabricated along with the maxillary complete denture to ensure an integrated occlusion. In **E** a similar clinical and laboratory strategy has enabled the dentist to provide an optimally balanced occlusion and cosmetic result.

the dentist's control over an optimal occlusal plane.

A problem that may be encountered is the increased risk of fracture of the maxillary denture base, which can result from adverse occlusal stress on the denture by the opposing dentition with possible enhancement of denture base flexure. A cast metal base is therefore frequently recommended for these patients.

Clinical and laboratory procedures

In the case of a single maxillary denture, an impression is made of both arches and a maxillary occlusion rim is fabricated. If a cast metal base (Stellite alloy or gold) is prescribed, this is now made in a full palatal coverage design with mesh extensions over the edentulous ridges and extending to the posterior palatal seal area. If bilateral or a tripod of stable centric stops can be established on this rim, a CR record is made in wax or fast-setting plaster. When stable centric stops are not feasible because of a depleted mandibular dentition, a partial mandibular occlusion rim must be employed for the CR record. A face-bow registration is made, and the casts are mounted on a semiadjustable articulator. The condylar guidances on the articulator are set to either an average value or the protrusive records.

The incisal guidance is set at the angle considered necessary for occlusion of the denture. The more nearly horizontal it is, the more the inclines will be reduced and the more stable the denture will be. Esthetics will influence the angle of the incisal guide because the vertical position of the anterior teeth varies with the amount of vertical overlap used.

The teeth are arranged with the proper inclinations and vertical overlaps and without the exact contours of the mandibular occlusal plane or intercuspation of the natural teeth being followed. The occlusal plane is oriented, and the teeth are inclined, with the anticipated necessary arrangement for occlusal balance.

However, there are many dips in the occlusal plane of natural teeth because of tipping if any teeth of the arch have been lost. The mandibular first molar is the tooth most frequently missing, with resultant drifting of the second and third molars (Fig. 27-1). This causes extremely steep inclines, so the maxillary molars should not be set down into contact with these malpositioned teeth. The denture teeth are prepared with reduced inclines to diminish lateral stress and ensure stability from the standpoint of occlusion. The posterior teeth are set to occlude in the hard baseplate-wax occlusion rim.

The articulator is moved into the various eccentric positions for study of the occlusal balancing contacts. The teeth are rearranged for the best possible occlusal balancing contacts. However, it may be found that the natural teeth will prevent this balancing, and it will then be necessary to grind the stone cast to remove these interferences. After arrangement of the denture is complete, grinding of the interferences of the mandibular teeth on the stone cast is done by moving the maxillary teeth over the mandibular stone teeth.

If an opposing fixed or removable partial denture is part of the treatment, it is waxed up at this stage. The objective is to insert all prostheses (fixed or removable partial dentures or the complete denture) at the same appointment to ensure optimal control and development of occlusal relations.

After the denture has been processed, it is placed in the mouth and tested for retention, and its borders are checked for height.

A comparison of the natural teeth with the stone cast is made for the surfaces to be ground. Preliminary grinding is done with diamond stones, preferably on the teeth at the locations suggested by the stone cast.

Thin articulating paper is placed over the mandibular teeth, and an opening and closing movement is made to indicate the surfaces to be ground in CR. These surfaces are then reduced with a fine soft Carborundum stone.

Next, simulated parafunctional or excursive movements are performed and gross discrepan-

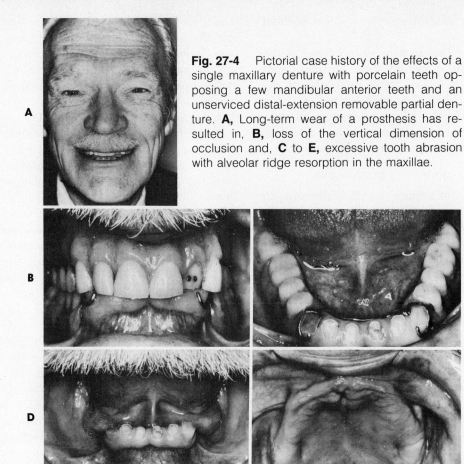

Fig. 27-4 Pictorial case history of the effects of a single maxillary denture with porcelain teeth opposing a few mandibular anterior teeth and an unserviced distal-extension removable partial denture. **A,** Long-term wear of a prosthesis has resulted in, **B,** loss of the vertical dimension of occlusion and, **C to E,** excessive tooth abrasion with alveolar ridge resorption in the maxillae.

cies are reduced with diamond stones and refined with fine soft Carborundum stones.

Some dentists elect to place Carborundum grinding paste over the maxillary teeth and then instruct the patient to make all excursive movements. Care must be taken then, however, to prevent the grinding from producing an error in CO. This grinding is continued until it is felt that the minor interferences have been removed. The final grinding with Carborundum paste (such as Kerr's abrasive) is done for removal of slight interferences.

Subsequent problems with single dentures against natural teeth

One of the major problems with dentures opposing natural teeth is abrasion.

The use of maxillary porcelain teeth, especially when ground during occlusal correction, will lead to rapid wear of the opposing natural teeth. If this is allowed to continue, the pulps may even be exposed (Fig. 27-4, *E*).

Gold inlays or crowns and silver alloy restorations wear away more rapidly than tooth enamel when opposed by porcelain complete

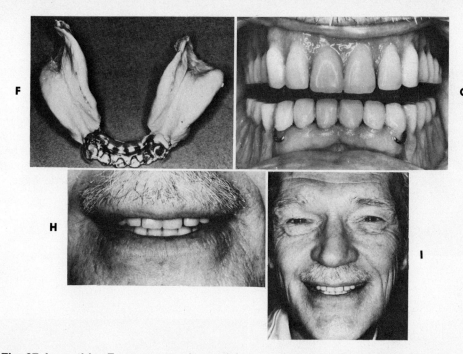

Fig. 27-4, cont'd   Treatment used a partial-type overdenture, **F,** which restored the vertical dimension, **G,** and permitted development of an incisal guidance that would discourage anterior tooth contacts except in excessive protrusion. Compare the final appearance, **H** and **I,** with the pretreatment photograph.   (From Zarb GA, et al: Prosthodontic treatment for partially edentulous patients, St Louis, 1978, The CV Mosby Co.)

denture teeth, and this can destroy a fine effort at occlusal reconstruction of the lower teeth that might have been done to develop the ideal occlusal plane and curvature. The use of acrylic resin teeth in the single denture in this situation has become a popular compromise. However, natural teeth or silver restorations also wear away the occlusal surfaces of the resin teeth in a relatively short time. Thus the obvious course is to examine prosthetically treated patients at regular intervals to ensure that any abraded teeth are replaced. Such replacement can be carried out easily and inexpensively.

Although modern resin teeth demonstrate excellent wear and hardness, some dentists still prefer to use gold occlusal surfaces if the denture teeth will oppose gold restorations or natural teeth (Fig. 27-5). When one or more gold occlusal surfaces are provided on each side of the single complete denture, they will stop the abrasion between unlike materials and protect the other teeth from abrasion.

Formation of gold occlusal surfaces. The procedure for making gold occlusal surfaces in-

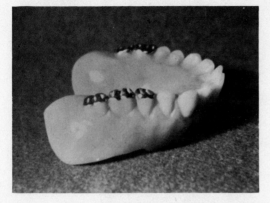

Fig. 27-5 Gold occusal surfaces on acrylic resin teeth serve as protection after the teeth have been set in occlusion. The resin is a toothcolored acrylic of the type used in fixed partial dentures.

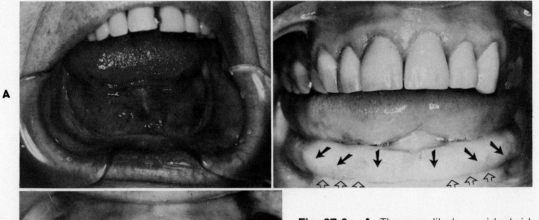

Fig. 27-6 **A,** The mandibular residual ridge has been destroyed by long-term, unserviced wear of a mandibular denture opposed by a natural dentition. In **B** and **C** a similar situation exists, a pseudo–Class III occlusion. Mandibular denture stability is further compromised in this patient by a high floor of the mouth attachment *(dark arrows)* and a resorbed ridge *(light arrows).*

volves arranging the plastic posterior teeth where their gold surfaces will be most protective.

Once the occlusion has been balanced and perfected after the tryin, the plastic teeth to be converted are removed from the trial denture base. Their occlusal surfaces are cut off with a separating disk at right angles to the long axis of each tooth. A wax retention loop is attached to the cut surface, and the sprue for casting is attached to this surface also. The wax and resin patterns are invested, burned out, and cast, and the castings are polished. White inlay wax is used to restore the original buccal and lingual contours of the teeth. Then the gold occlusal surfaces with their wax buccal and lingual patterns are invested, and tooth-colored acrylic resin is processed to the gold occlusal surfaces. The gold-and-acrylic-resin teeth are replaced in the positions they occupied when they were made only of acrylic resin. Since the occlusal surfaces have been corrected before the castings were made, the gold will assist in their being replaced in the original positions as guided by the opposing occlusion.

MANDIBULAR SINGLE DENTURES

The single mandibular denture opposing a restored complete or partial maxillary arch poses an even greater challenge. This situation is frequently compounded by advanced residual ridge resorption of the edentulous mandible, and it is tempting to conclude that such patients are better off with all their remaining teeth extracted and complete upper and lower dentures constructed. Fig. 27-6 shows an example of the terrific destruction of bone from the lower jaw caused by such a complete mandibular denture. The mandibular ridge was destroyed in a relatively short time.

A useful analogy can be presented: the force concentration encountered when a small hammer is violently swung against a large anvil. The edentulous mandible (small hammer) is the force-generating part of the equation; the dentate maxillae (large anvil) is the recipient of the force. The arm holding the hammer is vulnerable in such a situation, as is the edentulous mandible in such a context, since the action of force generation (that is, the functional and parafunctional contacts) can only lead to denture dislodgment and/or tissue trauma.

It is not always possible to convince the patient whose edentulous mandible opposes an intact or a restored maxillary dentition that the remaining maxillary teeth should be extracted. Although the potential for advanced residual ridge resorption of the mandible must be emphasized, along with the difficulties in denture stability that will be encountered, the dentist is frequently forced to compromise and attempt prosthodontic treatment of such patients without further extractions.

The clinical and laboratory procedures are almost identical to those described earlier in this chapter. Experience suggests, however, that a resilient denture liner in the mandibular denture is most useful. At the conclusion of Chapter 1 (see Fig. 1-8) the possible significance of employing permanent resilient (or, for that matter, a series of temporary resilient) liners to reduce stresses on the residual alveolar ridges was propounded. The premise was that a stress-breaking or stress-reducing material might compensate for the gross imbalance of available areas in an edentulous mandible to cope with the functional and parafunctional pressures—somewhere in the region of 45 cm^2 of periodontal ligament for the maxillary dentition versus 12 cm^2 or less for the mucosa-cov-

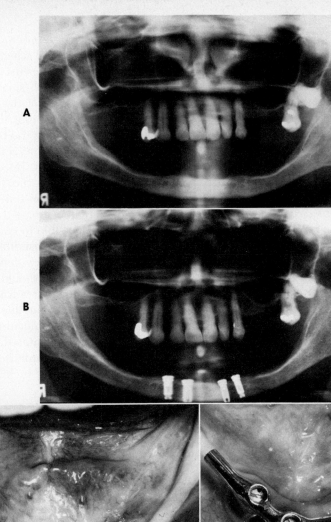

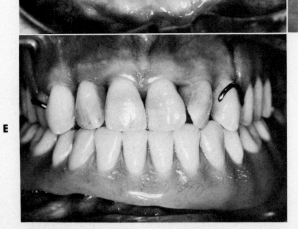

Fig. 27-7 This patient's maladaptive experience with a complete mandibular denture opposed by a partially restored maxillary dentition was resolved by prescribing an implant-supported mandibular overdenture. **A,** Preoperative and, **B,** postoperative radiographs underscore the pre- and post-treatment clinical appearances, **C** and **D,** of the edentulous mandibular ridge. The dentist's judgment is what dictated the number of clips to be incorporated in the mandibular prosthesis, **E,** for retentive purposes.

ered alveolar bone. We and several of our colleagues have adopted this approach for most of our patients in this predicament, with consistently acceptable results. In recent years patients in this dental morphologic predicament have been treated with implant-supported fixed or overdenture prostheses (Fig. 27-7). The availability of osseointegrated implants, together with their predictable therapeutic effectiveness, has ushered in a new era of expanded treatment options for these patients.

BIBLIOGRAPHY

Beyli MS, von Fraunhofer JA: An analysis of causes of fracture of acrylic dentures, J Prosthet Dent **46**:238-241, 1981.

Curtis TA, Langer Y, Curtis DA, Carpenter R: Occlusal consideration for partially or completely edentulous skeletal class II patients. II, Treatment concepts, J Prosthet Dent **60**:334-342, 1988.

Koper A: The maxillary complete denture opposing natural teeth: problems and some solutions, J Prosthet Dent **57**:704-707, 1987.

Schneider RL: Diagnosing functional complete denture fractures, J Prosthet Dent **54**:809-814, 1985.

Yurkstas AA: The single denture. In Clark's Clinical dentistry, vol 5, Philadelphia, 1988, JB Lippincott Co, Chapter 16, pp 1-16.

Supplemental prosthodontic procedures for the edentulous patient

CHAPTER 28

Relining or rebasing of complete dentures

The materials used in complete denture prosthodontics are vulnerable to change, insofar as the denture base may discolor or deteriorate and the artificial teeth can fracture or become abraded. However, the potential for irreversible change is greatest in the tissues supporting the prostheses. This point was emphasized in Section I as an insidious and unavoidable sequela of the edentulous state. Meticulous attention and care in the construction of complete dentures (Sections II and III) will minimize adverse changes in the supporting tissues and in associated facial structures as well. However, these changes cannot be entirely avoided, and the need for "servicing" complete dentures to keep pace with the changing foundations becomes mandatory. The clinical efforts that aim at prolonging the useful life of complete dentures involve a refitting of the impression surface of the denture by means of a reline or a rebase procedure.

TREATMENT RATIONALE

The foundation that supports a denture changes adversely as a result of varying degrees and rates of residual ridge resorption. These changes may be insidious or rapid, but they are progressive and inevitable, and they usually are accompanied by one or more of the features shown in Fig. 28-1. The resultant spatial reorientation of the dentures on their supporting tissues and occlusal surfaces leads to changes in circumoral support and, consequently, in the patient's appearance. The changes in occlusal relationships also induce more adverse stresses on the supporting tissues, which heightens the risk of further ridge resorption.

One compelling conclusion that can be drawn from clinical experience and research involving denture-wearing patients is that dentures need regular attention for maintenance purposes. Such attention can be achieved only by patient education and a regular recall schedule. During the recall appointments the dentist reconciles a patient's reports on his/her denture experiences with information derived from clinical examinations. The magnitude of the observed changes allows a decision to be made as to whether the prescribed resurfacing will necessitate a laboratory reline or a rebase. From a clinical standpoint, the terms are synonymous; however, the adjunctive laboratory techniques differ and may consist of simply relining or actually remaking the denture.

The clinical procedure in *relining* involves adding a small amount of impression material to the denture base. This can be done without adversely affecting the occlusal relationships or the esthetic support of the lips and face. When minimal or moderate changes are evident, it is the treatment of choice. A thin layer of impression material is added to compensate for changes that have occurred in the basal seat. Then, in the dental laboratory, the material is replaced by a new layer of acrylic resin, which bonds to the original fitting surface of the denture.

If extensive changes are encountered, the dentist must compensate not only for the re-

577

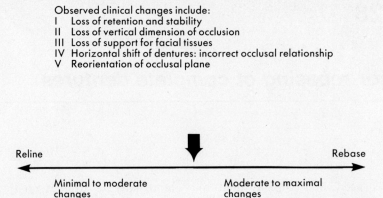

Observed clinical changes include:
I   Loss of retention and stability
II   Loss of vertical dimension of occlusion
III Loss of support for facial tissues
IV Horizontal shift of dentures: incorrect occlusal relationship
V   Reorientation of occlusal plane

Reline   Rebase

Minimal to moderate   Moderate to maximal
changes   changes

Fig. 28-1   A number of changes can occur in the tissues that support complete dentures. They are more common under mandibular than under maxillary dentures, but they may be encountered under either, particularly when an upper denture is opposed by the natural dentition. The magnitude of the changes is what determines whether a resurfacing or a refitting will be prescribed. If a new thin layer of resin is added to the denture base, the resurfacing is called a *reline*. If more material is added (as for a maxillary denture resting on severely resorbed residual ridges), a refitting is necessary and this is called a *rebase*.

duced supporting tissue but also for the reorientation of the dentures, and this necessitates a simultaneous refitting of the impression surface of the denture with a reorienting of its vertical and horizontal position in the mouth. The resultant bulky denture base will likely require a thinner palatal section in the maxillary denture; hence, the dental laboratory description of a *rebasing procedure*.

Quite clearly, relines can be done simply, accurately, and inexpensively. It is readily conceded, however, that rebasing a complete denture involves all the problems of making new dentures plus the restriction that the teeth cannot be moved around as easily as with a new denture. Nevertheless, socioeconomic realities dictate that rebasing must be provided quite frequently, and clinical experience justifies its routine use.

DIAGNOSIS

A thorough diagnosis of the changes that have occurred must be made before any clinical procedures are started. It is necessary to determine the nature of the changes as well as their extent and location. The dentist must therefore understand what changes are possible and what their symptoms are.

Patients who have worn dentures successfully for a long time often return for further service because of looseness, soreness, chewing inefficiency, or esthetic changes. These difficulties may have been caused by (1) an incorrect or unbalanced occlusion that existed at the time the dentures were inserted or (2) changes in the structures supporting the dentures that may or may not have been associated with a disharmonious occlusion. It is essential that the cause or causes of the difficulties be determined before any attempt is made to correct them.

Dentures with built-in errors in occlusion may not need relining. They may need only to have the occlusion corrected. Simple tests of the individual denture bases may show that stability and retention have not been lost even though the patient reports that the dentures are loose. In this situation the supporting tissues may show more irritation or inflammation on one side of the mouth than on the other. The apparent looseness results from uneven occlusal contact that was not discernible at first, and treatment involves keeping the dentures out of the mouth for 1 to 2 days or using a tissue conditioner to allow the supporting tissues to become healthy. If the occlusion has induced a gradual loss of retention, tissue rest followed by a new CR record with remounting and regrinding will eliminate the cause and make the dentures comfortable and serviceable without relining.

A change in the basal seats of the dentures may be obvious by comparison of the tissues in the mouth with the contours of the tissue surfaces of the dentures; or it may be revealed by looseness, general soreness and inflammation, loss of the occlusal vertical dimension and esthetics, or disharmonious occlusal contacts. An examination of the oral mucosa that supports the dentures will disclose the state of its health. When this tissue is badly irritated, occlusal disharmony associated with loss of the vertical dimension should be suspected. Unsatisfactory changes in esthetics indicate a loss of the vertical dimension even though the teeth may seem to occlude properly. If the supporting tissue is badly destroyed, surgical correction to eliminate the hyperplasia may be necessary before relining impressions are made.

The amount of change in the occlusal vertical dimension that has resulted from the loss of supporting structure must be carefully noted. The problem is not simply a change in the occlusal vertical dimension; it also can be a change in the horizontal relations of the dentures to each other and to their basal seats. A loss of vertical dimension will automatically cause the mandible to have a more forward position in relation to the maxillae than it would at the original occlusal vertical dimension. This situation exists even though the jaws are maintained in CR (Fig. 28-2).

Shrinkage of the bone of the maxillae usually permits the upper denture to move up and back in relation to its original position. However, the occlusion may force the maxillary denture forward. The lower denture usually moves down and forward, but it may move down and back relative to the mandible as shrinkage occurs. Concurrently the mandible moves to a higher position when the teeth are in occlusion than it occupied with the teeth in occlusion before the shrinkage occurred. This movement is rotary around a line approximately through the condyles. Since the occlusal plane and the body of the mandible are located below the level of this axis of rotation, the mandible moves forward as the space between the maxillae and mandible is reduced from that existing when the dentures were constructed originally. Such forward movement of the body of the mandible is not necessarily a change in CR, because CR may be retained despite the movement.

The effects of this rotary movement vary from patient to patient and appear to result from a complex interaction of several features—the duration and magnitude of bone resorption, the mandibular postural habit, tooth morphology, and the amount of material present. The mandible's rotation may be associated with a number of consequences:

1. A loss of centric occlusion in the dentures

     The lower teeth may assume a protruded position relative to the upper teeth; thus if cusped teeth are used, the contacts that occur in CR will be between the mesial inclines of the lower cusps and the distal inclines of the upper cusps. This effect may progress so far as to allow the lower teeth to contact the upper teeth a full cusp width anterior to the relation in which they were originally arranged (Fig. 28-2).

2. Changes in the structures that support the upper denture

     The upper denture may be forced anteriorly on the upper ridge, rather than

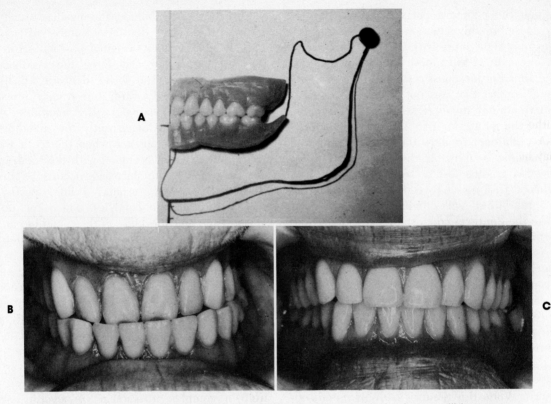

Fig. 28-2   A, Loss of bone structure under both dentures permits the mandible to move upward a corresponding amount. As the mandible rotates to a closed position without translation of the condyles, it moves forward. The problem is to determine the amount of change that has occurred in both basal seats. The occlusion may not appear to be correct when observed in the mouth, **B,** or it may appear deceptively adequate, **C.** The extraoral close-mouthed appearance will be almost identical in both cases.

posteriorly, because of heavy contacts between the mesial inclines of lower cusps and the distal inclines of upper cusps. These occlusal forces can cause destruction of the anterior maxillary denture foundation.

3. Forcing the lower denture backward so it impinges on the lower ridge

The changed relation of the inclined planes of the cusps may do this. The forces of centric closures can move the denture distally and cause destruction of

the labial side of the lower ridge (Fig. 28-3).

4. Forcing the lower denture anteriorly until one cusp occludes forward of its intended contact

The inclined planes of the teeth when the vertical dimension is reduced by shrinkage can do this. The contacts are made between the distal inclines of the lower cusps and the mesial inclines of the upper; they direct the occlusal forces posteriorly on the upper denture and anteri-

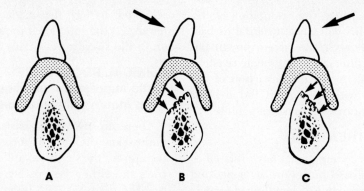

Fig. 28-3   Effect of a reduced vertical dimension of occlusion on the mandibular residual ridge. **A,** Cross section of the ridge when the denture was made. **B,** The inclined plane of the cusps forces the mandibular denture posteriorly *(large arrow)* and causes destruction of the labial side of the ridge *(small arrows).* **C,** The direction of force is altered when the lower denture moves forward enough *(large arrow)* to allow contact between the distal of the lower cusp and the mesial of the upper cusp. This force may destroy the lingual side of the ridge *(small arrows).*

orly on the lower (Fig. 28-3), tending to destroy the bone on the lingual side of the lower ridge.

It appears, then, that mandibular rotation can elicit severe damage in the denture-supporting tissues over a long period of unsupervised denture wear. The stresses are probably augmented by the use of cusped posterior teeth and by the resultant incisal guidance, which now locks the mandibular denture into the maxillary denture. Although proponents of the "noncusp" school of thought frequently indict cusped teeth as accelerating tissue damage in such situations, *no research evidence is available to support either school's claim that their tooth choice minimizes changes in the denture-supporting tissues.*

The horizontal position of each denture in relation to its own supporting ridge must be considered so a determination can be made as to whether the denture has moved forward or backward because of occlusal forces applied to it. Furthermore, one or both dentures may have rotated in relation to the supporting structures. The occlusion in the mouth must therefore not be used as a guide to the horizontal repositioning of either denture. A new determination of the vertical dimension of the face must be made by reestablishing a normal interocclusal distance. Again, the principles employed in the construction of complete dentures (Chapters 12 to 14) are called upon. Examination of the esthetics in profile, as far as the support of the lips in an anteroposterior direction is concerned, will serve to guide the orientation of the dentures in relation to their respective foundations. The relation of the teeth to the ridges must be observed for accuracy. If shrinkage has been only in the vertical direction (allowing the jaws to approach each other more closely than they should when occlusal contacts are made), the occlusion cannot be correct even though there has been no anterior or posterior movement of the dentures.

It must also be determined whether shrinkage of the jaws has been uniform under both dentures or whether one ridge has been destroyed more than the other. Greater shrinkage in one arch will change the orientation of the occlusal plane. This will cause occlusal disharmony in eccentric occlusions even though the occlusal vertical dimension has been reestablished by relining. A visual comparison of the size of the ridge with the size of the alveolar groove in the denture will serve as a guide.

PRELIMINARY TREATMENT

Most of the preceding points have related to the need for a rebase procedure as suggested in Fig. 28-1. Their clinical handling demands some preliminary steps before the actual procedure itself is undertaken. These steps aim at the following objectives: (1) reestablishing the height, orientation, and esthetics of the occlusal plane by manipulation of the mandibular denture (usually, though not necessarily, done first) and (2) relating the maxillary to the mandibular denture while the correct occlusal and esthetic position of the maxillary denture is being established. Both objectives can be achieved more or less automatically by use of a tissue conditioner, particularly if the adverse changes to be corrected are mild to moderate. On the other hand, more severe changes necessitate using combinations of compound stops, tissue conditioners, occlusal adjustment, and autopolymerizing augmentation of the denture's occlusal surfaces. This is routinely done to provide relief from mandibular dysfunction, which can follow vertical occlusal changes in complete denture wearers.

The obvious advantages of using tissue conditioners include those referred to in Chapter 6—simultaneous restoration of a healthy basal seat and the ease with which the liners can be modified for maximal function and cosmetic result.

After making certain that the tissues are healthy, the dentist looks for errors in the occlusion and occlusal vertical dimension that should be corrected as well as other changes that might be made before the final procedure is undertaken.

The clinical relining or rebasing can be achieved by (1) the static impression technique, (2) the functional impression technique, or (3) the so-called chairside technique.

CLINICAL PROCEDURES
Static impression technique: closed and open mouth relines/rebases

There are two major variations on the static impression theme. In one, the *closed mouth* technique, the dentures are used as impression trays and either the existing CO is employed to seat the dentures with lining impression material or else the CR is recorded (in the registration medium of choice) *before* the impressions are made. In the other, the so-called *open mouth* technique described by Boucher (1973), the following information is pertinent:

1. Relining/rebasing of both maxillary and mandibular dentures can be done at the same appointment.
2. The dentures are used essentially as trays for making the new impressions.
3. The existing CO is not utilized, and a new CR record is obtained *after* the impressions are made.

This is a demanding and laborious technique but apparently quite a good one.

We prefer the closed mouth reline/rebase technique when using the static impression method. Several variations have been suggested, all based on the same theme: using the denture as an impression tray with the denture occlusion (corrected in preliminary treatment or stabilized intraorally by wax or compound) holding the tray steady while the impression material sets. Table 28-1 presents three frequently used techniques that, if meticulously followed, will produce repeatably good results. The dentures are sent to the laboratory with an accompanying work authorization form that contains specific directions to the laboratory technician and other information—such as the specifications for alterations, materials, finish, remount casts, and remounting of the upper denture.

For many years it was believed that the

Table 28-1 Steps that can be considered as an integral part of a closed mouth reline technique

Centric relation	Existing intercuspation used to stabilize dentures
	Interocclusal record made by use of wax or compound
	Corrected during reestablishment of a new vertical dimension of occlusion by grinding or use of autopolymerizing resin
Denture preparations	Large undercuts relieved
	Hard resin surfaces relieved 1.5 to 2 mm
	Tissue conditioner removed or relieved
	"Escape" holes drilled, particularly in maxillary base; this will also assist easy removal of palatal portion during packing and processing
	Denture periphery shortened to create flat border
Impression procedure	Border molding achieved with low-fusing compound material
	Posterior palatal seal achieved with low-fusing compound
	Border molding retained from polymerized tissue-conditioning material
	Border molding achieved by choosing impression material that is soft and yet viscous enough to support and register peripheral detail (one of the polyether impression materials)

strains inherent in the processed denture base would be released by subsequent processing and cause some degree of warpage. However, it has now been found that dentures can be adequately relined with one of the autopolymerizing resins by a technique that offers the advantages of a simplified and less costly laboratory procedure.

The processed dentures are usually ready to be inserted on the same day the impressions are made. The protocol described in Chapter 24 is followed, and occlusal refinement is done intraorally or on the articulator. Follow-up instructions are similar to those provided at the time the new dentures are inserted.

Functional impression technique

The functional impression technique is both simple and practical and has gained considerable support during the past several years. It is the one we routinely use in our practice. It depends on a thorough understanding of the versatile properties of tissue conditioners as functional impression materials. The relative ease with which these temporary soft liners can be employed as functional impression materials has led to their abuse and to criticism by many dentists. However, they are excellent for refitting complete dentures when used carefully and meticulously. Improvements in these materials include their retaining compliance for many weeks, their good dimensional stability, and their excellent bonding to the resin denture base.

When a denture needs to be refitted, the patient's complaint or the dentist's oral prosthetic evaluation usually indicates undermined retention. Often one may see a variable hyperemia of the mucosa accompanied by sore spots in the denture-bearing mucosa. The denture is observed intraorally to assess the need for peripheral reduction or extension, and a posterior palatal seal extension is developed with modeling compound on maxillary dentures. (Occasionally, if extensive ridge resorption and overt loss of vertical dimension of occlusion have occurred, three compound stops may be required on the impression surface of the denture to reestablish a proper occlusal relationship or to improve the occlusal plane orientation.) A treatment liner is next placed inside the denture. The lining material should flow evenly to cover the whole impression surface and the borders of the denture with a thin layer. If voids are evident, they should be filled with a fresh mix of liner material. Unsupported parts of the liner may occur on the borders of the denture, and this indicates that localized border molding with stick modeling compound will be needed before the placement of a fresh mix of liner. Occasionally borders are formed that are low and narrow, and this too is indica-

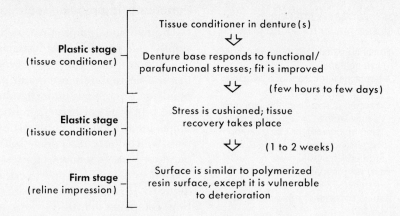

Plastic stage
(tissue conditioner)

Tissue conditioner in denture(s)

⇩

Denture base responds to functional/
parafunctional stresses; fit is improved

⇩   (few hours to few days)

Elastic stage
(tissue conditioner)

Stress is cushioned; tissue
recovery takes place

⇩   (1 to 2 weeks)

Firm stage
(reline impression)

Surface is similar to polymerized
resin surface, except it is vulnerable
to deterioration

Fig. 28-4   The physical stages of tissue conditioners/treatment liners allow the dentist to use them for different objectives.

tive of inadequate peripheral extension of the denture. Again, the borders must be corrected by border molding with compound or one of the autopolymerizing resins before they are covered with the lining material. Remember: These materials have a tendency to slump during setting unless they are adequately supported. This slumping phenomenon probably accounts for the undermined peripheral integrity that can reduce denture retention. The patient's mandible is guided into a retruded position, which is (hopefully) one of maximum intercuspation, to help stabilize the denture while the lining material is setting. Excess material is trimmed away with a hot scalpel. Most of the materials used for this purpose progress through plastic and then elastic stages before hardening, which can take several days (Fig. 28-4). The plastic stage permits movement of the denture base or bases so they are more compatible with the existing occlusion. This also allows the displaced tissues to recover and assume their original position. The patient is instructed regarding care of the prosthesis and its lining material.

Research has shown that a number of denture cleansers and other preparations that may be helpful in the control of plaque on dentures

can cause significant deterioration of tissue conditioners in a short time. Apparently simple rinsing of the temporarily lined denture and gentle brushing with a soft toothbrush are good interim measures to minimize damage to the lining. Clinical experience indicates that 10 to 14 days should elapse before the material is firm enough to proceed with the clinical reline sequence, however.

At the next appointment the temporarily relined denture will usually be well retained, with well-rounded peripheral borders and a healthy-appearing mucosa. It has been observed that the tissue-conditioning materials can create problems when used for impressions. The gradually increasing elasticity of the material in the mouth can lead to a recovery of the compressed material when the load is removed, that is, when the impression is removed from the mouth; hence the importance of pouring the cast when the material has reached the firm stage (Fig. 28-4).

Furthermore, these materials tend to deteriorate in some mouths, which precludes their use in this manner. If the dentist has any doubt about the quality of the surface appearance of the hardened liner, the reline procedure can be carried out as described earlier in the chapter, after the interim treatment liner has been removed. If the surface or peripheral deterioration is slight, these areas can be trimmed with a carbide bur, and the denture or dentures prepared for a secondary, or wash, impression with a light-bodied material.

The stone cast must be poured immediately after removal of the relined denture base from the mouth. The material should not be plastic, or "self-flow," because the material's own weight may deform the impression. It is also possible that the weight of the stone poured into the impression surface will cause distortion of the impression. Maxillary casts may have to be scored in the selected posterior palatal seal area, since the long period of plasticity of the material may not create sufficient displacement action in this area. Alternatively, a thin bead of compound material may be used to augment the posterior palatal seal.

It must be emphasized that the making of a new CR record and the remount procedure are almost always necessary to ensure an optimal prosthodontic occlusion. Researchers have demonstrated that the functional status of dentures relined with treatment liners used as impression materials is as good as the status of dentures relined by border molding and then refined with a light-bodied impression material.

The recent introduction of visible light–cured (VLC) resin systems has produced initially promising results when used in a wide range of prosthodontic activities. Biologic testing indicates that they are nontoxic and biocompatible. Ongoing research also appears to have improved their properties (such as fit, strength, ability to polymerize without residual components, ease of fabrication and manipulation, patient acceptance, ability to bond with other denture base resins, and low bacterial adherence).

One promising application of VLC resin material is its use for chairside relining. It is employed in a similar manner as a tissue conditioner, with all the possibilities of instant modifications since the flow of the material can be regulated by selection of appropriate viscosity, warming and cooling measures, and partial intraoral polymerization with a hand-held curing light. The relined denture is then taken to the laboratory for immediate light-curing of the new layer of material. Although long-term clinical results on treatment effectiveness and material integrity maintenance are not available, the VLC materials seem to hold considerable promise.

Both the static technique (or versions of it) and the functional impression technique are well accepted and experience-proved procedures. They can be used for simple situations (denture settling is minimal) and complicated situations (excessive tissue changes have taken place). It appears that the choice between the two methods is based on the dentist's and the patient's convenience.

Chairside technique

Several attempts have been made to produce an acrylic or other plastic material that could be added to the denture and allowed to set in the mouth to produce an instant chairside reline/rebase. These have met with failure for several reasons: (1) the materials have often produced a chemical burn on the mucosa; (2) the result was often porous and subsequently developed a bad odor; (3) color stability was poor; and (4) if the denture was not positioned correctly, the material could not be removed easily to start again. Until recently the chairside technique has been of little use in clinical practice because of these attendant difficulties and it has, therefore, been largely discarded.

BIBLIOGRAPHY

Boucher CO: The relining of complete dentures, J Prosthet Dent **30**:521-526, 1973.

Braden M: Tissue conditioners, I. Composition and structure, J Dent Res **49**:145-148, 1970.

Erhardson S, Johansson EG: Jämförande laboratorieundersökning av COE-comfort, COE-soft och Ivoseal som avtrycksmaterial, Svensk Tandlak Tidskr **63**:633-645, 1970.

Javid NS, Michael CG, Mohammed HA, Colaizzi FA: Three dimensional analysis of maxillary denture displacement during reline impression procedure, J Prosthet Dent **54**:232-237, 1985.

Kazanji MNM, Watkinson AC: Influence of thickness, boxing, and storage on the softness of resilient denture lining materials, J Prosthet Dent **59**:677-680, 1988.

Klinger SM, Lord JL: Effect of common agents on intermediary temporary soft reline materials, J Prosthet Dent **30**:749-755, 1973.

Nassif J, Jumbelic R: Current concepts for relining complete dentures: a survey, J Prosthet Dent **51**:11-15, 1984.

Newsome PRH, Basker RM, Bergman B, Glantz PO: The softness and initial flow of temporary soft lining materials, Acta Odontol Scand **46**:9-17, 1988.

Osle RE, Sorensen SE, Lewis EA: A new visible light–cured resin system applied to removable prosthodontics, J Prosthet Dent **56**:497-506, 1986.

Rantanen T, Siirilä HS: Fast and slow setting functional impression materials used in connection with complete denture relinings, Suom Hammaslaak Toim **68**:175-180, 1972.

Smith DE, Lord JL, Bolender CL: Complete denture relines with autopolymerizing resin processed in water under air pressure, J Prosthet Dent **18**:103-115, 1967.

Starcke EN, Marcroft KR, Fischer TE, Sweeney WT: Physical properties of tissue-conditioning materials as used in functional impressions, J Prosthet Dent **27**:111-119, 1972.

Wilson HJ, Tomlin HR, Osborne J: Tissue conditioners and functional impression materials, Br Dent J **121**:9-16, 1966.

CHAPTER 29

Repair of complete dentures and duplication of casts

REPAIR OF DENTURES

The repair of dentures can be a puzzling and difficult part of prosthesis construction. This problem can be handled as a laboratory procedure, but a knowledge of the preparation and of the technical phase is essential whether it is handled in the office or sent outside the office. Often this service is required by patients on an emergency basis because tooth and denture fractures seem to occur at most inopportune times.

It is well for the dentist to be aware of the hazards in repairing a denture. Many repairs are difficult to assemble correctly so they will not cause the dentures to be ill-fitting. If a second process of curing by heat is necessary, changes will occur because the old resin's physical properties change during processing. These changes may alter the occlusion and the fit of the denture over the basal seat. For this reason it is advisable to make a new CR record, mount the denture, and refine the occlusion after the repair has been completed.

The availability of autopolymerizing or cold-curing resins simplifies the repair procedure. The technique avoids the warpage of dentures that can result from reprocessing, and the entire operation is completed in much less time than by the heat-curing method. It is not necessary to flask the denture to cure the new resin.

Fracture of individual teeth or of the entire denture may be caused by trauma (dropping the denture), by a change in the occlusal relations, or by numerous other mishaps. It is im-possible with current laboratory procedures to return a perfectly adjusted occlusion. It is also well to advise the patient that the tissues will change during the time the denture is not worn but that they will readjust shortly. The patient must not think that the denture is entirely to blame if it does not feel the same immediately on insertion.

Maxillary and mandibular fracture repair

The broken edges of the denture are cleaned of food and material debris and other interferences, so the two parts will fit together well (Fig. 29-1). The two halves are held together by means of an old bur, which is luted to the denture teeth and the adjacent resin surface with sticky wax (Fig. 29-2). No wax is placed over the fracture, lest it prevent the halves

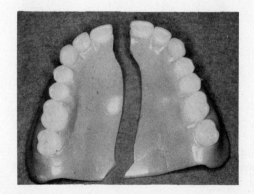

Fig. 29-1 When a denture is broken, the parts should be placed together to test for distortion and/or loss of material.

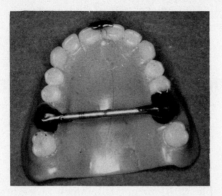

Fig. 29-2 The assembled parts can be held with sticky wax or modeling compound and an old bur.

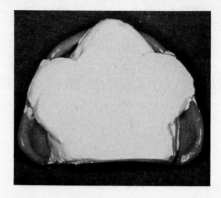

Fig. 29-3 Impression plaster is poured inside the denture to retain the parts after undercuts in the acrylic have been blocked out.

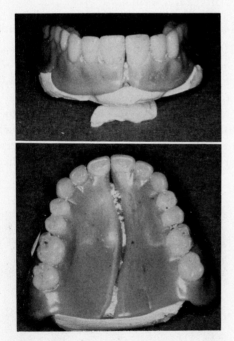

Fig. 29-4 Resin is cut away from the fracture line, and the denture is reassembled on the plaster matrix after tinfoil has been placed over it.

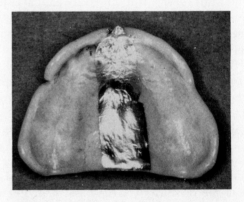

Fig. 29-5 Tinfoil over the fracture line.

from being examined for correct apposition.

Plaster is then gently vibrated onto the palatal surface of the denture, avoiding air bubble formation, and the remainder of the plaster is set on this to form the cast (Fig. 29-3).

Repairs using cold-curing resin

When a denture is to be repaired by use of cold-curing resins (Figs. 29-4 to 29-8), the same care is necessary in assembling the broken and replacement parts accurately.

The fitting surfaces of the fracture site must

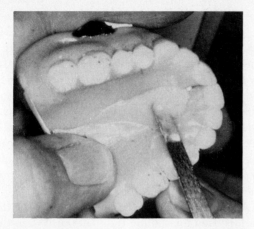

Fig. 29-6 Cold-curing acrylic resin is flowed into the open fracture over the tinfoil.

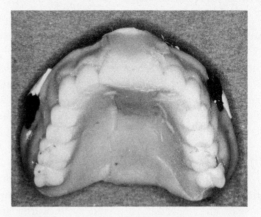

Fig. 29-7 The repair resin has polymerized.

be cleaned and brought tightly together, held with sticky wax or modeling compound and a matchstick (or bur). The cast is removed from the denture, and the resin on both sides of the break is cut away and beveled. Then the cast is replaced, acrylic resin monomer is painted on the cut surfaces, and a cold-curing repair resin is placed in the break (Fig. 29-6). The pre-mixed monomer and polymer are carefully flowed into the space until the area to be repaired is filled. The area should be slightly overfilled to allow for finishing.

Curing under air pressure. Pressure can be maintained on the cold-curing resin while it cures by immersing the denture in water in a pressure cooker after the resin has been forced into place. The water is preferably at 104° F (40° C) and the pressure cooker is used according to manufacturer's instructions; usually a minimum pressure of 20 to 25 psi (or 1.5 kg/cm^2) is employed. This condenses the repair resin. The curing can be done when the repair resin is added, in small increments of powder (polymer) and liquid (monomer). Without pressure, resin added in this manner will be less dense than that cured under pressure.

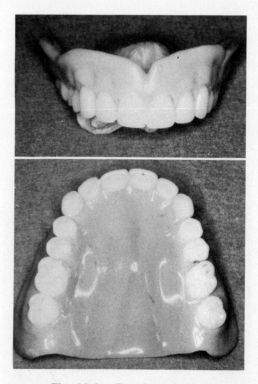

Fig. 29-8 Repair complete.

DUPLICATION OF CASTS

Duplicating casts has now become a comparatively simple and accurate process. These casts are necessary for a second set of (duplicate) dentures and for casts poured in a refractory investment material during partial and complete denture construction. The duplication is done by using (1) a reversible or (2) an irreversible hydrocolloid technique.

Reversible hydrocolloid technique

Several manufacturers supply hydrocolloid impression material for cast-duplicating purposes. The material is mixed with water according to recommendations and melted in a double boiler. The mixture is heated until it becomes smooth and homogeneous. In the meantime the cast is thoroughly soaked, which takes about 5 minutes. While it is cooling down, the cast is placed on the bottom plate of the special duplicating flask and held in position by two pieces of modeling compound (Plasticine) (Fig. 29-9). There are several types of duplicating flasks available, and the choice is based on laboratory convenience.

The bottom plate of the flask and the cast are immersed in warm water at 135° F (57° C) to ensure free flow of the material over the cast. If the cast is not warm and well soaked, it will dry and cool the hydrocolloid thus preventing a smooth surface. During the cooling process the hydrocolloid mixture in the double boiler is stirred to keep the mass at the same temperature throughout. It is cooled until a finger can be held in it without discomfort. This cooling is necessary to reduce shrinkage of the duplicating material and to prevent softening or melting of any wax relief that may be in place on the cast to be duplicated.

A pan that is deeper than the height of the flask is used for cooling the material. When the technician is ready to pour, the flask is assembled with the cast inside on the bottom plate, and the assembly is placed in the pan (Fig. 29-10). The material is poured into the flask through one of the openings until it flows out the other opening. By pouring all the material into one opening instead of using both openings, it is possible to avoid trapping air (Fig. 29-11). Ice and water are then placed in the pan to a level approximately half the height of the flask. After 20 minutes the water level is raised to cover the entire flask for another 20 minutes. (The latter step can also be accom-

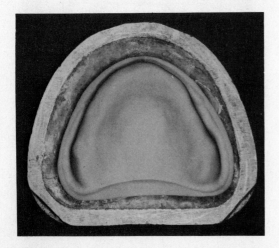

Fig. 29-9 The cast attached to the base of the duplicating flask with modeling compound (such as Plasticine).

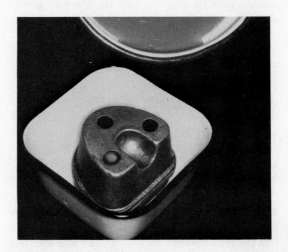

Fig. 29-10 The duplicating material ready to be poured into the flask over the cast.

plished by placing the flask under cold running water.)

The flask must not be opened until the mass is chilled thoroughly (Fig. 29-12). After chilling, the bottom plate is removed and the hydrocolloid mass is trimmed with a knife around the bottom of the cast to facilitate its removal (Fig. 29-13). This cutting away of hydrocolloid permits the cast to be grasped and gently withdrawn from the impression. The impression is now examined for incomplete flowing, spaces due to trapped air, and excessive scarring because of improper removal (Fig. 29-14).

If the impression is satisfactory, a mixture of stone or investment material is vibrated into the impression. The hydrocolloid has a high

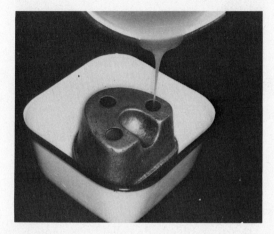

Fig. 29-11 Pouring the duplicating material into the flask.

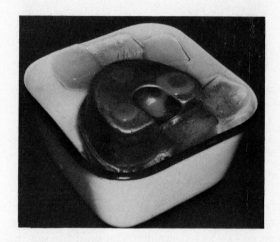

Fig. 29-12 Chilling the flask in ice water. The flask is submerged up to half its height for 20 minutes, and then totally for another 20 minutes.

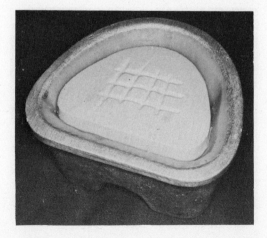

Fig. 29-13 Cutting away the duplicating material to facilitate removal of the cast.

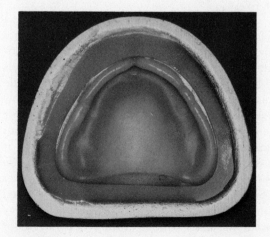

Fig. 29-14 Hydrocolloid impression of the cast in the flask.

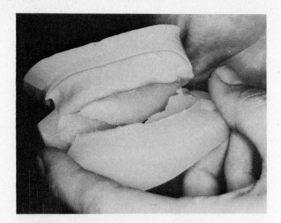

Fig. 29-15 Removal of the hydrocolloid and cast from the duplicating flask.

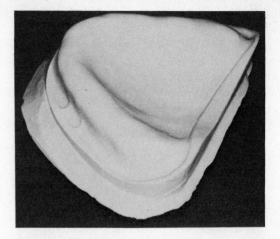

Fig. 29-16 The duplicated cast before trimming.

water content and tends to become dehydrated and distorted rapidly. The fluid leaving the hydrocolloid is acid in reaction and will neutralize the alkaline of the stone, thereby softening and roughening the surface of the cast. For this reason, the stone must be poured immediately.

In vibrating the stone into the impression, a mass about the size of a walnut is started on a mandibular impression in the area of the middle palate or between the ridges. It spreads when the impression is held at a sharp angle and flows to the other end. It is made to flow back and forth several times to keep the layer thin and thus prevent trapping of air. In this manner a smooth pitless surface of the cast is assured. Additional increments of stone are added until the impression is level full. After the stone has set, the hydrocolloid is slipped out of the flask and the material is peeled away from the cast. The hydrocolloid is saved for subsequent use. Rough edges are trimmed, and the cast is ready (Figs. 29-15 and 29-16).

Irreversible hydrocolloid technique

The irreversible hydrocolloid technique is an even simpler method and is economical in terms of time, equipment, and materials. The cast is carefully examined for defects (Fig. 29-

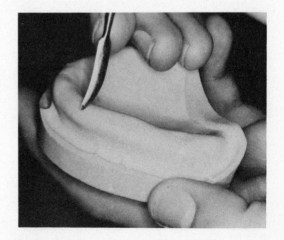

Fig. 29-17 The cast is carefully scrutinized for defects.

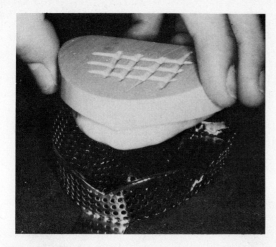

Fig. 29-18 An oversized stock tray is selected.

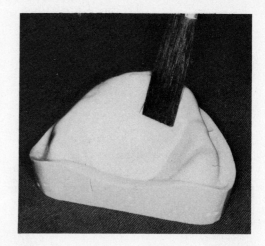

Fig. 29-19 Impression material being brushed onto the cast to ensure reproduction of detail.

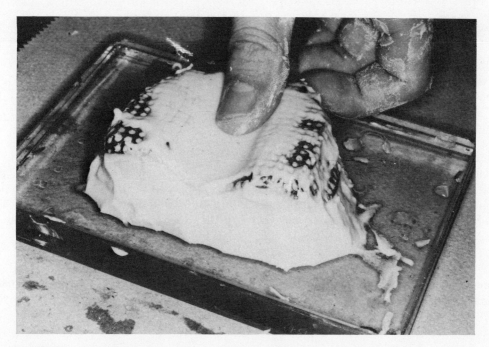

Fig. 29-20 The loaded impression tray is inverted onto the cast, which rests on a glass slab or other nonabsorbent smooth surface.

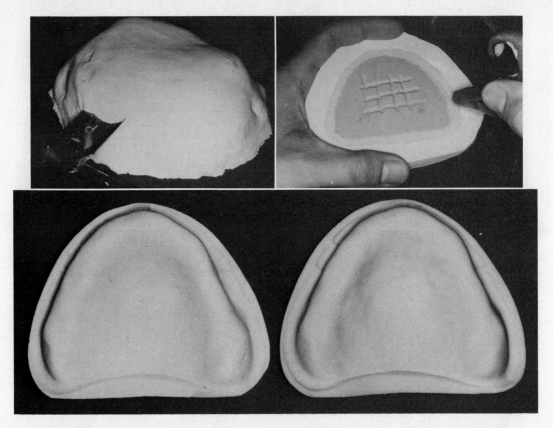

Fig. 29-21 Master and duplicate casts attest to the accuracy of the irreversible hydrocolloid technique.

17). Nodules of stone are removed, defects are filled with wax, and the cast is thoroughly soaked for about 5 minutes. An oversized rimlock impression tray is selected, a thin mix of irreversible hydrocolloid is prepared, and an impression of the cast is made (Figs. 29-18 and 29-19). The loaded tray is inverted on the cast (Fig. 29-20), care being taken to place additional amounts of hydrocolloid around the sides of the cast. After the impression has set, the cast is separated from the impression. If the impression is correct, a stone mix is poured into it and the duplicate cast is not separated until at least 45 minutes have elapsed. The result is usually indistinguishable from the original (Fig. 29-21).

BIBLIOGRAPHY

Sowter JB: Dental laboratory technology: prosthodontic techniques, Chapel Hill, 1968, University of North Carolina.

CHAPTER 30

Dental implants for the edentulous patient

It is tempting to conclude a text on the treatment of edentulous patients by suggesting that the applied content of the preceding chapters will ensure a happy complete denture experience for all persons. However, clinical experience demands the admission that some edentulous patients simply cannot tolerate complete dentures. Such failure is neither an indictment of one's professional skills nor necessarily a condemnation of the patient's response to the clinician's efforts. It must be accepted that many patients who wear complete dentures will experience considerable difficulty adapting to their prostheses. In fact, some patients simply cannot wear them at all, and their quality of life is profoundly affected by their predicament. Treatment for these patients usually entails considerable efforts of both the clinical technical variety and the emotional supportive variety. Regrettably, one may even be tempted at times to dismiss such patients as having difficult or "impossible" mouths or, worse, as lacking motivation or learning skills. These situations are very frustrating for both parties, especially when it becomes clear that conventional complete denture therapy is not the correct prescription.

MALADAPTIVE DENTURE BEHAVIOR

Diverse reasons are presented in the dental literature to explain the etiology, frequency, and duration of chronic inability to wear dentures. In the past, it was tempting to regard the maladaptive problem as resulting mainly from adverse anatomic changes in the denture-bearing surface. However, clinical experience and some research have confirmed that there are physiologic as well as psychologic contributions to such behavior. Apart from the extensive anecdotal evidence favoring denture construction techniques, the major treatment proposed for such patients has been preprosthetic surgery. This approach has usually sought to enlarge the denture-bearing area by deepening the sulcus and/or augmenting the ridge. (See Chapter 2.) Implicit in this prescription was the conviction that an enlarged denture-bearing surface would significantly increase the chances of denture stability, and therefore patient adaptation. Apart from the inherent morbidity risks associated with such procedures, however, longitudinal assessment has not produced a compelling therapeutic outcome. Dentists have therefore pioneered with other methods (such as dental implants) in an effort to treat or preclude maladaptive denture behavior. Implants are made of a variety of alloplastic materials and consist of diverse designs, from so-called blades to cylindrically shaped tooth root analogues, that are placed in selected edentulous host bone sites. A prosthetic superstructure is subsequently fitted onto transepithelial posts attached to the buried implants.

The objective of this chapter is to review the current status of dental implants in clinical dentistry.

USE OF DENTAL IMPLANTS

The predictably successful replacement of lost natural teeth by artificial tooth root analogues would advance dental treatment significantly. Both the dental literature and the presentations at dental meetings have reflected the profession's ongoing concern with such a technique. It is clearly an exciting one, and has fired the imagination of many dentists and researchers. However, the literature on oral implantology has until recently been dominated by anecdotal reports that misled dentists into thinking that implantology is a clinical treatment method to be readily incorporated into their practices. Insufficient data have become available to enable clinicians to predict the number of years of success of any alloplastic oral implant. Furthermore, premature dissemination of alloplastic implant materials, methods, and techniques has preceded scientific animal and clinical research. As a result there has been too much testing of dental implants in humans with too little evaluation of implant design and materials in laboratory animals. In addition, the biomechanical significance of the host tissue's interfacial response has not been adequately documented, and various misleading claims for a periodontal-like mechanism have been made (Fig. 30-1); nor has the longitudinal effectiveness of the attachment mechanism been conclusively established. Consequently, long-term criteria for implant success border on the specious. These early pioneering efforts in implant prosthodontics were, of course, necessary, since every technique undergoes a natural history of development, but a scientifically viable method of routine implant use has not been forthcoming, and thus many

of these past activities must be regarded only as halfway biotechnology.

THE SCIENTIFIC ERA

The routine clinical application of dental implants as an outgrowth of scientific research was ushered in by the work of Brånemark and his colleagues during the late 1970s. Starting in Sweden, and subsequently in various teaching centers around the world, several clinical researchers then began inserting threaded cylindrical titanium implants into mandibular and maxillary edentulous sites and using these to support a variety of prostheses. The titanium fixtures were implanted by a meticulous technique that aimed at direct contact between the implant material and living bone.

This direct contact, or the development of interfacial osteogenesis, had already been hypothesized by several authors. The belief was that certain implant materials possess a dynamic surface chemistry that induces histologic changes at the implant interface and these changes normally occur even when an implant is not present. Laboratory and clinical results have demonstrated the close spatial relationship between titanium and living bone, and this interface has been investigated by radiographs, histology, and scanning and transmission microscopy. Furthermore, no wear products have been found in the bone or soft tissues despite implant loading for up to 90 months. The observed "osseointegration" suggests a highly differentiated bone response to the careful placement of pure titanium tooth root ana-

Fig. 30-1 Comparison of the qualities of periodontal ligament and other "attachment" mechanisms induced with implants. **A** and **B,** The tooth or teeth are attached to bone via a highly differentiated mechanism (the PDL) that acts as a sensory organ, a shock absorber, and a participant in osteogenesis and bone remodeling. **C,** A pioneering type of implant (a blade) induces a poorly differentiated connective tissue–bone interface characterized by an unpredictable long-term functional outcome. **D,** The well-differentiated interface between titanium and bone is characterized by a predictably favorable long-term functional outcome, as shown by radiographic evidence of osseointegration, **E.**

CHAPTER 30

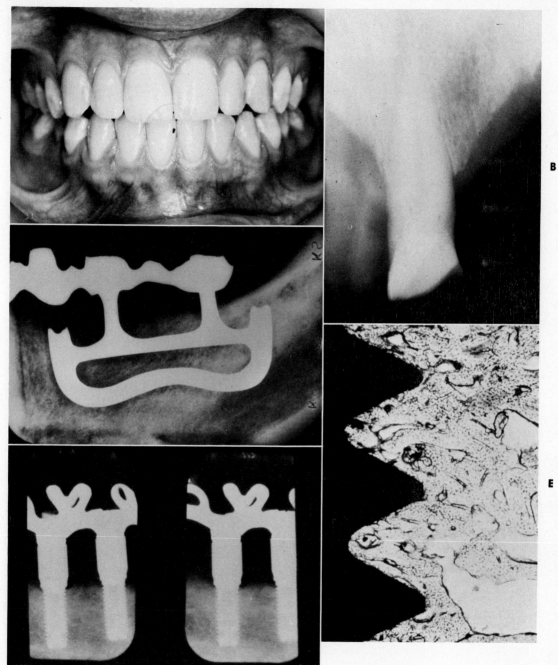

Fig. 30-1   For legend see opposite page.

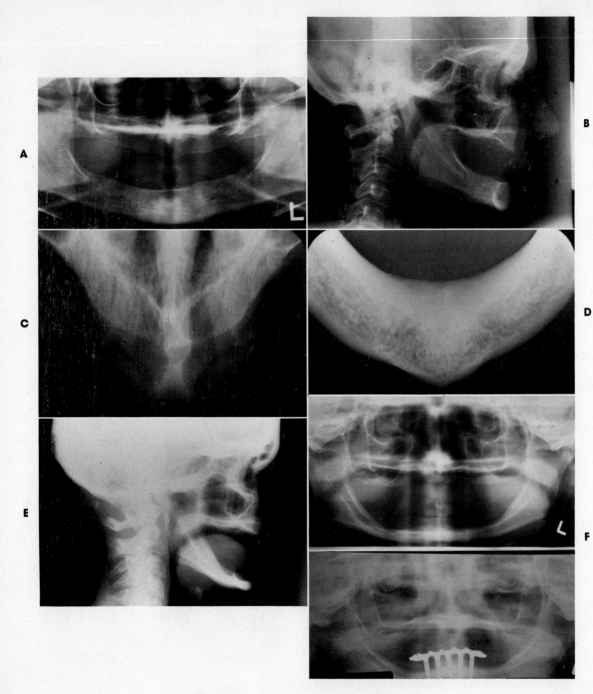

Fig. 30-2 For legend see opposite page.

logues. Moreover, this response appears to become organized according to functional demands (Fig. 30-1). It appears that osseointegration is also possible with stainless steel, vitallium, and tantalum as well as with titanium alloys. However, none of the former metals has demonstrated long-term clinical efficacy to date. Brånemark's clinical application has now been replicated in several centers and marks a very important advance in this field of tissue-integrated prostheses.

PATIENT CONSIDERATIONS

The psychologic reactions to various forms of bodily organ loss have been investigated in patients who have undergone a hysterectomy or mastectomy. However, remarkably little interest has been shown in the psychologic reaction to tooth loss. This apparent lack of interest is probably attributable to the prevalence of edentulism and the impressive success enjoyed by the dental profession in treating the condition. Furthermore, edentulism is neither fatal nor likely to elicit profound sympathy in a society preoccupied with youthful appearances. The sense of shame and inferiority that many edentulous patients feel is rendered even more poignant by the inability of some of them to tolerate a denture at all.

Patients who cannot wear dentures or who wear them with varying degrees of difficulty usually present with one or more of the following features:

1. Severe morphologic compromise of the denture-supporting areas that significantly undermines denture retention
2. Poor oral muscular coordination
3. Low tolerance of the mucosal tissues
4. Parafunctional habits leading to recurrent soreness and instability of the prosthesis
5. Unrealistic prosthodontic expectations
6. Active or hyperactive gag reflex elicited by a removable prosthesis
7. Psychologic inability to wear a denture, even if adequate denture retention or stability is present

Such patients are candidates for implant prescription. It should also be stated that even the most successful denture wearer frequently regrets his/her dependence on a removable prosthesis with all the attendant sequelae. These patients, too, could be added to the list, since longitudinal research in dental implants confirms the safe and easy availability of implant procedures. It is currently envisaged that this advance could well lead to therapeutic strategies in prosthodontics that will considerably reduce the conventional role of removable prostheses.

TISSUE INTEGRATION IN THE EDENTULOUS PATIENT (Figs. 30-2 to 30-4 and Plate 30-1)

The entire objective in prescribing implants is to provide the patient with an acceptable analogue for the lost periodontal ligament. If such

Fig. 30-2 A comprehensive radiographic survey of edentulous jaws will enable the dentist to ensure the presence of a healthy host bone site compatible with both quality and quantity considerations. More than one view is necessary if a three-dimensional assessment is to be made (unless there is access to a CT facility). All three views, **A,** panoramic, **B,** cephalometric, and, **C** and **D,** occlusal, provide magnified dimensions of differing degrees. **E** and **F** are the specific preoperative and postoperative films of the patient in Plate 30-1.

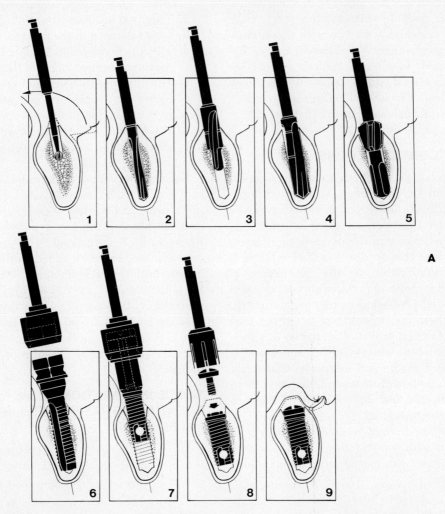

A

Fig. 30-3 A two-stage surgical procedure is required to bring about osseointegration. Both stages are performed under strict surgical and sterilization protocol, with a 4-to-6-month healing period in between. During the interval between stages the patient's old prosthesis is modified for use with tissue conditioners.

In the *first stage,* **A,** the following steps are needed to prepare the site for a titanium root analogue: *1* to *4,* flap preparation and gradual widening of the fixture site; *5* to *9,* countersinking for access to the fixture site, installation of the fixture, and placement of a cover screw under the mucoperiosteal flap. (Courtesy Dr. Ulf Lekholm, Institute of Applied Biotechnology, University of Göteborg, 1983.)

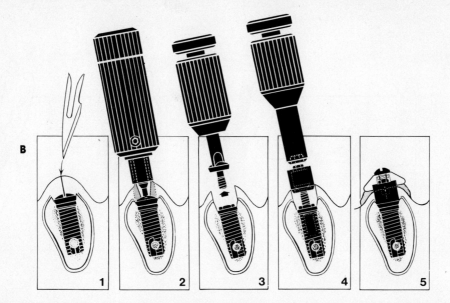

Fig. 30-3, cont'd   In the *second stage,* **B,** approximately 4 months later, the following steps are needed for the abutment connection: *1,* location of the cover screw; *2,* circular excision of the overlying mucosa; *3* and *4,* removal of the screw and connection of the abutment; *5,* abutment in place, with a surgical pack retained by means of a disposable healing cap. (Courtesy Dr. Ulf Lekholm, Institute of Applied Biotechnology, University of Göteborg, 1983.)

analogues are to be predictably safe and long-lasting, they should rely on a host bone response that is both highly differentiated and biomechanically adequate for functional and parafunctional stresses. The achievement of this appears to depend on several considerations:

1. Selection of patients whose systemic health does not preclude a minor oral surgical procedure

    Furthermore, the quality and quantity of the selected edentulous host bone sites must be surgically assessed by a careful and comprehensive radiographic evaluation (Fig. 30-2).

2. Careful surgical technique

    The predictability of a favorable healing response as manifested by subsequent tissue differentiation must not be compromised.

3. Use of an unalloyed titanium material

    The oxide layer that builds up over the metallic surface prevents actual contact between bone and metal, and this suggests that the implant behaves as if it were a ceramic surface. The layer is bound to affect the host tissue response, however, albeit in an imperfectly understood way.

4. Design of a root analogue that allows immediate stability of the implant and excellent stress distribution

5. Unloaded healing of the implant

    This is needed to ensure optimal healing of the tissue after treatment.

6. An impeccable fit of the prosthetic super-

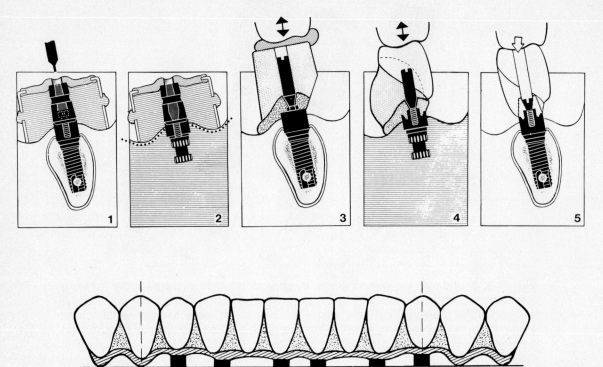

Fig. 30-4 The prosthodontic procedure: *1,* An impression of the transfer copings is screwed onto the osseointegrated abutment. *2,* Brass abutment analogues are screwed to the copings, and a stone cast is poured. *3,* Guide pins are used to stabilize a trial denture base for jaw relation—recording. *4,* The teeth are set up, tried in, indexed, and boiled out. *5,* A wax framework is designed to tie the teeth to the fixture analogue in a single cast unit, which allows for hygiene maintenance. *6,* The framework can be screwed into and out of the osseointegrated analogues as desired. (Courtesy Dr. Ulf Lekholm, Institute of Applied Biotechnology, University of Göteborg, 1983.)

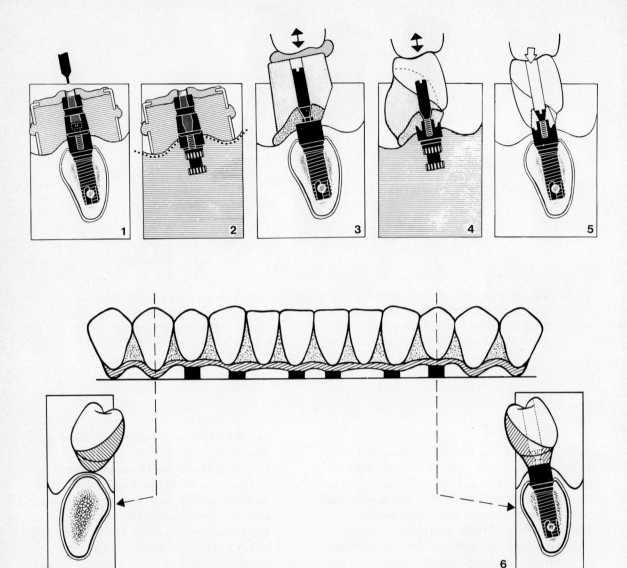

Fig. 30-4 The prosthodontic procedure: *1,* An impression of the transfer copings is screwed onto the osseointegrated abutment. *2,* Brass abutment analogues are screwed to the copings, and a stone cast is poured. *3,* Guide pins are used to stabilize a trial denture base for jaw relation—recording. *4,* The teeth are set up, tried in, indexed, and boiled out. *5,* A wax framework is designed to tie the teeth to the fixture analogue in a single cast unit, which allows for hygiene maintenance. *6,* The framework can be screwed into and out of the osseointegrated analogues as desired. (Courtesy Dr. Ulf Lekholm, Institute of Applied Biotechnology, University of Göteborg, 1983.)

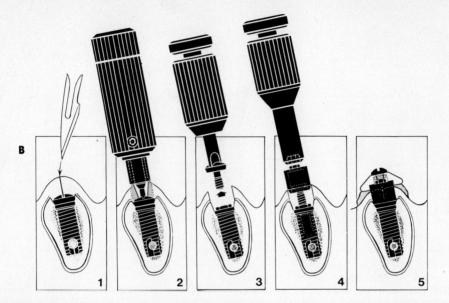

Fig. 30-3, cont'd   In the *second stage,* **B,** approximately 4 months later, the following steps are needed for the abutment connection: *1,* location of the cover screw; *2,* circular excision of the overlying mucosa; *3 and 4,* removal of the screw and connection of the abutment; *5,* abutment in place, with a surgical pack retained by means of a disposable healing cap. (Courtesy Dr. Ulf Lekholm, Institute of Applied Biotechnology, University of Göteborg, 1983.)

analogues are to be predictably safe and long-lasting, they should rely on a host bone response that is both highly differentiated and biomechanically adequate for functional and parafunctional stresses. The achievement of this appears to depend on several considerations:

1. Selection of patients whose systemic health does not preclude a minor oral surgical procedure

    Furthermore, the quality and quantity of the selected edentulous host bone sites must be surgically assessed by a careful and comprehensive radiographic evaluation (Fig. 30-2).

2. Careful surgical technique

    The predictability of a favorable healing response as manifested by subsequent tissue differentiation must not be compromised.

3. Use of an unalloyed titanium material

    The oxide layer that builds up over the metallic surface prevents actual contact between bone and metal, and this suggests that the implant behaves as if it were a ceramic surface. The layer is bound to affect the host tissue response, however, albeit in an imperfectly understood way.

4. Design of a root analogue that allows immediate stability of the implant and excellent stress distribution

5. Unloaded healing of the implant

    This is needed to ensure optimal healing of the tissue after treatment.

6. An impeccable fit of the prosthetic super-

structure and correct occlusal relationships

These are standard objectives in prosthodontics, but the absence of resilient periodontal ligament support in tissue-integrated prostheses indicates a need for technical prosthodontic accuracy that may very well exceed what is required for tooth abutments.

Figs. 30-3 and 30-4 and Plate 30-1 outline the salient features involved in the clinical application of the osseointegration method.

It must be pointed out that the precise nature of the interfacial titanium-bone relationship is not completely clear nor is information regarding the gingival response to the transepithelial part of the implant entirely known. Although there is evidence of epithelial attachment to the implant post, its significance or relationship to the oral environment is still under investigation. At present it is appropriate to suggest that the gingival cuff around an implant may not need to perform identically to the cuff surrounding the natural tooth.

It should also be pointed out that approximately 10% of individual implants fail to osseointegrate. The remainder, however, generally are sufficient to support a fixed prosthesis. Nevertheless, if the number of osseointegrated implants is three or less, treatment with an overdenture is usually prescribed and can be considered either a definite or a provisional treatment modality. In the latter instance, following placement of one or more additional implants, a final prosthesis can be inserted. With either treatment the patient's maladaptive experience is almost invariably solved. This underscores a most compelling conclusion: The osseointegration technique can be used to support different prosthetic designs that provide a solution to the denture wearing problems of practically all patients.

LONGITUDINAL CLINICAL CONSIDERATIONS

The most important reason for establishing criteria of success in any treatment method is to safeguard the oral health of the public. Each patient who receives an implant has the right to know the potential benefits and risks of its installation as well as an accurate prognosis of its usefulness. The scientific investigations into the use of osseointegrated implants have enabled clinical researchers to propose success criteria that can be used as a yardstick. These criteria protect the patient, whose informed consent before undertaking implant therapy should include an awareness of the highest standard of service currently available. The criteria for the success of implants that we endorse are

1. The individual unattached implant remains immobile when tested clinically.
2. No evidence of radiolucency around the implant is found on undistorted radiographs.
3. The mean vertical bone loss around the implant does not exceed 0.2 mm annually after the first year of service.
4. No persistent pain or discomfort is attributable to the implant.
5. The implant design does not preclude placement of a prosthesis that is esthetically satisfactory to both patient and dentist.
6. In the context of the foregoing criteria, an individual implant success rate of 85% at the end of a 5-year observation period and of 80% at the end of a 10-year period is the *minimum* level for success.

At the time of preparation of this text, only two implant systems for which an osseointegration response is claimed have received approval from the American Dental Association Council on Dental Materials, Instruments, and

Plate 30-1   Pre- and post-prosthodontic photographs, **A** and **B,** of a woman who exhibited chronic maladaptive complete denture behavior. Although this gratifying esthetic result might have been readily achieved with conventional complete dentures, in the present case a more stable support mechanism was required for the mandibular prosthesis, which was attained by the use of five osseointegrated implants, whose transepithelial abutment components are shown in **C.** The articulated working cast, **D,** incorporated brass implant abutment analogues to support a custom-designed rigid silver-palladium framework. With the addition of stock teeth, **E,** and a resin replacement for lost gingival tissues, **F,** a design was created that both facilitated home care procedures and enhanced the cosmetic effect.

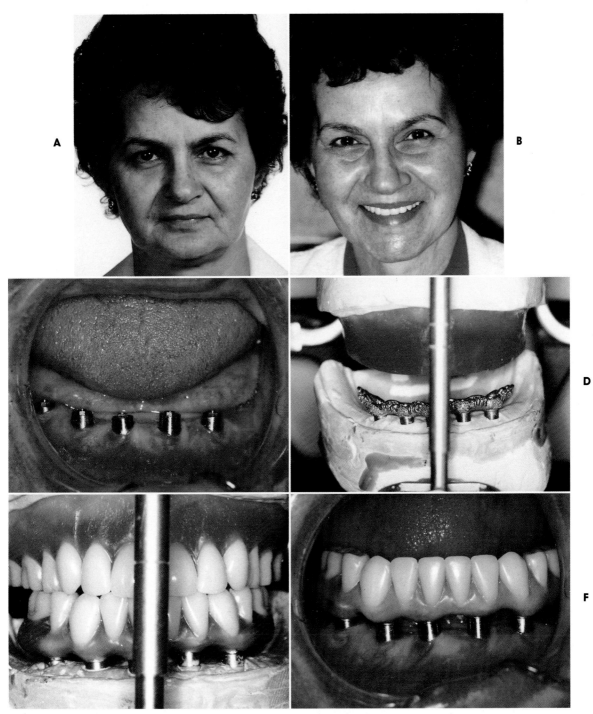

Plate 30-1 For legend see opposite page.

Equipment: Nobelpharma/Brånemark (full approval) and Interpore/IMZ (provisional approval).

This statement does not preclude the likelihood that other implant techniques and materials will achieve the same standards of scientific documentation. In fact, research over the next few years will most likely produce a new era in the treatment of edentulism that should prove both exciting and gratifying for patients and dentists alike.

It is tempting to suggest that Brånemark's work has led to the rapid development of different methods, materials, and applications in tissue integration. Clearly, however, clinical prosthodontics has entered a new era of therapy.

BIBLIOGRAPHY

Adell R: Clinical results of osseointegrated implants supporting fixed prostheses in edentulous jaws, J Prosthet Dent 50:251-254, 1983.

Adell R, Lekholm U, Rockler B, Brånemark PI: A 15-year study of osseointegrated implants in the treatment of the edentulous jaw, Int J Oral Surg 10:387-416, 1981.

Albrektsson T, Albrektsson B: Osseointegration of bone implants, Acta Orthop Scand 58:567-577, 1987.

Albrektsson T, Zarb GA, Worthington P, Eriksson AR: The long-term efficacy of currently used dental implants: a review and proposed criteria of success, Int J Oral Maxillofac Implants 1(1):11-25, 1986.

Babbush C, Kirsch A, Mentag PJ, Hill B: Intramobile cylinder (IMZ) two-stage osseointegrated implant system with the intramobile element (IME). I, Its rationale and procedure for use, Int J Oral Maxillofac Implants 2(4):203-216, 1987.

Blomberg S, Lindquist LW: Psychological reactions to edentulousness and treatment with jawbone-anchored bridges, Acta Psychiatr Scand 68:251-262, 1983.

Brånemark PI, Hansson BO, Adell R, Breine U, Lindstrom J, Hallen O, Ohman A: Osseointegrated implants in the treatment of the edentulous jaw—experience from a ten-year period. Monograph, Stockholm, 1977, Almquist & Wiksell.

Breine U, Brånemark PI: Reconstruction of alveolar jaw bone, Scand J Plast Reconstr Surg 14:23-48, 1980.

Brunski JB, Moccia AF Jr, Pollack SR, Korostoff E, Trachtenberg DI: The influence of functional use of endosseous dental implants on the tissue-implant interface. II, Clinical aspects, J Dent Res 58:1953-1969, 1979.

Dental implants: benefit and risk. An NIH-Harvard consensus development conference, Washington DC, December 1980, US Department of Health and Human Services.

Draft statement re National Guidelines for Health Planning, USA, Bethesda, National Institutes of Health, 1978.

Haraldson T: Functional evaluation of bridges on osseointegrated implants in the edentulous jaw. Thesis, 1979, University of Göteborg.

Henry PJ: Osseointegrated dental implants: two-year follow-up replication study. 24th Australian Dental Congress (Brisbane, May 1985), Aust Dent J 31(4):247-256, 1986.

Jemt T: Masticatory mandibular movements. Thesis, 1984, University of Göteborg.

Laney WR, Tolman DE, Keller EE, Desjardins RP, Van Roekel NB, Brånemark PI: Dental implants: tissue-integrated prosthesis utilizing the osseointegration concept. Mayo Clin Proc 61:91-97, 1986.

Lindquist LW: Prosthetic rehabilitation of the edentulous mandible. Thesis, 1987, University of Göteborg.

Smith D, Zarb GA: Criteria for success for osseointegrated endosseous implants, J Prosthet Dent 62:567-572, 1989.

van Steenberghe D, Quirynen M, Calberson L, Demanet M: A prospective evaluation of the fate of 697 consecutive intraoral fixtures modum Brånemark in the rehabilitation of edentulism, J Head Neck Pathol 6:53-58, 1987.

Worthington P, Bolender C, Taylor T: The Swedish system of osseointegrated implants: problems and complications encountered during a four-year trial period, Int J Oral Maxillofac Implants 2(2):77-84, 1987.

Zarb GA: The edentulous milieu. Toronto conference on osseointegration in clinical dentistry, J Prosthet Dent 49:825-831, 1983.

Zarb GA, Schmitt A: The longitudinal clinical effectiveness of osseointegrated implants: the Toronto study, J Prosthet Dent (In press, 1990.)

Index

Page numbers in *italics* indicate illustrations.

607